Math and Dosage Calculations for Healthcare Professionals

FIFTH EDITION

Math and Dosage Calculations for Healthcare Professionals

Kathryn A. Booth, RN, MS

Total Care Programming
Palm Coast, Florida

James E. Whaley, MS, RPh

Baker College
Owosso, Michigan

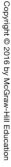

MATH AND DOSAGE CALCULATIONS FOR HEALTHCARE PROFESSIONALS, FIFTH EDITION

Published by McGraw-Hill Education, 2 Penn Plaza, New York, NY 10121. Copyright © 2016 by McGraw-Hill Education. All rights reserved. Printed in the United States of America. Previous editions © 2012, 2010, and 2007. No part of this publication may be reproduced or distributed in any form or by any means, or stored in a database or retrieval system, without the prior written consent of McGraw-Hill Education, including, but not limited to, in any network or other electronic storage or transmission, or broadcast for distance learning.

Some ancillaries, including electronic and print components, may not be available to customers outside the United States.

This book is printed on acid-free paper.

2 3 4 5 6 7 8 9 0 DOW/DOW 1 0 9 8 7 6 5

ISBN 978-0-07-351380-5
MHID 0-07-351380-6

Senior Vice President, Products & Markets: *Kurt L. Strand*
Vice President, General Manager, Products & Markets: *Marty Lange*
Vice President, Content Design & Delivery: *Kimberly Meriwether David*
Managing Director: *Chad Grall*
Brand Manager: *William Mulford*
Director, Product Development: *Rose Koos*
Senior Product Developer: *Christine Scheid*
Executive Marketing Manager: *Roxan Kinsey*
Digital Product Analyst: *Katherine Ward*
Director, Content Design & Delivery: *Linda Avenarius*
Program Manager: *Angela R. FitzPatrick*
Content Project Managers: *April R. Southwood/Sherry Kane*
Buyer: *Sandy Ludovissy*
Design: *Srdj Savanovic*
Content Licensing Specialists: *Lori Hancock/DeAnna Dausener*
Cover Image: © *ma-k, Getty images*
Compositor: *Laserwords Private Limited*
Printer: *R. R. Donnelley*

All credits appearing on page or at the end of the book are considered to be an extension of the copyright page.

Library of Congress Cataloging-in-Publication Data

Booth, Kathryn A., 1957-

Math & dosage calculations for healthcare professionals / Kathryn A. Booth, MS, RN, RMA (AMT), RPT, CPhT, facilitator/instructor, Military to Medicine INOVA Health System Falls Church, Virginia, James E. Whaley, RPh, MS, Baker College Owosso, Michigan, Susan Sienkiewicz, MA, RN, Community College of Rhode Island Warwick, Rhode Island, Jennifer F. Palmunen, MSN, RN, Community College of Rhode Island Warwick, Rhode Island. — [5th ed.].

　　pages cm

Includes bibliographical references and index.

　　ISBN 978-0-07-351380-5 (alk. paper)

1. Pharmaceutical arithmetic--Problems, exercises, etc. I. Whaley, James E. (James Earl)
II. Sienkiewicz, Susan. III. Palmunen, Jennifer F. IV. Title. V. Title: Math and dosage calculations for healthcare professionals.

　　RS57.H334 2015

　　615.1′401513--dc23

2014019158

The Internet addresses listed in the text were accurate at the time of publication. The inclusion of a website does not indicate an endorsement by the authors or McGraw-Hill Education, and McGraw-Hill Education does not guarantee the accuracy of the information presented at these sites.

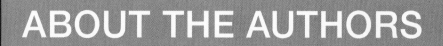

ABOUT THE AUTHORS

Kathryn A. Booth, RN-BSN, RMA (AMT), RPT, CPhT, MS, is a registered nurse (RN) with a master's degree in education as well as certifications in phlebotomy, pharmacy tech, and medical assisting. She is an author, educator, and consultant for Total Care Programming, Inc. She has over 30 years of teaching, nursing, and healthcare work experience that spans five states. As an educator, Kathy has been awarded the teacher of the year in three states where she taught nursing and various health sciences. She stays current in the field by practicing her skills in various settings as well as by obtaining and maintaining certifications. In addition, Kathy volunteers at a free healthcare clinic and teaches online. She is a member of advisory boards at two educational institutions. Her larger goal is to develop up-to-date, dynamic healthcare educational materials to assist other educators as well as to promote the healthcare professions. In addition, Kathy enjoys presenting innovative new learning solutions for the changing healthcare and educational landscape to her fellow professionals nationwide.

James E. Whaley, RPh, MS, is currently an associate professor of health sciences and chemistry at Baker College of Owosso (Michigan) and coordinator of the Pharmacy Technician Program, which is offered at nine Baker College campuses. He routinely teaches courses in the Pharmacy Technician Program in addition to anatomy and physiology, pathophysiology, and general chemistry. Mr. Whaley has taught at Baker College of Owosso since 1995 and was the first recipient of the college's prestigious Teacher of the Year award. He has been selected as a member of Who's Who among College Teachers numerous times. Prior to coming to Baker, Mr. Whaley was twice ranked in the top 10 percent of instructors at the University of Illinois, where he was awarded a fellowship in cellular and molecular biology from the National Institutes of Health. Mr. Whaley worked as a retail pharmacist before beginning his career as an educator, and he has been a registered pharmacist since 1981.

DEDICATION

To the future healthcare professionals using this book: may your career goals be achieved and the healthcare workforce be increased from your accomplishment.

To Kaylyn, Conner, JJ, Harleigh, Ian, Hunter, Delilah, Isaiah, and Harper, the true blessings in my life.

To my husband, Jim, for his enduring encouragement, love, friendship, and patience.

– K. Booth

To my wife, Jennie, who has provided unwavering love and support for over 40 years.

To Dennis and Cindy, our best friends, for sharing their family with us.

– J. Whaley

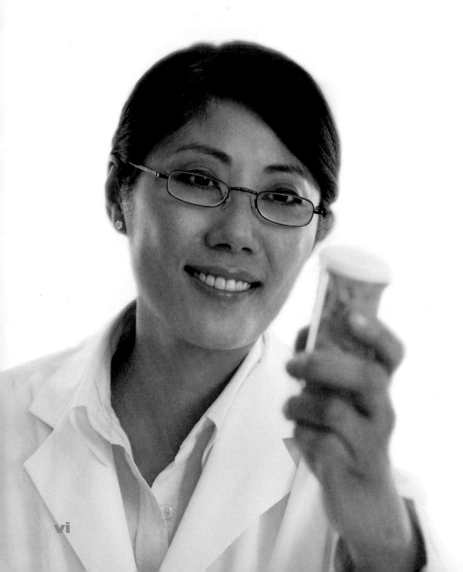

BRIEF CONTENTS

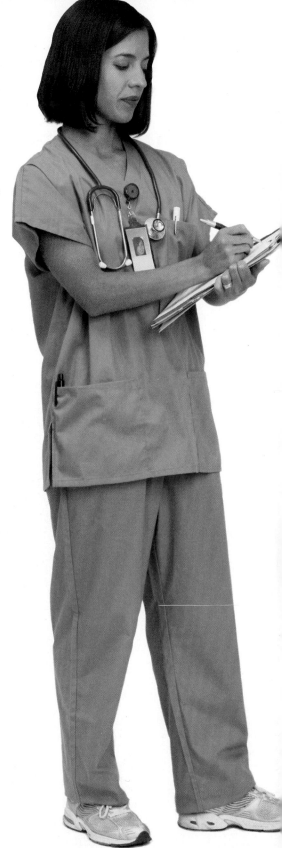

CONTENTS

Unit 1: Performing Basic Math

CHAPTER 1: FRACTIONS   2

CHAPTER 2: DECIMALS   37

CHAPTER 3: RELATIONSHIPS OF QUANTITIES: PERCENTS, RATIOS, AND PROPORTIONS   56

Unit 2: Using Systems of Measurement

Contents   ix

Unit 3: Identifying Information Needed for Dosage Calculations

Unit 5: Performing Advanced Dosage Calculations

Unit 6: Performing, Dispensing, and Compounding Calculations

CHAPTER 18: AMOUNT TO DISPENSE AND DAYS' SUPPLY 540

CHAPTER 19: CALCULATIONS FOR COMPOUNDING 563

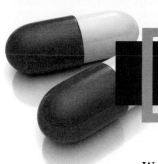

PREFACE

We've got you covered—from basic math skills to critical dosage calculations . . . from the print textbook to the digital supplements!

Welcome to the fifth edition of *Math and Dosage Calculations for Healthcare Professionals* (*M&DC*)! This product introduces students to the concepts and skills they will need to move forward within their chosen health profession or nursing curriculum. Students will need dynamic tools and multiple resources to ensure success and this product provides everything they need!

Here's what you and your students can expect from the new edition of *M&DC*:

- Reorganized content within chapters and units to allow for flexibility of utilizing the product across various healthcare and nursing curricula.
- Simplified dosage calculation steps and examples, and consistency throughout explanations.
- Continued comprehensive coverage of three methods of dosage calculation—proportion, formula, and dimensional analysis—to adapt to various learning styles.
- Updated learning outcomes based on the revised Bloom's taxonomy that serve as the framework for each chapter and are emphasized throughout the product assets to tie the concepts together.
- Tabular end-of-chapter summaries that are tied to the learning outcomes, along with page references—these reinforce key points for review.
- Comprehensive digital support with ALEKS Prep for Math & Dosage and Connect.
- Focus on the application of mathematics and accuracy of dosage calculations—the essential knowledge needed to prevent medication errors.

Here's How Your Colleagues Have Described the New Edition of *M&DC*:

"Math and Dosage Calculations is a well-written and current text with just the right amount of rigor and relevance.

This text covers all of the concepts required for medical assisting and nursing students in detail and with clarity and ease of use. Additionally, the use of three methods of dosage calculations and examples in each chapter provides students with the opportunities to work with the method they prefer. Real-life examples are given and students are required to extract information using critical thinking skills, rather than just completing exercises. Overall, this is an excellent product and I would highly recommend it to any medical program for the instruction of dosage calculation and administration of medications."

Amy Ensign
Baker College – Clinton Township

"Wow! This text is more than I expected. I am truly thrilled in all that it offers to me and my students."

Amanda Davis-Smith
Jefferson Community College – Louisville

"This is a very good book on the breakdown of dosage and calculations as it pertains to MAs and their future outcomes. I like the book as it is separate from pharmacology itself yet it is still a portion that could be added to the pharmacology course. Students will comprehend the math and calculations portions much better than what they are currently using."

Kathy Gaeng
Vatterott College

"Very easy to follow and teach, and it provides students with multiple opportunities to master the skills needed to administer and calculate medications accurately."

Lynnae Lockett
Bryant and Stratton College

"Excellent chapter layout and design. Easy to understand. Accurate. Good depth of information for our student population. Content that would be easy to build into Blackboard. Easy to understand while being appropriately challenging. I plan to recommend this to my math for health adjuncts."

Shawn Russell
University of Alaska – Fairbanks

Organization of *Math and Dosage Calculations for Healthcare Professionals,* Fifth Edition

M&DC is divided into 6 units:

UNIT	COVERAGE
1: Performing Basic Math	Chapters 1–3 focus on a review of basic math skills needed to perform dosage calculations.
2: Using Systems of Measurement	Chapters 4–7 focus on measurements used in dosage calculations and drug administration.
3: Identifying Information Needed for Dosage Calculations	Chapters 8–11 focus on equipment, interpreting medication orders and labels, and safe medication administration.
4: Calculating Dosages	Chapters 12–15 focus on basic dosage calculations, including three methods: proportion method, dimensional analysis, and formula method. These chapters include calculation methods and provide specific information for calculating oral, parenteral, and basic intravenous dosages.
5: Performing Advanced Dosage Calculations	Chapters 16–17 focus on advanced clinical calculations including special population calculations and critical IV calculations.
6: Performing Dispensing and Compounding Calculations	Chapters 18–19 focus on amount to dispense, estimated day's supply, compounding, and alligation.

New to the Fifth Edition!

Of the many improvements made to the fifth edition, key enhancements include:

- Chapters arranged into logical units of study for better organization and flexibility
- Changed titles to match the reorganized content for flexibility across healthcare and nursing curricula
- Icons throughout the first seven chapters to correlate chapter content to the ALEKS assessment system
- Updated Pretest that covers all of the learning outcomes in Chapters 1–7
- Updated Comprehensive Evaluation that covers all of the learning outcomes in Chapters 8–19

- Adherence to Institute for Safe Medication Practices (ISMP) error prevention guidelines
- Procedure Checklists that provide easy-to-follow, step-by-step instruction for common calculations
- Increased consistency among dosage calculation steps throughout the chapters
- Real and rendered labels that provide realistic practice of all types of calculations
- New algorithmic practice problems within Connect content

Chapter-by-chapter highlights include:

- Chapters 1–5: Content has been updated to provide clearer explanations of basic concepts and to explain ISMP number and unit formatting rules.
- Chapter 6: New Procedure Checklists were added to clarify the steps for writing conversion factors. The proportion method was separated into two distinct procedures: one for using fractions and one for using ratios.
- Chapter 7: The discussion of 12-hour and 24-hour time has been updated and clarified using consistent terminology.
- Chapter 8: Information was added regarding dropper standardization, calibration marks on syringes for IV lines, and clogged enteral tubes. The discussion of oral syringe safety was updated for accuracy, and information about other medication administration forms—such as drops, sprays, mists, inhalants, vaginal and rectal medications, topical medications, and transdermal systems—was moved to this chapter from former Chapter 14.
- Chapter 9: Information about prescriptions has been moved into this chapter from former Chapter 11.
- Chapter 10: New information was added regarding package inserts, including updated FDA regulations and when it is most necessary to consult the package insert.
- Chapter 11: Information about common look-alike and sound-alike medications and error-prone abbreviations was updated to reflect the latest ISMP guidelines. The new chapter emphasizes the importance of follow-up to ensure that authorized prescribers who give verbal orders provide an electronic or written signature. In addition, the information about the rights of medication administration was revised to emphasize the importance of following the procedures, rather than just memorizing the rights.
- Chapter 12: The rules in this chapter were revised to improve clarity, and Procedure Checklists were added to provide step-by-step guidance for dosage calculations. In Rule 12-2, Step A was changed from "Convert" to "Gather Information and Convert."
- Chapter 13: Repetitive content was replaced by a Learning Link that refers back to Chapter 12; both text and examples were revised to improve clarity.
- Chapter 14: Content was revised and reorganized to include calculations for subcutaneous administration of the high-alert medications heparin and insulin, as well as calculations for other parenteral forms. This chapter now includes calculations for all types of parenteral calculations, except IV. The discussion of methods of injection was revised and clarified, and a new figure was added to identify the various methods. A new Critical Thinking on the Job was added for insulin types, and the table in former Chapter 18 about timing of insulin action was updated and moved to this chapter.
- Chapter 15: Rules 15-6 and 15-7 pertaining to calculating flow rates were revised and simplified; a section was added about adjusting flow rates in mL/h; the photo showing primary and secondary solutions (Figure 15-8) was updated for clarity.

- Chapter 16: Procedure Checklists were added for rules that require step-by-step calculations. The key term for the third process in pharmacokinetics was changed from *biotransformation* to *metabolism* to conform with the often-used acronym ADME.
- Chapter 17: Information about calculating safe heparin IV dosages and performing heparin protocol calculations was merged in this chapter. Information about daily maintenance fluid needs (DMFN) was moved to this chapter. Step-by-step procedure checklists were added for calculating flow rates using DMFN, for determining safe dosage based on a patient's ideal weight, and for finding IV flow rate based on weight per time.
- Chapter 18: This completely new chapter was added to provide content for entry-level pharmacy technicians, including instructions for calculating the amount of medication to dispense and for calculating the days' supply of a medication.
- Chapter 19: Content from former Chapter 16 and Appendix A: Alligation Method were included in this new chapter targeted for entry-level pharmacy technicians. The chapter includes compounding calculations to determine quantities needed to make liquid, solid, or semisolid compounds, as well as to dilute stock products. In addition, the chapter includes new content to explain calculations using specific gravity.

Instructor Resources

McGraw-Hill knows how much effort it takes to prepare for a new course. Through focus groups, symposia, reviews, and conversations with instructors like you, we have gathered information about what materials you need in order to facilitate successful courses. We are committed to provide you with high-quality, accurate instructor support.

A one-stop spot to present, deliver, and assess digital assets available from McGraw-Hill:
McGraw-Hill *Connect* for Booth/Whaley: Math & Dosage Calculations

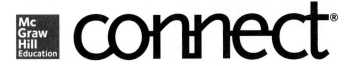

McGraw-Hill *Connect* for Math & Dosage Calculations provides online presentation, assignment, and assessment solutions. It connects your students with the tools and resources they'll need to achieve success. With *Connect* you can deliver assignments, quizzes, and tests online. A robust set of questions and activities, including all of the end-of-chapter questions, additional algorithmic math exercises focused on the three calculation methods, and interactives, are presented and aligned with the text's learning outcomes. As an instructor, you can edit existing questions and author entirely new problems. *Connect* enables you to track individual student performance—by question, by assignment, or in relation to the class overall—with detailed grade reports. You can integrate grade reports easily with Learning Management Systems (LMSs), such as Blackboard, Desire2Learn, or eCollege—and much more.

Connect for **Math & Dosage Calculations** provides students with all the advantages of *Connect* for Math & Dosage Calculations *plus* 24/7 online access to an eBook. This media-rich version of the textbook is available through the McGraw-Hill *Connect* platform and allows seamless integration of text, media, and assessments. To learn more, visit http://connect.mheducation.com.

A single sign-on with **Connect** *and your Blackboard course:* **McGraw-Hill Education and Blackboard—for a premium user experience**

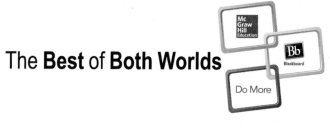

The **Best** of **Both Worlds**

Blackboard, the web-based course management system, has partnered with McGraw-Hill to better allow students and faculty to use online materials and activities to complement face-to-face teaching. Blackboard features exciting social learning and teaching tools that foster active learning opportunities for students. You'll transform your closed-door classroom into communities in which students remain connected to their educational experience 24 hours a day. This partnership allows you and your students access to McGraw-Hill's *Connect* and *Create* right from within your Blackboard course—all with a single sign-on. Not only do you get single sign-on with *Connect* and *Create*, but you also get deep integration of McGraw-Hill content and content engines right in Blackboard. Whether you're choosing a book for your course or building *Connect* assignments, all the tools you need are right where you want them—inside Blackboard. Gradebooks are now seamless. When a student completes an integrated *Connect* assignment, the grade for that assignment automatically (and instantly) feeds into your Blackboard grade center. McGraw-Hill and Blackboard can now offer you easy access to industry-leading technology and content, whether your campus hosts it or we do. Be sure to ask your local McGraw-Hill representative for details.

Want a single sign-on solution when using another Learning Management System?

See how **McGraw-Hill Campus** makes the grade by offering universal sign-on, automatic registration, gradebook synchronization, and open access to a multitude of learning resources—all in one place. MH Campus supports Active Directory, Angel, Blackboard, Canvas, Desire2Learn, eCollege, IMS, LDAP, Moodle, Moodlerooms, Sakai, Shibboleth, WebCT, BrainHoney, Campus Cruiser, and Jenzibar eRacer. Additionally, MH Campus can be easily connected with other authentication authorities and LMSs. Visit http://mhcampus.mhhe .com/ to learn more.

At-a-glance analysis on your class's progress: Connect Insight

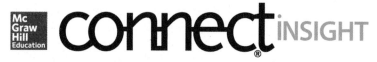

Connect Insight™ is the first and only analytics tool of its kind, which highlights a series of visual data displays—each framed by an intuitive question—to provide at-a-glance information regarding how your class is doing. As an instructor or administrator, you receive an instant, at-a-glance view of student performance on five key insights. It puts real-time analytics in your hands so you can take action early and keep struggling students from falling behind. It also empowers you by providing a more valuable, transparent, and productive connection between you and your students. Available on demand wherever and whenever it's needed, Connect Insight travels from office to classroom!

Create a textbook organized the way you teach: **McGraw-Hill** *Create*

With **McGraw-Hill** *Create,* you can easily rearrange chapters, combine material from other content sources, and quickly upload content you have written, such as your course syllabus or teaching notes. Find the content you need in *Create* by searching through thousands of leading McGraw-Hill textbooks. Arrange your book to fit your teaching style. *Create* even allows you to personalize your book's appearance by selecting the cover and adding your name, school, and course information. Order a *Create* book and you'll receive a complimentary print review copy in three to five business days or a complimentary electronic review copy (eComp) via email in minutes. Go to www.mcgrawhillcreate.com today and register to experience how McGraw-Hill *Create* empowers you to teach *your* students *your* way.

McGraw-Hill Tegrity records and distributes your class lecture with just a click of a button. Students can view it anytime and anywhere via computer, iPod, or mobile device. It indexes as it records your PowerPoint presentations and anything shown on your computer, so students can use keywords to find exactly what they want to study. Tegrity is available as an integrated feature of **McGraw-Hill** *Connect* for **Math & Dosage Calculations** and as a stand-alone product.

LEARNSMART® LearnSmart is one of the most effective and successful adaptive learning resources available on the market today and is now available for *Math and Dosage Calculations for Healthcare Professionals.* More than 2 million students have answered more than 1.3 billion questions in LearnSmart since 2009, making it the most widely used and intelligent adaptive study tool, one that has proven to strengthen memory recall, keep students in class, and boost grades. Studies show that students using LearnSmart are 13% more likely to pass their classes and are 35% less likely to drop out. This revolutionary learning resource is available only from McGraw-Hill Education. See the power of LearnSmart for yourself by trying it today at http://learnsmartadvantage.com/trial.

LEARNSMART™ ADVANTAGE New from McGraw-Hill Education, **LearnSmart Advantage** is a series of adaptive learning products fueled by LearnSmart, the most widely used and intelligent adaptive learning resource, which has been proven to improve learning since 2009. Developed to deliver demonstrable results in boosting grades, increasing course retention, and strengthening memory recall, the LearnSmart Advantage series spans the entire learning process from course preparation through final exams. LearnSmart Advantage also provides the first and only adaptive reading experience in SmartBook. Distinguishing what students know from what they don't, and honing in on concepts they are most likely to forget, each product in the series helps students study smarter and retain more knowledge. A smarter learning experience for students coupled with valuable reporting tools for instructors, and available in hundreds of course areas, LearnSmart Advantage is advancing learning like no other product in higher education today. **Go to** www.LearnSmartAdvantage.com for more information.

SMARTBOOK® **SmartBook** is the first and only adaptive reading experience available today. SmartBook personalizes content for each student in a continuously adapting reading experience. Reading is no longer a passive and linear experience, but an engaging and dynamic one where students are more likely to master and retain important concepts, coming to class better prepared. Valuable reports provide instructors with insight as to how students are progressing through textbook content, and are useful for shaping in-class time or assessment. As a result of the adaptive reading experience found in SmartBook, students are more likely to retain knowledge, stay in class, and get better grades. This revolutionary technology is available only from McGraw-Hill Education and for hundreds of courses—including *Math and Dosage Calculations for Healthcare Professionals*—as part of the LearnSmart Advantage series.

Best-in-Class Digital Support

Based on feedback from our users, McGraw-Hill Education has developed Digital Success Programs that will provide you and your students with the help you need, when you need it.

- Training for instructors: Get ready to drive classroom results with our **Digital Success Team**—ready to provide in-person, remote, or on-demand training as needed.
- Peer support and training: No one understands your needs like your peers. Get easy access to knowledgeable digital users by joining our Connect Community, or speak directly with one of our **Digital Faculty Consultants,** who are instructors using McGraw-Hill digital products.

- Online training tools: Get immediate, anytime/anywhere access to modular tutorials on key features through our **Connect Success Academy.**

Get started today. Learn more about McGraw-Hill Education's Digital Success Programs by contacting your local sales representative or visit http://connect.customer.mcgraw-hill .com/start.

Need help? Contact McGraw-Hill's Customer Experience Group (CXG)

Visit the CXG website at www.mhhe.com/support. Browse our FAQs and product documentation and/or contact a CXG representative. CXG is available Sunday through Friday.

ALEKS® (www.aleks.com)

ALEKS®   *Math and Dosage Calculations for Healthcare Professionals* also offers the integration of an **ALEKS** (**A**ssessment and **LE**arning in **K**nowledge **S**paces) "Prep Course" (see the three pages immediately before the beginning of Unit 1). Topics covered and remediated in **ALEKS** are noted by marginal icons throughout the first seven chapters.

    ALEKS is a dynamic online learning system for mathematics education, available over the Web 24/7. ALEKS assesses students knowledge, and then guides them to the material that they are most ready to learn. With a variety of reports, Textbook Integration Plus, quizzes, and homework assignment capabilities, ALEKS offers flexibility and ease of use for instructors.

- **ALEKS** uses artificial intelligence to determine exactly what each student knows and is ready to learn. **ALEKS** remediates student gaps and provides highly efficient learning and improved learning outcomes.
- **ALEKS** is a comprehensive curriculum that aligns with syllabi or specified textbooks. Used in conjunction with McGraw-Hill texts, it also provides students with links to text-specific videos, multimedia tutorials, and textbook pages.
- Textbook Integration Plus allows **ALEKS** to align automatically with syllabi or specified McGraw-Hill textbooks with instructor-chosen dates, chapter goals, homework, and quizzes.
- **ALEKS** with AI-2 gives instructors increased control over the scope and sequence of student learning. Students using **ALEKS** demonstrate a steadily increasing mastery of the course content.
- **ALEKS** offers a dynamic classroom management system that enables instructors to monitor and direct student progress toward mastery of course objectives.

ADDITIONAL INSTRUCTOR RESOURCES

- **Instructor's Manual** with course overview, lesson plans, answers to Review and Practice Sections, End-of-Chapter Homework Assignments and Chapter Reviews, Unit Assessments, competency correlations, sample syllabi, and more.
- **PowerPoint Presentations** for each chapter, containing teaching notes correlated to learning outcomes. Each presentation seeks to reinforce key concepts and provide an additional visual aid for students.
- **Test Bank** and answer key for use in class assessment. The comprehensive test bank includes a variety of question types, with each question linked directly to a learning outcome from the text. Questions are also tagged with relevant topic, Bloom's taxonomy level, difficulty level, and competencies, where applicable. The test bank is available in Connect; and the EZ Test version is also available.

- **Conversion Guide** with a chapter-by-chapter breakdown of how the content has been revised between editions. The guide is helpful whether you are a first-time adopter or are currently using *M&DC* and moving to the new edition.
- **Instructor Asset Map** to help you find the teaching material you need with a click of the mouse. These online chapter tables are organized by learning outcomes and allow you to find instructor notes, PowerPoint slides, and even test bank suggestions with ease! The Asset Map is a completely integrated tool designed to help you plan and instruct your courses efficiently and comprehensively. It labels and organizes course material for use in a multitude of learning applications.

All of these helpful materials can be found within your Connect course under the Instructor Resources.

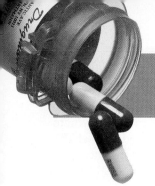

ACKNOWLEDGMENTS

Suggestions have been received from faculty and students throughout the country. This is vital feedback that is relied on with each edition. Each person who has offered comments and suggestions has our thanks.

The efforts of many people are needed to develop and improve a product. Among these people are the reviewers and consultants who point out areas of concern, cite areas of strength, and make recommendations for change. In this regard, the reviewers listed below provided feedback that was enormously helpful in preparing the fifth edition of *M&DC*.

Book Reviews

Over 100 instructors reviewed the fourth edition and the fifth edition manuscript, providing valuable feedback that directly affected the development of the fifth edition.

Fifth Edition Reviewers and Accuracy Checkers

Annette Baer—CMA, Ridley-Lowell School of Business

William Butler—MHA

Kevin Chakos—National College

Amanda Davis-Smith—Jefferson Community College—Louisville

Amy Ensign—CMA (AAMA), RMA (AMT), Baker College—Clinton Township

Kathy Gaeng—RMA, AHI, CPR/1st Aid, MA Vatterott College

Rhonda Johns—CMA (AAMA), Baker College—Allen Park

Lynnae Lockett—RN, RMA, CMRS, MSN Bryant and Stratton College

Frances Nicholson—CPhT, BFA National College

Denise Pruitt—Ed.D., Middlesex Community College

Shawn Russell—MPA, CPC University of Alaska—Fairbanks

Dawn Surridge—Ridley Lowell Business and Technology

Teresa Twomey—EdD, MSN, RN Goodwin College

Barbara Worley—DPM, BS, RMA (AMT) King's College—Charlotte

Deborah Zenzal—RN, BSN, AAPC, RMA Penn Foster College

Previous Edition Reviewers:

Karen Amsden—RN, BSN, MSHA, Jefferson College

Michele B. Bach—MS, BA, Kansas City Kansas Community College

Ilene Borze—RN, MS, Gateway Community College

Elicia S. Collins—BSN, MSN, Atlanta Technical College

Amy Ensign—CMA, RMA, Baker College

Rhonda Evans—AND, BSN, MSN, Central Carolina Community College

Timothy Feltmeyer—MS, Erie Business Center

Thomas Fridley—CPhT, Sanford Brown Institute

Margaret Gingrich—Harrisburg Area Community College

Sheldon Guenther—BS, DC, Kansas City Kansas Community College

Betty Hassler—RMA, AS, National College

Donna J. Headrick—FNP, Barstow Community College

Elizabeth Hoffman—MA, Ed., CMA, CPT, Baker College

Pilar Perez-Jackson—CPhT, Sanford Brown Institute

Jackie H. Jones—Kennesaw State University

DeLoris P. Larson—MSNNE, Northland College

Elizabeth Laurenz—CMA, LPN, MBA, National College

Larry M. Liggan—M.Ed, PA, RMA, AHI-C, National College

Jennifer Lipke—Hibbing Community College

Ralph C. Lucki—MA, CRT, RRT, EMT-P, West Virginia Northern Community College

Sheri Lee Martin—RN, BSN, LMT, BLS, Central Georgia Technical College

Belva J. Matherly—CPhT, National College

Keith A. Monosky—PhD, MPM, EMT-P, Central Washington University

Linda W. Moore—BA, Georgia Military College

Anne F. Mullenniex—BA, MA, Ph. C, Skagit Valley College

Donna M. Olafson—MA, Kansas City Community College

Gail P. Orr—MA, RMA, National College

Peggy A. Radke—MSN, Central Community College

Ramona Gail Rice—BS, MS, Ph.D, Georgia Military College

Helen Reid—EdD, MSN, BS, BA, Trinity Valley Community College

Katherine Lippitt-Seibert—RN, Mercy College of Health Sciences

Kathleen Sheehan—AS, BS, MSN, Elms College

Kristin M. Spencer—AAS, BHS, MBA, Baker College

George W. Strothmann Jr.—CPhT, Sanford Brown Institute

Jue-Ling Tai—MS, Danville Community College

Joseph A. Tinervia—CPhT, MBA, Tulsa Job Corps Center/Tulsa Community College

Debra J. Tymcio—RT, RMA, National College

Scott David Vaillancourt—Master Certified Novell Instructor, Certified Cisco Academy Instructor, Microsoft Certified Trainer, Ultimate Medical Academy

Jane K. Walker—BBA, MSN, PhD, Walters State Community College

Olma L. Weaver—LVN, Coastal Bend College-Beeville Campus

Janet M. Westhoff—Mott Community College

Denise York—BSN, MS, Med, Columbus State Community College

Technical Editing/Accuracy Checking

Kristin Brandemuehl—Washtenaw Community College

Kevin Chakos—National College

Rhonda Johns—Baker College-Allen Park

Teresa Twomey—Goodwin College

Sherrell Williams—Everest Institute

Connie Williams—Pinnacle Career Institute

Barbara Worley—King's College

LearnSmart Subject Matter Experts

Amy Ensign—Baker College

Tammy Vannatter—Baker College

Danielle Wilken—Goodwin College

Acknowledgments from the Authors

We would like to thank the many individuals who helped develop, critique, and shape our textbook and ancillary package. Suggestions have been received from faculty and students throughout the country. This is vital feedback that we rely on for content and product development. Each person who has offered comments, suggestions, and assistance has our thanks. We also want to thank the extraordinary efforts of individuals at McGraw-Hill, although we have had lots of hurdles, you have made all of this come together. A special thank you to Jody James for her enduring assistance through the entire process.

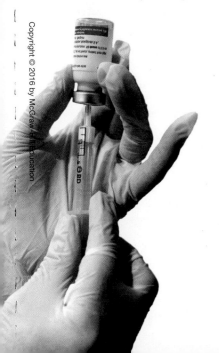

GUIDED TOUR

Chapter Opener

The **chapter opener** sets the stage for what will be learned in the chapter.

    Learning Outcomes are written to reflect the revised version of Bloom's Taxonomy and to establish the key points the student should focus on in the chapter. In addition, major chapter heads are structured to reflect the Learning Outcomes and are numbered accordingly.

    Key terms are first introduced in the chapter opener so the student can see them all in one place.

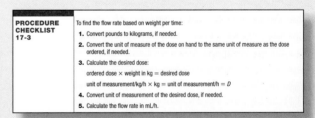

Rules and Examples

Rules state important formulas and facts for completing calculations. The **Examples** that follow illustrate these rules.

RULE 2-1	To write a decimal number:
	1. Write the whole-number part to the left of the decimal point.
	2. Write the decimal fraction part to the right of the decimal point. Decimal fractions are equivalent to fractions that have denominators of 10, 100, 1,000, and so forth.
	3. Use zero as a placeholder to the right of the decimal point just as you use zero for whole numbers. The decimal number 1.203 represents 1 ones, 2 tenths, 0 hundredths, and 3 thousandths.

Example 1	**Decimal**	**Description**	**Mixed Number**
	12.5	Twelve and five tenths	$12\frac{5}{10}$
	206.34	Two hundred six and thirty-four hundredths	$206\frac{34}{100}$

RULE 13-1	Always question and verify any calculation that indicates you should give a portion of a tablet when the tablet is not scored.
	• Do not administer $\frac{1}{2}$ of an unscored tablet.
	• Do not administer $\frac{1}{3}$ or $\frac{1}{4}$ of a tablet scored for division in two.

Procedure Checklists

Procedure Checklists provide easy-to-follow, step-by-step guidelines for performing dosage calculations.

PROCEDURE CHECKLIST 17-3	To find the flow rate based on weight per time:
	1. Convert pounds to kilograms, if needed.
	2. Convert the unit of measure of the dose on hand to the same unit of measure as the dose ordered, if needed.
	3. Calculate the desired dose: ordered dose × weight in kg = desired dose unit of measurement/kg/h × kg = unit of measurement/h = D
	4. Convert unit of measurement of the desired dose, if needed.
	5. Calculate the flow rate in mL/h.

Methods of Dosage Calculations

Three methods of dosage calculation are included; proportion, formula, and dimensional analysis. The methods are color-coded so you can easily find the method of problem solving that best fits your learning style or has been specified by your instructor.

PROPORTION METHOD

EXAMPLE 1   The order is to give the patient 15 mg codeine PO now. You have 30 mg scored tablets available.

STEP A: GATHER INFORMATION AND CONVERT

The dosage ordered is 15 mg. The dose on hand H is 30 mg, and the dosage unit Q is 1 tablet. Because the dosage ordered and the dose on hand have the same units, no conversion is needed and the dosage ordered is the desired dose D.

STEP B: CALCULATE
Follow Procedure Checklist 12-1.

1. Set up the proportion.

$$\frac{H}{Q} = \frac{D}{A} \quad \text{or} \quad \frac{\text{Dose on hand}}{\text{Dosage unit}} = \frac{\text{Desired dose}}{\text{Amount to administer}}$$

$$\frac{30 \text{ mg}}{1 \text{ tablet}} = \frac{15 \text{ mg}}{A}$$

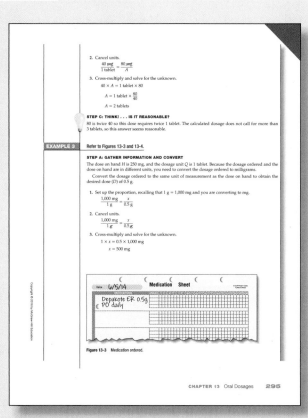

2. Cancel units.
$$\frac{40\ \cancel{mg}}{1\ \text{tablet}} = \frac{80\ \cancel{mg}}{A}$$

3. Cross-multiply and solve for the unknown.
$$40 \times A = 1\ \text{tablet} \times 80$$
$$A = 1\ \text{tablet} \times \frac{80}{40}$$
$$A = 2\ \text{tablets}$$

STEP C: THINK! . . . IS IT REASONABLE?
80 is twice 40 so this dose requires twice 1 tablet. The calculated dosage does not call for more than 3 tablets, so this answer seems reasonable.

EXAMPLE 3 Refer to Figures 13-3 and 13-4.

STEP A: GATHER INFORMATION AND CONVERT
The dose on hand H is 250 mg, and the dosage unit Q is 1 tablet. Because the dosage ordered and the dose on hand are in different units, you need to convert the dosage ordered to milligrams.
Convert the dosage ordered to the same unit of measurement as the dose on hand to obtain the desired dose (D) of 0.5 g.

1. Set up the proportion, recalling that 1 g = 1,000 mg and you are converting to mg.
$$\frac{1,000\ \text{mg}}{1\ \text{g}} = \frac{x}{0.5\ \text{g}}$$

2. Cancel units.
$$\frac{1,000\ \text{mg}}{1\ \cancel{g}} = \frac{x}{0.5\ \cancel{g}}$$

3. Cross-multiply and solve for the unknown.
$$1 \times x = 0.5 \times 1,000\ \text{mg}$$
$$x = 500\ \text{mg}$$

Medication Sheet
Date 6/5/14
Depakote ER 0.5g
PO daily

Figure 13-3 Medication ordered.

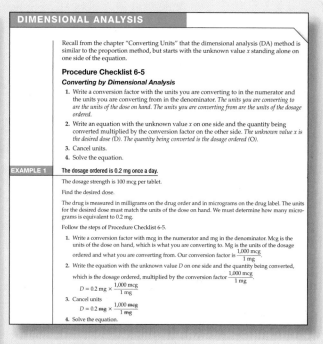

DIMENSIONAL ANALYSIS

Recall from the chapter "Converting Units" that the dimensional analysis (DA) method is similar to the proportion method, but starts with the unknown value x standing alone on one side of the equation.

Procedure Checklist 6-5
Converting by Dimensional Analysis
1. Write a conversion factor with the units you are converting to in the numerator and the units you are converting from in the denominator. *The units you are converting to are the units of the dose on hand. The units you are converting from are the units of the dosage ordered.*
2. Write an equation with the unknown value x on one side and the quantity being converted multiplied by the conversion factor on the other side. *The unknown value x is the desired dose (D). The quantity being converted is the dosage ordered (O).*
3. Cancel units.
4. Solve the equation.

EXAMPLE 1 The dosage ordered is 0.2 mg once a day.

The dosage strength is 100 mcg per tablet.

Find the desired dose.

The drug is measured in milligrams on the drug order and in micrograms on the drug label. The units for the desired dose must match the units of the dose on hand. We must determine how many micrograms is equivalent to 0.2 mg.

Follow the steps of Procedure Checklist 6-5.
1. Write a conversion factor with mcg in the numerator and mg in the denominator. Mcg is the units of the dose on hand, which is what you are converting to. Mg is the units of the dosage ordered and what you are converting from. Our conversion factor is $\frac{1,000\ \text{mcg}}{1\ \text{mg}}$.
2. Write the equation with the unknown value D on one side and the quantity being converted, which is the dosage ordered, multiplied by the conversion factor $\frac{1,000\ \text{mcg}}{1\ \text{mg}}$.
$$D = 0.2\ \text{mg} \times \frac{1,000\ \text{mcg}}{1\ \text{mg}}$$
3. Cancel units
$$D = 0.2\ \cancel{mg} \times \frac{1,000\ \text{mcg}}{1\ \cancel{mg}}$$
4. Solve the equation.

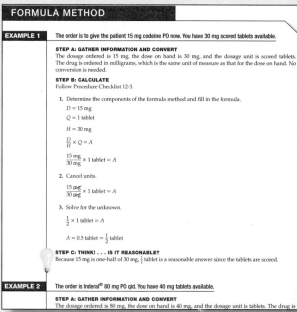

FORMULA METHOD

EXAMPLE 1 The order is to give the patient 15 mg codeine PO now. You have 30 mg scored tablets available.

STEP A: GATHER INFORMATION AND CONVERT
The dosage ordered is 15 mg, the dose on hand is 30 mg, and the dosage unit is scored tablets. The drug is ordered in milligrams, which is the same unit of measure as that for the dose on hand. No conversion is needed.

STEP B: CALCULATE
Follow Procedure Checklist 12-3.
1. Determine the components of the formula method and fill in the formula.
$$D = 15\ \text{mg}$$
$$Q = 1\ \text{tablet}$$
$$H = 30\ \text{mg}$$
$$\frac{D}{H} \times Q = A$$
$$\frac{15\ \text{mg}}{30\ \text{mg}} \times 1\ \text{tablet} = A$$

2. Cancel units.
$$\frac{15\ \cancel{mg}}{30\ \cancel{mg}} \times 1\ \text{tablet} = A$$

3. Solve for the unknown.
$$\frac{1}{2} \times 1\ \text{tablet} = A$$
$$A = 0.5\ \text{tablet} = \frac{1}{2}\ \text{tablet}$$

STEP C: THINK! . . . IS IT REASONABLE?
Because 15 mg is one-half of 30 mg, $\frac{1}{2}$ tablet is a reasonable answer since the tablets are scored.

EXAMPLE 2 The order is Inderal® 80 mg PO qid. You have 40 mg tablets available.

STEP A: GATHER INFORMATION AND CONVERT
The dosage ordered is 80 mg, the dose on hand is 40 mg, and the dosage unit is tablets. The drug is

Learning Aids

Learning Links refer students to an earlier chapter for a quick review when concepts are repeated.

LEARNING LINK Recall the components of a medication order addressed in the chapter "Interpreting Medication Orders": name of patient, patient's date of birth, date and time the order is written, drug name, drug dose, route, time and/or frequency of medication administration, and signature of authorized prescriber (AP).

PATIENT EDUCATION

Healthcare workers often educate patients about the proper way to take drugs at home. This responsibility may be the duty of the pharmacy technician, the nurse, or the certified medical assistant. If you are authorized to provide patient education, you should take the following steps:

1. Ensure there is no language barrier. If a language barrier exists, obtain a healthcare interpreter.
2. Be sure the patient or caretaker can read and understand the label. Some patients cannot see the fine print on labels. Others do not have the necessary literacy skills.
3. Ask the patient about drug allergies and any medications that he or she may be taking. Check the label or the package insert for drug interactions. Also

Patient Education boxes teach students about clear and accurate communication with their patients.

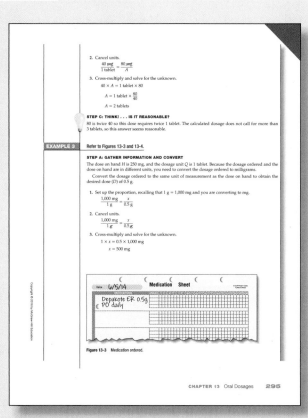

Error Alert! boxes point out common errors to students so they can focus on avoiding them and doing correct calculations instead.

Critical Thinking on the Job boxes contain real-world scenarios that help students apply math and dosage calculations to the healthcare profession. Students must read the scenarios and then answer critical thinking questions to determine what they would do to solve the scenario presented.

Review and Practice

Review and Practice exercises follow every section in each chapter, giving students an immediate opportunity to apply new concepts.

A **three-step solution process** has been included for the dosage calculation problems—Gather Information and Convert, Calculate, and "Think! . . . Is It Reasonable?" This process is used throughout the book to encourage critical thinking skills.

End-of-Chapter Resources

End-of-chapter summaries are tied to the learning outcomes and reinforce key points for the students to review. Page numbers are included for easy reference.

    Homework Assignments provide at least one of every type of problem introduced in the chapter. Answers are *not* provided in the back of the book so that instructors can assign these as an introduction, a review, or even a chapter quiz.

    The **Chapter Review** section offers additional exercises for reinforcement of the chapter content. It falls into these categories: Check Up, Critical Thinking Applications, Case Study, and Internet Activities.

    Unit Assessments are presented at the end of each of the 6 units. In each chapter, all of the calculations have been grouped together to allow students the opportunity to practice a specific skill. In the "real world," however, students will be faced with a variety of situations in which they will need to use each of these skills at various times throughout the day. This assessment requires students to use skills practiced in each of the chapters in the unit. If they have trouble with some of these calculations, it will help them to identify areas where more practice is needed. If they do well, they can move forward with the confidence that they are prepared for the next unit.

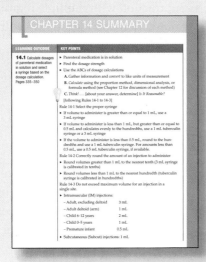

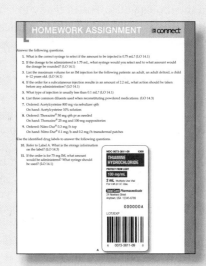

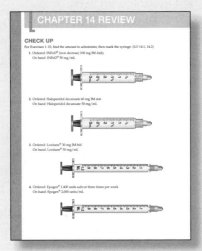

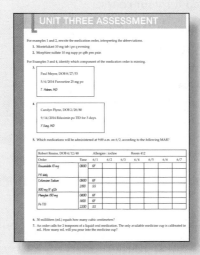

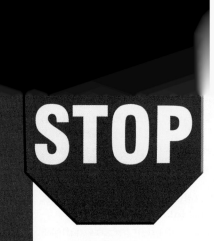

What is ALEKS?

Assessment and Learning in Knowledge Spaces, or ALEKS, is a Web-based, artificially intelligent assessment and learning system. **ALEKS** uses adaptive questioning to quickly and accurately determine exactly what you know and don't know and then instructs you on the topics you are most ready to learn. As you work through a course, **ALEKS** periodically reassesses your understanding to ensure that topics learned are also retained. **ALEKS** courses are very complete in their topic coverage. If you show a high level of mastery of an **ALEKS** course, odds are you will be successful in the actual course you are taking.

For **Booth & Whaley,** *Math and Dosage Calculations for Healthcare Professionals,* a "prep" course has been developed to coincide with the first seven chapters of basic math, measurement, and conversion in the text so that you can refresh your memory as well as brush up on the math skills needed for dosage calculation.

Your instructor can decide to include ALEKS for everyone, or you can also decide to purchase it on your own. See your instructor for information about what is provided for your course.

This course covers the topics shown below.

Prep for Math and Dosage

Whole Numbers (36 topics)

Place Value (2 topics)

- Whole number place value: Problem type 1
- Numeral translation: Problem type 1

Adding and Subtracting Whole Numbers (11 topics)

- Adding a two-digit number and a one-digit number with carry
- Addition without carry
- Addition with carry
- Addition with carry to the hundreds place
- Addition of large numbers
- Subtracting a one-digit number from a two-digit number
- Subtraction without borrowing
- Subtraction with borrowing
- Adding or subtracting 10, 100, or 1,000
- Subtraction with multiple regrouping steps
- Subtraction and regrouping with zeros

Multiplying and Dividing Whole Numbers (16 topics)

- One-digit multiplication
- Multiplication by 10, 100, and 1,000
- Multiplication without carry
- Multiplication with carry
- Introduction to multiplication of large numbers
- Multiplication with trailing zeros: Problem type 1
- Multiplication with trailing zeros: Problem type 2
- Multiplication of large numbers
- Division facts
- Division without carry
- Division with carry
- Division with trailing zeros: Problem type 1
- Division with trailing zeros: Problem type 2
- Division involving quotients with intermediate zeros
- Quotient and remainder: Problem type 1
- Quotient and remainder: Problem type 2

Rounding (2 topics)

- Rounding to tens or hundreds
- Rounding to thousands, ten thousands, or hundred thousands

Factors and Divisibility Rules (5 topics)

- Divisibility rules for 2, 5, and 10
- Divisibility rules for 3 and 9
- Prime numbers
- Greatest common factor of two numbers
- Least common multiple of two numbers

Fractions and Mixed Numbers (32 topics)

Equivalent Fractions (5 topics)

- Introduction to fractions
- Understanding equivalent fractions
- Equivalent fractions
- Introduction to simplifying a fraction
- Simplifying a fraction

Mixed Numbers (3 topics)

- Writing a mixed number and an improper fraction for a shaded region
- Writing an improper fraction as a mixed number
- Writing a mixed number as an improper fraction

Ordering and Plotting Fractions (5 topics)

- Ordering fractions with the same denominator
- Ordering fractions with the same numerator
- Using a common denominator to order fractions
- Fractional position on a number line
- Plotting fractions on a number line

Adding and Subtracting Fractions and Mixed Numbers (8 topics)

- Addition or subtraction of fractions with the same denominator
- Addition or subtraction of unit fractions
- Introduction to addition or subtraction of fractions with different denominators
- Addition or subtraction of fractions with different denominators
- Addition or subtraction of mixed numbers with the same denominator
- Addition of mixed numbers with the same denominator and carry
- Subtraction of mixed numbers with the same denominator and borrowing
- Addition or subtraction of mixed numbers with different denominators

Multiplying and Dividing Fractions and Mixed Numbers (11 topics)

- Product of a unit fraction and a whole number
- Product of a fraction and a whole number: Problem type 1
- Introduction to fraction multiplication
- Fraction multiplication
- The reciprocal of a number
- Division involving a whole number and a fraction
- Fraction division
- Complex fraction without variables: Problem type 1
- Mixed number multiplication: Problem type 1
- Mixed number multiplication: Problem type 2
- Mixed number division

Decimals (23 topics)

Decimal Place Value (6 topics)

- Writing a decimal and a fraction for a shaded region
- Decimal place value: Tenths and hundredths
- Decimal place value: Hundreds to ten thousandths
- Rounding decimals
- Introduction to ordering decimals
- Ordering decimals

Converting between Decimals and Fractions (7 topics)

- Converting a decimal to a fraction: Basic
- Converting a decimal to a proper fraction in simplest form: Advanced
- Converting a fraction with a denominator of 10, 100, or 1,000 to a decimal
- Converting a fraction to a terminating decimal
- Converting a fraction to a repeating decimal
- Converting a decimal to a mixed number
- Converting a mixed number to a decimal

Adding and Subtracting Decimals (3 topics)

- Addition of aligned decimals
- Decimal addition with three numbers
- Subtraction of aligned decimals

Multiplying and Dividing Decimals (7 topics)

- Multiplication of a decimal by a power of 10
- Multiplication of a decimal by a whole number
- Decimal multiplication: Problem type 1
- Division of a decimal by a power of 10
- Division of a decimal by a whole number
- Division of a decimal by a two-digit decimal
- Word problem with powers of 10

Percents, Ratios, and Proportions (7 topics)

Percents (4 topics)

- Finding the percentage of a grid that is shaded
- Converting between percentages and decimals
- Converting a percentage to a fraction in simplest form
- Converting a fraction to a percentage: Denominator of 20, 25, or 50

Ratios (1 topic)

- Writing a ratio as a percentage

Proportions (2 topics)

- Writing a ratio proportion as a fraction proportion
- Finding the missing value in a proportion

Measurements and Conversions (6 topics)

Metric System (4 topics)

- Metric distance conversion with whole number values
- Metric mass or capacity conversion with whole number values
- Metric distance conversion with decimal values
- Metric conversion with decimal values: Two-step problem

Converting Units (1 topic)

- Converting units

Temperature (1 topic)

- Converting between temperatures in Fahrenheit and Celsius

You can test-drive ALEKS yourself at:
http://www.aleks.com/free_trial/consumer
If your instructor has provided you with information and access cards, you'll want to log in at www.aleks.com as soon as possible and begin.

Click "Free Trial" in the "HIGHER EDUCATION" box.

If you're looking to purchase **ALEKS** on your own, go to "Independent Use" on the top of the home screen, from there select "Students" in the left hand side menu item, and then click on the "Getting Started" tab: http://www.aleks.com/independent/students/getting_started

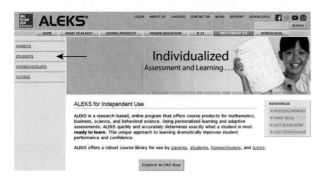

Then, click on the "Buy **ALEKS** Now" to begin to purchase the **Prep for Math and Dosage.** Be sure to choose Higher Education/Math for the Market, and Prep for Math and Dosage as the course.

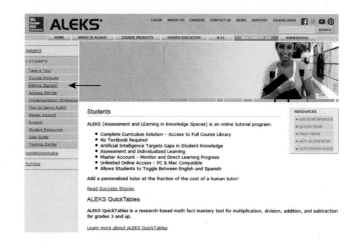

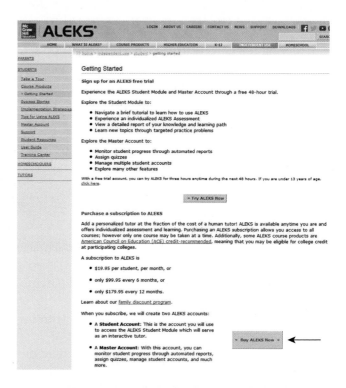

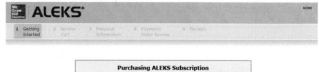

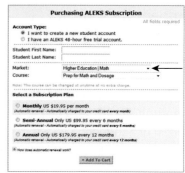

The following test covers basic mathematical concepts that you will need to understand in order to calculate dosages. This test will help you determine which concepts you need to review before continuing. You should already be able to perform basic operations—addition, subtraction, multiplication, and division—with whole numbers. The test covers fractions, decimals, percents, ratios, and proportions.

Take 2 hours to answer the following 75 questions. Review the questions you answered incorrectly to learn more about any basic math weaknesses. Then, as needed, review that content in Chapters 1 through 3. Each question (or group of questions) has an "LO" listed to indicate the learning outcome addressed by the question. If you need to review, these LO indicators will help you find the appropriate material in the text.

1. Convert $\frac{14}{3}$ to a mixed number. (LO 1.1)

2. Convert $3\frac{7}{8}$ to an improper fraction. (LO 1.1)

3. Convert $\frac{8}{5}$ to a mixed number. (LO 1.1)

4. Convert $2\frac{3}{4}$ to an improper fraction. (LO 1.1)

Find the missing numerator in the following proportions. (LO 1.2, 3.4)

5. $\frac{2}{7} = \frac{x}{21}$

6. $1\frac{1}{8} = \frac{x}{16}$

7. Reduce $\frac{40}{100}$ to lowest terms. (LO 1.3)

8. Which fraction has the greater value, $\frac{3}{8}$ or $\frac{2}{6}$? (LO 1.5)

9. Reduce $\frac{48}{10}$ and rewrite the answer as a mixed number. (LO 1.1, 1.3)

10. Which number has a greater value, $3\frac{1}{3}$ or $3\frac{1}{4}$? (LO 1.5)

Calculate the following. Reduce fractions to lowest terms and rewrite fractions greater than 1 as mixed numbers. (LO 1.1, 1.2, 1.3, 1.4, 1.6, 1.7, 1.8, 1.9)

11. $\frac{4}{5} + \frac{3}{8}$	12. $1\frac{1}{3} + \frac{5}{7}$	13. $\frac{7}{10} - \frac{1}{4}$	14. $8\frac{1}{4} - 2\frac{1}{3}$
15. $\frac{3}{5} \times \frac{1}{9}$	16. $3\frac{1}{5} \times 4\frac{3}{8}$	17. $\frac{2}{3} \div \frac{4}{5}$	18. $5\frac{1}{4} \div 2\frac{5}{8}$
19. $\frac{1}{4} + \frac{1}{3}$	20. $2\frac{3}{8} - \frac{3}{4}$	21. $7\frac{1}{2} \times \frac{3}{4}$	22. $3\frac{1}{3} \div 2$

23. Which number has the lesser value, 1.01 or 1.009? (LO 2.1)

24. Round 14.42 to the nearest whole number. (LO 2.2)

25. Round 6.05 to the nearest tenth. (LO 2.2)

26. Round 19.197 to the nearest hundredth. (LO 2.2)

27. Convert $3\frac{4}{5}$ to a decimal number. If necessary, round to the nearest tenth. (LO 2.3)

28. Convert 0.045 to a fraction or a mixed number. Reduce to lowest terms. (LO 2.4)

29. Which number has a greater value, 1.015 or 1.0105?

30. Convert $7\frac{1}{8}$ to a decimal number.

31. Round 3.08 to the nearest whole number.

32. Convert 3.6 to a fraction or mixed number. Reduce to lowest terms.

Calculate the following. (LO 2.5, 2.6, 2.7)

33. $7.289 + 8.011$

34. $0.012 + 0.9 + 4.2$

35. $19.1 - 4.4$

36. $100.03 - 0.6$

37. 0.07×3.2

38. $0.4 \div 0.02$

39. $6 - 1.025$

40. 1.4×1.5

41. $1.05 \div 2$

42. Convert 0.8% to a decimal number. (LO 3.1)

43. Convert 0.99 to a percent. (LO 3.1)

44. Convert 260% to a fraction or mixed number. (LO 3.1)

45. Convert $1\frac{1}{8}$ to a percent. (LO 2.3, 3.1)

46. Convert 7 : 12 to a fraction. Reduce to lowest terms. (LO 3.2)

47. Convert $\frac{10}{50}$ to a ratio. Reduce to lowest terms. (LO 3.2)

48. Convert 1 : 12 to a decimal. Round to the nearest hundredth, if necessary. (LO 3.2)

49. Convert 0.4 to a ratio. Reduce to lowest terms. (LO 3.2)

50. Convert 3 : 8 to a percent. Round to the nearest percent, if necessary. (LO 3.1)

51. Convert 0.5% to a ratio. Reduce to lowest terms. (LO 3.2)

52. Convert 8:3 to a mixed number. (LO 3.2)

53. Convert 0.15 to a ratio. Reduce to lowest terms. (LO 3.2)

54. Convert 1.05 to a percent. (LO 3.1)

55. Convert 1.5% to a fraction. Reduce to lowest terms. (LO 3.1)

Find the missing value in the following proportions. (LO 3.4)

56. $8 : 16 = x : 8$

57. $\frac{5}{9} = \frac{x}{27}$

58. $8 : 12 = x : 9$

59. $\frac{2}{7} = \frac{x}{28}$

60. $\frac{x}{4} = \frac{8}{32}$

61. A healthcare professional is instructed to give a patient $1\frac{1}{2}$ teaspoons of cough syrup 4 times a day. How many teaspoons of cough syrup will be given each day? (LO 3.4)

62. A healthcare professional tries to keep the equivalent of 12 bottles of a medication on hand. The hospital's first floor has $1\frac{1}{2}$ bottles, the second floor has $1\frac{3}{4}$ bottles, the third floor has $3\frac{1}{4}$ bottles, and the supply closet has 3 bottles. Is there enough medication on hand? If not, how much should be ordered? (LO 1.6)

63. A bottle contains 75 milliliters (mL) of a liquid medication. Since the bottle was opened, one patient has received 3 doses of 2.5 mL. A second patient has received 4 doses of 2.2 mL. How much medication remains in the bottle? (LO 2.5, 2.6)

64. A tablet contains 0.125 milligram (mg) of medication. A patient receives 3 tablets a day for 5 days. How many milligrams of medication does the patient receive over the 5 days? (LO 2.6)

65. An IV bag contained 1,000 mL of a liquid. The liquid was administered to a patient, and after 3 hours, 400 mL remain in the bag. How much IV fluid did the patient receive each hour? (LO 3.4)

66. The patient is taking 0.5 mg of medication 4 times a day. How many milligrams would the patient receive after $1\frac{1}{2}$ days? (LO 2.6, 3.4)

67. The patient took 0.88 microgram (mcg) every morning and 1.2 mcg each evening for 4 days. What was the total amount of medication taken? (LO 2.5, 2.6)

68. Write a ratio that represents that 500 mL of solution contains 5 mg of drug. Reduce to lowest terms. (LO 3.3)

69. Write a ratio that represents that every tablet in a bottle contains 25 mg of drug. Reduce to lowest terms. (LO 3.3)

70. Write a ratio that represents that 3 mL of solution contains 125 mg of drug. Reduce to lowest terms. (LO 3.4)

71. A patient takes 5 mL of a medication twice a day. How long will 120 mL last? (LO 3.4)

72. Write a ratio that represents 2 mg of drug in 1 mL of a liquid. Reduce to lowest terms. (LO 3.2)

73. If a patient has to take 2 tablets a day for 10 days, how many tablets will he need to fill his prescription? (LO 3.4)

74. If each 5 mL of a solution contains 15 mg of medication, how many mL of solution will a patient need to take to get 60 mg of medication? (LO 3.4)

75. If a solution has 80 mg of medication in 500 mL, how much solution is needed to get 40 mg of medication? (LO 3.4)

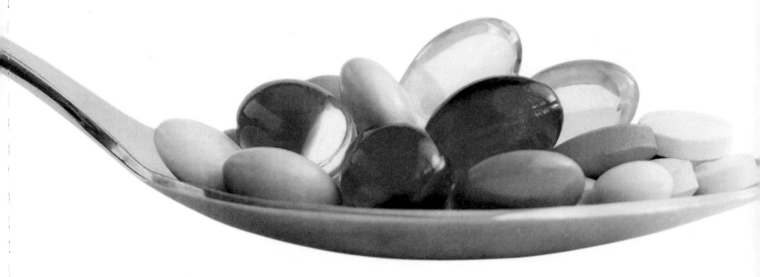

UNIT 1

Performing Basic Math

Fractions

CHAPTER 1

He who is ashamed of asking is ashamed of learning.

DANISH PROVERB

LEARNING OUTCOMES

When you have completed Chapter 1, you will be able to:

1.1 Produce fractions and mixed numbers in the proper form.

1.2 Identify and produce equivalent fractions.

1.3 Determine the simplest form of a fraction.

1.4 Find the least common denominator.

1.5 Compare the values of fractions.

1.6 Add fractions.

1.7 Subtract fractions.

1.8 Multiply fractions.

1.9 Divide fractions.

KEY TERMS

Complex fraction
Denominator
Equivalent fractions
Least common denominator
Mixed number
Numerator
Prime number
Reciprocal
Reduce
Simplify

INTRODUCTION

Basic math skills, such as working with fractions, are the building blocks for accurate dosage calculations. To prepare yourself mathematically, you must be confident in your math skills; so do not be afraid to ask for help while you are learning these important concepts. Remember that a minor mistake in basic math can mean major errors in the patient's medication.

1.1 Fractions and Mixed Numbers

Fractions measure a portion or part of a whole amount. They are written in two ways: as common fractions or as mixed numbers. In medical settings, it is sometimes necessary to convert from one type of fraction to another.

ALEKS®

GO TO . . .

Fractions and Mixed Numbers–Equivalent Fractions–Introduction to Fractions.

Common Fractions

A common fraction represents parts of a whole. It consists of two numbers and a fraction bar, and it is written in the form:

$$\frac{\text{Numerator}}{\text{Denominator}}$$

2

The **denominator**—the bottom part of the fraction—represents the whole. It can *never* equal zero. Suppose the whole is 1 yard (yd). You could express the denominator as 3 (the yard as 3 feet) or 36 (the yard as 36 inches).

The **numerator**—the top part of the fraction—represents parts of the whole. If you buy 2 feet (ft) of fabric out of a yard, you can express the numerator as 2 feet (ft) with the denominator as 3 feet (ft). The fraction $\frac{2}{3}$ represents how much of a yard of fabric you buy, or 2 of 3 ft.

Suppose you are working with a medicine tablet that is scored (marked) for division in two parts, and you must administer one part of that tablet each day. The denominator represents the whole tablet. The numerator represents one part, the amount that you administer each day. The fraction, or part, of the tablet that you must administer each day is written as:

$$\frac{\text{Numerator}}{\text{Denominator}} = \frac{1 \text{ part}}{2 \text{ parts}} = \frac{1}{2}$$

This number is read *one-half*. The denominator is 2, since two parts make up the whole. If you administer 1 part each day, you administer $\frac{1}{2}$ of the tablet.

If you have trouble remembering which number is the numerator and which is the denominator, note that the words *denominator* and *down* begin with the letter d. The <u>d</u>enominator is <u>d</u>own, under the fraction bar.

The fraction $\frac{2}{3}$, read as *two-thirds*, means two parts out of the three parts that make up the whole. The fraction bar also means *divided by*. Thus, $\frac{2}{3}$ can be read as "two divided by three," or $2 \div 3$. This definition is important when you change fractions to decimals.

Sometimes fractions show the relationship between part of a group and the whole group. For example, in a group of 15 patients with hyperthyroidism, 9 patients respond well to a medication. The other 6 patients show no change. The number of patients in the full group, 15, is the whole, or the denominator. You write the fraction of patients who respond well to the medication as:

$$\frac{\text{Part}}{\text{Whole}} = \frac{\text{respond well}}{\text{whole group}} = \frac{9}{15}$$

Similarly, the fraction of patients who show no change is:

$$\frac{\text{Part}}{\text{Whole}} = \frac{\text{show no change}}{\text{whole group}} = \frac{6}{15}$$

RULE 1-1	When the denominator is 1, the fraction equals the number in the numerator.
Example	$\frac{4}{1} = 4 \qquad \frac{100}{1} = 100$ Check these equations by treating each fraction as a division problem. $4 \div 1 = 4 \qquad 100 \div 1 = 100$

Mixed Numbers

Fractions with a value greater than 1 are more properly written as mixed numbers. A **mixed number** combines a whole number with a fraction. Examples include $2\frac{2}{3}$ (two and two-thirds), $1\frac{7}{8}$ (one and seven-eighths) and $12\frac{31}{32}$ (twelve and thirty-one thirty-seconds).

RULE 1-2	If the numerator of the fraction is less than the denominator, the fraction has a value less than ($<$) 1.
	If the numerator of the fraction is equal to the denominator, the fraction has a value equal to ($=$) 1.
	If the numerator of the fraction is greater than the denominator, the fraction has a value greater than ($>$) 1. Fractions with a value greater than 1 may be written as a mixed number.
Example 1	Is $\frac{8}{9}$ less than, greater than, or equal to 1?
	The fraction $\frac{8}{9}$ is less than 1 because the numerator (8) is less than the denominator (9). This can be written $\frac{8}{9} < 1$.
Example 2	Is $\frac{12}{12}$ less than, greater than, or equal to 1?
	$\frac{12}{12}$ is equal to 1 because the numerator (12) is equal to the denominator (12). This can be written $\frac{12}{12} = 1$.
Example 3	Is $\frac{8}{5}$ less than, greater than, or equal to 1?
	$\frac{8}{5}$ is greater than 1 because the numerator (8) is greater than the denominator (5). This can be written $\frac{8}{5} > 1$.

RULE 1-3	To convert a fraction to a mixed number:
ALEKS®	**1.** Divide the numerator by the denominator. The result will be a whole number plus a remainder.
GO TO . . .	**2.** Write the remainder as the numerator over the original denominator.
Mixed Numbers– Writing an Improper Fraction as a Mixed Number.	**3.** Combine the whole number and the fractional remainder. This mixed number equals the original fraction.
	Reminder: This rule is only applied when the numerator is greater than the denominator.
Example 1	Convert $\frac{11}{4}$ to a mixed number.
	1. Divide the numerator by the denominator.
	$11 \div 4 = 2$ R3 (R3 means a *remainder* of 3.)
	The result is the whole number 2 with a remainder of 3.

2. Write the remainder as the numerator over the original denominator of 4.

$$\frac{\text{Remainder}}{\text{Denominator}} = \frac{3}{4}$$

3. Combine the whole number and the fractional remainder.

$$2 + \frac{3}{4} = 2\frac{3}{4}$$

The mixed number $2\frac{3}{4}$ equals the original fraction $\frac{11}{4}$.

Example 2	Convert $\frac{23}{7}$ to a mixed number.

1. $23 \div 7 = 3 \text{ R2}$

The result is the whole number 3 with a remainder of 2.

2. $\dfrac{\text{Remainder}}{\text{Denominator}} = \dfrac{2}{7}$

3. $3 + \dfrac{2}{7} = 3\dfrac{2}{7}$

The fraction $\frac{23}{7}$ equals the mixed number $3\frac{2}{7}$.

You can also convert mixed numbers to fractions. This is often necessary before you use the number in a calculation.

RULE 1-4

ALEKS®

GO TO . . .
Mixed Numbers–
Writing a Mixed
Number as an
Improper Fraction.

To convert a mixed number to a fraction:

1. Multiply the whole number by the denominator of the fraction.

2. Add the product from step 1 to the numerator of the fraction.

3. Write the sum from step 2 over the original denominator. The result is a fraction equal to the original mixed number.

You can also use this equation for converting a mixed number to a fraction:

$$\text{Mixed number} = \frac{(\text{whole number} \times \text{denominator}) + \text{numerator}}{\text{denominator}}$$

Example 1

Convert $5\frac{1}{3}$ to a fraction.

The whole number is 5. The denominator of the fraction is 3. The numerator of the fraction is 1.

1. Multiply the whole number by the denominator of the fraction.

$$5 \times 3 = 15$$

2. Add the product from step 1 to the numerator of the fraction.

$$15 + 1 = 16$$

3. Write the sum from step 2 over the original denominator.

$$\frac{16}{3}$$

Thus, $5\frac{1}{3} = \frac{16}{3}$.

Example 2	Convert $10\frac{7}{8}$ to a fraction.

The whole number is 10. The denominator is 8. The numerator is 7.

1. $10 \times 8 = 80$

2. $80 + 7 = 87$

3. $\frac{87}{8}$

Thus, $10\frac{7}{8} = \frac{87}{8}$.

CRITICAL THINKING ON THE JOB

While performing a calculation, a healthcare professional adds the following numbers $21\frac{3}{4}$, $12\frac{1}{2}$, and $1\frac{1}{2}$. He calculates an answer of $49\frac{1}{4}$. Before he accepts this answer as correct, however, he asks himself "Is this reasonable?" In order to answer this question, he does a quick estimation. First, he adds the whole numbers from each of the mixed numbers in the problem: $21 + 12 + 1 = 34$. Then he rounds each mixed number up to a whole number and adds them: $22 + 13 + 2 = 37$. He recognizes that the correct answer to the problem must be between 34 and 37, so his original answer is incorrect. He likely entered one of the numbers into his calculator incorrectly. When he repeats the original calculation, he comes up with an answer of $35\frac{3}{4}$. This is between the values that he expected based on his estimate, so it is a reasonable answer to the problem.

 Think! . . . Is It Reasonable? Many types of errors can occur during a dosage calculation. In this case, a number had been entered incorrectly into a calculator. While errors like this can happen to anyone, they can usually be detected by performing a quick check to see if the answer is reasonable. Throughout this text you will be asked to "Think! . . . Is It Reasonable?" on a number of examples in each chapter. This question is included as a reminder, but you should develop the habit of asking yourself the same question *every time you perform a calculation*. When performing a calculation, analyze the problem and try to estimate a reasonable range for the answer. This critical thinking skill can help you to detect errors and should become a part of every calculation you perform.

REVIEW AND PRACTICE

1.1 Fractions and Mixed Numbers

1. What is the numerator in $\frac{17}{100}$?

2. What is the numerator in $\frac{8}{3}$?

3. What is the denominator in $\frac{4}{100}$?

4. What is the denominator in $\frac{60}{1}$?

5. Twelve patients are in a hospital ward. Four have type A blood.
   a. What fraction of the patients have type A blood?
   b. What fraction of the patients do not have type A blood?

6. Twenty patients are in a hospital ward. Six have diabetes.
   a. What fraction of the patients have diabetes?
   b. What fraction of the patients do not have diabetes?

7. Write this expression as a fraction: $16 \div 3$

8. Write this expression as a fraction: $4 \div 15$

9. Write this expression as a fraction: $3 \div 4$

10. Insert $<$, $>$, or $=$ to make a true statement, where $<$ means less than, $>$ means greater than, and $=$ means equal to.

    a. $\frac{14}{14}$ 1
    b. $\frac{24}{32}$ 1
    c. $\frac{125}{100}$ 1

11. Insert $<$, $>$, or $=$ to make a true statement, where $<$ means less than, $>$ means greater than, and $=$ means equal to.

    a. $\frac{24}{3}$ 1
    b. $\frac{75}{100}$ 1
    c. $\frac{18}{18}$ 1

Convert the following fractions to mixed or whole numbers.

12. $\frac{43}{6}$
13. $\frac{17}{3}$
14. $\frac{100}{20}$
15. $\frac{50}{50}$

16. $\frac{8}{5}$
17. $\frac{167}{25}$
18. $\frac{16}{12}$

Convert the following mixed numbers to fractions.

19. $2\frac{16}{17}$
20. $8\frac{8}{9}$
21. $1\frac{1}{10}$
22. $4\frac{1}{8}$

23. $103\frac{2}{3}$
24. $6\frac{7}{8}$
25. $8\frac{1}{5}$

1.2 Equivalent Fractions

Two fractions may have the same value even when they are written differently. These are known as **equivalent fractions**. Suppose you and a friend are sharing an orange equally, dividing it in half. If the orange has eight sections, you will each get four pieces, or $\frac{4}{8}$ of the whole orange. If the orange has six sections, you will each get three pieces, or $\frac{3}{6}$. And if the orange only has four sections, you will each get two pieces, or $\frac{2}{4}$. Whether you get $\frac{4}{8}$, $\frac{3}{6}$, or $\frac{2}{4}$

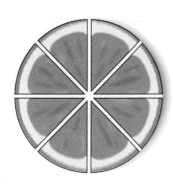 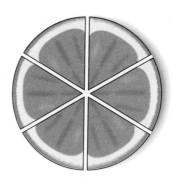 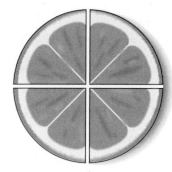

Figure 1-1 Equivalent fractions.

of the orange, you still have the same amount: one-half or $\frac{1}{2}$ of the orange (see Figure 1-1). Thus, $\frac{4}{8} = \frac{3}{6} = \frac{2}{4} = \frac{1}{2}$. These four fractions are equivalent fractions.

CONVERTING FRACTIONS Equivalent fractions help you compare measurements more easily. They also help you add and subtract fractions that have different denominators.

RULE 1-5 **ALEKS**® **GO TO . . .** Fractions and Mixed Numbers– Equivalent Fractions.	To find an equivalent fraction, multiply or divide both the numerator and denominator by the same number. *Exception:* The numerator and denominator cannot be multiplied or divided by zero.
Example 1	Find equivalent fractions for $\frac{2}{4}$. $\dfrac{2 \times 2}{4 \times 2} = \dfrac{4}{8}$ $\dfrac{2 \times 3}{4 \times 3} = \dfrac{6}{12}$ $\dfrac{2 \div 2}{4 \div 2} = \dfrac{1}{2}$ $\dfrac{2 \times 10}{4 \times 10} = \dfrac{20}{40}$ Thus, $\frac{2}{4} = \frac{4}{8} = \frac{6}{12} = \frac{1}{2} = \frac{20}{40}$. These are equivalent fractions.
Example 2	Find equivalent fractions for $\frac{4}{7}$. $\dfrac{4 \times 3}{7 \times 3} = \dfrac{12}{21}$ $\dfrac{4 \times 5}{7 \times 5} = \dfrac{20}{35}$ $\dfrac{4 \times 10}{7 \times 10} = \dfrac{40}{70}$ $\dfrac{4 \times 100}{7 \times 100} = \dfrac{400}{700}$ Thus, $\frac{4}{7} = \frac{12}{21} = \frac{20}{35} = \frac{40}{70} = \frac{400}{700}$. These are equivalent fractions. **Think! . . . Is It Reasonable?** In this case, the original numerator was more than half of the denominator. Since this was true for the original fraction, it should also be true for all of the equivalent fractions.
Example 3	Find some equivalent fractions for 4. To find equivalent fractions for a whole number, first write the whole number as a fraction. Then proceed as before. $4 = \dfrac{4}{1}$ $\dfrac{4 \times 2}{1 \times 2} = \dfrac{8}{2}$ $\dfrac{4 \times 3}{1 \times 3} = \dfrac{12}{3}$ $\dfrac{4 \times 4}{1 \times 4} = \dfrac{16}{4}$ $\dfrac{4 \times 5}{1 \times 5} = \dfrac{20}{5}$ Thus, $4 = \frac{4}{1} = \frac{8}{2} = \frac{12}{3} = \frac{16}{4} = \frac{20}{5}$. These are some equivalent fractions.

The **GO TO . . .** note at the left of the rule box reads:

ALEKS®

GO TO . . .
Fractions and Mixed Numbers– Equivalent Fractions– Understanding Equivalent Fractions.

| **Example 4** | Find some equivalent fractions for $1\frac{4}{6}$. |

To find equivalent fractions for a mixed number, first convert the mixed number to a fraction.

1. $1 \times 6 = 6$

2. $6 + 4 = 10$

3. $1\frac{4}{6} = \frac{10}{6}$

Now follow the same steps used in Examples 1 through 3.

$$\frac{10 \times 2}{6 \times 2} = \frac{20}{12} \qquad \frac{10 \times 3}{6 \times 3} = \frac{30}{18} \qquad \frac{10 \div 2}{6 \div 2} = \frac{5}{3} \qquad \frac{10 \times 10}{6 \times 10} = \frac{100}{60}$$

Thus, $1\frac{4}{6} = \frac{10}{6} = \frac{20}{12} = \frac{30}{18} = \frac{5}{3} = \frac{100}{60}$.

FINDING MISSING NUMERATORS   Suppose you want to convert a fraction into an equivalent one with a specific denominator. To convert $\frac{1}{5}$ to tenths, find the missing value in $\frac{1}{5} = \frac{x}{10}$. The x stands for the number you want to find.

In this case, multiply the numerator in the original fraction by the denominator in the new fraction. Then divide the result by the original denominator. The original numerator is 1 and the denominator is 10.

$$1 \times 10 = 10$$

The original denominator is 5.

$$10 \div 5 = 2$$

$$x = 2 \quad \text{The numerator for the new fraction is 2.}$$

| **RULE 1-6** | To find the missing numerator in an equivalent fraction: |

1. Multiply the original numerator by the denominator of the new fraction.

2. Divide the product from step a by the original denominator.

| **Example 1** | $\frac{2}{3} = \frac{x}{12}$ |

1. Multiply the original numerator by the denominator of the new fraction.

$$2 \times 12 = 24$$

2. Divide the product from step a by the original denominator.

$$24 \div 3 = 8$$

Thus, $x = 8$ and $\frac{2}{3} = \frac{8}{12}$.

Example 2

$$\frac{28}{60} = \frac{x}{15}$$

1. Multiply the original numerator by the denominator of the new fraction.

$28 \times 15 = 420$

2. Divide the product from step a by the original denominator.

$420 \div 60 = 7$

Thus, $x = 7$ and $\frac{28}{60} = \frac{7}{15}$.

Think! . . . Is It Reasonable? In the original fraction, the numerator (28) was slightly less than half the value of the denominator (60). Based on this observation, is 7 a reasonable answer?

Example 3

$$2\frac{1}{2} = \frac{x}{6}$$

First convert the mixed number into a fraction.

$$2\frac{1}{2} = \frac{(2 \times 2) + 1}{2} = \frac{5}{2}$$

The equation is now $\frac{5}{2} = \frac{x}{6}$.

1. Multiply the original numerator by the denominator of the new fraction.

$5 \times 6 = 30$

2. Divide the product from step a by the original denominator.

$30 \div 2 = 15$

Thus, $x = 15$ and $2\frac{1}{2} = \frac{15}{6}$.

REVIEW AND PRACTICE

1.2 Equivalent Fractions

Find three equivalent fractions for each of the following.

1. $\frac{4}{5}$
2. $\frac{1}{10}$
3. $\frac{4}{2}$
4. $\frac{15}{9}$
5. 9

6. 24
7. $2\frac{1}{3}$
8. $3\frac{6}{9}$
9. $\frac{7}{12}$
10. $4\frac{1}{4}$

Find the missing numerator in the following equations.

11. $\frac{3}{8} = \frac{x}{16}$
12. $\frac{1}{3} = \frac{x}{27}$
13. $\frac{16}{24} = \frac{x}{6}$
14. $\frac{18}{15} = \frac{x}{5}$
15. $3 = \frac{x}{4}$

16. $5 = \frac{x}{12}$
17. $1\frac{5}{16} = \frac{x}{160}$
18. $4\frac{2}{8} = \frac{x}{4}$
19. $\frac{8}{12} = \frac{x}{24}$
20. $\frac{32}{16} = \frac{x}{4}$

1.3 Reducing Fractions

To **reduce** (or **simplify**) a fraction means to divide the numerator and denominator by a common factor. This results in an equivalent fraction with a lower numerator and denominator. Reduced or simplified equivalent fractions are often easier to use when you are performing a calculation. It is considered proper form to express your final answer in a fraction that is reduced to its lowest terms.

To reduce a fraction to its lowest terms, find the largest whole number that divides evenly into both the numerator and the denominator. When no whole number except 1 divides evenly into them, the fraction is reduced to its lowest terms.

Example 1

Reduce $\frac{10}{15}$ to its lowest terms.

Both 10 and 15 are divisible by 5.

$$\frac{10 \div 5}{15 \div 5} = \frac{2}{3}$$

No whole number other than 1 divides evenly into *both* 2 and 3. Thus, $\frac{10}{15}$ has been reduced to its lowest terms, $\frac{2}{3}$.

Example 2

Reduce $\frac{24}{30}$ to its lowest terms.

Both 24 and 30 are divisible by 6.

$$\frac{24 \div 6}{30 \div 6} = \frac{4}{5}$$

No whole number other than 1 divides evenly into *both* 4 and 5. Thus, $\frac{24}{30}$ has been reduced to its lowest terms, $\frac{4}{5}$.

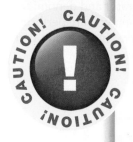

Reducing a Fraction Does Not Automatically Mean You Have

Simplified It to Its Lowest Terms

More than one number may divide evenly into both the numerator and the denominator. For example, both 18 and 42 are even numbers. To reduce $\frac{18}{42}$, you can divide by 2, so that:

$$\frac{18 \div 2}{42 \div 2} = \frac{9}{21}$$

You are not done, though. Both 9 and 21 are divisible by 3, so that:

$$\frac{18}{42} = \frac{9}{21} = \frac{9 \div 3}{21 \div 3} = \frac{3}{7}$$

Some fractions are easy to reduce. Looking at $\frac{2}{4}$, you can guess that 2 divides evenly into both the numerator and the denominator, so that $\frac{2 \div 2}{4 \div 2} = \frac{1}{2}$. In other cases, you may have to use several steps. See Table 1-1 for numbers divisible by 2, 3, 4, 5, 6, 8, 9, or 10.

Prime numbers are whole numbers other than 1 that can be evenly divided only by themselves and 1. The first 10 prime numbers are 2, 3, 5, 7, 11, 13, 17, 19, 23, and 29. If either the numerator or the denominator of a fraction is a prime number, and if the other term is not divisible by that prime number, then the fraction is in lowest terms. For example, $\frac{17}{24}$ is in lowest terms. However, you can simplify $\frac{17}{34}$ to $\frac{1}{2}$, dividing both the numerator and denominator by 17.

TABLE 1-1 Is a Number Divisible by 2, 3, 4, 5, 6, 8, 9, or 10?		
NUMBER	**HINT**	**EXAMPLE**
2	Even numbers (numbers ending with 2, 4, 6, 8, or 0) are divisible by 2.	112; 734; 2,936; 10,118; 356,920
3	If the sum of the digits of a number is divisible by 3, then the number is divisible by 3.	37,887 The sum of the digits is $3 + 7 + 8 + 8 + 7 = 33$; 33 is divisible by 3.
4	If the last two digits of a number are divisible by 4, the entire number is divisible by 4.	126,936 The last two digits form a number, 36, that is divisible by 4.
5	Any number that ends with 5 or 0 is divisible by 5.	735 12,290
6	Combine the rules for 2 and 3: If a number is even *and* the sum of its digits is divisible by 3, then the number is divisible by 6.	582 The number is even. The sum of its digits, $5 + 8 + 2 = 15$, is divisible by 3.
8	If the last three digits are divisible by 8, then the entire number is divisible by 8.	42,376 Here, 376 is divisible by 8.
9	If the sum of the digits is a multiple of 9, the number is divisible by 9.	42,705 $4 + 2 + 7 + 0 + 5 = 18$, which is divisible by 9.
10	If a number ends with 0, then the number is divisible by 10.	640

1.3 Reducing Fractions

Reduce the following fractions to their lowest terms.

1. $\dfrac{10}{12}$ 2. $\dfrac{3}{6}$ 3. $\dfrac{27}{81}$ 4. $\dfrac{11}{22}$ 5. $\dfrac{10}{100}$

6. $\dfrac{55}{100}$ 7. $\dfrac{4}{5}$ 8. $\dfrac{6}{17}$ 9. $\dfrac{21}{27}$ 10. $\dfrac{35}{50}$

11. $\dfrac{48}{90}$ 12. $\dfrac{49}{84}$ 13. $\dfrac{10}{28}$ 14. $\dfrac{5}{8}$ 15. $\dfrac{33}{99}$

16. $\dfrac{25}{35}$ 17. $\dfrac{18}{48}$ 18. $\dfrac{49}{77}$ 19. $\dfrac{8}{32}$ 20. $\dfrac{24}{44}$

1.4 Finding Common Denominators

A *common denominator* is any number that is a common multiple of all the denominators in a group of fractions. The **least common denominator** (LCD) is the smallest of these numbers. Before you can compare, add, or subtract fractions with different denominators, you must first convert them to equivalent fractions with a common denominator.

RULE 1-8	To find the least common denominator (LCD) of a group of fractions:
	1. List the multiples of each denominator.
	2. Compare the lists. Any numbers that appear on all lists are common denominators.
	3. The smallest number that appears on all the lists is the LCD.
	Once you have found the LCD, you can convert each fraction to an equivalent fraction with the LCD as the denominator.
Example 1	Find the least common denominator of $\frac{1}{3}$ and $\frac{1}{2}$. Then convert each to an equivalent fraction with the LCD.
	1. The number 3 divides evenly into 3, <u>6</u>, 9, <u>12</u>, 15, <u>18</u>, and 21. The number 2 divides evenly into 2, 4, <u>6</u>, 8, 10, <u>12</u>, 14, 16, and <u>18</u>.
	2. The numbers 6, 12, and 18 are common denominators.
	3. The smallest number that appears on both lists is 6. It is the least common denominator and is divisible by both 3 and 2.
	Now convert $\frac{1}{3}$ and $\frac{1}{2}$ to equivalent fractions with 6 as the denominator.

4. To convert $\frac{1}{3}$ to the equivalent fraction $\frac{x}{6}$:

$$\frac{1}{3} = \frac{x}{6}$$

$$6 \div 3 = 2$$

$$\frac{1}{3} = \frac{2}{6}$$

5. To convert $\frac{1}{2}$ to the equivalent fraction $\frac{x}{6}$:

$$6 \div 2 = 3$$

$$\frac{1}{2} = \frac{3}{6}$$

The least common denominator is 6. Using this denominator, the equivalent fractions are $\frac{1}{3} = \frac{2}{6}$ and $\frac{1}{2} = \frac{3}{6}$.

Example 2

Find the least common denominator of $\frac{1}{4}$, $\frac{1}{6}$, and $\frac{1}{8}$. Then convert each to an equivalent fraction with the LCD.

1. The number 4 divides evenly into 4, 8, 12, 16, 20, and <u>24.</u>

The number 6 divides evenly into 6, 12, 18, and <u>24.</u>

The number 8 divides evenly into 8, 16, and <u>24.</u>

2. The number 24 is a common denominator.

3. In this case, 24 is the LCD.

4. $\frac{1}{4} = \frac{x}{24}$

$$24 \div 4 = 6$$

$$\frac{1}{4} = \frac{6}{24}$$

5. $\frac{1}{6} = \frac{x}{24}$

$$24 \div 6 = 4$$

$$\frac{1}{6} = \frac{4}{24}$$

6. $\frac{1}{8} = \frac{x}{24}$

$$24 \div 8 = 3$$

$$\frac{1}{8} = \frac{3}{24}$$

The least common denominator is 24. Using this denominator, we see the equivalent fractions are:

$$\frac{1}{4} = \frac{6}{24}$$

$$\frac{1}{6} = \frac{4}{24}$$

$$\frac{1}{8} = \frac{3}{24}$$

You may find it difficult to find common denominators of fractions with large denominators. However, you can simply multiply the individual denominators to find a common denominator.

RULE 1-9	To convert fractions with large denominators to equivalent fractions with a common denominator: **1.** List the denominators of all the fractions. **2.** Multiply the denominators. The product is a common denominator. Convert each fraction to an equivalent one with the common denominator.
Example 1	Convert $\frac{1}{7}$ and $\frac{1}{19}$ to equivalent fractions with a common denominator. **1.** The denominators are 7 and 19. **2.** Multiply 7×19. The common denominator is 133. $$\frac{1}{7} = \frac{1 \times 19}{7 \times 19} = \frac{19}{133} \qquad \text{and} \qquad \frac{1}{19} = \frac{1 \times 7}{19 \times 7} = \frac{7}{133}$$ The equivalent fractions are $\frac{19}{133}$ and $\frac{7}{133}$.
Example 2	Convert $\frac{2}{37}$ and $\frac{7}{90}$ to equivalent fractions with a common denominator. **1.** The denominators are 37 and 90. **2.** $37 \times 90 = 3{,}330$ $$\frac{2 \times 90}{37 \times 90} = \frac{180}{3{,}330} \qquad \text{and} \qquad \frac{7 \times 37}{90 \times 37} = \frac{259}{3{,}330}$$ The equivalent fractions are $\frac{180}{3{,}330}$ and $\frac{259}{3{,}330}$.

REVIEW AND PRACTICE

1.4 Finding Common Denominators

For each set of fractions, find the least common denominator. Then convert each fraction to an equivalent fraction with the LCD.

1. $\frac{1}{3}$ and $\frac{1}{7}$ 2. $\frac{1}{5}$ and $\frac{1}{8}$ 3. $\frac{1}{25}$ and $\frac{1}{40}$ 4. $\frac{1}{24}$ and $\frac{1}{36}$ 5. $\frac{1}{2}$ and $\frac{1}{12}$

6. $\frac{1}{6}$ and $\frac{1}{18}$ 7. $\frac{5}{6}$ and $\frac{4}{7}$ 8. $\frac{3}{4}$ and $\frac{5}{8}$ 9. $\frac{1}{9}$ and $\frac{1}{36}$ 10. $\frac{5}{24}$ and $\frac{9}{96}$

11. $\frac{4}{5}$ and $\frac{9}{11}$ 12. $\frac{5}{6}$ and $\frac{7}{12}$ 13. $\frac{11}{30}$ and $\frac{21}{80}$ 14. $\frac{5}{48}$ and $\frac{7}{72}$ 15. $\frac{1}{2}, \frac{1}{3},$ and $\frac{1}{4}$

16. $\frac{1}{6}, \frac{4}{9},$ and $\frac{13}{24}$ 17. $\frac{2}{3}, \frac{4}{9},$ and $\frac{7}{15}$ 18. $\frac{1}{4}, \frac{5}{6},$ and $\frac{7}{16}$ 19. $\frac{1}{5}, \frac{3}{10},$ and $\frac{7}{20}$ 20. $\frac{1}{6}, \frac{5}{24},$ and $\frac{9}{40}$

1.5 Comparing Fractions

ALEKS®

GO TO . . .
Ordering and
Plotting Fractions–
Ordering Fractions
with the Same
Denominator.

Suppose a home patient is to take $\frac{3}{4}$ tablespoon (tbs) of medication with lunch. You learn that the patient took $\frac{2}{3}$ tbs. Did the patient take too little, too much, or just the right amount?

To determine this answer, convert the fractions to equivalent fractions with a common denominator, and then compare the numerators. For this example the equivalent fractions are:

$$\frac{3}{4} = \frac{9}{12} \qquad \frac{2}{3} = \frac{8}{12}$$

$\frac{9}{12}$ is more than $\frac{8}{12}$, so the patient did not take enough.

RULE 1-10	To compare fractions:
ALEKS® GO TO . . . Ordering and Plotting Fractions– Using a Common Denominator to Order Fractions.	1. Write all fractions as equivalent fractions with a common denominator. 2. Write the fractions in order by the size of the numerator. The fraction with the largest numerator is the largest in the group. 3. Restate the comparisons with the original fractions.
Example 1	Order from smallest to largest: $\frac{1}{5}, \frac{4}{5},$ and $\frac{3}{10}$. 1. Write the fractions as equivalent fractions with a common denominator. The least common denominator of $\frac{1}{5}, \frac{4}{5},$ and $\frac{3}{10}$ is 10. $$\frac{1}{5} = \frac{2}{10}$$

$$\frac{4}{5} = \frac{8}{10}$$

$$\frac{3}{10} = \frac{3}{10}$$

If you have difficulty with this step, review "Equivalent Fractions" and "Finding Common Denominators" in this chapter.

2. Order the fractions by the size of their numerators, in this case, from smallest to largest.

$$\frac{2}{10} \quad \frac{3}{10} \quad \frac{8}{10}$$

Insert the proper comparison signs.

$$\frac{2}{10} < \frac{3}{10} < \frac{8}{10}$$

3. Restate with the original equivalent fractions.

$$\frac{1}{5} < \frac{3}{10} < \frac{4}{5}$$

Example 2

Order from largest to smallest $1\frac{7}{8}, \frac{6}{3}, 2, \frac{2}{8}$.

First, convert all whole and mixed numbers to fractions.

$$1\frac{7}{8} = \frac{15}{8}$$

$$2 = \frac{2}{1}$$

If you have difficulty with this step, review "Fractions and Mixed Numbers" in this chapter.

1. Write all fractions as equivalent fractions with a common denominator. The LCD for this set of fractions is 24.

$$1\frac{7}{8} = \frac{15}{8} = \frac{45}{24}$$

$$\frac{6}{3} = \frac{48}{24}$$

$$2 = \frac{48}{24}$$

$$\frac{2}{8} = \frac{6}{24}$$

2. Write the fractions in descending order by the size of their numerator.

$$\frac{48}{24} \quad \frac{45}{24} \quad \frac{6}{24}$$

Insert the proper comparison signs.

$$\frac{48}{24} > \frac{45}{24} > \frac{6}{24}$$

3. Restate with the original equivalent fractions.

$$\frac{6}{3} > 1\frac{7}{8} > \frac{2}{8}$$

1.5 Comparing Fractions

Insert $>$, $<$, or $=$ to make a true statement.

1. $\dfrac{1}{5}$ $\dfrac{3}{5}$ 2. $\dfrac{7}{9}$ $\dfrac{4}{9}$ 3. $\dfrac{2}{8}$ $\dfrac{1}{4}$ 4. $\dfrac{7}{10}$ $\dfrac{7}{20}$ 5. $\dfrac{3}{24}$ $\dfrac{1}{8}$

6. $\dfrac{11}{3}$ $\dfrac{13}{9}$ 7. 1 $\dfrac{2}{3}$ 8. $\dfrac{9}{4}$ 2 9. $\dfrac{3}{12}$ $\dfrac{13}{36}$ 10. $1\dfrac{1}{12}$ $1\dfrac{5}{12}$

11. $3\dfrac{3}{5}$ $3\dfrac{2}{5}$ 12. $1\dfrac{3}{4}$ $1\dfrac{7}{8}$ 13. $2\dfrac{1}{10}$ $2\dfrac{1}{8}$ 14. $3\dfrac{1}{5}$ $2\dfrac{5}{8}$ 15. $\dfrac{9}{5}$ $1\dfrac{8}{10}$

Place in order from largest to smallest.

16. $\dfrac{3}{4}, \dfrac{2}{5}, \dfrac{5}{6}, \dfrac{4}{7}$ 17. $\dfrac{1}{3}, \dfrac{4}{7}, \dfrac{5}{9}, \dfrac{1}{2}$ 18. $1\dfrac{3}{16}, \dfrac{9}{8}, \dfrac{5}{2}, 2\dfrac{1}{10}$ 19. $2\dfrac{1}{2}, \dfrac{5}{3}, \dfrac{12}{9}, 1\dfrac{5}{6}$ 20. $\dfrac{1}{2}, \dfrac{3}{5}, \dfrac{6}{7}, \dfrac{5}{8}$

21. A home patient is supposed to take $\dfrac{2}{3}$ tbs of medication with lunch. You learn that the patient took $\dfrac{1}{2}$ tbs. Did the patient take too little, too much, or just the right amount?

22. You want to prepare 150 units of a solution that consists of 25 units of medication mixed with 125 units of water. You find an already prepared solution that has 1 unit of medication for every 5 units of water. Can you use 150 units of the already prepared solution? Explain your answer.

23. Of 12 patients in the north wing, 8 have high blood pressure. Of 15 patients in the east wing, 9 have high blood pressure. Which wing has a larger portion of patients with high blood pressure?

24. You give George his medication once every 8 hours (h). You give Martha the same medication 4 times a day. Who receives medication more often? (In this problem, a day means 24 h.)

25. You have $1\dfrac{3}{4}$ h until your shift starts. Your friend has $1\dfrac{7}{12}$ h. Who has more time before his or her shift starts?

1.6 Adding Fractions

ALEKS®

GO TO . . .
Adding and
Subtracting
Fractions and
Mixed Numbers–
Introduction to
Addition and
Subtraction
of Fractions
with Different
Denominators.

Suppose you gave a patient $\dfrac{1}{2}$ tbs of medication with breakfast, $\dfrac{3}{8}$ tbs with lunch, $\dfrac{3}{4}$ tbs with dinner, and another $\dfrac{3}{8}$ tbs at bedtime. To determine the total amount of medication you have given the patient, you must add the fractions. Before you can add fractions, however, you must convert them to equivalent fractions with a common denominator. For this example, the equivalent fractions are:

$$\frac{1}{2} = \frac{4}{8} \quad \frac{3}{8} = \frac{3}{8} \quad \frac{3}{4} = \frac{6}{8} \quad \frac{3}{8} = \frac{3}{8}$$

$$\frac{4}{8} + \frac{3}{8} + \frac{6}{8} + \frac{3}{8} = \frac{16}{8} = 2$$

You have given the patient a total of 2 tbs of medication.

RULE 1-11 **ALEKS**® **GO TO ...** Adding and Subtracting Fractions and Mixed Numbers– Addition and Subtraction of Fractions with Different Denominators.	To add fractions: **1.** Rewrite any mixed numbers as fractions. **2.** Write equivalent fractions with common denominators. The LCD will be the denominator of your answer. **3.** Add the numerators. The sum will be the numerator of your answer. *Reminder:* Answers should be reported in the proper form. If the answer has a value greater than 1, convert it to a mixed number. If you can reduce the fraction in the answer to lower terms, do so.
Example 1 **ALEKS**® **GO TO ...** Adding and Subtracting Fractions and Mixed Numbers– Addition and Subtraction of Fractions with the Same Denominator.	Add $\frac{2}{6} + \frac{3}{6}$. **1.** There are no mixed numbers. **2.** The fractions already have a common denominator. The denominator of the answer is 6. **3.** Add the numerators: $2 + 3 = 5$. The numerator of the answer is 5. The answer is $\frac{5}{6}$. It is already in the proper form.
Example 2 **ALEKS**® **GO TO ...** Adding and Subtracting Fractions and Mixed Numbers– Addition and subtraction of mixed numbers with different denominators.	Add $3\frac{1}{4} + 2\frac{1}{2}$. **1.** Rewrite any mixed numbers as fractions. $$3\frac{1}{4} = \frac{13}{4} \quad 2\frac{1}{2} = \frac{5}{2}$$ **2.** Write equivalent fractions with common denominators. The LCD of the fractions is 4. The denominator of the answer is 4. You don't need to change $\frac{13}{4}$. An equivalent fraction for $\frac{5}{2}$ is $\frac{10}{4}$. **3.** Add the numerators. $13 + 10 = 23$ The numerator of the answer is 23. The answer is $\frac{23}{4}$. The proper form for this answer is $5\frac{3}{4}$. **Think! ... Is It Reasonable?** The mixed numbers being added in this example were a little greater than 3 and 2. The answer should be a little greater than 5 because $3 + 2 = 5$. The answer is between 5 and 6, so it is reasonable.

Example 3   Add $1\frac{7}{8} + \frac{2}{3}$.

    1. Rewrite any mixed numbers as fractions.

       $1\frac{7}{8} = \frac{15}{8}$ $\frac{2}{3}$ is not a mixed number.

    2. Write equivalent fractions with common denominators.

       The LCD of the fractions is 24.

       The denominator of the answer is 24.

       An equivalent fraction for $\frac{15}{8}$ is $\frac{45}{24}$.

       An equivalent fraction for $\frac{2}{3}$ is $\frac{16}{24}$.

    3. Add the numerators.

       $45 + 16 = 61$

       The numerator of the answer is 61.

       The answer is $\frac{61}{24}$. The proper form for this answer is $2\frac{13}{24}$.

Example 4   Add $1\frac{2}{5} + \frac{1}{2}$.

    1. Rewrite any mixed numbers as fractions.

       $1\frac{2}{5} = \frac{7}{5}$ $\frac{1}{2}$ is not a mixed number.

    2. Write equivalent fractions with common denominators.

       The LCD of the fractions is 10.

       The denominator of the answer is 10.

       An equivalent fraction for $\frac{7}{5}$ is $\frac{14}{10}$.

       An equivalent fraction for $\frac{1}{2}$ is $\frac{5}{10}$.

    3. Add the numerators.

       $14 + 5 = 19$

       The numerator of the answer is 19.

The answer is $\frac{19}{10}$. The proper form for this answer is $1\frac{9}{10}$.

1.6 Adding Fractions

Find the following sums. (Rewrite answers in the proper form.)

1. $\frac{1}{8} + \frac{3}{8}$ 2. $\frac{1}{7} + \frac{3}{7}$ 3. $\frac{1}{7} + \frac{2}{14}$ 4. $\frac{2}{5} + \frac{4}{15}$ 5. $\frac{1}{6} + \frac{3}{8}$

6. $\frac{4}{10} + \frac{2}{25}$ 7. $\frac{5}{8} + \frac{7}{12}$ 8. $\frac{5}{6} + \frac{7}{9}$ 9. $2 + \frac{4}{5}$ 10. $\frac{8}{11} + 3$

11. $1\frac{1}{2} + \frac{1}{3}$ 12. $2\frac{3}{8} + \frac{1}{5}$ 13. $\frac{7}{9} + \frac{9}{12}$ 14. $1\frac{2}{5} + 4\frac{3}{7}$ 15. $2\frac{1}{8} + 1\frac{1}{2}$

16. $\frac{1}{2} + \frac{1}{5} + \frac{1}{8}$ 17. $\frac{1}{3} + \frac{1}{4} + \frac{1}{5}$ 18. $\frac{3}{4} + \frac{3}{8} + \frac{7}{12}$ 19. $\frac{1}{2} + \frac{2}{3} + \frac{3}{5}$ 20. $\frac{1}{4} + \frac{2}{5} + \frac{3}{10}$

21. The patient's chart indicates that he weighed 158 pounds (lb) at the end of April. He then gained $\frac{3}{4}$ lb in May and $1\frac{1}{2}$ lb in June. What did he weigh at the end of June?

22. $2\frac{1}{2}$ ounces (oz), $3\frac{3}{4}$ oz, and 5 oz were used from a bottle of solution in the office laboratory. What is the total amount of solution used?

23. Since breakfast, Kelly drank $1\frac{1}{4}$ cups of water, $\frac{2}{3}$ cup of juice, and $\frac{3}{4}$ cup of milk. How much liquid has Kelly had since breakfast?

24. During the day, you gave one of your patients $\frac{1}{2}$ tbs of medication with breakfast, $\frac{3}{8}$ tbs with lunch, $\frac{3}{4}$ tbs with dinner, and $\frac{3}{8}$ tbs at bedtime. What is the total amount of medication you gave your patient?

25. You are observing your patient's sleep pattern over the past 24 h. She slept $7\frac{1}{2}$ h at night, $1\frac{3}{4}$ h after breakfast, and $2\frac{1}{4}$ h after lunch. She also had a $\frac{1}{4}$ h nap before lunch and a $\frac{1}{4}$ h nap after dinner. How many hours did she sleep?

1.7 Subtracting Fractions

Subtracting fractions is similar to adding fractions. Before fractions can be subtracted they must be converted to equivalent fractions with common denominators.

RULE 1-12

ALEKS

GO TO . . .
Adding and
Subtracting
Fractions and
Mixed Numbers–
Addition and
Subtraction
of Fractions
with Different
Denominators.

To subtract fractions:

1. Rewrite any mixed numbers as fractions.

2. Write equivalent fractions with common denominators. The LCD will be the denominator of your answer.

3. Subtract the numerators. The difference will be the numerator of your answer.

Reminder: Answers should be reported in the proper form. If the answer has a value greater than 1, convert it to a mixed number. If you can reduce the fraction in the answer to lower terms, do so.

Example 1

Subtract $\frac{2}{6} - \frac{3}{12}$.

1. There are no mixed numbers.

2. Write equivalent fractions with common denominators.

   The LCD of the fractions is 12.

   The denominator of the answer is 12.

   An equivalent fraction for $\frac{2}{6}$ is $\frac{4}{12}$.

   You don't need to change $\frac{3}{12}$.

3. Subtract the numerators.

   $4 - 3 = 1$

   The numerator of the answer is 1.

   The answer is $\frac{1}{12}$. It is already in the proper form.

Example 2

ALEKS®

GO TO . . .
Adding and
Subtracting
Fractions and
Mixed Numbers–
Addition and
Subtraction of
Mixed Numbers
with Different
Denominators.

Subtract $3\frac{1}{4} - 2\frac{1}{2}$.

1. Rewrite any mixed numbers as fractions.

   $3\frac{1}{4} = \frac{13}{4} \qquad 2\frac{1}{2} = \frac{5}{2}$

2. Write equivalent fractions with common denominators.

   The LCD of the fractions is 4.

   The denominator of the answer is 4.

   You don't need to change $\frac{13}{4}$.

   An equivalent fraction for $\frac{5}{2}$ is $\frac{10}{4}$.

3. Subtract the numerators.

   $13 - 10 = 3$

   The numerator of the answer is 3.

   The answer is $\frac{3}{4}$. It is already in the proper form.

Example 3

Subtract $9\frac{3}{4} - 2\frac{3}{8}$.

1. Rewrite any mixed numbers as fractions.

   $9\frac{3}{4} = \frac{39}{4} \qquad 2\frac{3}{8} = \frac{19}{8}$

2. Write equivalent fractions with common denominators.

   The LCD of the fractions is 8.

   The denominator of the answer is 8.

   An equivalent fraction for $\frac{39}{4}$ is $\frac{78}{8}$.

   You don't need to change $\frac{19}{8}$.

3. Subtract the numerators.

$$78 - 19 = 59$$

The numerator of the answer is 59.

The answer is $\frac{59}{8}$. Written as a mixed number, this is $7\frac{3}{8}$.

Think! . . . Is It Reasonable? The mixed numbers being subtracted in this example were a little less than 10 and a little greater than 2. Since $10 - 2 = 8$, the answer 7 3/8, which is a little greater than 7, is reasonable.

Example 4

Subtract $6 - 1\frac{1}{2}$.

1. Rewrite any mixed numbers as fractions.

6 is not a mixed number.

$$1\frac{1}{2} = \frac{3}{2}$$

2. Write equivalent fractions with common denominators.

The LCD of the fractions is 2.

The denominator of the answer is 2.

An equivalent fraction for 6 is $\frac{12}{2}$.

You don't need to change $\frac{3}{2}$.

3. Subtract the numerators.

$$12 - 3 = 9$$

The numerator of the answer is 9.

The answer is $\frac{9}{2}$. The proper form for the answer is $4\frac{1}{2}$.

REVIEW AND PRACTICE

1.7 Subtracting Fractions

Find the following differences. Reduce the answers to lowest terms.

1. $7\frac{7}{15} - 4\frac{4}{15}$ 2. $\frac{7}{25} - \frac{2}{25}$ 3. $\frac{11}{3} - \frac{2}{6}$ 4. $\frac{4}{7} - \frac{3}{21}$ 5. $\frac{5}{6} - \frac{4}{9}$

6. $\frac{3}{4} - \frac{1}{6}$ 7. $1\frac{7}{8} - \frac{1}{4}$ 8. $2\frac{5}{8} - \frac{1}{2}$ 9. $6\frac{1}{3} - \frac{5}{6}$ 10. $4\frac{1}{2} - \frac{3}{4}$

11. $14\frac{9}{10} - 3\frac{1}{3}$ 12. $6\frac{6}{7} - 2\frac{3}{5}$ 13. $24\frac{1}{8} - 3\frac{3}{16}$ 14. $8\frac{7}{10} - 3\frac{3}{4}$ 15. $6 - \frac{2}{3}$

16. $7 - \frac{3}{7}$ 17. $5 - \frac{3}{5}$ 18. $\frac{2}{3} - \frac{1}{2}$ 19. $10\frac{1}{5} - \frac{7}{15}$ 20. $7\frac{2}{3} - \frac{7}{12}$

21. You give a patient $\frac{3}{4}$ cup (c) of juice, but he only drinks $\frac{3}{8}$ c. How much juice remains?

22. You give a patient $1\frac{1}{4}$ c of water to drink before supper. When you bring in the meal, you see that $\frac{5}{8}$ c remains in the glass. How much water did the patient drink?

23. At the beginning of the day, you have $6\frac{1}{2}$ bottles of a medication on hand. At the end of the day, $2\frac{3}{4}$ bottles remain. How much of the medication was used during the day?

24. Brenda weighed $153\frac{1}{2}$ lb when she began a diet. The first month she lost $2\frac{3}{4}$ lb. The second month she lost $4\frac{1}{2}$ lb. The third month she lost $2\frac{1}{2}$ lb. What does she weigh now? (*Hint:* You can subtract each month separately, or you can calculate her total weight loss first.)

25. The patient's temperature is $101\frac{1}{2}$ degrees. The patient's normal temperature is $98\frac{3}{4}$ degrees. How many degrees above normal is this patient's temperature?

1.8 Multiplying Fractions

ALEKS

GO TO . . .
Multiplying
and Dividing
Fractions and
Mixed Numbers–
Introduction
to Fraction
Multiplication.

Unlike adding and subtracting fractions, multiplying fractions does not need a common denominator. Think about what $\frac{2}{3} \times \frac{1}{2}$ means. This problem could be read as "two-thirds times one-half" or "two-thirds of one-half." In Figure 1-2a, a pizza is divided into six slices. Half of the pizza (three slices) has green peppers. When you look for $\frac{2}{3}$ of $\frac{1}{2}$ of the pizza, you are looking for two-thirds of the green peppers half.

In Figure 1-2b, two-thirds of the green peppers half also has mushrooms. The mushroom slices represent $\frac{2}{3}$ of $\frac{1}{2}$ of the pizza, or $\frac{2}{3} \times \frac{1}{2}$. They also represent $\frac{2}{6}$ of the entire pizza. Thus, $\frac{2}{3} \times \frac{1}{2} = \frac{2}{6} = \frac{1}{3}$.

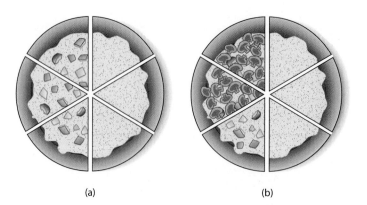

(a)   (b)

Figure 1-2   Multiplying fractions.

RULE 1-13 **ALEKS** **GO TO . . .** Multiplying and Dividing Fractions and Mixed Numbers–Fraction Multiplicaton.	To multiply fractions: **1.** Convert any mixed or whole numbers to improper fractions. **2.** Multiply the numerators of the fractions. **3.** Multiply the denominators of the fractions. **4.** Reduce the product to its lowest terms.
Example 1	Multiply $\frac{1}{6} \times \frac{3}{4}$. There are no mixed or whole numbers. The product of the numerators is $1 \times 3 = 3$. The product of the denominators is $6 \times 4 = 24$. Thus, $\frac{1}{6} \times \frac{3}{4} = \frac{3}{24}$. $\frac{3}{24}$ reduces to $\frac{1}{8}$.
Example 2	Multiply $\frac{1}{2} \times \frac{7}{3} \times \frac{4}{9}$. The only difference from Example 1 is that now you are multiplying three numerators and three denominators. $$\frac{1}{2} \times \frac{7}{3} \times \frac{4}{9} = \frac{1 \times 7 \times 4}{2 \times 3 \times 9} = \frac{28}{54}$$ $\frac{28}{54}$ reduces to $\frac{14}{27}$.
Example 3 **ALEKS** **GO TO . . .** Multiplying and Dividing Fractions and Mixed Numbers–Mixed Number Multiplication: Problem Type 1.	Multiply $1\frac{4}{7} \times 2\frac{3}{5}$. First convert the mixed numbers to improper fractions. $$1\frac{4}{7} = \frac{11}{7} \qquad \text{and} \qquad 2\frac{3}{5} = \frac{13}{5}$$ Now multiply the numerators and denominators. $$1\frac{4}{7} \times 2\frac{3}{5} = \frac{11}{7} \times \frac{13}{5} = \frac{11 \times 13}{7 \times 5} = \frac{143}{35}$$ $\frac{143}{35}$ converts to $4\frac{3}{35}$.
Example 4 **ALEKS** **GO TO . . .** Multiplying and Dividing Fractions and Mixed Numbers–Product of a Fraction and a Whole Number: Problem Type 1.	Multiply $3 \times \frac{2}{3}$. First convert 3 to the improper fraction $\frac{3}{1}$. Now solve. $$3 \times \frac{2}{3} = \frac{3}{1} \times \frac{2}{3} = \frac{3 \times 2}{1 \times 3} = \frac{6}{3}$$ $\frac{6}{3}$ reduces to 2.

Reducing terms provides a shortcut that makes multiplying fractions easier. It lets you work with smaller numbers, decreasing the potential for arithmetic errors. If you divide both the numerator and the denominator of a fraction by the same number, you have not changed the fraction's value. You already use this rule to reduce a fraction. This rule also applies to two or more fractions that are being multiplied.

To multiply $\frac{8}{21} \times \frac{7}{16}$, you could multiply the numerators and multiply the denominators.

$$\frac{8}{21} \times \frac{7}{16} = \frac{8 \times 7}{21 \times 16} = \frac{56}{336}$$

$\frac{56}{336}$ reduces to $\frac{1}{6}$, although that may not be immediately clear to you. By reducing terms before multiplying, however, you work with smaller numbers.

RULE 1-14	To reduce terms when you are multiplying fractions, divide both a numerator and a denominator by the same number. You may reduce terms only if a numerator and denominator can both be divided evenly.
Example 1	Reduce terms to solve $\frac{8}{21} \times \frac{7}{16}$. Both the numerator 8 and the denominator 16 can be divided evenly by 8. You can now write the problem as: $\dfrac{\overset{1}{\cancel{8}}}{21} \times \dfrac{7}{\underset{2}{\cancel{16}}}$ which is equivalent to $\dfrac{1}{21} \times \dfrac{7}{2}$ The slash marks indicate that 8 and 16 were reduced. In this case, they were divided by 8, reducing 8 and 16 to 1 and 2, respectively. Both the numerator 7 and the denominator 21 are divisible by 7. After you reduce again, you can rewrite the problem as: $\dfrac{\overset{1}{\cancel{8}}}{\underset{3}{\cancel{21}}} \times \dfrac{\overset{1}{\cancel{7}}}{\underset{2}{\cancel{16}}}$ which is equivalent to $\dfrac{1}{3} \times \dfrac{1}{2}$ Now when you solve, the answer will already be in lowest terms. $\dfrac{8}{21} \times \dfrac{7}{16} = \dfrac{\overset{1}{\cancel{8}}}{\underset{3}{\cancel{21}}} \times \dfrac{\overset{1}{\cancel{7}}}{\underset{2}{\cancel{16}}} = \dfrac{1}{3} \times \dfrac{1}{2} = \dfrac{1}{6}$
Example 2	$\dfrac{27}{36} \times \dfrac{4}{5}$ In this problem, one of the fractions has not been reduced to lowest terms. Both 27 and 36 are divisible by 9. $\dfrac{\overset{3}{\cancel{27}}}{\underset{4}{\cancel{36}}} \times \dfrac{4}{5}$ becomes $\dfrac{3}{4} \times \dfrac{4}{5}$

Copyright © 2016 by McGraw-Hill Education

26   **UNIT 1**   Performing Basic Math

You can also reduce the numerator 4 and what had begun as the denominator 36. The problem now becomes:

$$\frac{\overset{3}{\cancel{27}}}{\underset{1}{\cancel{36}}} \times \frac{\overset{1}{\cancel{4}}}{5} = \frac{3}{\cancel{4}} \times \frac{\overset{1}{\cancel{4}}}{5} = \frac{3}{1} \times \frac{1}{5} = \frac{3}{5}$$

The answer $\frac{3}{5}$ is already reduced to lowest terms.

Example 3

ALEKS®

GO TO . . .
Multiplying and Dividing Fractions and Mixed Numbers–Mixed Number Multiplication: Problem Type 2.

$$2\frac{1}{2} \times \frac{8}{15} \times \frac{45}{4}$$

First convert the mixed number $2\frac{1}{2}$ to the improper fraction $\frac{5}{2}$. Now the problem becomes:

$$\frac{5}{2} \times \frac{8}{15} \times \frac{45}{4}$$

Both the numerator 45 and the denominator 15 are divisible by 15. Both the numerator 8 and the denominator 2 are divisible by 2.

$$\frac{5}{\underset{1}{\cancel{2}}} \times \frac{\overset{4}{\cancel{8}}}{\underset{1}{\cancel{15}}} \times \frac{\overset{3}{\cancel{45}}}{4} = \frac{5}{1} \times \frac{4}{1} \times \frac{3}{4}$$

You have another opportunity to reduce both a numerator and a denominator by 4. The problem now becomes:

$$\frac{5}{\underset{1}{\cancel{2}}} \times \frac{\overset{4}{\cancel{8}}}{\underset{1}{\cancel{15}}} \times \frac{\overset{3}{\cancel{45}}}{4} = \frac{5}{1} \times \frac{\overset{1}{\cancel{4}}}{1} \times \frac{3}{\underset{1}{\cancel{4}}} = \frac{5}{1} \times \frac{1}{1} \times \frac{3}{1} = \frac{15}{1} = 15$$

If you are not sure what numbers will divide evenly into both the numerator and the denominator, review Table 1-1.

ERROR ALERT!

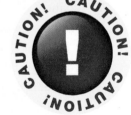

Avoid Reducing Too Many Terms

A term that you plan to reduce may be a factor in more than one numerator or more than one denominator. Each time you reduce a term, you must reduce it from *one numerator **and** one denominator.*

Suppose you are multiplying $\frac{7}{12} \times \frac{8}{20}$. You can reduce 4 from the numerator 8. You can also reduce either of the denominators (12 or 20) by 4, but not both. Either of the following is correct.

$$\frac{7}{\underset{3}{\cancel{12}}} \times \frac{\overset{2}{\cancel{8}}}{20} \qquad \text{or} \qquad \frac{7}{12} \times \frac{\overset{2}{\cancel{8}}}{\underset{5}{\cancel{20}}}$$

Continued

However, *you cannot reduce by 4 as shown below.*

$$\frac{7}{\overset{}{\underset{3}{\cancel{12}}}} \times \frac{\overset{2}{\cancel{8}}}{\overset{}{\underset{5}{\cancel{20}}}}$$

If the problem were $\frac{5}{12} \times \frac{9}{24}$, where the numerator can be reduced by 3 twice, then you could reduce 3 twice in the denominators. Thus,

$$\frac{5}{12} \times \frac{9}{24} = \frac{5}{\underset{4}{\cancel{12}}} \times \frac{\overset{1}{\cancel{9}}}{\underset{8}{\cancel{24}}} = \frac{5}{4} \times \frac{1}{8} = \frac{5}{32}$$

REVIEW AND PRACTICE

1.8 Multiplying Fractions

Find the following products. (Rewrite answers in the proper form.)

1. $\frac{1}{6} \times \frac{1}{8}$ 2. $\frac{2}{7} \times \frac{3}{5}$ 3. $\frac{1}{2} \times \frac{6}{8}$ 4. $\frac{6}{9} \times \frac{1}{6}$ 5. $\frac{3}{8} \times \frac{4}{9}$

6. $\frac{5}{12} \times \frac{6}{15}$ 7. $\frac{10}{14} \times \frac{7}{5}$ 8. $\frac{5}{3} \times \frac{9}{10}$ 9. $\frac{9}{8} \times \frac{8}{2}$ 10. $\frac{4}{3} \times \frac{15}{8}$

11. $1\frac{7}{8} \times \frac{4}{5}$ 12. $3\frac{1}{3} \times \frac{9}{15}$ 13. $3\frac{6}{8} \times 5\frac{2}{9}$ 14. $1\frac{5}{6} \times 7\frac{4}{5}$ 15. $\frac{7}{16} \times \frac{4}{3} \times \frac{1}{2}$

16. $\frac{5}{7} \times \frac{3}{10} \times \frac{3}{4}$ 17. $\frac{11}{32} \times \frac{4}{22} \times 12$ 18. $5 \times \frac{7}{15} \times \frac{3}{14}$ 19. $\frac{12}{25} \times \frac{8}{9} \times \frac{15}{16}$ 20. $\frac{49}{20} \times \frac{12}{7} \times \frac{5}{21}$

21. A bottle of liquid medication contains 24 doses. If the hospital has a supply of $9\frac{3}{4}$ bottles of the medication, how many doses are available?

22. A tablet contains $\frac{1}{4}$ grain (gr) of a medication. If you give a patient $1\frac{1}{2}$ tablets 3 times per day, how many grains of the medication are you giving to the patient each day?

23. A patient is supposed to take $\frac{1}{3}$ teaspoon (tsp) of medicine 4 times per day. However, the patient misunderstood the directions and took $\frac{1}{4}$ tsp of medicine 3 times per day.
    a. How much medicine should the patient have taken per day?
    b. How much medicine did the patient take per day?
    c. What is the difference per day between the two amounts?

24. For 4 days, you give a patient $1\frac{1}{2}$ oz of a medication 5 times per day. How much medication did you give the patient over the 4 days?

25. One tablet contains 500 milligrams (mg) of medication. How many milligrams are in $3\frac{1}{2}$ tablets?

1.9 Dividing Fractions

ALEKS®

GO TO . . .
Multiplying and
Dividing Fractions
and Mixed
Numbers–The
Reciprocal of a
Number.

You have now learned most of the steps needed to divide fractions. Suppose you have $\frac{3}{4}$ bottle of liquid medication available. The regular dose you would give a patient is $\frac{1}{16}$ bottle, and you want to know how many doses remain in the bottle. You solve this problem by dividing fractions.

You want to solve $\frac{3}{4} \div \frac{1}{16}$, where $\frac{3}{4}$ is the dividend, $\frac{1}{16}$ is the divisor, and your answer is the quotient. The problem is read, "three-quarters divided by one-sixteenth," where you are finding out how many times $\frac{1}{16}$ goes into $\frac{3}{4}$.

To solve this problem, multiply the dividend $\frac{3}{4}$ by the reciprocal of the divisor $\frac{1}{16}$. You find the **reciprocal** of a fraction by inverting it—flipping it so that the numerator becomes the denominator and the denominator becomes the numerator. The reciprocal of $\frac{1}{16}$ is $\frac{16}{1}$. Thus,

$$\frac{3}{4} \div \frac{1}{16} = \frac{3}{4} \times \frac{16}{1}$$

You now solve this as a multiplication problem.

$$\frac{3}{\overset{}{\underset{1}{4}}} \times \frac{\overset{4}{16}}{1} = \frac{3}{1} \times \frac{4}{1} = \frac{12}{1} = 12$$

The bottle has 12 doses remaining.

RULE 1-15 ALEKS® GO TO . . . Multiplying and Dividing Fractions and Mixed Numbers–Fraction Division.	To divide fractions: **1.** Convert any mixed or whole numbers to improper fractions. **2.** Invert (flip) the divisor to find its reciprocal. **3.** Multiply the dividend by the reciprocal of the divisor and reduce.
Example 1	Divide $\frac{1}{2} \div \frac{1}{4}$. **1.** The problem has no mixed or whole numbers. **2.** Invert (flip) the divisor $\frac{1}{4}$ to find its reciprocal $\frac{4}{1}$. **3.** Multiply the dividend by the reciprocal of the divisor. $$\frac{1}{2} \div \frac{1}{4} = \frac{1}{2} \times \frac{4}{1} = \frac{1}{\underset{1}{2}} \times \frac{\overset{2}{4}}{1} = \frac{2}{1} = 2$$
Example 2 ALEKS® GO TO . . . Multiplying and Dividing Fractions and Mixed Numbers–Mixed Number Division.	Divide $1\frac{1}{2} \div \frac{1}{4}$. **1.** Convert the mixed number to a fraction. $$1\frac{1}{2} = \frac{3}{2}$$ **2.** Invert (flip) the divisor $\frac{1}{4}$ to find its reciprocal $\frac{4}{1}$. **3.** Multiply the dividend by the reciprocal of the divisor. $$1\frac{1}{2} \div \frac{1}{4} = \frac{3}{2} \div \frac{1}{4} = \frac{3}{\underset{1}{2}} \times \frac{\overset{2}{4}}{1} = \frac{3}{1} \times \frac{2}{1} = \frac{6}{1} = 6$$

Example 3 **ALEKS** GO TO . . . Multiplying and Dividing Fractions and Mixed Numbers– Complex Fraction without Variables: Problem Type 1.	You may have to simplify a **complex fraction**, in which the numerator and the denominator are themselves fractions. The main fraction bar will often be wider and darker than the fraction bars within the numerator and the denominator. You can simply rewrite a complex fraction as an ordinary division problem and proceed. Simplify $\dfrac{\frac{7}{10}}{\frac{3}{5}}$. Here $\frac{7}{10}$ is the numerator and $\frac{3}{5}$ is the denominator. Rewrite the complex fraction as a regular division problem, then solve. $$\dfrac{\frac{7}{10}}{\frac{3}{5}} = \frac{7}{10} \div \frac{3}{5} = \frac{7}{10} \times \frac{5}{3} = \frac{7}{\overset{2}{\cancel{10}}} \times \frac{\overset{1}{\cancel{5}}}{3} = \frac{7}{2} \times \frac{1}{3} = \frac{7}{6} = 1\frac{1}{6}$$
Example 4	Divide $20\frac{1}{6} \div 4$. **1.** Convert $20\frac{1}{6}$ to $\frac{121}{6}$. Change the whole number 4 to $\frac{4}{1}$. **2.** $\dfrac{121}{6} \div \dfrac{4}{1}$ Flip (invert) the divisor $\frac{4}{1}$ to find its reciprocal $\frac{1}{4}$. **3.** Multiply $\frac{121}{6} \times \frac{1}{4} = \frac{121}{24}$. Reduce answer to proper form $5\frac{1}{24}$.

ERROR ALERT!

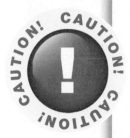

Write Division Problems Carefully to Avoid Mistakes

Be sure to find the reciprocal of the correct fraction. You want the reciprocal of the divisor when you convert the problem from division to multiplication.

$$\frac{2}{3} \div \frac{4}{5} = \frac{2}{3} \times \frac{5}{4} \qquad \text{not} \qquad \frac{3}{2} \times \frac{4}{5}$$

1.9 Dividing Fractions

Find the following quotients. (Rewrite the answers in proper form.)

1. $\dfrac{4}{9} \div \dfrac{5}{7}$

2. $\dfrac{3}{11} \div \dfrac{4}{5}$

3. $\dfrac{3}{8} \div \dfrac{1}{2}$

4. $\dfrac{1}{6} \div \dfrac{3}{4}$

5. $\dfrac{3}{5} \div \dfrac{2}{8}$

6. $\dfrac{6}{9} \div \dfrac{5}{11}$

7. $\dfrac{9}{10} \div \dfrac{3}{5}$

8. $\dfrac{7}{12} \div \dfrac{21}{36}$

9. $1\dfrac{3}{4} \div \dfrac{2}{3}$

10. $\dfrac{7}{8} \div 1\dfrac{3}{4}$

11. $4\dfrac{2}{9} \div 2\dfrac{3}{8}$

12. $3\dfrac{1}{2} \div 1\dfrac{1}{4}$

13. $1\dfrac{7}{8} \div 9$

14. $6 \div \dfrac{5}{8}$

15. $\dfrac{\frac{9}{12}}{\frac{4}{6}}$

16. $\dfrac{\frac{2}{9}}{\frac{1}{8}}$

17. $\dfrac{2}{7} \div \dfrac{1}{4}$

18. $\dfrac{7}{10} \div \dfrac{3}{5}$

19. $5 \div \dfrac{4}{5}$

20. $\dfrac{\frac{4}{5}}{\frac{3}{8}}$

21. A bottle of pills has 40 tablets scored so that each tablet can be divided into four pieces. If a typical dose is $\frac{1}{4}$ tablet, how many doses does the bottle contain?

22. A healthcare professional administered doses of $2\frac{1}{2}$ milliliters (mL) of medication from a bottle that contained 150 mL. How many $2\frac{1}{2}$ mL doses was the healthcare professional able to give from the bottle?

23. A patient is told to drink the equivalent of 8 glasses of water each day. How many times must the patient drink $\frac{1}{2}$ glass of water to reach the daily goal?

24. A healthcare professional opens a case that has a total of 84 oz of medication. If each vial in the case holds $1\frac{3}{4}$ oz, how many vials are in the case?

25. How many $\frac{2}{3}$ h periods of time are in $8\frac{1}{2}$ h?

CHAPTER 1 SUMMARY

LEARNING OUTCOME	KEY POINTS
1.1 Produce fractions and mixed numbers in the proper form. Pages 2–7	▶ The numerator of a proper fraction is always smaller than the denominator. • Examples of proper fractions are $\frac{1}{2}, \frac{2}{3}, \frac{4}{15}$. ▶ A mixed number is made up of a number and a fraction. • Examples of mixed numbers are $3\frac{1}{2}, 2\frac{5}{8}, 12\frac{3}{4}$. ▶ A fraction with a numerator greater than the denominator is called an improper fraction. • Examples of improper fractions are $\frac{12}{5}, \frac{7}{3}, \frac{5}{2}$. ▶ It is sometimes necessary to use an improper fraction while performing calculations, but the answer should always be reported as a proper fraction or a mixed number. • For example, an answer of $\frac{5}{2}$ should be rewritten as $2\frac{1}{2}$.
1.2 Identify and produce equivalent fractions. Pages 7–11	▶ In order to perform calculations with fractions, it is sometimes necessary to convert a fraction to an equivalent fraction. ▶ Equivalent fractions are fractions that have the same value but that are written in different ways. • The fractions $\frac{1}{3}, \frac{2}{6}, \frac{3}{9}$, and $\frac{4}{12}$ are all equivalent. ▶ Changing a fraction to an equivalent may be necessary before adding or subtracting fractions.
1.3 Determine the simplest form of a fraction. Pages 11–13	▶ The simplest form of a fraction is the equivalent fraction with the lowest numerator and denominator. ▶ After performing calculations involving fractions, the answer should always be reduced to its simplest form. • For example, if you perform a calculation and come up with an answer of $\frac{4}{8}$, the proper answer would be this fraction reduced to its simplest form, which is $\frac{1}{2}$.
1.4 Find the least common denominator. Pages 13–16	▶ Fractions must be converted into equivalent fractions with the same denominator before they can be added or subtracted. • Before subtracting $\frac{1}{3}$ from $\frac{5}{6}$ you will need to find a common denominator. ▶ The least common denominator is the lowest multiple of all denominators in the problem.

LEARNING OUTCOME	KEY POINTS
1.5 Compare the values of fractions. Pages 16–18	▶ Changing a fraction to an equivalent fraction can make it easier to compare the values of fractions. • It is easier to compare $\frac{5}{8}$ and $\frac{6}{8}$ than it is $\frac{5}{8}$ and $\frac{3}{4}$.
1.6 Add fractions. Pages 18–21	▶ Change mixed numbers to improper fractions before adding them. • For example, before adding $3\frac{2}{5} + 1\frac{4}{5}$, rewrite the problem as $\frac{17}{5} + \frac{9}{5}$. ▶ Convert fractions to equivalent fractions with a common denominator before adding them. • For example, before adding $\frac{2}{3} + \frac{1}{4}$, rewrite the problem as $\frac{8}{12} + \frac{3}{12}$.
1.7 Subtract fractions. Pages 21–24	▶ Change mixed numbers to improper fractions before subtracting them. • For example, before subtracting $3\frac{2}{5} - 1\frac{4}{5}$, rewrite the problem as $\frac{17}{5} - \frac{9}{5}$. ▶ Convert fractions to equivalent fractions with a common denominator before subtracting them. • For example, before subtracting $\frac{2}{3} - \frac{1}{4}$, rewrite the problem as $\frac{8}{12} - \frac{3}{12}$.
1.8 Multiply fractions. Pages 24–28	▶ Fractions do NOT need common denominators when they are multiplied. ▶ Change mixed numbers to improper fractions before multiplying. • Before multiplying $1\frac{2}{3} \times \frac{3}{8}$, rewrite the problem as $\frac{5}{3} \times \frac{3}{8}$. ▶ To multiply fractions, you multiply the numerators and then the denominators. • $\frac{5}{6} \times \frac{7}{8}$ is equal to 5×7 (the numerators) over 6×8 (the denominators).
1.9 Divide fractions. Pages 29–30	▶ Fractions do NOT need common denominators when they are divided. ▶ Change mixed numbers to improper fractions before dividing. • Before dividing $1\frac{2}{3} \div \frac{3}{8}$, rewrite the problem as $\frac{5}{3} \div \frac{3}{8}$. ▶ To divide fractions, you multiply the fraction you are dividing into (the dividend) by the *reciprocal* of the fraction that you are dividing by (the divisor). • $\frac{5}{6} \div \frac{7}{8}$ is equal to $\frac{5}{6} \div \frac{8}{7}$

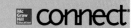

Convert the following mixed numbers to fractions. (LO 1.1)

1. $3\frac{1}{5}$ **2.** $5\frac{2}{3}$ **3.** $8\frac{5}{8}$

Reduce the following fractions to their lowest terms. Convert improper fractions to mixed numbers when necessary. (LO 1.3)

4. $\frac{14}{42}$ **5.** $\frac{12}{45}$ **6.** $\frac{42}{8}$

Find the least common denominator for each set of fractions, and then write equivalent fractions that use the common denominator. (LO 1.2, 1.4)

7. $\frac{3}{4}$ and $\frac{5}{6}$ **8.** $\frac{3}{5}, \frac{2}{3},$ and $\frac{3}{4}$

Place >, <, or = between the following pairs of fractions to make a true statement. (LO 1.5)

9. $\frac{4}{9}$ $\frac{2}{5}$ **10.** $\frac{14}{25}$ $\frac{3}{5}$

Perform the following calculations. Give the answer in the proper form. (LO 1.6 to 1.9)

11. $\frac{3}{2} + \frac{1}{3}$ **12.** $\frac{5}{8} \times \frac{4}{9}$ **13.** $3\frac{2}{5} - 1\frac{1}{5}$ **14.** $\frac{5}{7} + \frac{11}{14} + \frac{16}{21}$

15. $\frac{3}{8} \div \frac{2}{3}$ **16.** $\frac{5}{9} \times \frac{3}{10}$ **17.** $\frac{4}{9} - \frac{1}{3}$ **18.** $\frac{7}{15} \div 1\frac{5}{9}$

CHECK UP

Convert the following mixed numbers to fractions. (LO 1.1)

1. $2\frac{3}{8}$
2. $1\frac{2}{7}$
3. $9\frac{9}{10}$
4. $12\frac{11}{12}$

Reduce the following fractions to their lowest terms. Convert improper fractions to mixed numbers when necessary. (LO 1.1, 1.3)

5. $\frac{12}{36}$
6. $\frac{39}{48}$
7. $\frac{45}{9}$
8. $\frac{58}{8}$

Find the least common denominator. Then write an equivalent fraction for each. (LO 1.2, 1.4)

9. $\frac{3}{10}$ and $\frac{4}{5}$
10. $\frac{5}{6}$ and $\frac{4}{9}$
11. $\frac{3}{8}, \frac{3}{4}$, and $\frac{1}{6}$
12. $\frac{7}{10}, \frac{1}{4}$, and $\frac{2}{3}$

Place >, <, or = between the following pairs of fractions to make a true statement. (LO 1.5)

13. $\frac{3}{10}$ $\frac{3}{16}$
14. $\frac{3}{2}$ $\frac{8}{5}$
15. $1\frac{2}{3}$ $1\frac{16}{24}$
16. $\frac{4}{25}$ $\frac{16}{75}$

Perform the following calculations. Give the answer in the proper form. (LO 1.1, 1.6 to 1.9)

17. $\frac{9}{4} + \frac{2}{3}$
18. $\frac{3}{5} + \frac{12}{5}$
19. $\frac{2}{10} + \frac{1}{100} + \frac{4}{50}$
20. $6 + \frac{5}{8} + \frac{1}{3} + \frac{5}{12}$

21. $\frac{11}{9} - \frac{1}{3}$
22. $\frac{4}{5} - \frac{3}{4}$
23. $3\frac{1}{4} - 1\frac{7}{8}$
24. $3 - \frac{2}{7}$

25. $\frac{5}{6} \times \frac{2}{3}$
26. $\frac{7}{9} \times \frac{3}{14}$
27. $2\frac{2}{5} \times \frac{10}{3}$
28. $\frac{3}{8} \times 11$

29. $\frac{1}{7} \div \frac{3}{4}$
30. $\frac{12}{13} \div \frac{3}{52}$
31. $2\frac{5}{8} \div \frac{1}{6}$
32. $\frac{1}{3} \div 1\frac{1}{4}$

33. A medical unit has 18 patients. Eight have type O blood. Five have type A blood. Two have type AB blood. Three have type B blood. Write the fractions that describe the portions of the medical unit patients that have each blood type. (LO 1.1)

34. A patient is supposed to receive $\frac{1}{2}$ cup (c) of medication 3 times per day. Instead, the patient receives 1/3 c twice per day. During the day, how much medicine does the patient receive? How does that amount compare with the amount ordered? (LO 1.2, 1.4 to 1.6)

35. During the day, Brian drank $\frac{3}{4}$ c of water 7 times, 1 c of milk 2 times, and $\frac{1}{2}$ c of juice 3 times. How much liquid did Brian consume? (LO 1.2, 1.4, 1.6)

36. A bottle contains 48 mL of liquid medication. If the average dose is $\frac{3}{4}$ mL, how many doses does the bottle contain? (LO 1.9)

CRITICAL THINKING APPLICATIONS

A healthcare professional is asked to arrange a set of instruments on a tray in order from smallest to largest on the basis of the instruments' diameters. The diameters are marked $\frac{1}{4}, \frac{7}{16}, \frac{1}{2}, \frac{1}{8}, \frac{1}{16}, \frac{3}{16}$, and $\frac{5}{16}$. How should the healthcare professional arrange the instruments? Look at the pattern of increase in these measurements. Are any instruments missing in the sequence? If so, which ones? (LO 1.2, 1.4, 1.5)

CASE STUDY

A healthcare professional is tracking the weight of a patient who is retaining fluids because of congestive heart failure. On day 3, the patient is given a diuretic. Here is a summary of the weight changes that occurred. In the column marked "change," write the amount of weight change since the previous measurement. Use a plus (+) sign to indicate weight gained and a minus sign (−) to indicate weight lost. Day 2 has been completed as an example. (LO 1.2, 1.4, 1.6, 1.7)

time	weight in pounds	change
Day 1, 8:00 a.m.	$142\frac{1}{2}$	n/a
Day 2, 8:00 a.m.	144	$+1\frac{1}{2}$
Day 3, 8:00 a.m.	$145\frac{3}{4}$	
Day 3, 8:00 a.m.	Patient receives diuretic Lasix (furosemide) 40 mg	
Day 3, 2:00 p.m.	$144\frac{3}{4}$	
Day 3, 4:00 p.m.	Lasix 40 mg	
Day 4, 8:00 a.m.	$142\frac{3}{4}$	
Day 4, 8:00 a.m.	Lasix 20 mg	
Day 4, 4:00 p.m.	$140\frac{1}{2}$	

connect

Now that you have completed the materials in the chapter text, go to CONNECT and complete any chapter activities you have not yet done.

Decimals

*Learning is not attained by chance, it must be sought
for with ardor and attended to with diligence.*

ABIGAIL ADAMS

LEARNING OUTCOMES

When you have completed Chapter 2, you will be able to:

2.1 Write decimals and compare their value.

2.2 Apply the rules for rounding decimals.

2.3 Convert fractions into decimals.

2.4 Convert decimals into fractions.

2.5 Add and subtract decimals.

2.6 Multiply decimals.

2.7 Divide decimals.

KEY TERMS

Leading zero
Trailing zero

INTRODUCTION

In the "Fractions" chapter you were asked to review your mathematical skills for writing and using fractions. In this chapter you will be practicing many of the same skills for numbers containing decimals. As was true with fractions, it is important that you be comfortable working with decimals before learning how to perform dosage calculations.

2.1 Writing and Comparing Decimals

The decimal system provides another way to represent whole numbers and their fractional parts. Healthcare professionals use decimals in their daily work. The metric system, which is decimal based, is used in dosage calculations, instrument calibrations, and general charting work. You must be able to work with decimals and convert fractions and mixed numbers to decimals.

In the decimal system, the location of a digit relative to the decimal point determines its value. The decimal point separates the whole number from the decimal fraction.

Writing Decimals

Each position in a decimal number has a place value. You already know values to the left of a decimal point. The places to the right of a decimal point represent fractions.

The number 1,542.567 is read "one thousand five hundred forty-two *and* five hundred sixty-seven thousandths." Note that when you are writing decimal numbers using words or speaking decimal numbers, the word *and* replaces the decimal point. All numbers to the right of the decimal point are read and written as whole numbers with the place value of the decimal number written last. See Table 2-1.

GO TO . . .
Decimal Place
Value–Decimal
Place Value:
Tenths and
Hundredths
AND Decimal
Place Value:
Hundreds to Ten
Thousandths

TABLE 2-1 Decimal Place Values

The number 1,542.567 can be represented as follows:

WHOLE NUMBER				DECIMAL POINT	DECIMAL FRACTION		
Thousands	Hundreds	Tens	Ones	.	Tenths	Hundredths	Thousandths
1	5	4	2	.	5	6	7

RULE 2-1

To write a decimal number:

1. Write the whole-number part to the left of the decimal point.

2. Write the decimal fraction part to the right of the decimal point. Decimal fractions are equivalent to fractions that have denominators of 10, 100, 1,000, and so forth.

3. Use zero as a placeholder to the right of the decimal point just as you use zero for whole numbers. The decimal number 1.203 represents 1 ones, 2 tenths, 0 hundredths, and 3 thousandths.

Example 1

Decimal	Description	Mixed Number
12.5	Twelve and five tenths	$12\frac{5}{10}$
206.34	Two hundred six and thirty-four hundredths	$206\frac{34}{100}$
0.33	Thirty-three hundredths	$\frac{33}{100}$
1.125	One and one hundred twenty-five thousandths	$1\frac{125}{1,000}$

Example 2

Write $3\frac{4}{10}$ in decimal form.

$3\frac{4}{10}$ is 3 ones and 4 tenths. In decimal form, $3\frac{4}{10} = 3.4$.

Example 3

Write $20\frac{7}{100}$ in decimal form.

$20\frac{7}{100}$ is 2 tens, 0 ones, 0 tenths, and 7 hundredths. In decimal form, $20\frac{7}{100} = 20.07$.

RULE 2-2	Always write a zero to the left of the decimal point when the decimal number has no whole-number part. This zero is known as a **leading zero**, and failure to use it is a violation of standards established by The Joint Commission (TJC). Using the leading zero makes the decimal point more noticeable. Never place a trailing zero after the decimal point when working with medication dosages. A **trailing zero** is a zero found to the right of the decimal that follows the last nonzero digit. Trailing zeros are also on TJC's "Do Not Use" list. Using zeros correctly helps to prevent medication errors.

Examples

ALEKS

GO TO . . .
Converting
Between Decimals
and Fractions–
Converting
Fraction with a
Denominator of
10, 100, or 1,000
to a Decimal

Write the following fractions in decimal form.

a. $\frac{4}{10}$

$\frac{4}{10} = 0.4$ Do *not* write .4 or 0.40.

b. $\frac{25}{1,000}$

$\frac{25}{1,000} = 0.025$ Do *not* write .25 or 0.250.

c. 100/25

$\frac{100}{25} = 4$ Do not write 4.0.

ALEKS

GO TO . . .
Decimal Place
Value–Introduction
to Ordering
Decimals

Comparing Decimals

The more places a number is to the right of the decimal point, the smaller its value. For example, 0.3 is $\frac{3}{10}$ or three tenths; 0.03 is $\frac{3}{100}$ or three hundredths; and 0.003 is $\frac{3}{1,000}$ or three thousandths. Think of it like this: $\frac{3}{10}$ is similar to three dimes and $\frac{3}{100}$ is similar to three cents.

RULE 2-3	To compare the values of a group of decimal numbers:
ALEKS **GO TO . . .** Decimal Place Value–Ordering Decimals	**1.** Look first at the whole-number part. The decimal number with the greatest whole number is the greatest decimal number. **2.** If the whole numbers of two decimals are equal, compare the digits in the tenths place. The tenths place is the first place to the right of the decimal point. **3.** If the tenths places are equal, move to the right and compare the hundredths place digits. **4.** Continue moving to the right, comparing digits until one is greater than the other. This will be the larger number. Zeros added to the right of the last nonzero digit after the decimal point do not change the value of the number.

Example 1	Which is larger, 2.1 or 2.3? The whole number 2 is the same in both numbers. Move one space to the right of the decimal. Compare the tenths digits. Because 3 > 1, $\qquad$ 2.3 > 2.1
Example 2	Which is larger, 0.3 or 0.05? There is no whole number. Move one space to the right of the decimal. Compare the tenths digits. Because 3 > 0, $\qquad$ 0.3 > 0.05
Example 3	Which is larger, 0.121 or 0.13? There is no whole number. Move one space to the right of the decimal. Compare the tenths digits. These digits are equal. Move one space to the right and compare the hundredths digits. Because 3 > 2, $\qquad$ 0.3 > 0.121 $\qquad$ 0.13 > 0.121

REVIEW AND PRACTICE

2.1 Writing and Comparing Decimals

Write the following fractions in decimal form.

1. $\frac{2}{10}$ $\qquad$ 2. $\frac{17}{100}$ $\qquad$ 3. $6\frac{5}{10}$ $\qquad$ 4. $7\frac{19}{100}$

5. $\frac{3}{1,000}$ $\qquad$ 6. $\frac{23}{1,000}$ $\qquad$ 7. $5\frac{67}{1,000}$ $\qquad$ 8. $7\frac{151}{1,000}$

Place > or < between each pair of decimals to make a true statement.

9. 4.27   4.02 $\qquad$ 10. 12.25   12.18 $\qquad$ 11. 0.4   0.6 $\qquad$ 12. 2.22   2.20

13. 0.0170   0.0172 $\qquad$ 14. 0.3001   0.2998 $\qquad$ 15. 5.41   5.34 $\qquad$ 16. 34.58   34.85

17. 0.7   0.9 $\qquad$ 18. 0.67   0.53 $\qquad$ 19. 0.0542   0.0524 $\qquad$ 20. 0.6891   0.8619

2.2 Rounding Decimals

In healthcare settings, you will usually round decimals to the nearest tenth or hundredth, especially if you use a calculator. The answer you get may contain many more decimal places than you need, and you must round the answer. In healthcare settings, you will usually round decimals to the nearest tenth or hundredth. For example, standard syringes are calibrated in tenths of a milliliter, while tuberculin syringes are calibrated in hundredths. Suppose you calculate a dosage using a calculator and the calculator shows the answer is 1.666666667. You cannot measure the medication more accurately than the calibrations on the syringe, so you will need to round the answer to match the calibrations. In this case, if you were using a standard syringe, you would round to the nearest tenth, which is 1.7. If you were using a tuberculin syringe, you would round the answer to the nearest hundredth, which is 1.67.

RULE 2-4 **ALEKS** GO TO . . . Decimal Place Value–Rounding Decimals	To round decimals: **1.** Underline the place value to which you want to round. **2.** Look at the digit to the right of this target place value. If this digit is 4 or less, do not change the digit in the target place value. If this digit is 5 or more, round the digit in the target place value up one unit. **3.** Drop all digits to the right of the target place value.
Example 1	Round 2.42 to the nearest tenth. **1.** Underline the tenths place (the target place value): 2.4̲2. **2.** The digit to the right of the tenths place is 2, which is less than 4. Do not change the digit in the tenths place. **3.** Drop the digits to the right of the tenths place. The number 2.42 rounded to the nearest tenth equals 2.4.
Example 2	Round 0.035 to the nearest hundredth. **1.** 0.03̲5 **2.** The digit to the right of the hundredths place is 5. Round the digit in the hundredths place up one unit: 0.04. **3.** Drop the digits to the right of the target (hundredths) place. The number 0.035 rounded to the nearest hundredth equals 0.04.
Example 3	Round 3.99 to the nearest tenth. **1.** 3.9̲9 **2.** The digit to the right of the tenths place is 9. Round the digit in the tenths place up one unit. When 9 is rounded up, it becomes 10. Place the 0 in the tenths place, and carry the 1 to the ones place. When 1 is added to the ones place, 3 becomes 4 and the rounded number becomes 4.0̲0. **3.** The number 3.99 rounded to the nearest tenth equals 4.0. (Note that this number has a trailing zero and violates Rule 2-2. The proper way to write this number, therefore, would be as 4, not 4.0.)

Rounding Errors with 9

A healthcare professional is calculating how much medication to administer. The patient should receive 4.95 mL, but the syringe being used is calibrated (marked) in tenths. He must round the calculation to the nearest tenth.

The healthcare professional looks at the 5 in the hundredths place and rounds the tenths place up from 9 to 0. However, the healthcare professional neglects to carry the unit to the ones place and draws 4 mL of medication into the syringe.

 Think! . . . Is It Reasonable? What mistake was made and how could it have been avoided?

REVIEW AND PRACTICE

2.2 Rounding Decimals

Round to the nearest tenth.

1. 14.34   **2.** 3.45   **3.** 0.86   **4.** 0.19

5. 1.007   **6.** 0.2083   **7.** 152.68

Round to the nearest hundredth.

8. 9.293   **9.** 55.168   **10.** 4.0060   **11.** 2.2081

12. 5.5195   **13.** 11.999   **14.** 767.4562

Round to the nearest whole number.

15. 11.493   **16.** 19.98   **17.** 2.099   **18.** 50.505

19. You are preparing a syringe to administer 3.75 mL of medication. The syringe is calibrated in tenths. How much medication should you draw into the syringe?

20. A healthcare professional is preparing a syringe for an injection. The calculations indicate that 0.38 mL should be given to the patient. The syringe is calibrated in hundredths. How much medication should the healthcare professional draw into the syringe?

2.3 Converting Fractions into Decimals

Conversions between fractions and decimals is important in healthcare settings. For example, a medication order may be written using decimals when the medication is labeled using a fraction. When you convert fractions to decimals, think of the fractions as division problems. You can write $\frac{1}{4}$ as $1 \div 4$. Reducing fractions first (if possible) often makes the division easier.

RULE 2-5	To convert a fraction to a decimal, divide the numerator by the denominator.
Example 1 **ALEKS®** GO TO . . . Converting Between Decimals and Fractions– Converting a Fraction to a Terminating Decimal	Convert $\frac{3}{4}$ to a decimal. Divide the numerator by the denominator. $$\begin{array}{r} 0.75 \\ 4\overline{)3.00} \\ \underline{28} \\ 20 \\ \underline{20} \end{array} \qquad \frac{3}{4} = 0.75$$
Example 2	Convert $\frac{2}{3}$ to a decimal. $$\begin{array}{r} 0.666 \\ 3\overline{)2.000} \\ \underline{18} \\ 20 \\ \underline{18} \\ 20 \\ \underline{18} \\ 2\ldots \end{array}$$ Sometimes the decimal repeats rather than terminates, as with $\frac{2}{3}$. In such cases, you round, for example, to the nearest hundredth. $\frac{2}{3} = 0.67$
Example 3	Convert $\frac{8}{5}$ to a decimal. $$\begin{array}{r} 1.6 \\ 5\overline{)8.0} \\ \underline{5} \\ 3.0 \\ \underline{3.0} \end{array} \qquad \frac{8}{5} = 1.6$$
Example 4 **ALEKS®** GO TO . . . Converting Between Decimals and Fractions– Converting a Mixed Number to a Decimal	Convert $1\frac{7}{8}$ to a decimal. When converting a mixed number to a decimal, you first convert the fraction and then add the whole number. $$\begin{array}{r} 0.875 \\ 8\overline{)7.000} \\ \underline{64} \\ 60 \\ \underline{56} \\ 40 \\ \underline{40} \end{array} \qquad 1\frac{7}{8} = 1 + \frac{7}{8} = 1 + 0.875 = 1.875$$

REVIEW AND PRACTICE

2.3 Converting Fractions into Decimals

Convert the following numbers into decimals. Where necessary, round to the nearest thousandth.

1. $\frac{2}{5}$

2. $\frac{7}{20}$

3. $\frac{9}{12}$

4. $\frac{12}{24}$

5. $\frac{1}{3}$

6. $\frac{4}{9}$

7. $\frac{15}{27}$

8. $\frac{21}{36}$

9. $\frac{12}{8}$

10. $\frac{11}{5}$

11. $\frac{7}{3}$

12. $\frac{9}{8}$

13. $1\frac{4}{5}$

14. $2\frac{1}{10}$

15. $6\frac{3}{4}$

16. $3\frac{1}{2}$

17. $\frac{7}{8}$

18. $\frac{9}{45}$

19. $\frac{20}{7}$

20. $7\frac{2}{3}$

2.4 Converting Decimals into Fractions

Sometimes you need to convert a decimal to a fraction, especially when you use a calculator that provides decimals, but you need a fraction. When you work with decimals, treat the number to the left of the decimal point as a whole number and the number to the right of the decimal point as a fraction. For example, 12.5 is twelve and five tenths, or $12\frac{5}{10}$. The place value of the digit farthest to the right of the decimal point is the denominator. For 12.5, this place value is the tenths place. The denominator is 10. The numerator is 5, the number to the right of the decimal point.

RULE 2-6 **ALEKS** GO TO . . . Converting Between Decimals and Fractions– Converting a Decimal to a Fraction: Basic	To convert a decimal to a fraction or mixed number: 1. Write the digit to the left of the decimal point as the whole number. 2. Write the digit to the right of the decimal point as the numerator of the fraction. 3. Use the place value of the digit farthest to the right of the decimal point as the denominator. 4. Reduce the fraction part to its lowest terms.
Example 1 **ALEKS** GO TO . . . Converting Between Decimals and Fractions– Converting a Decimal to a Mixed Number	Convert 3.75 to a mixed number. 1. Write the digit to the left of the decimal point, 3, as the whole number. 2. Write the digit to the right of the decimal point, 75, as the numerator of the fraction. 3. The digit farthest to the right of the decimal point, 5, is in the hundredths place. Thus, the denominator is 100. The mixed number is $3\frac{75}{100}$. 4. Reduce to lowest terms: $3\frac{75}{100} = 3\frac{3}{4}$.

Example 2

Convert 0.015 to a fraction.

1. The digit to the left of the decimal point is 0, so 0.015 has no whole number.

2. The digits 015 are to the right of the decimal point. Because 015 = 15, write 15 as the numerator of the fraction.

3. The digit farthest to the right of the decimal point is 5, in the thousandths place. The denominator is 1,000. The fraction is $\frac{15}{1,000}$.

4. $\frac{15}{1,000} = \frac{3}{200}$

ERROR ALERT!

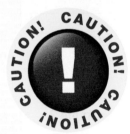

Always Write a Zero to the Left of the Decimal When Writing a Number That Is Less Than Zero

When converting a fraction such as 1/5 to a decimal, you might be tempted to write the answer as .2 instead of 0.2. After all, the zero does not change the value of the number. By doing this, however, you will run the risk of missing the decimal point when referring to the number at a later time and reading the number as a 2. While including a zero does not change the value, it does serve a purpose. It brings attention to the decimal, which could otherwise be mistaken for a stray mark. This can lead to avoidable errors.

REVIEW AND PRACTICE

2.4 Converting Decimals into Fractions

Convert the following decimals to fractions or mixed numbers. Reduce the answer to its lowest terms.

1. 1.2	**2.** 98.6	**3.** 0.3	**4.** 0.442	**5.** 5.03
6. 0.301	**7.** 100.04	**8.** 206.070	**9.** 10.68	**10.** 7.44

2.5 Adding and Subtracting Decimals

When you add or subtract decimals, you align them by their place value, just as you do to add or subtract whole numbers. Be sure to align the decimal points vertically.

RULE 2-7

ALEKS®

GO TO . . .
Adding and
Subtracting
Decimals–Addition
of Aligned
Decimals

To add or subtract decimals:

1. Write the problem vertically, as you would with whole numbers. Align the decimal points.

2. Add or subtract, starting from the right. Include the decimal point in your answer.

Example 1

Add 2.47 + 0.39.

1. Write the problem vertically.
Align the decimal points.

$$
\begin{array}{r}
2.47 \\
+\ 0.39 \\
\end{array}
$$

2. Add.

$$
\begin{array}{r}
2.47 \\
+\ 0.39 \\
\hline
2.86 \\
\end{array}
$$

Example 2

Subtract 52.04 − 14.31.
Align the decimal points.

$$
\begin{array}{r}
52.04 \\
-14.31 \\
\hline
37.73 \\
\end{array}
$$

Example 3

ALEKS®

GO TO . . .
Adding and
Subtracting
Decimals–Decimal
Addition with
Three Numbers

Add 14.3 + 1.56 + 9 + 0.352.

Align the numbers. (Rewrite 9 as 9.0 to help you align it properly.) When the decimals have an unequal number of places, add zeros to the end of the decimal fraction so that all numbers are the same length past the decimal point. Writing zeros after the last digit to the right of the decimal point does not change the number's value. Including these zeros helps prevent errors in calculations. Then add.

$$
\begin{array}{r}
14.3 \\
1.56 \\
9.0 \\
+\ 0.352 \\
\end{array}
\qquad
\begin{array}{r}
14.300 \\
1.560 \\
9.000 \\
+\ 0.352 \\
\hline
25.212 \\
\end{array}
$$

Think! . . . Is It Reasonable? Estimate the range that the answer should fall into. To do this, round all numbers down to whole numbers and add: 14 + 1 + 9 + 0 = 24. Then round all of the numbers up and add: 15 + 2 + 9 + 1 + 27. The answer must be between 24 and 27, and the answer is 25.212.

Example 4

ALEKS®

GO TO . . .
Adding and
Subtracting
Decimals–
Subtraction of
Aligned Decimals

Subtract 7.3 − 1.005.

Align the numbers. Fill in zeros so that all decimal fractions are of equal length. Then subtract.

$$
\begin{array}{r}
7.3 \\
-\ 1.005 \\
\end{array}
\qquad
\begin{array}{r}
7.300 \\
-\ 1.005 \\
\hline
6.295 \\
\end{array}
$$

Example 5

Subtract 10 − 0.75.

$$
\begin{array}{r}
10.00 \\
-\ 0.75 \\
\hline
9.25 \\
\end{array}
$$

2.5 Adding and Subtracting Decimals

Add or subtract the following pairs of numbers.

1. 7.58 + 3.24	**2.** 143.05 + 22.07	**3.** 13.561 + 0.099	**4.** 24.102 + 2.410	**5.** 2.01 + 0.5
6. 2.30 + 0.005	**7.** 0.075 + 0.73	**8.** 4 + 0.025	**9.** 31.64 − 17.39	**10.** 16.250 − 1.625
11. 5.66 − 0.09	**12.** 14.7 − 0.9	**13.** 1.22 − 0.4	**14.** 12.2 − 0.972	**15.** 8 − 0.076
16. 12 − 0.02	**17.** 8.67 + 0.93	**18.** 121.04 + 56.75	**19.** 70.22 − 4.23	**20.** 526.10 − 7.41

21. Steve's temperature on Wednesday morning was 101.4 degrees Fahrenheit (101.4°F). By Thursday afternoon, it was 99.5°F. By how many degrees had his temperature changed?

22. While waiting to see her father, Helene ate at the hospital cafeteria, where she spent $1.30 for a soda, $2.65 for a bowl of soup, and $3.50 for a garden salad. How much did Helene spend?

23. You are supposed to administer 9 grams (g) of a medication. You give the patient one tablet with 4.5 g and a second tablet with 2.25 g. How much more medication should you administer?

24. A bottle of liquid medication contains 50 mL. The following amounts are given to patients from the bottle: 2.5 mL, 3.1 mL, 1.75 mL, 3 mL, and 2.25 mL. How much medication remains in the bottle?

25. Your patient weighed 70.57 kilograms (kg) 2 months ago. His weight then increased by 2.3 kg one month and 1.75 kg the next month. What is this patient's current weight in kilograms?

2.6 Multiplying Decimals

Multiplying decimals is similar to multiplying whole numbers, except you must determine where to place the decimal point.

RULE 2-8

ALEKS®

GO TO . . .
Multiplying
and Dividing
Decimals–Decimal
Multiplication:
Problem Type 1

To multiply decimals:

1. When you are multiplying, the decimal points *do not* need to line up as they do for adding and subtracting. First multiply without considering the decimal points, as if the numbers were whole numbers.

2. Count the total number of places to the right of the decimal points in *both* numbers.

3. To place the decimal point in the answer, start at its right end. Move the decimal point to the left the same number of places as the answer from step 2.

Example 1

Multiply 3.42 × 2.5.

1. First multiply without considering the decimal points.

```
  3.42
× 2.5
  1710
  684
  8550
```

2. Count the total number of decimal places (to the right of the decimal point) in the numbers. The number 3.42 has two decimal places; 2.5 has one decimal place. The numbers have a total of three decimal places.

3. Place the decimal point in the answer. Start at the right of the answer 8550. Move the decimal point three places to the left: 8.550. *After* placing the decimal point, you can drop the final zero so that the answer is 8.55.

 Think! . . . Is It Reasonable? Estimate the range that the answer should fall into. To do this, multiply the whole numbers: 3 × 2 = 6. Then round both numbers up and multiply: 4 × 3 = 12. The answer must be between 6 and 12, and the answer is 8.55.

Example 2

Multiply 0.001 × 0.02.

1. Multiply.

```
  0.001
× 0.02
  2
```

2. The number 0.001 has three decimal places, and 0.02 has two decimal places. The numbers have a total of five decimal places.

3. Start to the right of the answer 2. Move the decimal point five places to the left. Insert zeros to the left of 2 in order to correctly place the decimal point. The correct answer is 0.00002.

CRITICAL THINKING ON THE JOB

Placing Decimals Correctly

A practitioner was instructed to give 0.25 gram (g) of medication for every 1.0 kilogram (kg) of body weight. A baby she was treating weighed 6.25 kg. She set up this calculation:

```
  6.25
× 0.25
  3125
  1250
  156.25
```

 Think! . . . Is It Reasonable? What mistake did the healthcare professional make? What could have happened if the mistake was not corrected?

2.6 Multiplying Decimals

Multiply the following numbers.

1. 7.4×8.2 **2.** 8.21×1.1 **3.** 4.2×0.3 **4.** 3.04×0.04 **5.** 0.55×0.5

6. 0.027×0.4 **7.** 0.003×0.02 **8.** 0.25×0.75 **9.** 1.03×14 **10.** 12×0.09

11. 0.004×15.5 **12.** 0.004×40.01 **13.** 5.2×3.1

14. A patient is given 7.5 mL of liquid medication 5 times per day. How many milliliters does she receive per day?

15. A small syringe is used to give a patient 0.28 mL of medication 4 times per day for 4 days. How much medication does he receive over the 4 days?

16. A tablet has a strength of 0.25 milligram (mg) of medication. You give the patient $1\frac{1}{2}$ tablets 3 times per day. How many milligrams of medication do you give the patient each day? (Hint: Convert $1\frac{1}{2}$ to decimal form first.)

17. A tablet has a strength of 0.4 mg of medication. If you give the patient $\frac{1}{4}$ tablet twice a day, how many milligrams of medication does the patient receive per day?

18. A case of isopropyl alcohol contains 12 bottles. Each bottle contains 15.95 oz. How many ounces of alcohol are in each case?

2.7 Dividing Decimals

The key to dividing decimals correctly is to place the decimal point properly. Recall that the dividend is the number that will be divided. If the divisor is a decimal, you want to convert the problem to one in which the divisor is a whole number.

RULE 2-9

To divide decimals:

1. Move the decimal point to the right the same number of places in both the divisor (the number you are dividing by) and the dividend (the number you are dividing into) until the divisor is a whole number. Insert zeros as necessary.

3. Complete the division as you would with whole numbers. Align the decimal point of the quotient with the decimal point of the dividend if needed.

| **Example 1** | Divide 0.8 ÷ 0.02. |
| | $\underset{\text{(dividend)}}{0.8} \div \underset{\text{(divisor)}}{0.02}$ |

ALEKS

GO TO . . .
Multiplying
and Dividing
Decimals–Division
of a Decimal by a
Two-Digit Decimal

1. Move the decimal point two places to the right in both the divisor and the dividend. The divisor is now a whole number.

$0.02\overline{)\,.80}$

2. Complete the division.

$$2\overline{)80} = 40$$
$$\underline{80}$$

so $0.8 \div 0.02 = 40$

Think! . . . Is It Reasonable? When performing division, a quick check for "reasonable" is to compare the values of the numbers.

- If the divisor is greater than the dividend, your answer should be less than 1.
- If the dividend is greater than the divisor, your answer should be greater than 1.

The dividend is greater than the divisor, so the answer should be greater than 1 and the answer is 40.

Example 2

Divide 0.066 ÷ 0.11.

1. $0.11\overline{)\,0.06.6}$

Move the decimal point two places to the right so that the divisor is a whole number.

2. $11\overline{)6.6}$ gives 0.6, $\underline{6.6}$

Align the decimal point of the quotient with the decimal point of the dividend. Here, $0.066 \div 0.11 = 0.6$

REVIEW AND PRACTICE

2.7 Dividing Decimals

Divide the following numbers. When necessary, round to the nearest thousandth.

1. $3.2 \div 1.6$
2. $48.6 \div 1.8$
3. $24.5 \div 0.2$
4. $0.004 \div 0.002$

5. $1.25 \div 0.5$
6. $0.32 \div 0.8$
7. $0.05 \div 4$
8. $12.6 \div 4$

9. $40 \div 0.8$
10. $0.44 \div 4.4$
11. $29.05 \div 100$
12. $3.48 \div 1000$

13. $39.666 \div 0.03$
14. $54.54 \div 0.009$
15. $59.48 \div 66.93$
16. $84.3 \div 68.48$

17. A bottle holds 60 mL of medication. If the average dose is 0.75 mL, how many doses does the bottle hold?

18. A bottle contains 32 oz of medication. If the average dose is 0.4 oz, how many doses does the bottle contain?

19. A patient received a total of 2.25 g of a medication. If the patient received the total over a 3-day period and was given 3 doses per day, what was the strength of each dose?

20. A patient weighs 197.5 lb. The patient's goal is to weigh 152.5 lb a year from now. How much weight should the patient lose per month to be successful?

CHAPTER 2 SUMMARY

LEARNING OUTCOME	KEY POINTS
2.1 Write decimals and compare their value. Pages 37–40	▶ The places to the right of a decimal represent fractions, and each position has a place value. • For example, digits in the first position after the decimal represent a fraction with a denominator of 10. If there are two places after the decimal, they represent a fraction with a denominator of 100. ▶ When comparing numbers that contain decimals, you first compare the value of the digits to the left of the decimal. • For example, when comparing the value of 3.15 and 5.65 it is not necessary to look at the digits to the right of the decimal; 5 is greater than 3, so 5.65 is greater than 3.15. ▶ When the digits to the left of the decimal are the same, compare values to the right of the decimal. Move to the right one place at a time until you find one value greater than another. • For example, when comparing 25.025 and 25.04, you would compare values starting at the first place after the decimal. The first place after the decimal contains the same value in both numbers, so you proceed to the second, where 4 is greater than 2. Therefore, 25.04 is greater than 25.025.
2.2 Apply the rules for rounding decimals. Pages 41–42	▶ When rounding, you must look at the first digit to the right of the place value that you are rounding to. If this digit is 5 or more, round up. If it is less than 5, round down. • For example, to round 2.7384 to the hundredths place, you look at the digit to the right of the 3. This digit, 8, is greater than 5, so you round the number up to 2.74.

LEARNING OUTCOME	KEY POINTS
2.3 Convert fractions into decimals. Pages 42–44	▶ To convert a fraction to a decimal, divide the numerator by the denominator. • For example, to convert 1/5 to a decimal you would divide 1 by 5:1 ÷ 5 = 0.2.
2.4 Convert decimals into fractions. Pages 44–45	▶ To convert a decimal to a fraction, write the digits to the right of the decimal as the numerator and the place value of the digit furthest to the right as the denominator. • For example, to convert 0.12 to a fraction, the numerator is 12 (the digits to the right of the decimal) and the denominator is 100 (the place value of the 2). The equivalent fraction for 0.12 is $\frac{12}{100}$.
2.5 Add and subtract decimals. Pages 46–47	▶ To add and subtract decimals, it is first necessary to align the decimals vertically before adding or subtracting. • For example, to add 10.3 + 3.05: $$\begin{array}{r} 10.3 \\ + 3.05 \\ \hline 13.35 \end{array}$$
2.6 Multiply decimals. Pages 47–49	▶ To multiply decimals, first multiply the numbers, then determine the position of the decimal. The decimal in your answer should be placed so that the number of digits to the right of the decimal is equal to the total number of decimal places in the numbers that were multiplied. • For example, to multiply 1.05 × 3.1 you first multiply 105 × 31 = 3255. You then determine the position of the decimal. Since the numbers that were multiplied contained a total of three decimal places, the decimal should be placed three places from the right in your answer. The answer is 3.255.
2.7 Divide decimals. Pages 49–51	▶ To divide decimals, first move the decimal to the right the same number of places in both the divisor and dividend until the divisor is a whole number. • Example: 3.2 ÷ 0.4 = 32 ÷ 4 = 8

Place >, <, or = between the following pairs of fractions to make a true statement. (LO 2.1)

1. 0.017   0.09
                2. 3.092   3.27

Round to the nearest hundredth. (LO 2.2)

3. 1.1834
                   4. 17.526

Round to the nearest tenth. (LO 2.2)

5. 6.158
                   6. 0.135

Round to the nearest whole number. (LO 2.2)

7. 12.185
                   8. 1.518

Convert the following fractions to decimals. (LO 2.3)

9. $2\frac{1}{8}$
                   10. $\frac{12}{5}$

Convert the following decimals to fractions. Reduce the answers to lowest terms. (LO 2.4)

11. 1.35
                   12. 0.025

Perform the following calculations. (LO 2.5 to 2.7)

13. 4.25×1.2 **14.** $1.86 \div 0.3$ **15.** $3.26 + 0.015$ **16.** 0.325×2.8

17. $12.05 - 7.6$ **18.** $10.5 \div 1.5$ **19.** $0.321 + 0.0075$ **20.** $3.65 - 0.125$

21. During the day, a patient drank the following quantities of fluid: $1\frac{1}{2}$ cups, 2.4 cups, $1\frac{3}{4}$ cups, and 1.2 cups.

     a. Convert each of the measurements into fractions. Add the fractions to find the total volume of fluid.

     b. Convert each of the measurements into decimals. Add the decimals to find the total volume of fluid.

CHECK UP

Place >, <, or = between the following pairs of decimals to make a true statement. (LO 2.1)

1. 5.7   5.09   **2.** 0.04   0.004   **3.** 6.3   6.300   **4.** 9.033   9.303

Round to the nearest hundredth. (LO 2.2)

5. 0.229   **6.** 7.091   **7.** 46.001   **8.** 9.885

Round to the nearest tenth. (LO 2.2)

9. 4.34   **10.** 3.65   **11.** 6.991   **12.** 0.073

Round to the nearest whole number. (LO 2.2)

13. 8.96   **14.** 20.6   **15.** 0.931   **16.** 12.449

Convert the following fractions to decimals. (LO 2.3)

17. $\dfrac{7}{14}$ **18.** $\dfrac{5}{8}$ **19.** $2\dfrac{3}{5}$ **20.** $\dfrac{32}{4}$

Convert the following decimals to fractions. Reduce the answers to lowest terms. (LO 2.4)

21. 0.82   **22.** 0.65   **23.** 3.5   **24.** 1.001

Perform the following calculations. (LO 2.4 to 2.7)

25. $7.23 + 12.38$ **26.** $4.59 + 0.2$ **27.** $0.031 + 0.99$ **28.** $12 + 0.004 + 1.7$

29. $7.49 - 0.38$ **30.** $4.28 - 3.39$ **31.** $0.852 - 0.61$ **32.** $14.01 - 0.788$

33. 2.3×4.9 **34.** 0.33×0.002 **35.** 5×0.999 **36.** 12.01×1.005

37. $38.85 \div 2.1$ **38.** $4.875 \div 3.25$ **39.** $2.2 \div 0.11$ **40.** $1.4 \div 0.07$

41. A bottle contains 48 mL of liquid medication. If the average dose is 1.2 mL, how many doses does the bottle contain?

CRITICAL THINKING APPLICATIONS

A healthcare professional is asked to arrange a set of instruments in order from smallest to largest on the basis of each instrument's diameter. The diameters are marked 0.875, 0.25, 0.625, 1.0, 0.75, 0.125, and 0.375. How should the healthcare professional arrange the instruments? Look at the pattern of increase in these measurements. Are any missing in the sequence? If so, which ones? (LO 2.1)

CASE STUDY

A healthcare professional is tracking the weight of a patient who is retaining fluids because of congestive heart failure. On day 3, the patient is given a diuretic. Here is a summary of the weight changes that occurred. In the column marked "Change," write the amount of weight change since the previous measurement. Use a plus (+) sign to indicate weight gained and a minus sign (−) to indicate weight lost. Day 2 has been completed as an example. (LO 2.3, 2.4)

time	weight in pounds	change
Day 1, 8:00 a.m.	142.5	n/a
Day 2, 8:00 a.m.	144	+1.5
Day 3, 8:00 a.m.	145.75	
Day 3, 8:00 a.m.	Patient receives diuretic Lasix (furosemide) 40 mg	
Day 3, 2:00 p.m.	144.75	
Day 3, 4:00 p.m.	lasix 40 mg	
Day 4, 8:00 a.m.	142.75	
Day 4, 8:00 a.m.	Lasix 20 mg	
Day 4, 4:00 p.m.	140.5	

To check your answers, see the Answer section at the end of the book, which starts on page A-1.

connect

Now that you have completed the materials in the chapter text, go to CONNECT and complete any chapter activities you have not yet done.

Relationships of Quantities: Percents, Ratios, and Proportions

CHAPTER 3

If what you're working for really matters, you'll give it all you've got.

Nido Qubein

LEARNING OUTCOMES

When you have completed Chapter 3, you will be able to:

3.1 Convert values to and from a percent.

3.2 Convert values to and from a ratio.

3.3 Write proportions.

3.4 Use proportions to solve for an unknown quantity.

INTRODUCTION

As a healthcare professional, you will need to know how to determine the amount of drug contained in a quantity of a product such as a tablet or a solution. For example, you may need to calculate how much drug is in $2\frac{1}{2}$ tablets, or in 300 mL of an IV solution. To do this, you must have a keen understanding of percents, ratios, and proportions. So in preparation for your health career, give Chapter 3 all you've got!

3.1 Percents

Percents, like decimals and fractions, provide a way to express the relationship of parts to a whole. Indicated by the symbol %, **percent** literally means "per 100" or "divided by 100." On a test that has 100 questions, for example, a grade of 75% means that 75 of 100 questions are answered correctly. Table 3-1 shows the same number expressed as a decimal, a fraction, and

TABLE 3-1 COMPARING Decimals, Fractions, and Percents

WORDS	DECIMAL	FRACTION	PERCENT
Eight hundredths	0.08	$\frac{8}{100}$	8%
Twenty-three hundredths	0.23	$\frac{23}{100}$	23%
Seven-tenths	0.7	$\frac{7}{10}$	70%
One		$\frac{1}{1}$	100%
One and five-tenths or one and one-half	1.5	$1\frac{5}{10}$ or $1\frac{1}{2}$	150%

ALEKS

GO TO . . .

Percents–
Converting
Between
Percentages and
Decimals

a percent. A number less than 1 is expressed as less than 100 percent. A number greater than 1 is expressed as greater than 100 percent. Any expression of 1 (for instance, 1.0 or $\frac{5}{5}$) equals 100 percent.

Converting Values to and from a Percent

Converting between percents and decimals requires dividing and multiplying by 100. Converting a percent to a decimal is similar to dividing a number by 100—you move the decimal point two places to the left. If the percent is a fraction or a mixed number, first convert it to a decimal (see the "Decimals" chapter for review). Then divide by 100, moving the decimal point two places to the left.

RULE 3-1	To convert a percent to a decimal, remove the percent symbol. Then divide the remaining number by 100 by moving the decimal point two places to the left.
Example 1	Convert 42 percent to a decimal. $42\% = 42.\% = .42. = 0.42$ Insert the zero before the decimal point for clarity.
Example 2	Convert 175 percent to a decimal. $175\% = 175.\% = 1.75. = 1.75$
Example 3	When you move the decimal point to the left, you may need to insert zeros. Convert 0.3 percent to a decimal. $0.3\% = 000.3\% = 0.00.3 = 0.003$
Example 4	Convert $25\frac{1}{2}$ percent to a decimal. $25\frac{1}{2}\% = 25\frac{5}{10}\% = 25.5\% = .25.5 = 0.255$ Add a zero in front of the decimal point for clarity.
Example 5	Convert $\frac{3}{4}$ percent to a decimal. First convert $\frac{3}{4}$ to a decimal. $\frac{3}{4} = 4\overline{)3.00}^{\,0.75} = 0.75$ $\frac{3}{4}\% = 0.75\% = 000.75\% = 0.00.75 = 0.0075$ **Think! . . . Is It Reasonable?** When dividing a number by 100, you move the decimal point two places to the left and insert zeros when necessary. In this case, 0.75% = 0.0075. Since converting from a percent involves dividing by 100, your answer should be a smaller number than the percentage was. Here, 0.0075 is smaller than 0.75, so the answer is reasonable.

Converting a decimal to a percent is similar to multiplying a number by 100—you move the decimal point two places to the right. Because 100% = 1.00, multiplying a number by 100 percent does not change its value.

RULE 3-2	To convert a decimal into a percent, multiply the decimal by 100. Then add the percent symbol.
Example 1	Convert 1.42 to a percent. $1.42 \times 100\% = 142\%$ You can write this as $1.42 = 1.42.\% = 142\%$.
Example 2	Convert 0.02 to a percent. $0.02 \times 100\% = 2\%$ You can write this as $0.02 = 0.02.\% = 2\%$.
Example 3	When you move the decimal point to the right, you may need to insert zeros. Convert 0.8 to a percent. $0.8 \times 100\% = 80\%$ You can write this as $0.8 = 0.80 = 0.80.\% = 80\%$. **Think! . . . Is It Reasonable?** When you multiply a number by 100, you move the decimal point two places to the right. Since percents are based on hundredths, numbers must be written with at least two decimal places (hundredths) before you can move the decimal and express them as a percent. In this example, 0.8 is first rewritten with an extra zero (0.80) and then as 80%.

ALEKS®

GO TO . . .
Percents–
Converting a
Percentage to
a Fraction in
Simplest Form

Because percent means "per 100" or "divided by 100," you can easily convert percents to equivalent fractions.

RULE 3-3	To convert a percent to an equivalent fraction, write the value of the percent as the numerator and 100 as the denominator. Then reduce the fraction to its lowest terms.
Example 1	Convert 8 percent to an equivalent fraction. $8\% = \dfrac{8}{100} = \dfrac{\overset{2}{\cancel{8}}}{\underset{25}{\cancel{100}}} = \dfrac{2}{25}$
Example 2	Convert 130 percent to an equivalent mixed number. $130\% = \dfrac{130}{100} = \dfrac{\overset{13}{\cancel{130}}}{\underset{10}{\cancel{100}}} = \dfrac{13}{10} = 1\dfrac{3}{10}$
Example 3	Change 0.6 percent to an equivalent fraction. $0.6\% = \dfrac{0.6}{100}$ To reduce a fraction, it must not include a decimal point. To eliminate the decimal point, multiply it by $\dfrac{10}{10}$. (Remember that a fraction with the same number in the numerator and denominator is equal to 1.) $\dfrac{0.6}{100} \times \dfrac{10}{10} = \dfrac{6}{1,000} = \dfrac{3}{500}$

Example 4	Change $\frac{3}{4}$ percent to an equivalent fraction.
	$$\frac{3}{4}\% = \frac{3}{4} \div 100 = \frac{3}{4} \times \frac{1}{100} = \frac{3}{400}$$
	For a review of division with fractions, see Chapter 1.

RULE 3-4	To convert a fraction to a percent, first convert the fraction to a decimal. Round the decimal to the nearest hundredth. Then follow the rule for converting a decimal to a percent.
Example 1	Convert $\frac{1}{2}$ to a percent.
	First convert $\frac{1}{2}$ to a decimal.
	$$\frac{1}{2} = 1 \div 2 = 0.5$$
	Now convert the decimal to a percent.
	$$\frac{1}{2} = 0.5 = 0.5 \times 100\% = 50\%$$
	You can write this as $0.5 = 0.50 = 0.50.\% = 50\%$.
Example 2	Convert $\frac{2}{3}$ to a percent.
	Convert $\frac{2}{3}$ to a decimal. Round to the nearest hundredth.
	$$\frac{2}{3} = 2 \div 3 = 0.666 = 0.67$$
	Now convert to a percent.
	$$\frac{2}{3} = 0.67 = 0.67 \times 100\% = 67\%$$
	You can write this as $0.67 = 0.67.\% = 67\%$.
Example 3	Convert $1\frac{3}{4}$ to a percent.
	$$1\frac{3}{4} = \frac{7}{4} = 1.75 = 1.75 \times 100\% = 175\%$$
	You can write this as $1\frac{3}{4} = 1.75.\% = 175\%$.
Example 4	Convert $\frac{1}{2}$ to a percent.
	$$\frac{1}{2} \times 100\%$$
	$$\frac{1}{2} \times \frac{100\%}{1} = \frac{100\%}{2} = 50\%$$
	An alternative method for converting a fraction to a percent is to multiply the fraction by 100 percent.
Example 5	Convert $\frac{2}{3}$ to a percent.
	$$\frac{2}{3} \times \frac{100\%}{1} = \frac{200\%}{3} = 66.66\% \text{ rounded to } 67\%.$$

Example 6	Convert $1\frac{3}{4}$ to a percent.
	Change $1\frac{3}{4}$ to the fraction $\frac{7}{4}$.
	$\frac{7}{4} \times \frac{100\%}{1} = \frac{700\%}{4} = 175\%$

REVIEW AND PRACTICE

3.1 Percents

Convert the following percents to decimals. Round to the nearest thousandth.

1. 14%   **2.** 30%   **3.** 2%   **4.** 9%   **5.** 103%

6. 300%   **7.** 0.21%   **8.** 0.4%   **9.** $42\frac{1}{2}\%$ **10.** $3\frac{4}{5}\%$

11. 4.5%   **12.** 250.75%   **13.** $23\frac{2}{3}\%$ **14.** $1\frac{5}{6}\%$ **15.** $14\frac{1}{2}\%$

Convert the following decimals to percents.

16. 4.04   **17.** 2.3   **18.** 0.7   **19.** 0.33   **20.** 0.06

21. 0.013   **22.** 15   **23.** 32   **24.** 121

Convert the following percents to fractions. Reduce the answers to their lowest terms.

25. 22%   **26.** 4%   **27.** 158%   **28.** 300%   **29.** 0.1%

30. 0.8%   **31.** $\frac{9}{10}\%$ **32.** $1\frac{2}{5}\%$ **33.** 0.3%

Convert the following fractions to percents. Round to the nearest percent.

34. $\frac{6}{8}$ **35.** $\frac{4}{5}$ **36.** $\frac{1}{6}$ **37.** $\frac{5}{9}$ **38.** $1\frac{1}{10}$

39. $2\frac{1}{4}$ **40.** $\frac{175}{100}$ **41.** $\frac{40}{100}$ **42.** $5\frac{2}{3}$

3.2 Ratios

Ratios, like fractions, express the relationship of a part to the whole. They may relate a quantity of liquid drug to a quantity of a solution, such as an injection or an IV. Ratios can also be used to express how much drug is in a tablet or a capsule.

Like a fraction, a ratio has two parts. The first part of the ratio is like the numerator of a fraction, and represents parts of the whole. The second part of the ratio is like the denominator of a fraction, and represents the whole. The two parts are separated by a colon. For example, if a tablet contains 250 mg of drug, the ratio 250 mg : 1 tablet could be used to represent the tablet. This same tablet could also be expressed as a fraction: 250 mg of drug would be the numerator, 1 tablet would be the denominator: $\frac{250 \text{ mg}}{1 \text{ tablet}}$.

Converting Values to and from a Ratio

You use only whole numbers when you write a ratio. Correct ratios include 8 : 1, 2 : 5, and 1 : 100. Incorrect ratios include 2.5 : 10, 1 : 4.5, and $3\frac{1}{2}$: 100.

Ratios are sometimes expressed in lowest terms. Just as $\frac{4}{100}$ reduces to $\frac{1}{25}$, the ratio 4 : 100 can be written 1 : 25. Similarly, you can reduce 2 : 10 to 1 : 5 and 10 : 12 to 5 : 6.

RULE 3-5	Reduce a ratio as you would a fraction. Find the largest whole number that divides evenly into both values *A* and *B*.
Example 1	Reduce 2 : 12 to its lowest terms. Both values 2 and 12 are divisible by 2. $2 \div 2 = 1 \qquad 12 \div 2 = 6$ Thus, 2 : 12 is written 1 : 6.
Example 2	Reduce 10 : 15 to its lowest terms. Both values 10 and 15 are divisible by 5. $10 \div 5 = 2 \qquad 15 \div 5 = 3$ 10 : 15 = 2 : 3

Because a ratio relates two quantities, value *A* and value *B*, ratios can be written as fractions. Within this textbook for simplicity when two numbers are expressed as *A* : *B*, this is a ratio. When two numbers are expressed as $\frac{A}{B}$ or A/B, this is a fraction.

RULE 3-6	To convert a ratio to a fraction, write value *A* (the first number) as the numerator and value *B* (the second number) as the denominator, so that $A : B = \frac{A}{B}$.
Examples	**a.** Convert 4 : 5 to a fraction. $4 : 5 = \frac{4}{5}$ **b.** Convert 1 : 100 to a fraction. $1 : 100 = \frac{1}{100}$ **c.** Convert 7 : 3 to a fraction. $7 : 3 = \frac{7}{3}$

RULE 3-7	To convert a fraction to a ratio, write the numerator as the first value (A) and the denominator as the second value (B). $$\frac{A}{B} = A : B$$ Convert a mixed number to a ratio by first writing the mixed number as a fraction.
Examples	**a.** Convert $\frac{7}{12}$ to a ratio. **b.** Convert $\frac{3}{2}$ to a ratio. **c.** Convert $2\frac{1}{2}$ to a ratio. $$\frac{7}{12} = 7 : 12 \qquad\qquad \frac{3}{2} = 3 : 2 \qquad\qquad 2\frac{1}{2} = \frac{5}{2} = 5 : 2$$

RULE 3-8	To convert a ratio to a decimal: **1.** Write the ratio as a fraction. **2.** Convert the fraction to a decimal. (See the "Decimals" chapter.)
Example 1	Convert 1 : 10 to a decimal. **1.** Write the ratio as a fraction. $$1 : 10 = \frac{1}{10}$$ **2.** Convert the fraction to a decimal. $$\frac{1}{10} = 1 \div 10 = 0.1$$ Thus, $1 : 10 = \frac{1}{10} = 0.1$.
Example 2	Convert 3 : 2 to a decimal. **1.** $3 : 2 = \frac{3}{2}$ **2.** $\frac{3}{2} = 3 \div 2 = 1.5$ Thus, $3 : 2 = \frac{3}{2} = 1.5$.

RULE 3-9	To convert a decimal to a ratio: **1.** Write the decimal as a fraction. (See the "Decimals" chapter.) **2.** Reduce the fraction to lowest terms. **3.** Restate the fraction as a ratio by writing the numerator as value A and the denominator as value B; in the form A : B.

Example 1   Convert 0.8 to a ratio.

    1. Write the decimal as a fraction.

       $0.8 = \dfrac{8}{10}$

    2. Reduce the fraction to lowest terms.

       $\dfrac{8}{10} = \dfrac{\overset{4}{\cancel{8}}}{\underset{5}{\cancel{10}}} = \dfrac{4}{5}$

    3. Restate the number as a ratio.

       $\dfrac{4}{5} = 4 : 5$

Thus, $0.8 = \dfrac{8}{10} = \dfrac{4}{5} = 4 : 5$.

Example 2   Convert 0.05 to a ratio.

    1. $0.05 = \dfrac{5}{100}$

    2. $\dfrac{5}{100} = \dfrac{\overset{1}{\cancel{5}}}{\underset{20}{\cancel{100}}} = \dfrac{1}{20}$

    3. $\dfrac{1}{20} = 1 : 20$

Thus, $0.05 = \dfrac{1}{20} = 1 : 20$.

Example 3   Convert 2.5 to a ratio.

    1. $2.5 = 2\dfrac{5}{10} = \dfrac{25}{10}$

    2. $\dfrac{25}{10} = \dfrac{\overset{5}{\cancel{25}}}{\underset{2}{\cancel{10}}} = \dfrac{5}{2}$

    3. $\dfrac{5}{2} = 5 : 2$

Thus, $2.5 = \dfrac{5}{2} = 5 : 2$.

LEARNING LINK   Recall from Rule 3-3 that you can write a percent as a fraction with the denominator of 100. This step helps you to convert a ratio to a percent and a percent to a ratio.

RULE 3-10	To convert a ratio to a percent:
ALEKS®	**1.** Convert the ratio to a decimal.
GO TO . . . Ratios–Writing a Ratio as a Percentage	**2.** Write the decimal as a percent by multiplying the decimal by 100 and adding the percent symbol.

Example 1

Convert 1 : 50 to a percent.

    1. Convert the ratio to a decimal.

$$1 : 50 = \frac{1}{50} = 0.02$$

    2. Multiply 0.02 by 100 and add the percent symbol.

$$0.02 = 100\% = 2\%$$

Thus, $1 : 50 = \frac{1}{50} = 0.02 = 2\%$

Example 2

Convert 2 : 3 to a percent.

    1. $2 : 3 = \frac{2}{3} = 0.67$

    2. $0.67 \times 100\% = 67\%$

Thus, $2 : 3 = \frac{2}{3} = 0.67 = 67\%$

Example 3

Convert 5 : 2 to a percent.

    1. $5 : 2 = \frac{5}{2} = 2.5 = 2.50$

    2. $2.50 \times 100\% = 250\%$

Thus, $5 : 2 = \frac{5}{2} = 2.50 = 250\%$

 Think! . . . Is It Reasonable? When a fraction or ratio with a value of less than 1 is converted to a percent, it will be less than 100 percent. If the fraction or ratio is greater than 1, it will equal over 100 percent.

RULE 3-11	To convert a percent to a ratio:
	1. Write the percent as a fraction.
	2. Reduce the fraction to lowest terms.
	3. Write the fraction as a ratio by writing the numerator as value A and the denominator as value B, in the form $A : B$.
Example 1	Convert 25 percent to a ratio.
	1. Write the percent as a fraction.
	$25\% = \frac{25}{100}$
	2. Reduce the fraction.
	$\frac{25}{100} = \frac{1}{4}$
	3. Restate the fraction as a ratio. Write the numerator as value A and the denominator as value B.
	$\frac{1}{4} = 1 : 4$
	Thus, $25\% = \frac{1}{4} = 1 : 4$.
Example 2	Convert 450 percent to a ratio.
	1. $450\% = \frac{450}{100}$
	2. $\frac{450}{100} = \frac{45}{10} = \frac{9}{2}$
	3. $\frac{9}{2} = 9 : 2$
	Thus, $450\% = \frac{9}{2} = 9 : 2$.
Example 3	Convert 0.3 percent to a ratio.
	1. Write the percent as a fraction. In this case, rewrite the fraction without decimal points.
	$0.3\% = \frac{0.3}{100} = \frac{3}{1,000}$
	2. $\frac{3}{1,000}$ is reduced to lowest terms.
	3. $\frac{3}{1,000} = 3 : 1,000$
	Thus, $0.3\% = \frac{3}{1,000} = 3 : 1,000$.

3.2 Ratios

Convert the following ratios to fractions or mixed numbers.

1. $3:4$ **2.** $4:9$ **3.** $5:3$ **4.** $10:1$ **5.** $1:20$

6. $1:250$ **7.** $4:12$

Convert the following fractions to ratios.

8. $\frac{2}{3}$ **9.** $\frac{6}{7}$ **10.** $\frac{5}{4}$ **11.** $\frac{7}{3}$ **12.** $1\frac{7}{8}$

13. $3\frac{1}{3}$ **14.** $\frac{6}{10}$ **15.** $\frac{18}{27}$ **16.** $\frac{1}{50}$ **17.** $\frac{1}{75}$

18. $5\frac{4}{5}$

Convert the following ratios to decimals. Round to the nearest hundredth, if necessary.

19. $1:4$ **20.** $1:8$ **21.** $3:4$ **22.** $2:5$ **23.** $50:1$

24. $25:2$ **25.** $8:3$ **26.** $5:6$ **27.** $5:75$

Convert the following decimals to ratios.

28. 0.9 **29.** 0.3 **30.** 0.01 **31.** 0.45 **32.** 6

33. 2.4 **34.** 8 **35.** 9.8

Convert the following ratios to percents. If necessary, round to the nearest percent.

36. $1:4$ **37.** $1:25$ **38.** $2:9$ **39.** $7:17$ **40.** $20:1$

41. $15:2$ **42.** $3:8$

Convert the following percents to ratios.

43. 14% **44.** 65% **45.** 400% **46.** 175% **47.** 0.6%

48. 0.18% **49.** 84% **50.** 0.57%

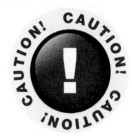

Do Not Forget the Units of Measurement

Including units in the dosage strength will help you to avoid some common errors. Consider the case in which we have two solutions of a drug. One of the solutions contains 1 g of drug in 50 mL; the other contains 1 mg of drug in 50 mL. While both of these solutions have ratio strengths of 1 : 50, they are obviously different from each other. To distinguish between them, the first solution could be written as 1 g : 50 mL while the second is written 1 mg : 50 mL.

3.3 Proportions

A **proportion** is a mathematical statement that two ratios are equal. Because ratios are often written as fractions, a proportion is also a statement that two fractions are equal.

Writing Proportions

You have learned that 2 : 3 is read "two to three." The proportion 2 : 3 = 4 : 6 reads "two is to three as four is to six." A double colon in a proportion means "as" and can be used in place of the equals sign. For example, the proportion 2 : 3 :: 4 : 6 would also read, "two is to three as four is to six." In this text we will use the = sign when writing proportions. This proportion states that the relationship of 2 to 3 is the same as the relationship of 4 to 6. By now, you know that 2 divided by 3 is the same as 4 divided by 6. *When you write proportions, do not reduce the ratios to their lowest terms.*

You can write proportions by using either ratios or fractions. Thus, 2 : 3 = 4 : 6 is the same as $\frac{2}{3} = \frac{4}{6}$.

RULE 3-12	To change a proportion from ratios to fractions, convert both ratios to fractions.
Example 1 **ALEKS®** **GO TO . . .** Proportions– Writing a Ratio Proportion as a Fraction Proportion	Write 3 : 4 = 9 : 12 as a proportion using fractions. Convert both ratios to fractions. Here 3 : 4 becomes $\frac{3}{4}$ and 9 : 12 becomes $\frac{9}{12}$, so that: $3 : 4 = 9 : 12 \rightarrow \frac{3}{4} = \frac{9}{12}$
Example 2	Write 5 : 10 = 50 : 100 as a proportion using fractions. $5 : 10 = 50 : 100 \rightarrow \frac{5}{10} = \frac{50}{100}$
Example 3	Write 8 : 6 = 4 : 3 as a proportion using fractions. $8 : 6 = 4 : 3 \rightarrow \frac{8}{6} = \frac{4}{3}$

RULE 3-13	To change a proportion from fractions to ratios, convert each fraction to a ratio.
Example 1	Write $\frac{5}{6} = \frac{10}{12}$ using ratios. Convert each fraction to a ratio. $\frac{5}{6} = 5:6$ and $\frac{10}{12} = 10:12$ so $5:6 = 10:12$
Example 2	Write $\frac{3}{8} = \frac{9}{24}$ using ratios. $\frac{3}{8} = 3:8$ and $\frac{9}{24} = 9:24$, so that $3:8 = 9:24$
Example 3	Write $\frac{10}{2} = \frac{5}{1}$ using ratios. $\frac{10}{2} = 10:2$ and $\frac{5}{1} = 5:1$ so that $10:2 = 5:1$

REVIEW AND PRACTICE

3.3 Proportions

Write the following proportions using fractions.

1. $4:5 = 8:10$

2. $5:12 = 10:24$

3. $1:10 = 100:1,000$

4. $2:3 = 20:30$

5. $50:25 = 10:5$

6. $6:4 = 18:12$

7. $5:24 = 10:48$

8. $75:100 = 150:200$

9. $4:16 = 16:64$

10. $125:100 = 375:300$

Write the following proportions using ratios.

11. $\frac{3}{4} = \frac{75}{100}$

12. $\frac{1}{5} = \frac{3}{15}$

13. $\frac{8}{4} = \frac{2}{1}$

14. $\frac{8}{7} = \frac{24}{21}$

15. $\frac{18}{16} = \frac{9}{8}$

16. $\frac{10}{1} = \frac{40}{4}$

17. $\frac{5}{7} = \frac{15}{21}$

18. $\frac{45}{5} = \frac{9}{1}$

19. $\frac{1}{100} = \frac{100}{10,000}$

20. $\frac{36}{12} = \frac{72}{24}$

3.4 Using Proportions to Solve for an Unknown Quantity

You often work with proportions to calculate dosages. When you know three of four values of a proportion, you can solve the proportion to determine the unknown quantity. The proportion can be set up using either ratios or fractions—both methods lead to the same answer. Which method you select is a matter of personal preference.

It is not enough to learn to find the unknown quantity. You must also learn to set up the proportion correctly. If you set up the proportion incorrectly, you could give the wrong amount of medication, with serious consequences for the patient. Use critical thinking skills to select the appropriate information and set up the proportion. In later chapters, you will learn to read physician's orders and drug labels, the sources for the information that goes into the proportion. The remainder of this chapter focuses on finding unknown quantities.

Means and Extremes

When you set up a proportion in the form $A : B = C : D$, the values A and D are the **extremes**. The values B and C are the **means**. If you have trouble remembering which is which, think, "<u>E</u>xtremes are on the <u>e</u>nds. <u>M</u>eans are in the <u>m</u>iddle."

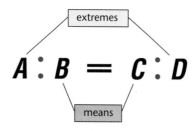

In any true proportion, the product of the means always equals the product of the extremes.

RULE 3-14	To determine if a proportion is true:
	1. Multiply the means.
	2. Multiply the extremes.
	3. Compare the product of the means with the product of the extremes. If the products are equal, the proportion is true.
Example 1	Determine if $1 : 2 = 3 : 6$ is a true proportion.
	1. Multiply the means: $2 \times 3 = 6$
	2. Multiply the extremes: $1 \times 6 = 6$
	3. Compare the products of the means and the extremes.
	$6 = 6$
	The statement $1 : 2 = 3 : 6$ is a true proportion.
Example 2	Determine if $100 : 40 = 50 : 20$ is a true proportion.
	1. $40 \times 50 = 2,000$
	2. $100 \times 20 = 2,000$
	3. $2,000 = 2,000$
	The proportion $100 : 40 = 50 : 20$ is true.

Example 3	Determine if $100 : 20 = 5 : 4$ is a true proportion.
	1. $20 \times 5 = 100$
	2. $100 \times 4 = 400$
	3. $400 \neq 100$
	The proportion $10 : 20 = 5 : 4$ is not a true proportion.

By definition, both sides of an equation are equal. If you perform the same calculation on both sides of an equation, the two sides will still be equal. For instance, consider the equation:

$$4 \times 2 = 8$$

You can add 3 to both sides or subtract 5 from both sides of the equation, and the resulting equations are still true.

$$(4 \times 2) + 3 = 8 + 3 \quad (4 \times 2) - 5 = 8 - 5$$
$$11 = 11 \qquad\qquad 3 = 3$$

You can also multiply or divide both sides by the same nonzero number and the sides remain equal.

$$(4 \times 2) \times 6 = 8 \times 6 \quad (4 \times 2) \div 4 = 8 \div 4$$
$$48 = 48 \qquad\qquad 2 = 2$$

Now you can use the means and extremes to help you find an unknown quantity in a proportion. Suppose you have the proportion:

$$2 : 4 = x : 12$$

where x represents the unknown quantity. The product of the means equals the product of the extremes.

$$4 \times x = 2 \times 12$$
$$4 \times x = 24$$

To find the value of x, you must write the equation so that x stands alone on one side of the equal sign. Here you simply divide both sides by the number before x, or 4, since any number divided by itself equals 1.

$$4 \times x = 24$$
$$\frac{4 \times x}{4} = \frac{24}{4}$$
$$x = 6$$

Check that the proportion is now true:

$$2 : 4 = 6 : 12$$
$$4 \times 6 = 24 \quad \text{and} \quad 2 = 12 = 24$$

Because $4 \times 6 = 2 \times 12$, the proportion is true. *Remember,* taking the time to check your work will help you avoid errors.

RULE 3-15	To find the unknown quantity in a proportion:
ALEKS®	**1.** Write an equation setting the product of the means equal to the product of the extremes.
GO TO . . .	**2.** Solve the equation for the unknown quantity.
Proportions– Finding the Missing Value in a Proportion	**3.** Restate the proportion, inserting the unknown quantity.
	4. Check your work. Determine if the proportion is true.

Example

Find the unknown quantity in $25 : 5 = 50 : x$.

1. Write an equation setting the product of the means equal to the product of the extremes.

$$5 \times 50 = 25 \times x$$

$$250 = 25 \times x$$

2. Solve the equation. Here, divide both sides by 25.

$$\frac{250}{25} = \frac{25 \times x}{25}$$

$$10 = x$$

3. Restate the proportion, inserting the unknown quantity.

$$25 : 5 = 50 : 10$$

4. Check your work.

$$5 \times 50 = 25 \times 10$$

$$250 = 250$$

The unknown quantity is 10.

CANCELING UNITS IN PROPORTIONS It is important to include units when you are writing ratios and proportions. Including units, and learning how to cancel like units, will help you to determine the correct units for the answer when you solve problems using proportions. For example, you have a solution containing 200 mg of drug in 5 mL, and you are asked to determine how many milliliters of a solution contain 500 mg of drug. You can solve the problem by using the following two ratios.

200 mg : 5 mL

500 mg : x

If the units of the first parts of the two ratios are the same, they can be dropped or canceled. Likewise, if the units from the second part of the two ratios are the same, they can be canceled. In this case, the units for the first part of each ratio are milligrams. Canceling the units leaves us with the following proportion.

200 : 5 mL = 500 : x

The product of the means equals the product of the extremes.

$$5 \text{ mL} \times 500 = 200 \times x$$

We then divide both sides of the equation by 200 so that x stands alone.

$$\frac{5 \text{ mL} \times 500}{200} = \frac{200 \times x}{200}$$

$$12.5 \text{ mL} = x$$

There are 500 mg of the drug in 12.5 mL of the solution.

 Think! . . . Is It Reasonable? There is 200 mg for every 5 mL, and we need 500 mg of medication, which is $2\frac{1}{2}$ times the 200 mg. Our solution of 12.5 mL is $2\frac{1}{2}$ times the 5 mL of solution.

RULE 3-16	If the units in the first part of the ratios in a proportion are the same, the units can be canceled. If the units in the second part of the ratios in a proportion are the same, the units can be canceled.

Example 1	If 100 mL of solution contains 20 mg of drug, how many milligrams of the drug will be in 500 mL of the solution?
	Start by setting up the ratios.
	
	  20 mg : 100 mL and x : 500 mL
	
	Compare the units used in the two ratios to see if any can be canceled. In this case, the units for the second part of both ratios are milliliters. These can be canceled when we set up the proportion.
	
	  20 mg : 100 = x : 500
	
	Now solve for x, the unknown quantity.
	
	1. $100 \times x = 20 \text{ mg} \times 500$
	
	2. $\dfrac{100 \times x}{100} = \dfrac{20 \text{ mg} \times 500}{100}$
	
	3. $x = 100 \text{ mg}$
	
	The second solution will contain 100 mg of drug in 500 mL of solution.

Example 2	15 g of drug is dissolved in 300 mL of solution. If you need 45 g of the drug, how many milliliters of the solution do you need?
	Set up the ratios.
	
	  15 g : 300 mL and 45 g : x
	
	Cancel units and set up the proportion.
	
	  15 : 300 mL = 45 : x
	
	Solve for the unknown quantity.
	
	1. $300 \text{ mL} \times 45 = 15 \times x$
	
	2. $\dfrac{300 \text{ mL} \times 45}{15} = \dfrac{15 \times x}{15}$
	
	3. $900 \text{ mL} = x$
	
	You will need 900 mL of the solution to have 45 g of drug.

Setting Up the Correct Proportion

A physician's order calls for a patient to receive 250 mg of amoxicillin oral suspension 3 times a day. Amoxicillin oral suspension is a dry medication that is mixed with water before being given to the patient. Each 5 mL of suspension contains 125 mg of drug. The healthcare professional needs to calculate how many milliliters he will need to give the patient for each dose. He sets up the proportion as 5 mL/ 125 mg = 250 mg/x.

 Think! . . . Is It Reasonable? What mistake did the healthcare professional make? How should it be corrected? What dose should the patient receive?

Cross-Multiplying

When a proportion is written with fractions, you can use a method, known as **cross-multiplying** to determine if it is true. Cross-multiplying is multiplying the numerator from each fraction by the denominator of the other. If the proportion is true, the products must be equal.

$$\frac{A}{B} \bowtie \frac{C}{D}$$

Cross-multiplying

RULE 3-17	To determine if a proportion written with fractions is true:
	1. Cross-multiply. Multiply the numerator of the first fraction with the denominator of the second fraction. Then multiply the denominator of the first fraction with the numerator of the second fraction.
	2. Compare the products. The products must be equal.
Example 1	Determine if $\frac{2}{5} = \frac{10}{25}$ is a true proportion.
	1. Cross-multiply.
	$\frac{2}{5} \bowtie \frac{10}{25} \rightarrow 2 \times 25 = 5 \times 10$
	2. Compare the products on both sides of the equal sign.
	$50 = 50$
	$\frac{2}{5} = \frac{10}{25}$ is a true proportion.

Example 2

Determine if $\frac{100}{1,000} = \frac{500}{5,000}$ is a true proportion.

1. $\frac{100}{1,000} \diagdown \frac{500}{5,000} \rightarrow 100 \times 5,000 = 1,000 \times 500$

2. $500,000 = 500,000$

$\frac{100}{1,000} = \frac{500}{5,000}$ is a true proportion.

Example 3

Determine if $\frac{5}{8} = \frac{40}{72}$ is a true proportion.

1. $\frac{5}{8} \diagdown \frac{40}{72} \rightarrow 5 \times 72 = 8 \times 40$

2. $360 \neq 320$

The proportion $\frac{5}{8} = \frac{40}{72}$ is not true.

In the previous section, you learned to use means and extremes to find an unknown quantity in a proportion that was written using ratios. As you might expect, you can cross-multiply to find the unknown quantity in a proportion expressed with fractions.

RULE 3-18

To find the unknown quantity in a proportion written with fractions:

1. Cross-multiply. Write an equation setting the products equal to each other.

2. Solve the equation to find the unknown quantity.

3. Restate the proportion, inserting the unknown quantity.

4. Check your work. Determine if the proportion is true.

Example 1

Find the unknown quantity in $\frac{3}{5} = \frac{6}{x}$.

1. Cross-multiply.

$$\frac{3}{5} \diagdown \frac{6}{x} \rightarrow 3 \times x = 5 \times 6$$

$$3 \times x = 30$$

2. Solve the equation. Here, divide both sides by 3.

$$\frac{3 \times x}{3} = \frac{30}{3}$$

$$x = 10$$

3. Restate the proportion, inserting the unknown quantity.

$$\frac{3}{5} = \frac{6}{10}$$

4. Check your work by cross-multiplying.

$$3 \times 10 = 5 \times 6$$
$$30 = 30$$

The unknown quantity is 10.

Example 2

Find the unknown quantity in $\frac{25}{5} = \frac{50}{x}$.

1. $\frac{25}{5} \diagdown \frac{50}{x} \rightarrow 25 \times x = 5 \times 50$

$$25 \times x = 250$$

2. $\frac{25 \times x}{25} = \frac{250}{25}$

$$x = 10$$

3. $\frac{25}{5} = \frac{50}{10}$

4. $25 \times 10 = 5 \times 50$

$$250 = 250$$

The unknown quantity is 10.

CANCELING UNITS IN PROPORTIONS WRITTEN WITH FRACTIONS Just as we were able to cancel units in proportions written as ratios, we can cancel them in proportions written as fractions. Now, however, we need to compare the units used in the top and bottom of the two fractions in the proportion. For example, you have a solution containing 200 mg of drug in 5 mL, and you are asked to determine how many milliliters of a solution contain 500 mg of drug. You can solve the problem by using the following two fractions. Make sure that the labels are in like positions. In this case, mg is placed in the numerator in both fractions.

$$\frac{200 \text{ mg}}{5 \text{ mL}} = \frac{500 \text{ mg}}{x}$$

Because the units for both numerators of the fraction are milligrams, they can be canceled. Canceling the units leaves us with the following proportion.

$$\frac{200}{5 \text{ mL}} = \frac{500}{x}$$

The unknown quantity can now be found by cross-multiplying and solving the equation as before.

RULE 3-19	If the units of the numerator of the two fractions are the same, they can be dropped or canceled before you set up a proportion. Likewise, if the units from the denominator of the two fractions are the same, they can be canceled.

Example 1

If 100 mL of solution contains 20 mg of drug, how many milligrams of the drug will be in 500 mL of the solution?

Start by setting up the fractions.

$$\frac{20 \text{ mg}}{100 \text{ mL}} \quad \text{and} \quad \frac{x}{500 \text{ mL}}$$

Compare the units used in the two fractions to see if any can be canceled. In this case, the units for the denominators of both fractions are milliliters. These can be canceled when you set up the proportion.

$$\frac{20 \text{ mg}}{100} = \frac{x}{500}$$

Now solve for x, the unknown quantity.

1. $100 \times x = 20 \text{ mg} \times 500$

2. $\dfrac{100 \times x}{100} = \dfrac{20 \text{ mg} \times 500}{100}$

3. $x = 100 \text{ mg}$

The second solution will contain 100 mg of drug in 500 mL of solution.

Example 2

15 grams of drug is dissolved in 300 mL of solution. If you need 45 g of the drug, how many milliliters of the solution do you need?

Set up the fractions.

$$\frac{15 \text{ g}}{300 \text{ mL}} \quad \text{and} \quad \frac{45 \text{ g}}{x}$$

Cancel units and set up the proportion.

$$\frac{15}{300 \text{ mL}} = \frac{45}{x}$$

Solve for the missing value.

1. $300 \text{ mL} \times 45 = 15 \times x$

2. $\dfrac{300 \text{ mL} \times 45}{15} = \dfrac{15 \times x}{15}$

3. $900 \text{ mL} = x$

You will need 900 mL of the solution to have 45 g of drug.

Confusing Multiplying Fractions with Cross-Multiplying

A healthcare professional is preparing a 5% solution of dextrose in batches of 500 milliliters (mL). She sets up the calculation as follows: $\frac{5\,g}{100\,mL} = \frac{x}{500\,mL}$. Distracted by a call, she returns to the calculation and computes:

$5 \times x = 100 \times 500 = 50{,}000$

This calculation leads to:

$x = 10{,}000$

 Think! . . . Is It Reasonable? What mistake did the healthcare professional make? How could she have avoided this mistake?

REVIEW AND PRACTICE

3.4 Using Proportions to Solve for an Unknown Quantity

Determine if the following proportions are true.

1. $6:12 = 12:24$ **2.** $3:8 = 9:32$ **3.** $5:75 = 15:250$ **4.** $8:100 = 20:250$

5. $6:18 = 18:54$ **6.** $\frac{7}{16} = \frac{28}{48}$ **7.** $\frac{6}{9} = \frac{24}{36}$ **8.** $\frac{100}{250} = \frac{150}{375}$

9. $\frac{50}{125} = \frac{125}{300}$ **10.** $\frac{60}{96} = \frac{80}{108}$

Find the missing value.

11. $10:x = 5:8$ **12.** $10:4 = 20:x$ **13.** $4:25 = 16:x$ **14.** $x:15 = 100:75$

15. $21:27 = x:45$ **16.** $100:x = 50:2$ **17.** $3:12 = x:36$ **18.** $33:39 = 55:x$

19. $x:24 = 5:30$ **20.** $18:x = 27:6$ **21.** $\frac{3}{15} = \frac{x}{5}$ **22.** $\frac{2}{x} = \frac{8}{100}$

23. $\frac{x}{20} = \frac{120}{100}$ **24.** $\frac{50}{75} = \frac{100}{x}$ **25.** $\frac{10}{3} = \frac{x}{60}$ **26.** $\frac{x}{4} = \frac{4}{16}$

27. $\frac{25}{x} = \frac{75}{3}$ **28.** $\frac{2}{3} = \frac{6}{x}$ **29.** $\frac{x}{9} = \frac{18}{27}$ **30.** $\frac{25}{125} = \frac{x}{150}$

31. A patient must take 3 tablets per day for 14 days. How many tablets should the pharmacy supply to fill this order?

32. If 15 mL of solution contains 75 mg of drug, how many milligrams of drug are in 60 mL of solution?

33. A healthcare professional is instructed to administer 600 mL of a solution every 8 h. How many hours will be needed to administer 1,800 mL of the solution?

34. Two tablets contain a total of 50 mg of drug. How many milligrams of drug are in 10 tablets?

35. If 250 mL of solution contains 90 mg of drug, there is 450 mg of drug in how many milliliters of solution?

CHAPTER 3 SUMMARY

LEARNING OUTCOME	KEY POINTS

3.1 Convert values to and from a percent. Pages 56–60	▶ A value expressed as a percent represents the value divided by 100.
	  • Example: 15% is equal to 0.15 or 15 hundredths.
	▶ Fractions can be converted to percents by dividing the numerator by the denominator, multiplying by 100, and then adding the percent sign.
	  • Example: To convert $\frac{3}{4}$ to a percent, divide 3 by 4 and then multiply by 100%: $(3 \div 4) \times 100\% = 75\%$
	▶ Decimals can be converted into a percent by multiplying them by 100 and then adding the percent sign.
	  • Example: To convert 0.125 to a percent, multiply by 100%: $0.125 \times 100\% = 12.5\%$

3.2 Convert values to and from a ratio. Pages 60–67	▶ A ratio is another way to write a fraction. ▶ A ratio contains two numbers separated by a colon. The number before the colon is the numerator of the fraction; the number after the colon is the denominator. • Example: The fraction $\frac{5}{8}$ is equal to the ratio $5:8$.
3.3 Write proportions. Pages 67–68	▶ Proportions state that two fractions or two ratios are equal to each other. ▶ Proportions can be written using either ratios or fractions. • Example: $2:3 = 6:9$ and $\frac{2}{3} = \frac{6}{9}$ are the same proportion written in two different ways.

3.4 Use proportions to solve for an unknown quantity. Pages 68–77	▶ When three of the four values in a proportion are known, the unknown value can be calculated.
	▶ Proportions using ratios can be solved by multiplying means and extremes.
	  • Example: To solve for the unknown in $2:4 = 3:x$, multiply the means $(4 \times 3 = 12)$ then the extremes $(2 \times x = 2x)$. Write an equation using the products $(2x = 12)$ and then solve for the unknown $(x = 6)$.
	▶ Proportions using fractions are solved by cross-multiplying.
	  • Example: To solve for the unknown in $\frac{2}{3} = \frac{x}{12}$, cross-multiply $(3 \times x = 2 \times 12)$ and then solve for the unknown $(x = 8)$.

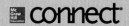

In each row of the table below, use the information to calculate the equivalent values. When necessary, round decimals to the nearest hundredth. Round percents to the nearest tenth of a percent. Do not reduce ratios or fractions. (LO 3.1, 3.2)

	fraction	decimal	ratio	percent
1		0.625		
2	$\frac{5}{2}$			
3			3 : 5	
4				35%
5	$\frac{1}{6}$			
6		11.4		
7				18.5%
8			6 : 20	

Find the missing value. (LO 3.3, 3.4)

9. $2 : x = 6 : 15$ **10.** $x : 8 = 3 : 12$ **11.** $5 : 8 = x : 40$

12. $\frac{1}{6} = \frac{x}{18}$ **13.** $\frac{4}{12} = \frac{2}{x}$ **14.** $\frac{15}{x} = \frac{6}{8}$

15. If 1 tablet contains 30 mg of drug, how many milligrams of drug do 5 tablets contain?

16. If 10 g of drug is in 250 mL of solution, how many grams of drug are in 1,000 mL of solution?

17. If 3 tablets contain 45 mg of drug, how many milligrams of drug are in 1 tablet?

18. If 60 mg of drug is in 500 mL of solution, how many milliliters of solution contain 36 mg of drug?

19. If 80 mg of drug is in 480 mL of solution, how many milliliters of solution contain 60 mg of drug?

20. If 3 capsules contain 60 mg of drug, how many capsules contain 100 mg of drug?

CHECK UP

In each row of the table below, use the information to calculate the equivalent values. For instance, in row 1, convert the ratio 2 : 3 to a fraction, a decimal, and a percent. Where necessary, round decimals to the nearest hundredth. Round percents to the nearest percent. Do not reduce ratios and fractions. (LO 3.1, 3.2)

	fraction	decimal	ratio	percent
1			2 : 3	
2	$\frac{5}{4}$			
3				28%
4		0.03		
5	$\frac{40}{8}$			
6			4 : 12	
7	$\frac{9}{27}$			
8		1.4		
9				0.5%
10			3 : 50	
11				25%
12		6		
13	$\frac{1}{9}$			
14				150%
15			6 : 97	
16		12.8		

Find the missing value. (LO 3.4)

17. $1 : 10 = 4 : x$ **18.** $3 : 27 = x : 9$ **19.** $x : 6 = 8 : 12$ **20.** $5 : x = 10 : 50$

21. $\frac{4}{8} = \frac{24}{x}$ **22.** $\frac{x}{14} = \frac{5}{70}$ **23.** $\frac{3}{x} = \frac{30}{20}$ **24.** $\frac{1}{25} = \frac{x}{125}$

25. If 1 tablet contains 25 mg of drug, how many milligrams of drug are in 3 tablets? (LO 3-3, 3-4)

26. If 100 mL of drug is in 600 mL of solution, how many milliliters of drug are in 1,800 mL of solution? (LO 3.3, 3.4)

27. A solution contains 5 g of dextrose in 100 mL of solution. How many grams of dextrose are in 500 mL of solution? (LO 3.3, 3.4)

28. A solution contains 1 g of drug for every 50 mL of solution. How much solution would you need to give a patient to administer 3 g of drug? (LO 3.3, 3.4)

29. 10 mL of a liquid medication contains 250 mg of drug. How many milliliters contain 50 mg of drug? (LO 3.3, 3.4)

30. If 30 g of drug is in 100 mL of solution, how many grams of drug are in 350 mL of solution? (LO 3.3, 3.4)

CRITICAL THINKING APPLICATIONS

A healthcare professional has just finished preparing 250 mL of a solution containing 6 grams of drug in every 100 mL when he learns that the physician wants a solution containing 8 grams of drug in 100 mL of solution. How many additional grams of drug should the healthcare professional add to the first solution he prepared? (LO 3.3, 3.4)

CASE STUDY

A physician's order calls for Ceclor® oral suspension 750 mg to be given daily for 14 days. The daily dosage is to be divided into 3 equal doses per day. Ceclor® oral suspension is a drug that is mixed with solvent before it is administered. (LO 3.3, 3.4)

1. How many milligrams of drug should be given in each dose?

2. If 5 mL of solution contains 125 mg of drug, how many milliliters should be given in each dose?

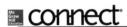

Now that you have completed the materials in the chapter text, go to CONNECT and complete any chapter activities you have not yet done.

UNIT ONE ASSESSMENT

Up until now, all of the calculations have been grouped together to allow you the opportunity to practice a specific skill. In one chapter, you focused on fractions; in another, decimals; and in another, percents, ratios, and proportions. In the "real world," however, you will be faced with a variety of situations in which you will need to use each of these skills at various times throughout the day. Problems will not be sorted by chapter. This assessment requires you to use skills practiced in each of the chapters in this unit. If you have trouble with some of these calculations, it will help you to identify areas where more practice is needed. Be sure to write your answer in the proper format: reduce fractions, include leading zeros, and delete trailing zeros. If you do well, you can move forward with the confidence that you are prepared for the next unit.

1. Place >, <, or = between the following pairs of numbers to make a true statement.

   a. $3\frac{1}{5}$ 3.25

   b. 135% $1\frac{1}{2}$

   c. 14.5 $\frac{29}{2}$

2. 0.57 = _____%

3. $2.4 \div 0.3 = x$

4. A bottle contains 60 mL of medication. How many 5 mL doses does it contain?

5. $1 : 6 = x : 18$

6. Write 7.4 as an improper fraction.

7. There are 250 mg of drug in 5 mL of a solution. How many milligrams of drug are there in 12 mL?

8. Write 0.4 as a ratio.

9. $3 : 50 =$ _____%

10. Write 3.5% as a decimal.

11. $\frac{3}{14} = \frac{9}{x}$

12. $\frac{x}{5} = \frac{15}{25}$

13. $\frac{1}{4} \div \frac{1}{3} = x$

14. $5\frac{1}{8} + 3\frac{1}{4} = x$

15. What is the least common denominator for $\frac{2}{5}$, $\frac{1}{3}$, and $\frac{1}{2}$?

16. $2 : 5 = 7 : x$

17. Reduce $\frac{18}{4}$ and rewrite it as a mixed number.

18. Write $\frac{23}{4}$ as a decimal.

19. If 3 tablets contain 150 mg of a drug, how much drug is there in 4 tablets?

20. $3.125 - 1.7 = x$

UNIT 2

Using Systems of Measurement

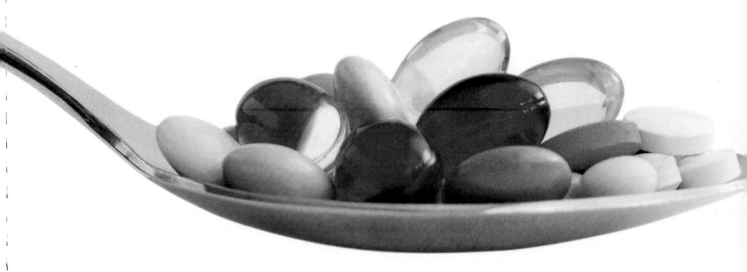

Metric System

Practice is the best instruction of them all.

PUBLILIUS SYRUS

LEARNING OUTCOMES

When you have completed Chapter 4, you will be able to:

4.1   Write measurements in metric notation.

4.2   Convert metric units by moving the decimal.

KEY TERMS

Centi (c)

Gram (g)

Kilo (k)

Liter (L)

Meter (m)

Micro (mc)

Milli (m)

INTRODUCTION

The metric system is the most commonly used system of measurement in the healthcare system. Drugs are most often labeled and ordered in milligrams, although some are measured in micrograms or **grams**. Injections are usually measured in milliliters. Intravenous solutions may be measured in liters. Knowing how to accurately convert units within the metric system is an essential skill for anyone performing dosage calculations. Practice these concepts until you are certain you understand.

4.1 Metric System

The metric system is the most widely used system of measurement in the world today. The system, which was defined in 1792, gets its name from the **meter**, the basic unit of length. A meter is approximately 3 inches (8.56 cm) longer than a yard. It may be helpful to visualize the relationship of the metric system to measurements you already know. (See Figure 4-1.)

Units of measurement in the metric system are sometimes referred to as SI units, an abbreviation for International System of Units. This system was established in 1960 to make units of measurement for the metric system standard throughout the world. Table 4-1 lists the basic metric units for length, weight, and volume.

Notice that meter and gram are abbreviated with lowercase letters, but **liter** is abbreviated with an uppercase L. Using the uppercase L minimizes the chance of confusing the lowercase letter L (l) with the digit 1. You will use length mostly when expressing measurements such as patient height, infant head circumference, and lesion or wound size. However, you

TABLE 4-1 Basic Units of Metric Measurement		
TYPE OF MEASURE	BASIC UNIT	ABBREVIATION
Length	meter	m
Weight (or mass)	gram	g (or gm)
Volume	liter	L

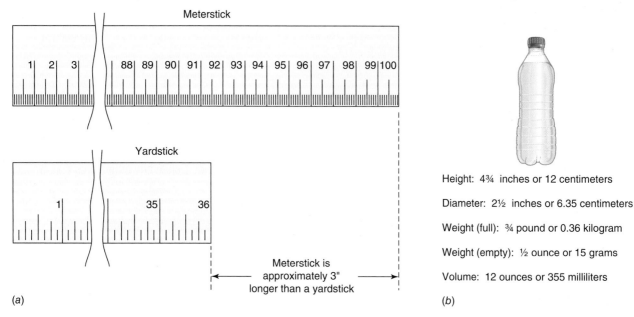

Meterstick

1 2 3 | 88 89 90 91 92 93 94 95 96 97 98 99 100

Yardstick

1 | 35 36

Meterstick is approximately 3" longer than a yardstick

Height: 4¾ inches or 12 centimeters

Diameter: 2½ inches or 6.35 centimeters

Weight (full): ¾ pound or 0.36 kilogram

Weight (empty): ½ ounce or 15 grams

Volume: 12 ounces or 355 milliliters

(a)

(b)

Figure 4-1 *(a)* Meter versus yard. *(b)* Metric and common measurements comparison.

will use weight and volume frequently when you calculate dosages. Most dosages and drug strengths are expressed using the metric system.

Metric Notation

ALEKS

GO TO . . .
Metric System–
Metric Distance
Conversion with
Whole Number
Values

Like the decimal system, the metric system is based on multiples of 10. The greater confidence you have working with decimals, the more comfortable you will be working with metric units. (To review decimals, see the "Decimals" chapter.)

A prefix before the basic unit indicates relative size. For example, **kilo**- indicates that you multiply the basic unit by 1,000. A kilometer is 1,000 meters, a kilogram is 1,000 grams, and a kiloliter is 1,000 liters. When you divide 1 meter into 1,000 equal lengths, each length is 1 millimeter. The prefix **milli**- means one-thousandth. A millimeter is one-thousandth of a meter, a milliliter is one-thousandth of a liter, and a milligram is one-thousandth of a gram.

As a healthcare provider, you will most often use the metric prefixes **kilo**-, **centi**-, **milli**-, and **micro**-. Table 4-2 shows how these prefixes are combined with the base units and their value relative to the base unit.

RULE 4-1	Use Arabic numerals with decimals to represent any fractions.
Example	Write 1.25 g to represent $1\frac{1}{4}$ g.

TABLE 4-2 Common Metric Prefixes

Prefix	kilo-	base unit	centi-	milli-	micro-
Value	×1,000	—	÷100	÷1,000	÷1,000,000
Length	kilometer km 1,000 m	meter m 1 m	centimeter cm 0.01 m	millimeter mm 0.001 m	micrometer mcm 0.000001 m
Weight (Mass)	kilogram kg 1,000 g	gram g 1 g	centigram cg 0.01 g	milligram mg 0.001 g	microgram mcg 0.000001 g
Volume	kiloliter kL 1,000 L	liter L 1 L	centiliter cL 0.01 L	millilimter mL 0.001 L	microliter mcm 0.000001 L

RULE 4-2	If the quantity is less than 1, include a zero before the decimal point. Delete any other zeros that are not necessary.
Example	Do not write .750; instead, write 0.75, adding a zero before the decimal point and deleting the unnecessary zero at the end.

RULE 4-3	Write the unit after the quantity with a space between them.
Example	Write 30 mg, not mg 30 or 30mg.

RULE 4-4	Use lowercase letters for metric abbreviations. However, use uppercase L to represent liter.
Example	Write mg, not MG. Write mL, not ml. While ml is technically correct, you will avoid errors if you use an uppercase L.

Considering Rules 4-1 to 4-4, we will determine the correct metric notation for six and two-eighths milliliters. First, $6\frac{2}{8}$ must be converted to decimals.

$$6\frac{2}{8} = 6.25$$

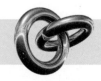

LEARNING LINK   Recall from the *Fractions* chapter (Rule 1-5) and the *Decimals* chapter (Rule 2-5) that $\frac{2}{8}$ can be reduced to $\frac{1}{4}$ and $\frac{1}{4} = 0.25$.

Next, write the unit after the quantity, leaving a space between them and using the abbreviation mL for milliliters. So:

6.25 mL is correct metric notation for six and two-eighths milliliters.

Now consider how you would write one-half milligram.

$$\frac{1}{2} = 0.50$$

Place a zero in front of the decimal point, and delete any unnecessary zeros.

0.5

Place the unit after the quantity with a space between them.

0.5 mg is correct metric notation for one-half milligram.

REVIEW AND PRACTICE

4.1 Metric System

In Exercises 1–10, select the correct metric notation.

1. Two and one-half kilograms
   a. 2.5 Kg   **b.** 2.05 kg   **c.** $2\frac{1}{2}$ kg   **d.** 2.5 kg

2. Seven-tenths of a milliliter
   a. $\frac{7}{10}$ mL   **b.** .7 mL   **c.** ml 0.7   **d.** 0.7 mL

3. Four-hundredths of a gram
   a. 400 G   **b.** 0.4 g   **c.** 0.04 g   **d.** .04 g

4. Thirty-one millimeters
   a. 31mm   **b.** 0.031 mm   **c.** 31.0 mlm   **d.** 31 mm

5. Eight liters
   a. 8.0 l   **b.** 8 L   **c.** 8.0 L   **d.** 0.8 l

6. One hundred twenty-five micrograms
   a. 125 mg   **b.** 0.125 mcg   **c.** 125 mcg   **d.** 125 mg

7. Seventy-eight centimeters
   a. 78 ctm   **b.** 78.0 Cm   **c.** 0.78 cm   **d.** 78 cm

8. Two hundred fifty microliters
   a. mcL 250   **b.** 250 mcL   **c.** 25.0 mcL   **d.** 250 mL

9. Nine and one-quarter milligrams
   a. $9\frac{1}{4}$ mg
   b. $9\frac{25}{100}$ mg
   c. 9.25 mg
   d. 9.25 mgm

10. Four-tenths of a liter
    a. 0.4 L
    b. $\frac{4}{10}$ L
    c. 0.40 L
    d. 0.40 l

In Exercises 11–20, write the indicated amounts with correct metric notation.

11. Four and one-half milliliters _____

12. Sixty-two hundredths of a gram _____

13. Three-quarters of a milliliter _____

14. Seven-tenths of a meter _____

15. Twelve liters _____

16. Nine-twelfths of a kilogram _____

17. One hundred fifty-seven kilometers _____

18. Seven and three-quarters centimeters _____

19. Ninety-three micrograms _____

20. Eight-hundredths of a milligram _____

4.2 Converting Within the Metric System

Recall from the "Decimals" chapter that when you multiply a decimal number by 100, you move the decimal point two places to the right and get a larger number. When you divide a decimal number by 100, you move the decimal point two places to the left and get a smaller number.

Converting one metric unit of measurement to another is similar to multiplying and dividing decimal numbers. For example, if you travel 1 kilometer, you travel 1,000 meters. When you convert from the larger unit of measurement (kilometer) to the smaller unit (meter), the quantity of units increases. Therefore, you multiply, moving the decimal point to the right.

If you convert from meters to kilometers, the quantity of units decreases. If you travel 1,000 meters, you travel 1 kilometer. When you convert from a smaller unit (meter) to a larger unit (kilometer), the quantity of units decreases. Therefore, you divide, moving the decimal point to the left.

When you calculate dosages, you will work most often with four metric units of weight and three metric units of volume. The four units of weight are kilogram (kg), gram (g), milligram (mg), and microgram (mcg). Two of the units of volume are liter (L) and milliliter (mL). The third is cubic centimeter (cc), which is equivalent to milliliter (mL). Although the abbreviation cc for cubic centimeter may be seen in practice, it should not be used. Instead use the abbreviation mL for milliliter.

RULE 4-5

ALEKS

GO TO . . .
Metric System–
Metric Conversion
with Decimal
Values: Two-Step
Problem

When you convert a quantity from one unit of metric measurement to another:

1. Move the decimal point to the right if you convert from a larger to a smaller unit.

2. Move the decimal point to the left if you convert from a smaller to a larger unit.

Table 4-3 and Figure 4-2 will help you determine both the direction and the number of places to move the decimal point when you convert between units of metric measurement. For example, milliliter is three places to the right of liter, the basic unit. To convert a quantity from liters (larger) to milliliters (smaller), move the decimal point three places to the right. Similarly, to convert a quantity from grams (smaller) to kilograms (larger), move the decimal point three places to the left.

TABLE 4-3 Metric System Place Values and Units

	KILO-	BASE UNIT	CENTI-	MILLI-	MICRO-
Meaning	1,000	1	$\frac{1}{100}$ 0.01	$\frac{1}{1,000}$ 0.001	$\frac{1}{1,000,000}$ 0.000001
Commonly used units and abbreviations	kilograms (kg)	grams (g) meters (m) liters (L)	centimeters (cm)	milligrams (mg) millimeters (mm) milliliters (mL)	micrograms (mcg)

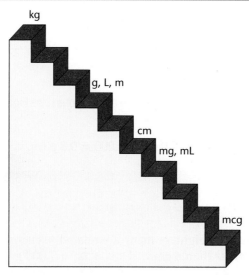

Figure 4-2 Metric steps.

Example 1	Convert 4 L to milliliters (mL).
	Move the decimal point for 4 (or 4.0) three places to the right to find the number of milliliters. Add zeros as necessary.
	4 L = 4.000 L = 4,000 mL
	Think! . . . Is It Reasonable? A milliliter (mL) is smaller than a liter (L); a quantity will have more milliliters than liters. Using Figure 4-2, you can see that milliliter is three steps to the right of liter.
Example 2 **ALEKS** ――――― **GO TO . . .** Metric System– Metric Mass or Capacity Conversion with Decimal Values	How many meters (m) are in 75 mm? A meter (m) is larger than a millimeter (mm); a quantity will have fewer meters than millimeters. Using Figure 4-2, you can see that meter is three steps to the left of millimeter. Write 75 as 75.0, and move the decimal point in 75 three places to the left. Add zeros as necessary. 75 mm = 75.0 mm = 0.075 m
Example 3	Convert 4.5 mcg to milligrams (mg). You are converting from a smaller unit to a larger one. Use Figure 4-2 or divide 4.5 by 1,000, moving the decimal point three places to the left. 4.5 mcg ÷ 1,000 = 0004.5 mcg ÷ 1,000 = 0.0045 mg

Example 4 **ALEKS** ─────────── **GO TO . . .** Metric System– Metric Mass or Capacity Conversion with Whole Number Values ───────────	Convert 62 kg to grams (g). You are converting from a larger unit to a smaller one. Use Figure 4-2 or multiply 62 by 1,000, moving the decimal point three places to the right. $$62 \text{ kg} \times 1{,}000 = 62.000 \text{ kg} \times 1{,}000 = 62{,}000 \text{ g}$$
Example 5	Convert 300 mg to grams (g). You are converting from a smaller unit to a larger one. Use Figure 4-2 or divide 300 by 1,000, moving the decimal point three places to the left. $$300 \text{ mg} \div 1{,}000 = 0300.0 \text{ mg} \div 1{,}000 = 0.3 \text{ g}$$

The four units of weight, or mass, are related to each other by a factor of 1,000. A kilogram is 1,000 times larger than a gram. Thus, 1 kg = 1,000 g. In turn, a gram is 1,000 times larger than a milligram, which is 1,000 times larger than a microgram. The same relationship is true for liters and milliliters; a liter is 1,000 times larger than a milliliter. Table 4-4 lists four of the most commonly used equivalent measurements. Because they are so important to dosage calculations, you should memorize them.

TABLE 4-4 Equivalent Metric Measurements	
1 kg = 1,000 g	1 mg = 1,000 mcg
1 g = 1,000 mg	1 L = 1,000 mL

ERROR ALERT!

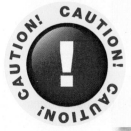

Remember: The Larger the Unit, the Smaller the Quantity; the Smaller the Unit, the Larger the Quantity

You may be tempted to multiply when you convert from a smaller unit to a larger unit, thinking that you are increasing in size. If you find yourself confused, think about conversions you have made all your life.

For example, a dollar bill is a larger unit of money than a quarter, which is a larger unit of money than a penny. When you write their relationship, look at how the quantity changes:

1 dollar bill = 4 quarters = 100 pennies

When you convert from the larger unit to the smaller one, the quantity increases. Writing the money relationship as:

100 pennies = 4 quarters = 1 dollar bill

shows you that as the unit increases in size, the quantity decreases. You see the same relationship with units of time and in the metric system:

1 hour = 60 minutes = 3,600 seconds

1 g = 1,000 mg = 1,000,000 mcg

CRITICAL THINKING ON THE JOB

Placing the Decimal Point Correctly

A child suffering from congestive heart failure is rushed into an emergency room. The physician orders 0.05 mg of Lanoxin® for the child. The healthcare professional quickly calculates that 0.05 mg = 500 mcg. Lanoxin® is available for injection in quantities of 500 mcg. The nurse hands the syringe to the doctor.

Fortunately, the doctor catches the error before the Lanoxin® is administered. The child should be given 50 mcg, not 500 mcg of Lanoxin®. As it turns out, Lanoxin® is available as an elixir in doses of 50 mcg. This quantity should be administered. The larger dose of 500 mcg could be fatal to the child.

 Think! . . . Is It Reasonable? How can the attending healthcare professional ensure that she converted the quantity correctly? How should the problem have been solved? Why is it important in this situation?

ERROR ALERT!

Converting Quantities for Medications

When you convert quantities from one unit of measure to another within the metric system, pay close attention to the decimal point. For example, when going from milligrams (mg) to micrograms (mcg), the quantity should be multiplied by 1,000; the decimal should move three places to the right. If you move the decimal the wrong direction a dangerous error can occur.

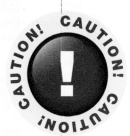

REVIEW AND PRACTICE

4.2 Converting Within the Metric System

In Exercises 1–20, complete the conversions.

1. 7 g = _____ mg
2. 1,200 mg = _____ g
3. 23 g = _____ kg
4. 8 kg = _____ g
5. 8.01 L = _____ mL
6. 100 mL = _____ L
7. 3.6 m = _____ mm
8. 5,233 mm = _____ m
9. 500 m = _____ km
10. 3.25 km = _____ m
11. 0.25 mg = _____ mcg
12. 462 mg = _____ mcg
13. 250 mcg = _____ mg
14. 75 mcg = _____ mg
15. 0.06 g = _____ mcg
16. 0.5 g = _____ mcg
17. 8,000 mcg = _____ g
18. 20,000 mcg = _____ g
19. 562 mm = _____ cm
20. 4.32 cm = _____ m

CHAPTER 4 SUMMARY

LEARNING OUTCOME	KEY POINTS
4.1 Write measurements in metric notation. Pages 84–88	▶ The base units of the metric system are the gram (for weight), liter (for volume), and meter (for length). ▶ Grams, liters, and meters are abbreviated using a single letter—g, L, or m. • The L is capitalized to avoid confusing it with the number 1. ▶ Metric prefixes can be combined with the base unit. • For example, milligram is written mg. This combines the prefix for milli- with the abbreviation for the base unit gram. ▶ The metric prefixes used in dosage calculations are kilo-, centi-, milli-, and micro-.
4.2 Convert metric units by moving the decimal. Pages 88–92	▶ When converting to a larger unit the decimal is moved to the left, giving you a smaller number. • When converting 250 mg to grams you are converting to a larger unit, so you move the decimal to the left: 250 mg = 0.25 g ▶ When converting to a smaller unit the decimal is moved to the right, giving you a larger number. • When converting liters to milliliters you are converting to a smaller unit, so you move the decimal to the right: 1.8 L = 1,800 mL

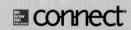

Write the indicated amounts using the proper abbreviations. (LO 4.1)

   1. Twenty-five micrograms _____

   2. Seven and one-half milliliters _____

   3. Eighty-two centimeters _____

   4. Three-hundredths of a gram _____

   5. Two and three-quarters liters _____

Perform the following conversions. (LO 4.2)

   6. 3.5 g = _____ mg

   7. 30 mg = _____ g

   8. 1.2 kg = _____ g

   9. 0.25 mg = _____ mcg

 10. 350 g = _____ kg

 11. 0.5 L = _____ mL

 12. 180 mL = _____ L

 13. 1.2 mm = _____ cm

 14. 5 mcg = _____ mg

 15. 36 cm = _____ m

CHECK UP

In Exercises 1–8, write the indicated amounts, using numerals and abbreviations. (LO 4.1)

1. Twenty-five and one-half kilograms

2. Forty-five hundredths of a centimeter

3. Forty micrograms

4. Three-quarters of a liter

5. Nine-tenths of a milligram

6. One and one-half millimeters

7. Three hundred seventy-five thousandths of a gram

8. Twelve milliliters

In Exercises 9–20, calculate the conversions. (LO 4.2)

9. 0.06 g = _____ mg

10. 125 mcg = _____ mg

11. 0.004 km = _____ m

12. 0.75 cm = _____ mm

13. 965 mL = _____ L

14. 0.008 L = _____ mL

15. 0.32 kg = _____ g

16. 0.05 mg = _____ mcg

17. 988 m = _____ km

18. 1,725 cm = _____ km

19. 368 mg = _____ g

20. 247 g = _____ kg

CRITICAL THINKING APPLICATIONS

A patient is given a prescription for 0.5 g of a medication. The medication is available in both 250 mg and 400 mg tablets. Which product should be used? How many tablets would the patient take for each dose? (LO 4.2)

CASE STUDY

A patient suffering from a cold is given a prescription for 15 mL of cough suppressant every 8 h for 10 days. (LO 4.2)

1. How many milliliters of medication will the patient take in one day?

2. If the medication is supplied in 0.5 L bottles, how many bottles will the patient need to complete the 10 days of treatment?

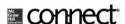

Now that you have completed the materials in the chapter text, go to CONNECT and complete any chapter activities you have not yet done.

Other Systems of Measurement

The purpose of learning is growth, and our minds, unlike our bodies, can continue growing as we continue to live.

MORTIMER ADLER

LEARNING OUTCOMES

When you have completed Chapter 5, you will be able to:

5.1 Write measurements and equivalent measures using the apothecary system.

5.2 Write measurements and equivalent measures using the household system.

5.3 Recognize equivalent measures used in dosage calculations.

INTRODUCTION

While the metric system is the most commonly used system, there are other systems of measurement that you will need to be familiar with when performing dosage calculations. Each of these systems is less common than they once were, but they are still used in some circumstances. In this chapter you will be introduced to the commonly used units for the apothecary and household systems of measurement. You will also learn how and when quantities are expressed using milliequivalents (mEq) and units. An understanding of each of these systems is essential to anyone dispensing or administering medications.

5.1 Apothecary System

The apothecary system is an old system of measurement. Used first by apothecaries (early pharmacists), it traveled across Europe from Greece and Rome to France and England. Eventually, it crossed the Atlantic to colonial America. The common measures of gallon, quart, pint, and fluid ounce are derived from the apothecary system. Certain medications, especially older ones such as aspirin and morphine, are sometimes labeled and ordered using apothecary units. Apothecary units are less familiar and can be confused with metric units, so they are infrequently used. Metric units are preferred for dosage calculations in most cases.

Units of Measure

The basic unit of weight in the apothecary system is the grain (gr). Originally, the grain was defined as the weight of a single grain of wheat, hence its name. Other units of weight used in the apothecary system include the ounce and pound, which are still commonly used. Table 5-1 shows the relationship between these units.

TABLE 5-1 Equivalent Apothecary Measurements	
WEIGHTS	**VOLUMES**
1 ounce = 480 grains	60 minims = 1 dram
16 ounces = 1 pound	8 drams = 1 fluid ounce

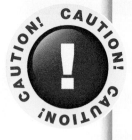

ERROR ALERT!

Do Not Confuse Grains and Grams

Because they have names and abbreviations that are similar, **grains** (gr) and grams (g) are easily confused. A grain is a measure in the apothecary system; a gram is a measure in the metric system. If you are not sure whether an order refers to grains or grams, check with the physician or pharmacist. For most conversions, 1 grain equals either 60 or 65 milligrams (mg), which means:

$$1 \text{ gr} = 60 \text{ mg} = 0.06 \text{ g} \quad \text{or} \quad 1 \text{ gr} = 65 \text{ mg} = 0.065 \text{ g}$$

In either case, 1 grain is significantly smaller than 1 gram. Medications that are measured in grains do not all use the same conversion. However, typically their labels list the metric units as well.

Three units of volume in the apothecary system are the **minim**, the **dram**, and the **ounce**. The symbols to represent these three units are error prone and should not be used. The minim was originally defined as the volume of a drop of wine. The apothecary ounce has become part of the common system of measures used in the United States. There are 8 ounces (oz) to 1 cup (c) in our commonly used household system of measures. Minims are seldom used these days, although many syringes continue to have marks that indicate minims.

ERROR ALERT!

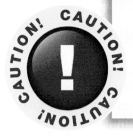

Do Not Confuse Symbols of the Apothecary System

Note that the symbols for dram (ℨ) and ounce (℥) are very similar to one another. These similarities are the reason the two symbols should NOT be used in practice and are considered error prone. If you see them on any order or document, check with the physician or other authorized prescriber before proceeding.

Apothecary Notation

The system of apothecary notation has special rules that combine fractions, Roman and Arabic numerals, symbols, and abbreviations. Even the order in which information is written differs from the order most familiar to you. Recall that Roman numerals may be written with a bar above them.

Converting from grains in the apothecary system to milligrams in the metric system is much like converting from minutes to seconds (see Figure 5-1).

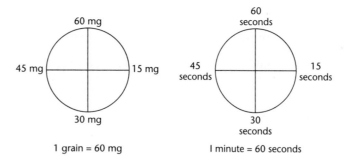

1 grain = 60 mg   I minute = 60 seconds

Figure 5-1 Converting from grains to milligrams is much like converting from minutes to seconds. One-quarter of a minute is 15 seconds, and one-quarter of a grain is 15 milligrams!

RULE 5-1	When you are writing a value in the apothecary system:
	• Write values with lowercase Roman numerals such as i or ii. Roman numerals are discussed in more detail in the chapter "Interpreting Medication Orders."
	• For values that are not whole numbers, use fractions or mixed numbers, not Roman numerals or decimals.
	• Use the abbreviation "gr" to represent grain. For ounces write either the term "ounce" or the abbreviation "oz". The units dram and minim should be written out and are not abbreviated.
	• When using the abbreviation for grain along with Roman numerals, the unit is written before the quantity.
Example 1	Write *four grains,* using apothecary notation. Use lowercase Roman numerals to represent four as iv. Abbreviate grains as gr, and place it before the quantity: gr iv.
Example 2	Write *two and one-half grains,* using apothecary notation. Use a mixed number to represent the value because it is not a whole number: gr $2\frac{1}{2}$.

REVIEW AND PRACTICE

5.1 Apothecary System

In Exercises 1–6, write the amounts using the units or abbreviations of the apothecary system.

1. Seven grains

2. Eight ounces

3. Five drams

4. Fourteen grains

5. One-half grain

6. Five and one-half ounces

In Exercises 7–10, write the equivalent apothecary measurement.

7. One ounce = _____ grain(s)

8. Sixty minims = _____ dram(s)

9. Eight drams = _____ fluid ounce(s)

10. One pound = _____ ounce(s)

5.2 Household System

Patients who take medication at home are more likely to use everyday household measures than metric ones. Many over-the-counter medications provide instructions for patients relying on household measures. For instance, a patient may be told to take 2 teaspoons of a cough syrup.

While the household system may be the most familiar one to patients, in practice it is the least accurate. For instance, patients who take a teaspoon of a syrup will often use everyday spoons that vary in size, rather than baking or other calibrated spoons. Instructions for over-the-counter medications can even invite inaccuracies. A patient may be told to mix a rounded teaspoon of powder with a quantity of water. The interpretation of *rounded* will vary from patient to patient.

Units of Measure

Basic units of volume in the household system, in increasing size, include the drop, teaspoon, tablespoon, ounce, cup, pint, quart, and gallon. Of these, the four smallest measures are most commonly used for medications. Table 5-2 summarizes the equivalent measures of the household measurements most likely to be encountered in a medical setting.

When one is specifically discussing medications, the word *ounce* generally implies volume; it represents fluid ounce. In other contexts, *ounce* may represent a unit of weight, as does *pound*.

Household Notation

As with the metric system, household notation places the quantity in Arabic numerals before the abbreviation for the unit. Table 5-3 summarizes the standard abbreviations.

Example 1	Write *six drops*, using household notation. Write the quantity with Arabic numerals before the abbreviation for the unit: 6 gtt.
Example 2	Write *twelve ounces*, using household notation. Write the quantity with Arabic numerals before the abbreviation for the unit: 12 oz.

TABLE 5-2 Equivalent Household Measurements

WEIGHTS	VOLUMES
1 pound = 16 ounces	1 cup = 8 fluid ounces
	1 pint = 16 fluid ounces
	1 ounce = 2 tablespoons
	1 tablespoon = 3 teaspoons

TABLE 5-3 Abbreviations for Household Measures	
UNIT OF MEASUREMENT	ABBREVIATION
Drop(s)	gt, gtt
Teaspoon	tsp or t
Tablespoon	tbsp, tbs, or T
Ounce	oz
Cup	cup or c
Pint	pt
Quart	qt
Gallon	gal
Pound	lb

REVIEW AND PRACTICE

5.2 Household System

In Exercises 1–6, write the quantity with the appropriate abbreviations.

1. Two teaspoons

2. Three and one-half tablespoons

3. Seventy-five pounds

4. Four fluid ounces

5. Two drops

6. One gallon

In Exercises 7–10, write the equivalent household measurement.

7. Two pints = _____ mL

8. Four tablespoons = _____ oz

9. Two tablespoons = _____ teaspoons

10. Thirty-two ounces = _____ pounds

5.3 Equivalent Measures

Units of measurement found in both the apothecary and the household systems are equal: an apothecary ounce equals a household ounce. Unlike the metric system, neither the apothecary system nor the household system is based on multiples of 10. When performing dosage

TABLE 5-4 Approximate Equivalent Measures for the Metric, Apothecary, and Household Systems

1 teaspoon = 5 mL*	1 tablespoon = 15 mL*	1 fl oz = 30 mL*
1 pint = 480 mL	1 pound = 454 g	1 gr = 60 mg*
1 kg = 2.2 lb	1 oz = 30 g*	15 gr = 1 g*
1 cup = 8 fl oz	1 fl oz = 2 tablespoons	

*Indicates approximation. See Error Alert for more information.

calculations, sometimes it will be necessary to convert units from one system to another. In order to do this, you must become familiar with their equivalent measures. Keep in mind that these equivalent measures are approximations (see Table 5-4).

ERROR ALERT!

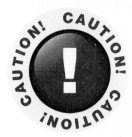

Equivalent Measure Approximations

The equivalent measures shown in Table 5-4 are approximations. The exact values of apothecary units are usually rounded when performing dosage calculations. Note the following:

- Household teaspoons and tablespoons are not uniform in size, although measuring spoons will have the volume indicated.
- A pint is actually equal to 473 mL, but 480 mL is used for most calculations.
- The ounce (weight) is slightly less than 30 g; the ounce (volume) is slightly less than 30 mL.
- One grain is actually equal to 64.8 mg. The conversion 1 grain = 60 mg is the one most often used when performing dosage calculations. For some medications (aspirin, acetaminophen, iron) the conversion that is typically used is 1 grain = 65 mg.

Example 1	How many teaspoons of solution are contained in 1 fluid ounce of solution? From Table 5-4, you can see that 1 fluid ounce contains 2 tablespoons. In turn, each tablespoon contains 3 teaspoons. Therefore, 1 fl oz = 2 × 1 tbsp = 2 × 3 tsp = 6 tsp One fluid ounce of solution contains six teaspoons of solution.
Example 2	How many tablespoons are in $\frac{1}{2}$ cup of solution? Convert 1 cup to fluid ounces, then ounces to tablespoons. From Table 5-4, you know that 1 cup = 8 fl oz and 1 fl oz = 2 tbsp: $\frac{1}{2}$ cup = $\frac{1}{2}$ × 1 cup = $\frac{1}{2}$ × 8 fl oz = 4 oz = 4 × 1 fl oz = 4 × 2 tbsp = 8 tbsp One-half cup of solution contains eight tablespoons of solution.

Milliequivalents and Units

Milliequivalents are a unit of measure based on the chemical combining power of a substance. One milliequivalent is defined as $\frac{1}{1,000}$ of the equivalent weight of a chemical. Electrolytes, such as sodium and potassium, are often measured in milliequivalents. Sodium bicarbonate and potassium chloride are examples of drugs that are prescribed in milliequivalents. You do not need to learn to convert from milliequivalents to another system of measurement.

Medications such as insulin, heparin, and penicillin are measured in *USP units*. A **unit** is the amount of a medication required to produce a certain effect. *The size of a unit varies for each drug.* Some medications, such as vitamins, are measured in standardized units called **international units**. These units represent the amount of medication needed to produce a certain effect, but they are standardized by international agreement. As with milliequivalents, you do not need to convert from units to other measures. Medications that are ordered in units will also be labeled in units.

REVIEW AND PRACTICE

5.3 Equivalent Measures

1. 3 kg = _____ lb

2. 30 mL = _____ tablespoons

3. 30 gr = _____ g

4. 180 mg = _____ gr

5. 3 pt = _____ mL

6. 2 teaspoons = _____ mL

7. 120 mL = _____ fl oz

8. 3 tablespoons = _____ mL

9. 1 lb = _____ g

10. 2 oz = _____ g

ERROR ALERT!

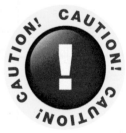

Milliequivalents (mEq) Conversions

Some minerals, especially potassium, are available as over-the-counter medications. Certain patients may elect to take the over-the-counter version to save money. Prescription potassium is ordered in mEq and the over-the-counter version is available in mcg or mg. Converting between mEq and mcg or mg is tricky and can lead to errors. There are several forms of potassium (potassium gluconate, potassium citrate, etc.) and each converts differently. Always check with the physician or pharmacist to ensure that the proper conversion is made based on the form of the medication.

CHAPTER 5 SUMMARY

LEARNING OUTCOME	KEY POINTS
5.1 Write measurements and equivalent measures using the apothecary system. Pages 95–98	▶ Units of volume for the apothecary system include the minim, dram, and fluid ounce. ▶ Units of weight for the apothecary system include the grain, ounce, and pound.
5.2 Write measurements and equivalent measures using the household system. Pages 98–99	▶ Units of volume for the household system include the drop, teaspoon, tablespoon, fluid ounce, cup, pint, and quart. ▶ Units of weight for the household system include the ounce and pound, which are the same as those used in the apothecary system.
5.3 Recognize equivalent measures used in dosage calculations. Pages 99–101	▶ While metric units are the most commonly used units in dosage calculations, other systems are sometimes used. ▶ In order to perform dosage calculations, it is essential to know the equivalent measures needed for converting between the systems of measurement.

HOMEWORK ASSIGNMENT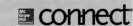

Write the equivalent measurement. (LO 5.1 to 5.3)

1. 1 oz = _____ gr

2. 1 lb = _____ g

3. 1 tsp = _____ mL

4. 1 c = _____ fl oz

5. 1 g = _____ gr

6. 1 gr = _____ mg

7. 1 kg = _____ lb

8. 1 fl oz = _____ tbsp

9. 1 lb = _____ oz

10. 1 T = _____ mL

CHECK UP

In Exercises 1–8, write the indicated amounts, using numerals and abbreviations. (LO 5.1, 5.2)

1. Fourteen and one-quarter ounces
2. Two tablespoons
3. Fifteen grains
4. Three and one-half gallons
5. Two drops
6. Seventy-five pounds
7. One and one-half teaspoons
8. Two pints

In Exercises 9–20, write the equivalent measurement. (LO 5.1 to 5.3)

9. 1 oz = _____ gr
10. 1 tbsp = _____ mL
11. 1 fl oz = _____ mL
12. 1 oz = _____ tbsp
13. 1 pt = _____ mL
14. 1 gr = _____ mg
15. 1 cup = _____ fl oz
16. 1 kg = _____ lb
17. 1 lb = _____ oz
18. 1 T = _____ t
19. 1 pt = _____ fl oz
20. 1 tsp = _____ mL

CRITICAL THINKING APPLICATIONS

A patient suffering from a cold is given a prescription for 2 teaspoons of cough suppressant every 6 h for 10 days. The patient will be using a teaspoon to measure the dose of medication. (LO 5.3)

1. How many teaspoons of cough suppressant should the patient take each day?

2. How many eight fluid ounce bottles of medication will the patient need to complete the order?

3. If the medication is supplied in pint bottles, how many bottles will the patient need during the 10 days?

CASE STUDY

The package insert for a medication states that the patient should be given 5 mL of medication for every 50 kg that she weighs. If the patient weighs 66 lb, how many mL of medication should she be given? (LO 5.3)

Mc Graw Hill Education connect®

Now that you have completed the materials in the chapter text, go to CONNECT and complete any chapter activities you have not yet done.

6 CHAPTER

Converting Units

Knowing is not enough; we must apply.
Willing is not enough; we must do.

GOETHE

LEARNING OUTCOMES

When you have completed Chapter 6, you will be able to:

6.1 Write conversion factors from equivalent measures.

6.2 Convert units.

KEY TERMS

Conversion factor
Dimensional analysis

INTRODUCTION
One of the most crucial skills needed for calculating dosages is the ability to perform conversions. Two methods for performing conversions will be presented in this chapter—the proportion method and dimensional analysis. You will notice that the methods are different only in the initial setup of the problem. While practicing these methods, you should decide which works best for you. In later chapters you will learn how to use these same methods for dosage calculations.

6.1 Writing Conversion Factors from Equivalent Measures

In the "Metric System" and "Other Systems of Measurement" chapters you learned the systems of measurement that are most commonly used in dosage calculations—the metric, apothecary, and household systems.

A **conversion factor** is a fraction or ratio made of two quantities that are equal to each other but expressed in different units. For example, if you wished to convert between days and weeks, you would start by recalling that 1 week is equal to 7 days. You can write four conversion factors from this relationship:

$$\frac{1 \text{ week}}{7 \text{ days}}$$

$$\frac{7 \text{ days}}{1 \text{ week}}$$

1 week : 7 days

7 days : 1 week

The conversion factor you choose depends on two factors—the method that you are using (fractions or ratios) and whether you are converting from days to weeks or from weeks to days. Table 6-1 shows many of the equivalent measures that you will need to use when writing the conversion factors used in dosage calculations.

TABLE 6-1 Equivalent Measures

WEIGHTS	VOLUMES
1 grain = 60 milligrams	1 teaspoon = 5 milliliters
1 grain = 0.06 gram	1 tablespoon = 15 milliliters
1 milligram = 1,000 micrograms	1 ounce = 2 tablespoons
1 gram = 1,000 milligrams	1 ounce = 30 milliliters
1 pound = 454 grams	1 cup = 240 milliliters
1 kilogram = 2.2 pounds	1 pint = 480 milliliters
	1 quart = 960 milliliters
	1 liter = 1,000 milliliters

USING CONVERSION FACTORS

[Fractions

Procedure Checklist 6-1

Writing Conversion Factors as Fractions

1. The two quantities in the conversion factor must be equal to each other. One of the quantities must be expressed in the units you are converting from; the other must have the units you are converting to.

2. Write the conversion factor as a fraction with the quantity containing the units that you are converting *to* in the numerator and the quantity containing the units you are converting *from* in the denominator.

EXAMPLE 1 | Write a conversion factor for converting to ounces from milliliters using proportions and fractions.

1. According to Table 6-1, 1 fluid ounce is equal to 30 milliliters.

   1 fl oz = 30 mL

2. Since you are converting to ounces, the quantity containing ounces (1 oz) will be the numerator of your conversion factor; the quantity containing milliliters (30 mL) will be the denominator.

   $\dfrac{1 \text{ oz}}{30 \text{ mL}}$

EXAMPLE 2 | Write a conversion factor for converting to grams from pounds using proportions and fractions.

1. According to Table 6-1, 1 pound is equal to 454 grams.

   1 lb = 454 g

2. Since you are converting to grams, the quantity containing grams (454 g) will be the numerator of your conversion factor; the quantity containing pounds (1 pound) will be the denominator.

   $\dfrac{454 \text{ g}}{1 \text{ pound}}$

[Ratios

Procedure Checklist 6-2
Writing Conversion Factors as Ratios

1. The two quantities in the conversion factor must be equal to each other. One of the quantities must be expressed in the units you are converting from; the other must have the units you are converting to.

2. Write the conversion factor as a ratio with the quantity containing the units that you are converting to *before* the colon and the quantity containing the units you are converting from *after* the colon.

EXAMPLE 1 | Write a conversion factor for converting to ounces from milliliters using proportions and ratios.

1. According to Table 6-1, 1 ounce is equal to 30 milliliters.

    1 oz = 30 mL

2. Since you are converting to ounces, the quantity containing ounces (1 oz) will go before the colon of the conversion factor; the quantity containing milliliters (30 mL) will go after the colon.

    1 oz : 30 mL

EXAMPLE 2 | Write a conversion factor for converting to grams from pounds using proportions and ratios.

1. According to Table 6-1, 1 pound is equal to 454 grams.

    1 pound = 454 g

2. Since you are converting to grams, the quantity containing grams (454 g) will go before the colon of the conversion factor; the quantity containing pounds (1 pound) will go after the colon.

    454 g : 1 pound

[REVIEW AND PRACTICE

6.1 Writing Conversion Factors from Equivalent Measures

Write conversion factors as fractions and ratios for the following conversions.

1. grains to milligrams

2. pounds to grams

3. milliliters to teaspoons

4. grams to milligrams

5. ounces to tablespoons

6. kilograms to pounds

7. milliliters to liters

8. cups to milliliters

9. milligrams to micrograms

10. tablespoons to milliliters

6.2 Converting Units

ALEKS®

GO TO . . .
Converting Units

If you know a conversion factor, you can set up a proportion and convert from one unit to another using methods you learned in previous chapters. If you are using fractions, you can cross-multiply. If you are using ratios, you can multiply means and extremes.

Another method of converting units is **dimensional analysis**. This method is similar to the proportion method, but starts with the unknown value x standing alone on one side of the equation.

You should try each of these methods and decide which one works best for you. Once you have selected a method, use it when you perform conversions.

LEARNING LINK Recall from the chapter "Relationships of Quantities: Percents, Ratios, and Proportions" you can solve proportions for an unknown value by cross-multiplying or multiplying the means and extremes.

PROPORTION METHOD

Fractions

Procedure Checklist 6-3

Converting by the Proportion Method Using Fractions

1. Write a conversion factor with the units needed in the answer in the numerator and the units you are converting from in the denominator.

2. Write a fraction with the unknown, x, in the numerator and the quantity that you are converting from in the denominator.

3. Set the two fractions up as a proportion.

4. Cancel units.

5. Cross-multiply and solve for the unknown value.

EXAMPLE 1 Convert 2 teaspoons to milliliters.

1. According to Table 6-1, 1 teaspoon is equal to 5 milliliters. Since you are converting to milliliters, milliliters must appear in the numerator of the conversion factor. The conversion factor is $\frac{5 \text{ mL}}{1 \text{ tsp}}$.

2. The other fraction for the proportion has the unknown x for a numerator and 2 teaspoons as the denominator: $\frac{x}{2 \text{ tsp}}$.

(Continued)

3. Setting up the two fractions as a proportion gives you the following equation:

$$\frac{x}{2\text{ tsp}} = \frac{5\text{ mL}}{1\text{ tsp}}$$

4. Cancel units.

$$\frac{x}{2\ \cancel{\text{tsp}}} = \frac{5\text{ mL}}{1\ \cancel{\text{tsp}}}$$

5. Solve for the unknown by cross-multiplying.

$$1 \times x = 5\text{ mL} \times 2$$

$$\frac{1 \times x}{1} = \frac{5\text{ mL} \times 2}{1}$$

$$x = 10\text{ mL}$$

EXAMPLE.2

Convert 75 pounds to kilograms. Round your answer to the nearest tenth.

1. According to Table 6-1, 1 kilogram is equal to 2.2 pounds. Since you are converting to kilograms, kilograms must appear in the numerator of the conversion factor. The conversion factor is $\frac{1\text{ kg}}{2.2\text{ lb}}$.

2. The other fraction for the proportion has the unknown x for a numerator and 75 pounds as the denominator: $\frac{x}{75\text{ lb}}$.

3. Setting up the two fractions as a proportion gives you the following equation:

$$\frac{x}{75\text{ lb}} = \frac{1\text{ kg}}{2.2\text{ lb}}$$

4. Cancel units.

$$\frac{x}{75\ \cancel{\text{lb}}} = \frac{1\text{ kg}}{2.2\ \cancel{\text{lb}}}$$

5. Solve for the unknown by cross-multiplying.

$$2.2 \times x = 1\text{ kg} \times 75$$

$$\frac{2.2 \times x}{2.2} = \frac{1\text{ kg} \times 75}{2.2}$$

$$x = 34.1\text{ kg}$$

PROPORTION METHOD

Ratios

Procedure Checklist 6-4
Converting by the Proportion Method Using Ratios

1. Write a conversion factor with the units needed in the answer before the colon and the units you are converting from after the colon.

2. Write a ratio with the unknown, x, before the colon and the quantity that you are converting from after the colon.

3. Set the two ratios up as a proportion.

4. Cancel units.

5. Multiply the means and extremes and solve for the unknown value.

EXAMPLE 1 **Convert 2 teaspoons to milliliters.**

1. According to Table 6-1, 1 teaspoon is equal to 5 milliliters. Since you are converting to milliliters, milliliters must appear before the colon of the conversion factor. The conversion factor is 5 mL : 1 tsp.

2. The other fraction for the proportion has the unknown x for a numerator and 2 teaspoons as the denominator: x : 2 tsp.

3. Setting up the two ratios as a proportion gives you the following equation:

$$x : 2 \text{ tsp} :: 5 \text{ mL} : 1 \text{ tsp}$$

4. Cancel units.

$$x : 2 \text{ \sout{tsp}} :: 5 \text{ mL} : 1 \text{ \sout{tsp}}$$

5. Solve for the unknown by multiplying the means and extremes.

$$1 \times x = 5 \text{ mL} \times 2$$

$$\frac{1 \times x}{1} = \frac{5 \text{ mL} \times 2}{1}$$

$$x = 10 \text{ mL}$$

EXAMPLE 2 **Convert 75 pounds to kilograms. Round your answer to the nearest tenth.**

1. According to Table 6-1, 1 kilogram is equal to 2.2 pounds. Since you are converting to kilograms, kilograms must appear before the colon of the conversion factor. The conversion factor is 1 kg : 2.2 lb.

2. The other ratio for the proportion has the unknown x before the colon and 75 pounds after the colon: x : 75 lb.

3. Setting up the two ratios as a proportion gives you the following equation:

$$x : 75 \text{ lb} :: 1 \text{ kg} : 2.2 \text{ lb}$$

4. Cancel units.

$$x : 75 \text{ \sout{lb}} :: 1 \text{ kg} : 2.2 \text{ \sout{lb}}$$

5. Solve for the unknown by multiplying the means and extremes.

$$2.2 \times x = 1 \text{ kg} \times 75$$

$$\frac{2.2 \times x}{2.2} = \frac{1 \text{ kg} \times 75}{2.2}$$

$$x = 34.1 \text{ kg}$$

DIMENSIONAL ANALYSIS

Dimensional

Procedure Checklist 6-5
Converting by Dimensional Analysis

1. Write a conversion factor with the units you are converting to in the numerator and the units you are converting from in the denominator.
2. Write an equation with the unknown value x on one side and the quantity being converted multiplied by the conversion factor on the other side.
3. Cancel units.
4. Solve the equation.

EXAMPLE 1   Convert 2 teaspoons to milliliters.

1. According to Table 6-1, 1 teaspoon is equal to 5 milliliters. Since you are converting to milliliters, milliliters must appear in the numerator of the conversion factor. The conversion factor is $\frac{5\,\text{mL}}{1\,\text{tsp}}$.

2. Write an equation with the unknown value x on one side and the quantity being converted multiplied by the conversion factor on the other side.
$$x = 2\ \text{tsp} \times \frac{5\,\text{mL}}{1\,\text{tsp}}$$

3. Cancel units.
$$x = 2\ \cancel{\text{tsp}} \times \frac{5\,\text{mL}}{1\,\cancel{\text{tsp}}}$$

4. Solve the equation.
$$x = 10\ \text{mL}$$

EXAMPLE 2   Convert 75 pounds to kilograms. Round your answer to the nearest tenth.

1. According to Table 6-1, 1 kilogram is equal to 2.2 pounds. Since you are converting to kilograms, kilograms must appear in the numerator of the conversion factor. The conversion factor is $\frac{1\,\text{kg}}{2.2\,\text{lb}}$.

2. Write an equation with the unknown value x on one side and the quantity being converted multiplied by the conversion factor on the other side.
$$x = 75\ \text{lb} \times \frac{1\,\text{kg}}{2.2\,\text{lb}}$$

3. Cancel units.
$$x = 75\ \cancel{\text{lb}} \times \frac{1\,\text{kg}}{2.2\,\cancel{\text{lb}}}$$

4. Solve the equation.
$$x = 34.1\ \text{kg}$$

ERROR ALERT!

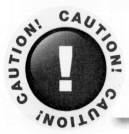

Always Include Units When Using Conversion Factors

It is important to always include units when you use conversion factors. Errors can be made by using the wrong form of the conversion factor. If you include units and follow the rules for canceling them, you will be able to recognize when the wrong form of the conversion factor was used. Never take shortcuts by leaving off units!

6.2 Converting Units

In Exercises 1–11, convert the measures from one unit of measurement to another.

1. 30 mL = _____ tbsp

2. 1.5 tsp = _____ mL

3. 120 mL = _____ tsp

4. 240 mL = _____ L

5. 15 mg = gr _____

6. gr 15 = _____ mg

7. 10 mg = _____ g

8. 2.5 g = gr _____

9. 42 kg = _____ lb

10. 44 lb = _____ kg

11. 6 fl oz = _____ mL

12. During the total course of his treatment, a patient will receive 720 mL of medication. How many pints will he receive?

13. If an order calls for the patient to receive 2 tsp of cough syrup, how many milliliters of syrup should the patient receive?

14. A patient weighs 65 kg. How many pounds does she weigh?

15. A patient weighs 187 lb. How many kilograms does he weigh?

16. A physician orders 2 fluid ounces of liquid medication. How many tablespoons should the patient take?

17. A patient drinks 4 c of liquid during the morning. How many milliliters did the patient drink?

18. An order is for gr iii of medication. How many milligrams should the patient be given?

19. A physician orders that a patient be given 10 mg of medication 3 times per day. How many grains of medication should the patient be given per day?

20. An order calls for 1.5 tbsp of medicated mouthwash. How many milliliters of medicated mouthwash should the patient receive?

Selecting the Correct Conversion Factor

Greg is teaching a patient how much liquid medication to take. The physician has ordered 30 mL of Milk of Magnesia, but the patient will be using teaspoons to measure her medication. Using a conversion chart, Greg confuses 1 tbsp with 1 tsp, and he reads 1 tsp = 15 mL. Using the incorrect information, he calculates the dose as follows:

$$\frac{x}{30 \text{ mL}} = \frac{1 \text{ tsp}}{15 \text{ mL}}$$

$$x \times 15 = 1 \text{ tsp} \times 30$$

$$x = 2 \text{ tsp}$$

Greg tells the patient to take 2 tsp of Milk of Magnesia. This amount is only one-third of the amount that the physician ordered; the patient does not get the relief desired.

 Think! . . . Is It Reasonable? What mistake did Greg make? How could the error have been avoided? What is the correct dose the patient should receive?

LEARNING OUTCOME	KEY POINTS
6.1 Write conversion factors from equivalent measures. Pages 104–107	▶ Conversion factors can be written as either fractions or ratios. • $\frac{1\,\text{tsp}}{5\,\text{mL}}$ and 1 tsp : 5 mL are the same conversion factor written in different ways. ▶ The two quantities in a conversion factor are equal to one another but written with different units. • The quantities in the conversion factors $\frac{1\,\text{tsp}}{5\,\text{mL}}$ and 1 tsp : 5 mL are equal to one another: 1 tsp = 5 mL.
6.2 Convert units. Pages 107–112	▶ Units can be converted using proportions expressed as either ratios or fractions. • When using fractions, you cross-multiply. • When using ratios, you use means and extremes. ▶ When using fractions, the conversion factor should have the unit being converted to in the numerator and the unit being converted from in the denominator. • To use fractions for converting to pounds from kilograms, use the conversion factor $\frac{2.2\,\text{lb}}{1\,\text{kg}}$. ▶ When using ratios, the conversion factor should have the unit being converted to before the colon and the unit being converted from after the colon. • To use ratios for converting to pounds from kilograms, use the conversion factor 2.2 lb : 1 kg. ▶ In order to avoid errors, it is important to always include units when setting up proportions for converting units. • $\frac{1\,\text{g}}{1{,}000}$ mg is a conversion factor. $\frac{1}{1{,}000}$ is a fraction but not a conversion factor. ▶ In dimensional analysis, the measurement to be converted is multiplied by a conversion factor that is expressed as a fraction. ▶ In order to avoid errors, it is important to always include units when setting up multiplication problems for converting units.

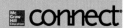
Perform the following conversions using either the proportion method or dimensional analysis. (LO 6.1, 6.2)

1. 3.5 g = _____ mg

2. 30 mg = gr _____

3. 3 tbsp = _____ mL

4. 0.25 mg = _____ mcg

5. 110 lb = _____ kg

6. 3 tsp = _____ mL

7. 180 mL = _____ oz

8. 1.2 mm = _____ cm

9. 5 gr = _____ mg

10. 600 mL = _____ L

CHAPTER 6 REVIEW

CHECK UP

In Exercises 1–8, write conversion factors as both fractions and ratios. (LO 6.1)

1. kilograms to pounds

2. fluid ounces to milliliters

3. micrograms to milligrams

4. grains to milligrams

5. teaspoons to milliliters

6. milliliters to liters

7. tablespoons to fluid ounces

8. tablespoons to milliliters

In Exercises 9–18, perform the conversions. (LO 6.2)

9. 8 g = gr _____

10. gr $2\frac{1}{2}$ = _____ mg

11. 90 mL = _____ tbsp

12. 5 tsp = _____ mL

13. 8 fl oz = _____ mL

14. 1,200 mL = _____ fl oz

15. 540 mg = gr _____

16. gr $\frac{3}{4}$ = _____ mg

17. 178.2 lb = _____ kg

18. 47 kg = _____ lb

19. An order is placed for gr v of medication. If the medication is supplied in milligrams, how many milligrams should be given? (LO 6.1, 6.2)

20. If a patient weighs 44 lb, how many kilograms does she weigh? (LO 6.1, 6.2)

21. A physician orders $\frac{1}{2}$ fl oz of medication for a patient. How many milliliters of medication should the patient be given? (LO 6.1, 6.2)

22. The maximum dose of a medication is 3 tbsp. What is the maximum number of milliliters that the patient should be given? (LO 6.1, 6.2)

23. A physician tells a patient to drink 2,400 mL of fluid per day. How many quarts of liquid should this patient drink? (LO 6.1, 6.2)

24. Several months ago, a patient weighed 95 kg. When he comes in for his next appointment, he tells you he has lost 11 lb. If he is correct, how many kilograms should he weigh? (LO 6.1, 6.2)

CRITICAL THINKING APPLICATIONS

A patient is given a prescription for 7.5 mL of cough suppressant every 4 h for 10 days. The patient will be using a device that is calibrated in teaspoons. (LO 6.1, 6.2)

1. How much medication should the patient take for each dose?

2. If the medication is supplied in 200 mL bottles, how many bottles will the patient need during the 10 days?

CASE STUDY

You are doing an inventory of medications on hand. For one product you have open bottles containing 350 mL, 85 mL, 220 mL, and 175 mL on hand. You also have a full pint bottle of the medication. (LO 6.1, 6.2)

1. How many milliliters total do you have available?

2. You need to order enough of the medication so that you have at least 2 liters on hand. How many pint bottles do you need to order?

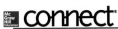

Now that you have completed the materials in the chapter text, go to CONNECT and complete any chapter activities you have not yet done.

Temperature and Time

Learning is not a spectator sport.

ANONYMOUS

LEARNING OUTCOMES

When you have completed Chapter 7, you will be able to:

7.1 Convert temperatures between the Celsius and Fahrenheit systems.

7.2 Convert times between conventional and 24-hour systems.

KEY TERMS

24-hour time

Celsius

Conventional time

Fahrenheit

INTRODUCTION

Temperature and time are both commonly expressed in two different ways. Temperature can be expressed using either the Fahrenheit scale or the Celsius scale. Time is usually given using the conventional system of AM and PM, but in certain settings (such as the military and when charting drug administration) the 24-hour clock is used. As a healthcare professional you must be able to convert accurately between these systems.

7.1 Converting Temperature

Both the **Fahrenheit** (F) and **Celsius** (C) temperature scales are used in healthcare settings. If you examine the two thermometers in Figure 7-1, you will notice that the Fahrenheit scale sets the temperature at which water freezes at 32 degrees, or 32°F. It also measures the temperature at which water boils as 212°F. On the Celsius scale, water freezes at 0°C and boils at 100°C. In Fahrenheit, average body temperature is 98.6°F. In Celsius, average body temperature is 37°C.

As a healthcare worker, you may need to convert between these two temperature scales. The following formula can be used for converting between the two systems:

$$5F - 160 = 9C$$

In this formula, F represents the temperature in degrees Fahrenheit and C represents the temperature in degrees Celsius.

You may also use these formulas to convert between temperature scales.
From Fahrenheit to Celsius use:

$$\frac{°F - 32}{1.8} = °C$$

From Celsius to Fahrenheit use:

$$(1.8 \times °C) + 32 = °F$$

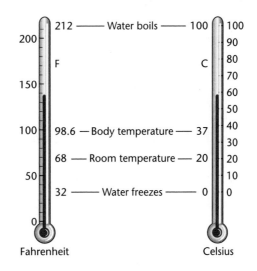

212 —— Water boils —— 100
200
F   C
150
98.6 — Body temperature — 37
68 — Room temperature — 20
50
32 —— Water freezes —— 0
0
Fahrenheit   Celsius

Figure 7-1 Fahrenheit and Celsius scales.

ALEKS

GO TO . . .
Temperature–Converting Between Temperatures in Fahrenheit and Celsius

RULE 7-1	To convert between temperature systems use any of the following formulas to convert a temperature from Fahrenheit to Celsius or Celsius to Fahrenheit.

$$5F - 160 = 9C \text{ (to convert between systems)}$$

$$\frac{°F - 32}{1.8} = °C \text{ (to convert from °F to °C)}$$

$$(1.8 \times °C) + 32 = °F \text{ (to convert from °C to °F)}$$

Example 1

Convert 98.6°F to degrees Celsius.

$$5F - 160 = 9C$$

$$(5 \times 98.6) - 160 = 9C \quad \text{(Multiply before subtracting.)}$$

$$493 - 160 = 9C$$

$$333 = 9C \quad \text{(Since } \tfrac{9}{9} \text{ equals 1, divide both sides by 9 to solve for } C.)$$

$$\frac{333}{9} = \frac{9C}{9}$$

$$37 = C$$

Thus 98.6°F = 37°C; both measures represent normal body temperature.

Example 2

Convert 100°C to degrees Fahrenheit.

$$5F - 160 = 9C$$

$$5F - 160 = 9 \times 100$$

$$5F - 160 = 900 \quad \text{(Add 160 to both sides.)}$$

$$5F = 900 + 160$$

$$\frac{5F}{5} = \frac{1,060}{5} \quad \text{(Since } \tfrac{5}{5} \text{ equals 1, divide both sides by 5 to solve for } F.)$$

$$F = 212$$

So 100°C = 212°F; both measures represent the boiling point of water.

Example 3	Convert 98.6°F to degrees Celsius. $$\frac{°F - 32}{1.8} = °C$$ $$\frac{98.6 - 32}{1.8} = \frac{66.6}{1.8} = 37$$ So 98.6°F = 37°C; both measures represent normal body temperature.
Example 4	Convert 37°C to degrees Fahrenheit. $$(1.8 \times °C) + 32 = °F$$ $$(1.8 \times 37) + 32 = 66.6 + 32 = 98.6$$ Thus 37°C = 98.6°F.

REVIEW AND PRACTICE

7.1 Converting Temperature

In Exercises 1–10, convert the temperatures. Round to the nearest tenth, when necessary.

1. 34°C = _____°F
2. 41°C = _____°F
3. 95°F = _____°C
4. 102°F = _____°C
5. 45.3°F = _____°C
6. 212°F = _____°C
7. 25°C = _____°F
8. 100°C = _____°F
9. 59°F = _____°C
10. 67°C = _____°F

7.2 Converting Time

Many healthcare facilities use the clock with 24 hours (h), known as military, international, or **24-hour time**. **Conventional time** uses a 12-hour clock and is a source of errors in administering medication. On the clock, each time occurs twice a day. For instance, the hour 10:00 is recorded as both 10:00 a.m. and 10:00 p.m. The abbreviation "a.m." means *ante meridian* or before noon; "p.m." means *post meridian* or after noon. If these abbreviations are not clearly marked, the patient could receive medication at the wrong time.

The 24-hour clock (military time) bypasses this opportunity for error. Each time occurs only once per day. In military time, 10:00 a.m. is written as 1000, whereas 10:00 p.m. is written as 2200. (See Figure 7-2.)

When you write the time using a 12-hour clock, you separate the hour from the minutes by a colon. You write a single digit for hours 1 through 9. You then add a.m. or p.m. to indicate before or after noon. When you write the time using a 24-hour clock, you use a four-digit number with no colon. The first two digits represent the hour; the last two digits, the minutes.

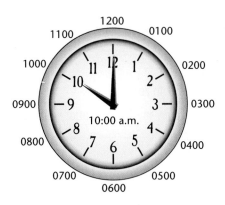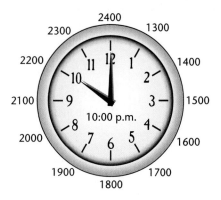

Figure 7-2   Military time is based on a 24-hour clock.

RULE 7-2	When you are using a 24-hour clock for time: **1.** Write 00 as the first two digits to represent the first hour after midnight. **2.** Write 01, 02, 03, . . . , 09 as the first two digits to represent the hours 1:00 a.m. through 9:00 a.m. **3.** Add 12 to the first two digits to represent the hours 1:00 p.m. through 11:00 p.m., so that 13, 14, 15, . . . , 23 represent these hours. **4.** Write midnight as either 2400 or 0000.
Example 1	Convert 9:00 a.m. to 24-hour time. Remove the colon and the abbreviation a.m. Write the hour 9 with two digits, starting with zero. 9:00 a.m. = 0900
Example 2	Convert 12:19 a.m. to 24-hour time. Remove the colon and the abbreviation a.m. Because this time occurs in the first hour after midnight, use 00 for the hour. 12:19 a.m. = 0019
Example 3	Convert 4:28 p.m. to 24-hour time. Remove the colon and the abbreviation p.m. Because this time is after noon, add 12 to the hour. 4:28 p.m. = 1628
Example 4	Convert 1139 to 12-hour (conventional) time. Insert a colon to separate the hour from the minutes. Because this time occurs before noon, add a.m. following the time. 1139 = 11:39 a.m.
Example 5	Convert 1515 to 12-hour (conventional) time. Insert a colon to separate the hour from the minutes. Subtract 12 from the hour, and add the abbreviation p.m. 1515 = 3:15 p.m.

RULE 7-3	To state the time using 24-hour time:
	1. Say *zero* if the first digit is a zero.
	2. Say *zero zero* if the first two digits are both zero.
	3. If the minutes are represented by 00, then say *hundred* after you say the hour.
Example 1	State the time 0900.
	Say *zero nine* for the hours and *hundred* for the minutes. Thus, 0900 is stated as *zero nine hundred*.
Example 2	State the time 1139.
	Say *eleven* for the hours and *thirty-nine* for the minutes. Thus, 1139 is stated as *eleven thirty-nine*.
Example 3	State the time 0023.
	Say *zero zero* for the hours and *twenty-three* for the minutes. Thus, 0023 is stated *zero zero twenty-three*.

REVIEW AND PRACTICE

7.2 Converting Time

In Exercises 1–10, convert the times to 24-hour time.

1. 2:35 a.m.
2. 7:57 a.m.
3. 12:08 a.m.
4. 12:55 a.m.
5. 1:49 p.m.
6. 3:14 p.m.
7. 11:54 p.m.
8. 10:19 p.m.
9. 6:59 p.m.
10. 4:26 a.m.

In Exercises 11–20, convert the times to 12-hour (conventional) time.

11. 0011
12. 0036
13. 0325
14. 0849
15. 1313
16. 1527
17. 2145
18. 2359
19. 2037
20. 1818

LEARNING OUTCOME	KEY POINTS
7.1 Convert temperatures between the Celsius and Fahrenheit systems. Pages 116–118	▶ Storage requirements for medications are usually indicated in Celsius; thermostats are often calibrated in Fahrenheit. It is therefore necessary to be able to convert temperatures accurately. ▶ There are many formulas for converting temperature. Learn the one that works best for you. • $5F - 160 = 9C$ • $\dfrac{(°F - 32)}{1.8} = °C$ • $(1.8 \times °C) + 32 = °F$
7.2 Convert times between conventional and 24-hour systems. Pages 118–120	▶ Conventional time uses a.m. and p.m. to indicate before noon or after noon. • 7:00 a.m. is in the morning, or before noon; 7:00 p.m. is in the evening, or after noon. ▶ When using the 24-hour clock, time is indicated with four digits and without the use of a.m. or p.m. • 7:00 in the morning is written 0700; 7:00 in the evening is 1900. ▶ The first two digits in 24-hour time indicate hours after midnight. The last two digits are for minutes. • 0415 is 4 hours and 15 minutes past midnight.

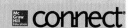
Perform the following conversions. Round to the nearest tenth, when necessary. (LO 7.1)

   1. 41°F = _____ °C

   2. 36°C = _____ °F

   3. 70°F = _____ °C

   4. 10°C = _____ °F

Convert the following times to 24-hour time. (LO 7.2)

   5. 5:30 p.m.

   6. 11:15 a.m.

Convert the following times to conventional time. (LO 7.2)

   7. 0730

   8. 1234

CHAPTER 7 REVIEW

CHECK UP

Convert the following temperatures to Celsius. Round to the nearest tenth, when necessary. (LO 7.1)

1. 97.6°F   **2.** 72°F   **3.** 57.4°F   **4.** 82.8°F

Convert the following temperatures to Fahrenheit. Round to the nearest tenth, when necessary. (LO 7.1)

5. 24°C   **6.** 43.8°C   **7.** 15.6°C   **8.** 8.8°C

Convert the following times to 24-hour time. (LO 7.2)

9. 3:21 a.m.   **10.** 4:42 p.m.   **11.** 10:47 p.m.   **12.** 11:20 a.m.

Convert the following times to conventinal time. (LO 7.2)

13. 0029   **14.** 1417   **15.** 2053   **16.** 0912

CRITICAL THINKING APPLICATIONS

A medication order calls for a drug to be given every 8 hours. The patient takes the first dose at 7:30 a.m. (LO 7.2)

1. At what times will the patient take the next two doses? (Use conventional time)

2. At what times will the patient take the next two doses? (Use 24-hour time)

CASE STUDY

The state health department requires that certain medications be stored between 36°F and 41°F. The refrigerator in the medication room has a Celsius thermometer. What temperature range is appropriate, using the Celsius thermometer? (LO 7.1)

Mc Graw Hill Education connect®

Now that you have completed the materials in the chapter text, go to CONNECT and complete any chapter activities you have not yet done.

1. 150 mcg = _____ mg

2. 44 lb = _____ kg

3. 15° C = _____ °F

4. 4 fl oz = _____ mL

5. $2\frac{1}{2}$ tsp = _____ mL

6. 2,400 mL = _____ L

7. 8 grains = _____ mg

8. 1530 = _____ (in conventional time)

9. 3.4 m = _____ cm

10. 2 oz = _____ tbsp

11. 8 kg = _____ g

12. 0.6 L = _____ oz

13. 55°F = _____ °C

14. 2:15 p.m. = _____ (in military time)

15. 2 cups = _____ mL

16. When Bill had a physical a year ago, he weighed 185 pounds. The clinic now weighs patients in kilograms, and Bill weighs 82.5 kg now. Did his weight change? If yes, how much has he lost or gained in the past year?

17. A patient receives a 4 oz bottle of cough syrup. The instructions are to take $1\frac{1}{2}$ teaspoons four times a day. How many days will the bottle of cough syrup last?

18. The label on a bottle of extra-strength aspirin states that there are 7.5 grains of aspirin in one tablet. Approximately how many milligrams of aspirin will a patient receive if he takes two tablets?

19. The following orders were filled from a 1 pt bottle of medication: 2 fl oz, 45 mL, 3 fl oz, and 180 mL. You receive an order for 4 ounces of the medication. Is there enough remaining in the bottle to fill the order?

20. A coworker shares a recipe with you for making lasagna. The recipe comes from a relative in Italy and says to bake the lasagna at 220°C for 90 minutes.
    a. What temperature (in °F) would you cook the lasagna at?
    b. If you start the lasagna at 5:45 p.m., what time will it be done (in military time)?

UNIT 3

Identifying Information Needed for Dosage Calculations

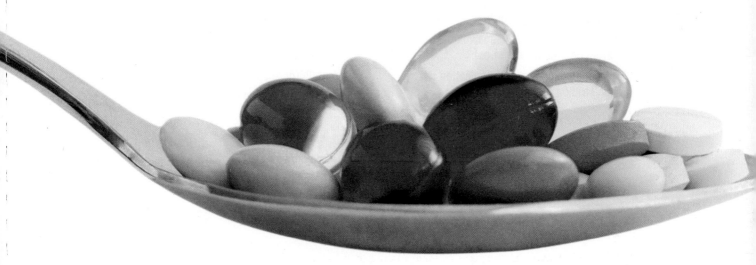

8

CHAPTER

Equipment for Dosage Measurement

Nothing will work unless you do.

MAYA ANGELOU

LEARNING OUTCOMES

When you have completed Chapter 8 you will be able to:

8.1 Recognize medication dosage volumes in different enteral equipment.

8.2 Recognize medication dosage volumes in different parenteral equipment.

8.3 Differentiate among other medication administration forms and equipment.

INTRODUCTION

To prepare the correct dosage of medications, you must know the equipment you will be using. You will be required to accurately select and read this equipment. This chapter will introduce you to common equipment used to prepare dosages and administer medications.

8.1 Enteral Medication Administration Devices

Many medications are available in liquid form and can be administered via the **enteral** route. Enteral medications are absorbed in the gastrointestinal tract. This includes medications that are administered orally or through a tube into the stomach or intestines. Several types of equipment are used to measure and administer enteral liquid medications. These include medicine cups, droppers, calibrated spoons, and oral syringes.

Each measuring device has a series of **calibrations**, or marks numbered at varying intervals. Calibrations enable you to measure the amount of liquid in the device. When you choose a measuring device, compare its calibrations with the desired dose of medication. They may represent different units of measurement. If your equipment does not match the order, then you will have to convert the order to the unit of measurement you will use to administer the medication. For example, a patient is required to take 10 mL of a medication. You have available a container that is marked in teaspoons only. In this case you will have to obtain a different container that is marked in milliliters or convert the amount of medication (10 mL) to teaspoons.

Medicine Cups

Medicine cups are used to measure oral liquid medications and administer them to patients. Cups provide a measured dose that is easy for most patients to swallow. Usually, medicine cups are plastic and measure up to 1 fluid ounce, or its equivalent. To make dose calculation easier, most cups are typically marked with metric, household, and apothecary systems of measurement. Thus, cups include units such as tablespoons (tbsp), teaspoons (tsp), milliliters (mL), drams (dr), and ounces (oz). Although sometimes marked on medication cups, the dram is an outdated unit of measurement and is rarely, if ever, used in medication administration.

Use the two views of a cup shown in Figure 8-1 to compare the different calibrations. In Figure 8-1A, milliliters are displayed in units of 5. Teaspoons and tablespoons are marked in units of 1 or $\frac{1}{2}$. On the other side of the cup in Figure 8-1B, ounces are displayed in units of $\frac{1}{8}$ or $\frac{1}{4}$, and drams are marked in units of 1 or 2. You can see that 5 mL is equivalent to 1 tsp.

The slight curve in the surface of a liquid is the **meniscus**. The quantity of liquid is measured at the bottom of the meniscus, not by the higher levels at the edges. (Refer to Figure 8-2.)

RULE 8-1	Do not use medicine cups for doses less than 5 mL, even if the cup has calibrations smaller than 5 mL. Instead, use a dropper, calibrated spoon, or oral syringe to ensure accuracy.

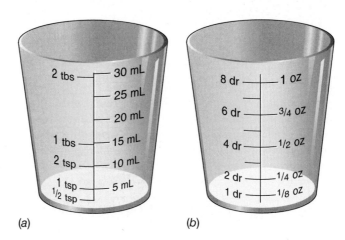

(a)   (b)

Figure 8-1   (a), (b) Two views of a medicine cup.

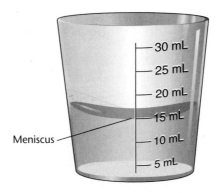

Figure 8-2   Fluid in a medicine cup should be measured at the bottom of the meniscus. This medicine cup contains 15 mL of liquid.

Droppers

Droppers help you measure and administer small amounts of oral liquid medication. You may also use them to deliver certain liquid medications to the eyes, ears, and nose. Droppers are especially helpful with oral pediatric doses. A product that requires a dropper is often packaged with a special dropper calibrated for the specified dose. The indicated units of measurement (calibrations) are usually milliliters (mL), cubic centimeters, drops, or even teaspoons. See Figure 8-3 for various types of droppers.

Although many droppers are standardized to 20 drops per milliliter, droppers frequently have different-size openings. The diameter of the opening affects the size of the individual drops. For example, 3 drops from a dropper with a large opening provides more medication than 3 drops from one with a smaller opening. So do not interchange droppers that are packaged with medications. However, separate calibrated droppers can be reused if properly cleaned between uses.

Calibrated Spoons

In some cases, you can deliver small amounts of medication by using **calibrated spoons** (see Figure 8-4). Spoons are often used with pediatric or elderly patients. They come in many sizes, calibrated to a variety of doses.

You can use the spoons to administer medication directly into the mouth. You can also use them to measure medication into food or a beverage for a child or elderly patient. Children who are used to being fed from a household spoon may accept medication if it comes from a calibrated spoon rather than from a dropper or a medicine cup. You can also use spoons for thick liquids that cannot be easily delivered through the small openings of a dropper.

Oral Syringes

For small quantities of liquid, especially less than 5 mL, oral syringes provide accurate readings. Generic oral syringes are often calibrated for milliliters and teaspoons, with additional

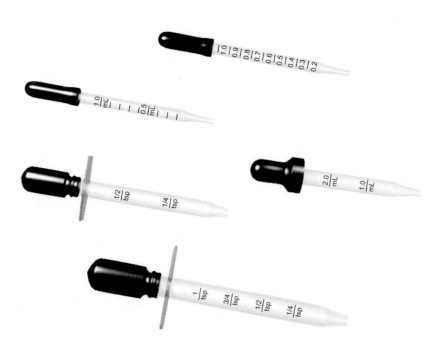

Figure 8-3 Droppers come in various sizes with different calibrations.

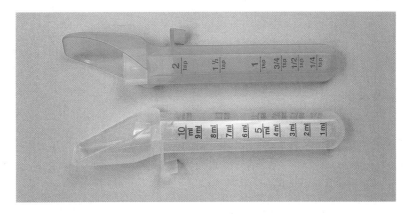

Figure 8-4 Calibrated spoons.

PATIENT EDUCATION

Patients who take oral medications at home need instruction in the proper use of medicine cups, droppers, and calibrated spoons.

1. To measure the correct dose by using a medicine cup, locate the appropriate calibration mark on the cup. While being careful not to tilt the cup, pour the liquid medication. The cup should be on a flat surface, such as a table, while you pour. If the flat surface is not already at eye level, then bend down to check the measurement at eye level for accuracy. The measurement should be read at the lowest level of the meniscus. Also check the expiration date of the medication and the medication itself for changes in clarity, color, or consistency.

2. Measure the proper amount using the marks on the calibrated dropper before delivery. Hold the dropper in a vertical position when delivering liquid. Count slowly, allowing drops to form fully.

3. Use the appropriate marks on calibrated spoons for medications that are measured by teaspoons, tablespoons, or milliliters. Do not measure medication with household spoons used for eating. They vary in size and are not reliable measures. Measuring spoons used for baking are acceptable, but not as accurate as calibrated spoons.

calibrations between these numbers (see Figure 8-5). Oral syringes are designed with safety features to keep them from being confused with hypodermic syringes. Oral syringes often have **eccentric**, or off-center, tips that have a different shape and size than the tips of hypodermic syringes. Oral syringes may be tinted, whereas hypodermic syringes are clear.

Oral syringes are not to be confused with hypodermic syringes. Oral syringes are not sterile. Some oral syringes include a small cap that must be removed before administering medication orally to prevent choking on the cap. To administer sterile medications, you must use a sterile syringe.

RULE 8-2

1. Never attach a needle to an oral syringe.

2. Never inject an oral dose.

3. In emergencies, you may use a hypodermic syringe without a needle to measure and administer liquid oral doses, but never while its needle is attached.

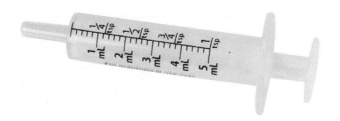

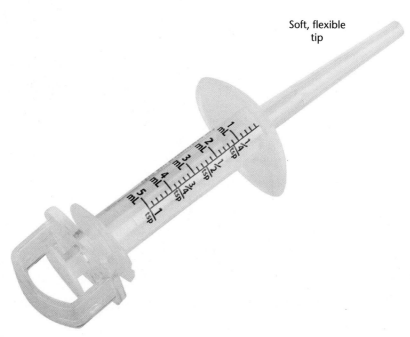

Soft, flexible
tip

Figure 8-5 Oral syringes.

Other Equipment for Enteral Medications

Sometimes oral medications, intended for absorption in the stomach or intestines, cannot be delivered orally. The patient may have difficulty swallowing or some condition or trauma that prevents taking the medication orally.

Liquid medications are preferred for **nasogastric tubes,** which deliver medication into the stomach (see Figure 8-6). Sometimes, you can crush a solid medication, adding water to transport it through the tube. Many solid oral medications, such as gelcaps and extended-release medications, may *not* be crushed. See the chapter "Oral Dosages" for further discussion about these medications.

There are other tubes used to deliver medications directly to the stomach or intestines. A **percutaneous** (through the skin) **endoscopic gastrostomy (PEG) tube** delivers medication and nutrients directly to the stomach. A **jejunostomy tube** delivers medication and nutrients directly to the small intestine.

No matter what equipment is used to administer medication, the medication must be measured accurately using the equipment's calibrations. In addition, enteral tubes can become clogged easily, so check the procedure at your facility before administering any medication.

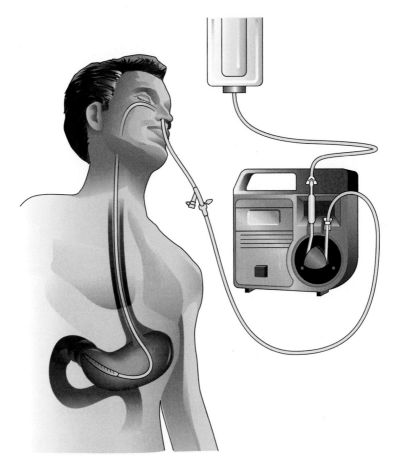

Figure 8-6 A nasogastric tube delivers medication into the stomach.

ERROR ALERT!

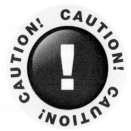

The Utensil You Use Must Provide the Calibration You Need to Accurately Measure the Dose

Suppose the volume of the dose is less than 0.5 mL. The calibrations on the utensil must measure increments of less than 0.5 mL. Otherwise, you cannot accurately measure the medication. Using a utensil that is marked in 1-mL increments and estimating the halfway point is not accurate.

CRITICAL THINKING ON THE JOB

Use the Correct Dropper

A baby with a fever is prescribed acetaminophen for home administration. The healthcare professional tells the baby's father that he will be given a bottle of liquid acetaminophen and a medicine dropper for measuring the prescribed number of drops. The father is told to give the baby 8 drops of medicine at regular intervals.

(Continued)

(Continued)

At home, the father accidentally drops and breaks the dropper. He remembers, though, that he has a dropper from another medication. He uses it instead to measure the acetaminophen. The second dropper is much smaller than the one that came with the acetaminophen. The baby receives a smaller dose than prescribed, even though the father administers the prescribed 8 drops.

Two nights later, the baby's symptoms are not relieved. The father calls the physician, who asks if he has been delivering the number of prescribed drops. The physician prescribes a stronger medication. The baby has suffered needlessly and now is exposed to a stronger medication for no reason.

 Think! . . . Is It Reasonable? How could this error have been avoided?

REVIEW AND PRACTICE

8-1 Enteral Medication Administration Devices

For Exercises 1–14, determine if the statement is true or false. If false, explain why it is incorrect.

1. You may use a syringe with a needle to administer oral medications.

_____

2. You may use a medicine cup to measure liquid doses of less than 1 mL for oral administration.

_____

3. Oral and hypodermic syringes are identical in appearance.

_____

4. When you measure liquid for oral administration, the bottom of the meniscus must be level with the corresponding calibration line on the device.

_____

5. If the dropper supplied by a drug manufacturer for a specific medication is not available, you may substitute a dropper supplied for another medication, as long as the replacement dropper has never been used.

_____

6. If a patient does not have a calibrated spoon, then any household spoon may be substituted.

_____

7. Measuring utensils are often calibrated with more than one system of measurement.

_____

8. A prescribed dose of liquid oral medication cannot be dispensed reliably without calibrated cups, spoons, oral syringes, or droppers.

_____

9. When you calculate volume and dosage, it is helpful to remember that 1 mL is equal to 1.5 cubic centimeters.

_____

10. If a prescribed dose and the calibrated device used for administering that dose use different systems of measurement, then the device cannot be used.

_____

11. Measure the quantity of liquid in a measuring cup by the higher levels at the edge.

_____

12. Droppers may be used to deliver certain liquid medications to the eyes and ears but not the nose.

_____

13. Measuring spoons used for baking are acceptable for measuring liquid medication.

_____

14. Gelcaps and extended-release medications may be delivered through a nasogastric tube as long as they are crushed and flushed with water.

_____

For Exercises 15–20, convert the dosage ordered to the same units as those marked on calibrated utensils. You may wish to refer to the conversion factors in the chapter "Other Systems of Measurement." There may be more than one correct answer for each conversion.

15. The prescribed dose is 2 tbs. Which of the following is *not* equivalent, as marked on the medicine cup?

   a. 30 mL **b.** 1 oz **c.** 6 tsp **d.** 15 mL

16. An oral medication comes in a bottle labeled 10 units per cubic centimeter. The dose to be administered is 50 units. Which of the following is a correct dose?

   a. 50 mL **b.** 500 mL **c.** 5 mL **d.** 0.5 mL

17. Which of the following statements about calibrated droppers is true?

   a. 0.25 mL equals 25 drops. **c.** 1 mL equals 10 drops.

   b. 0.25 mL equals 5 drops. **d.** The number of drops in each milliliter varies per dropper.

18. The dose to be given is 5 mL. The medicine cup is labeled in tablespoons, teaspoons, and ounces. Which of the following is a correct dose?

   a. 1 tsp **b.** $\frac{1}{3}$ tsp **c.** $\frac{1}{3}$ tsp **d.** $\frac{1}{3}$ oz

19. An oral medication comes in a bottle labeled 200 mg per 5 mL. The dose to be administered is 600 mg. Which of the following is a correct dose?

   a. 1 tsp **b.** 2 tsp **c.** 1 tbs **d.** 2 tbs

20. The dose to be given is 15 mL. The dose cup is labeled in tablespoons, teaspoons, and ounces. Which of the following is an incorrect dose?

   a. 3 tsp **b.** 1 tbs **c.** $\frac{1}{2}$ oz **d.** 1 oz

8.2 Parenteral Medication Administration Devices

Many medications must be administered **parenterally**, bypassing the digestive tract. (*Parenterally* means "outside the intestines.") While parenteral dosage forms include other medication forms discussed in the next section, the term most often refers to injections. The most common injection routes are *intravenous* (IV), *intramuscular* (IM), *intradermal* (ID), and *subcutaneous* (subcut). See the chapter "Parenteral Dosages" for more information about these methods of injection. Different **hypodermic syringes** are used to administer injections. These syringes are calibrated with different measurements. The type of syringe you use depends on the type and amount of medication to be administered. Remember 1 milliliter (mL) equals 1 cubic centimeter (cc). Although cc is an "error prone" abbreviation (see the chapter "Safe Medication Administration") you may see the abbreviation cc printed on a syringe.

Standard Syringes

The 3-mL syringe is one of the most common standard syringes used for parenteral administration. Standard syringes have scales calibrated in milliliters. Syringes with smaller capacities may have divisions of tenths, two-tenths, or even hundredths of a milliliter, allowing for measurement of small doses. The 3-mL syringe in Figure 8-7 is calibrated in tenths; it has 10 calibrations for each milliliter. Calibrations for half and whole milliliters are numbered. Standard syringes may also be marked with a minim scale from the apothecary system. However, the metric system is almost always used.

Any healthcare worker who uses a syringe must be familiar with its calibrations so that the correct dose is administered. On all syringes, the zero calibration is the edge of the barrel closest to the needle. The barrel is filled with liquid up to the point of the wide ring, known as the **leading ring**, on the tip of the plunger closest to the needle. Liquid in the barrel does not go past this ring. While the leading ring might have a raised middle, measure from the ring itself. Do *not* measure from the **trailing ring**, which is the ring farther from the needle.

Safety syringes have needles that are protected by plastic shields. These shields help prevent needlestick injury. Although safety syringes do not guarantee that healthcare workers will not receive accidental needlesticks, the syringes reduce the chances of such accidents. Some safety syringes have needles that retract into the syringe at the end of the injection. See Figures 8-8 and 8-9. Safety syringes come in all sizes with various calibrations. They are calibrated in milliliters or units. Smaller-capacity safety syringes are divided into tenths, two-tenths, and hundredths of a milliliter.

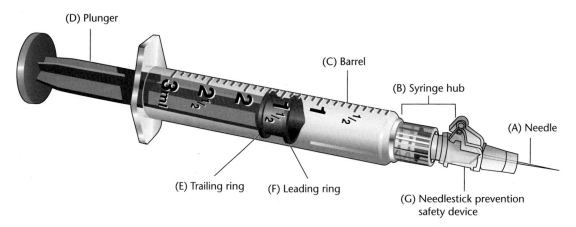

Figure 8-7 The parts of a standard syringe include (A) the needle, (B) the syringe hub, (C) the barrel that contains the liquid, (D) the plunger, (E) the trailing ring, (F) the plunger tip, also called the leading ring, and (G) the needlestick prevention safety device.

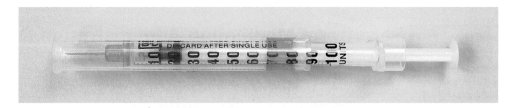

Figure 8-8 This 100-unit insulin safety syringe has a shield that covers the needle during transport and after the injection, minimizing needlestick injuries.

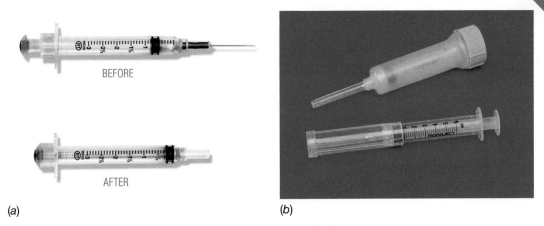

BEFORE

AFTER

(a)

(b)

Figure 8-9 All syringes should have a safe-needle device. Shown here are insulin syringes before activation. (*a*) VanishPoint® safety needles retract when the plunger is fully depressed. (*b*) The Monoject can be activated by the thumb, finger, or any flat surface.

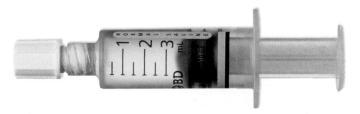

Figure 8-10 Prefilled syringe. Notice that the calibration marks indicate milliliters and the syringe is filled beyond the 3-mL mark.

Prefilled Syringes

Prefilled syringes are shipped from the manufacturer filled with a single dose of medication. If the patient is given only a portion of the dose, the remainder must be discarded before the medication is administered. Prefilled syringes have the same parts as a standard syringe: a needle, a syringe hub, a barrel, and a plunger (see Figure 8-8). Shown in Figure 8-10 is a syringe prefilled with normal saline. This syringe would most likely be used to flush an IV. Always check any prefilled syringe you use carefully. They may be marked in units other than milliliters (mL) and they may contain more medication than the markings indicate. You may need to perform a calculation and discard any excess before administration.

RULE 8-3

When you are using a prefilled syringe, always examine the markings to determine whether the syringe is calibrated in milliliters or milligrams and calculate the dose accordingly.

Insulin Syringes

Insulin syringes are used only to measure and administer insulin. Insulin is measured in units. Insulin syringes are unique. They are calibrated in the amount of medication in units rather than by volume (milliliters). Whether for adults or children, insulin doses are smaller than many other doses. In turn, insulin syringes are calibrated in smaller increments. The most common strength of insulin is U-100; it contains 100 units of insulin per 1 mL. Insulin syringes are marked with "U-100", indicating that they are calibrated for use with U-100 insulin only.

Figure 8-11 shows a standard U-100 insulin syringe. It can contain up to 100 units (1 mL) of U-100 insulin. The larger numbers mark increments of 10 units. The smaller calibrations indicate every 2 units. Many 100-unit syringes have two scales—one on the right showing the even number unit lines and one on the left showing the odd number unit lines. Not all insulin syringes are marked with these increments. Figure 8-12 shows a syringe that holds up to 50 units of U-100 insulin. The larger numbers show increments of 5 units, and the smaller calibrations show increments of 1 unit. This syringe is often used to measure and administer pediatric or adult doses of insulin that are less than 50 units. (See Figure 8-13 for a comparison.)

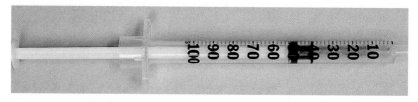

Figure 8-11 A standard insulin syringe can hold up to 100 units of insulin.

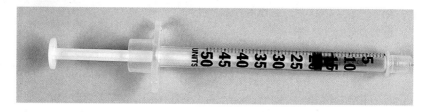

Figure 8-12 This insulin syringe can hold up to 50 units of insulin.

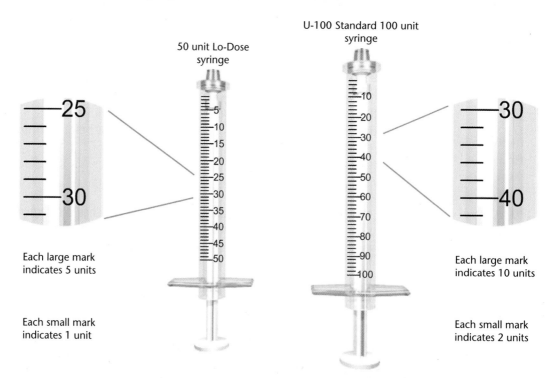

Figure 8-13 When comparing a 50-unit (0.5 mL) versus standard 100-unit (1 mL) insulin syringe, always check the calibrations carefully.

Tuberculin Syringes

Tuberculin syringes are used to administer subcutaneous injections as well as the intradermal purified protein derivative (PPD) skin test that determines if a person has been exposed to tuberculosis. More than that, they are simply small syringes used when small doses of medication—less than 1 mL—are administered. Vaccines, heparin, pediatric medicines, and allergen extracts are typically administered with a tuberculin syringe.

Tuberculin syringes usually hold a total volume of 1 mL and are calibrated in hundredths of a milliliter. The numbering is slightly different from that of the other syringes. In Figure 8-14, the marked numbers represent tenths of a milliliter. The first number, located on the tenth calibration, is 0.1 mL. Each smaller calibration represents one-hundredth (0.01) of a milliliter. Some syringes are even smaller. The tuberculin syringe in Figure 8-15 holds a total volume of 0.5 mL.

Measuring the correct dose with a tuberculin syringe requires extreme care. The calibrations are close together and marked with a number only at every one-tenth or two-tenths calibration. Be sure the leading ring is aligned with the proper calibration. See Figure 8-16 to become familiar with these calibrations. Sometimes tuberculin syringes are also calibrated with the apothecary scale in minims, although these calibrations are not used very often. You must always take great care when reading any syringe to ensure you are reading the correct scale.

Syringes for Established Intravenous Lines

Some syringes are used to administer medication through already established intravenous lines that deliver medication and fluids directly into a patient's veins. Figure 8-17 shows an example of such a syringe.

Adding medication through existing lines has several advantages. Using the injection ports, IV medications can be administered quickly without the patient being punctured repeatedly. Because the syringes do not have needles, accidental needlesticks to patients and healthcare workers are avoided. An intravenous system with needleless syringes allows more than one drug to be administered at a time, provided that the drugs are compatible. Needleless syringes also enable you to deliver drugs on a periodic basis and to dilute the medication. As with other syringes, reading the calibrations correctly when administering medication is essential.

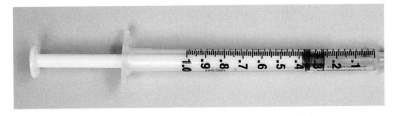

Figure 8-14   A 1-mL tuberculin syringe.

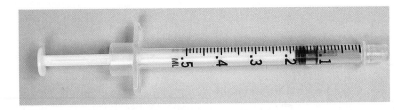

Figure 8-15   A 0.5-mL tuberculin syringe.

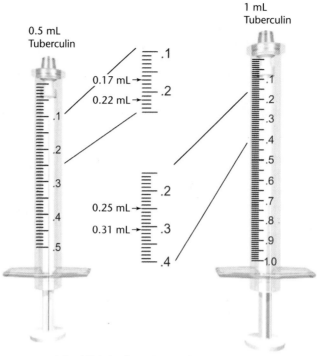

0.5 mL
Tuberculin

1 mL
Tuberculin

0.17 mL →
0.22 mL →

0.25 mL →
0.31 mL →

0.5 mL Tuberculin vs 1 mL Tuberculin syringe

Figure 8-16 Both syringes are calibrated to 0.01 mL. Each number indicates 0.1 mL.

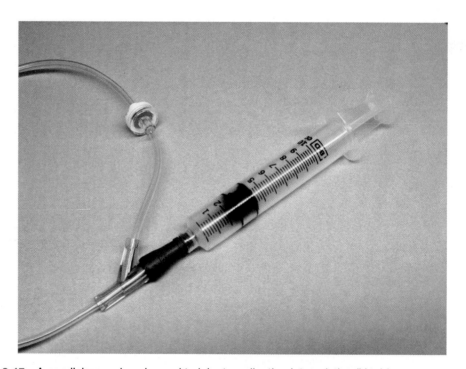

Figure 8-17 A needleless syringe is used to inject medication into existing IV tubing.

Large-Capacity Syringes

Although the maximal volume of an IM injection is 3 mL in any one site, not all medications can be delivered in doses of 3 mL or less. Larger volumes of medications may be added to IV infusions or administered IV push. Therefore, syringes with 5, 6, 10, and 12 mL or even more

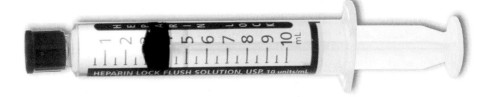

Figure 8-18   A large-capacity syringe.

are available (see Figure 8-18). As with other syringes, volume is measured in milliliters, and the number of calibrations between numbered milliliters varies. Because of this you must look carefully at the marks to measure an accurate amount of medication.

ERROR ALERT!

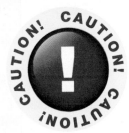

Pay Close Attention to the Calibration of Any Syringe You Use

Perhaps the most important aspect of a syringe is its calibration. If medication is not accurately measured, serious problems can result for the patient. Do not assume the calibration of any syringe you use. Check the marks carefully. After you determine the value of each calibration mark, align the plunger at the appropriate level. **Remember:** No matter what type of syringe you use, *the leading ring, closest to the needle, is the part that must be aligned with the calibration.*

Ampules, Vials, and Cartridges

Parenteral medications may be packaged in ampules, vials, or cartridges (see Figure 8-19). **Cartridges** are prefilled containers shaped like syringe barrels. They generally hold one dose of medication and fit a reusable syringe. Tubex® and Carpuject are examples of cartridges.

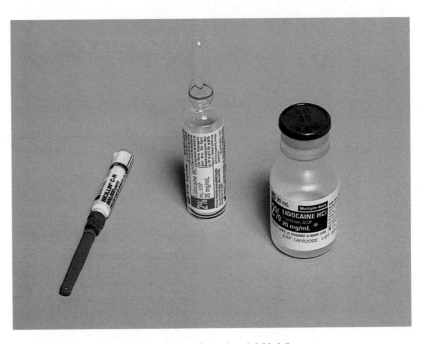

Figure 8-19   A cartridge (left), an ampule (center), and a vial (right).

Ampules are glass containers and usually hold one dose of liquid medication. You snap them open using care not to cut your fingers on the sharp edges. Sometimes a plastic protective sleeve is used when snapping the ampule, or an alcohol wipe package or 2 × 2 gauze is wrapped around the neck of the vial to avoid injury from the edge of the ampule. A filter needle (needle with a filter inside) should always be attached to the syringe to withdraw the medication from the ampule, and then the filter needle should be discarded and replaced by an appropriate needle for administration. By doing this, any glass fragments that may have been aspirated will be removed before patient use. **Vials** are containers covered with a rubber stopper, or diaphragm. They may hold more than a single dose of medication, in either liquid or powder form. If powder, then diluent is injected in the vial to reconstitute the medication. Vials are safer than ampules and are more commonly used.

Preparing the Syringe

If you fill a syringe, you must label it with the contents, including the strength of the contents. See Figure 8-20.

RULE 8-5	In most circumstances, the person who prepares a syringe for injection should deliver the injection. Exceptions include: • Pharmacy technicians who prefill syringes for nurses, medical assistants, or patients. • Nurses or medical assistants preparing a syringe for a physician. • Healthcare workers teaching a patient to administer his or her own medication. This last exception occurs, for instance, when you teach a patient with diabetes how to administer insulin.

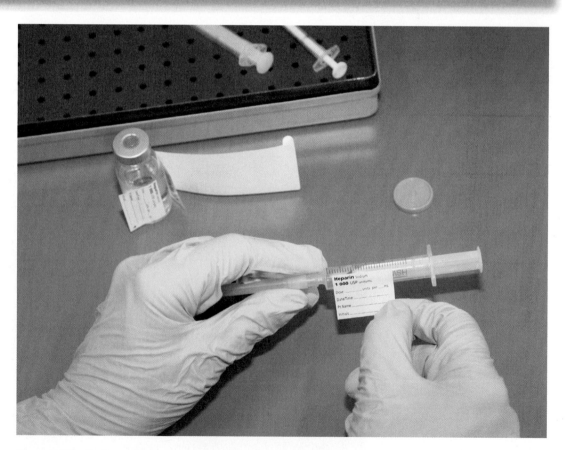

Figure 8-20 Syringes that are prepared before administration must be labeled with the medication and its dosage strength.

Needle Gauge and Length

When you administer an injection, you must choose a needle with an appropriate gauge. A needle's *gauge* is its interior diameter. Lower numbered gauges correspond to larger diameters; an 18-gauge needle is wider than a 22-gauge needle (see Figure 8-21). The gauge you use depends on the viscosity (thickness) of the medication as well as the injection site. More viscous drugs and deeper injections require larger needles (those with a lower gauge number), as seen in Table 8-1.

The injection site also determines the length of the needle. You should select a needle that is long enough to reach the area of tissue specified. However, the needle should not be so long that it penetrates beyond that area.

CRITICAL THINKING ON THE JOB

Finishing What You Start

A healthcare professional prepares to deliver a single dose of Valium® by injection. He has a prefilled syringe containing 2.5 mL, but the prescribed dose is 1.5 mL. Before he can administer the injection, his pager goes off and he rushes to another patient's room. As he does, he asks another healthcare professional to administer the Valium.

She administers the Valium®, assuming that the prefilled syringe contains the appropriate dose. As a result of receiving more Valium® than was prescribed, the patient's blood pressure drops. The first healthcare professional does not ask if the correct dose has been administered, and the patient undergoes tests to find the cause of the drop in blood pressure.

 Think! . . . Is It Reasonable? How could this error have been avoided?

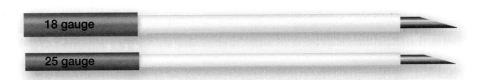

Figure 8-21 The gauge of the needle refers to the diameter. The larger the number, the narrower the needle diameter.

TABLE 8-1 Suggested Needle Gauge, Length, Injection Amount, and Location

AGE	NEEDLE SIZE	NEEDLE LENGTH	MAXIMUM INJECTION AMOUNT	LOCATION
		Intradermal (ID)		
All ages	25 to 26 gauge	$\frac{1}{4}$ to $\frac{5}{8}$ inch	0.1 mL	Interior aspect of forearm (most common)
				(Continued)

TABLE 8-1 Continued

AGE	NEEDLE SIZE	NEEDLE LENGTH	MAXIMUM INJECTION AMOUNT	LOCATION
		Subcutaneous (Subcut)		
1 to 12 months	23 to 27 gauge	$\frac{5}{8}$ inch	0.5 mL	Fatty tissue over anterior lateral thigh muscle
> 12 months to adults	23 to 27 gauge	$\frac{1}{2}$ to $\frac{3}{4}$, $\frac{5}{8}$ most common	0.5 to 1 mL	Fatty tissue over anterior lateral thigh muscle, triceps, or abdomen
		Intramuscular (IM)		
Infant to child	22 to 25 gauge	$\frac{5}{8}$ to 1 inch	0.5 to 1 mL	Vastus lateralis (anterior lateral thigh)
Adult	21 to 25 (very viscous medication may require 20 gauge)	1 to $1\frac{1}{2}$ inches	2 to 3 mL	Ventrogluteal (lateral hip)
	23 to 25 gauge		0.5 to 1 mL	Deltoid

REVIEW AND PRACTICE

8-2 Parenteral Medication Administration Devices

For Exercises 1–4, provide a brief answer.

1. What is the standard calibration of a 3-mL syringe?

2. What is the standard calibration of a 50-unit insulin syringe?

3. What is the standard calibration of a tuberculin syringe?

4. What is the standard calibration of a 100-unit syringe?

For Exercises 5–13, determine if the statement is true or false. If false, explain why it is incorrect.

5. Any extra medication in a syringe should be discarded before the injection is given.

6. The first calibration on any syringe is always zero (0).

7. When you are measuring a dose in a syringe, read the calibration that aligns with the trailing ring on the plunger.

8. Some prefilled syringes are overfilled with 0.1 to 0.2 mL of medication to allow for air expulsion from the needle.

9. Prefilled syringes may be calibrated in mg or mL.

10. You can use an insulin syringe to measure 6 mL of medication.

11. A patient is punctured each time a syringe is used with an established intravenous line.

12. Safety syringes are a guaranteed way to avoid accidental needlestick injuries.

13. Tuberculin syringes are used to administer the subcutaneous PPD skin test.

For Exercises 14–25, identify the type of syringe and the volume of the dosage it contains. Identify the correct units of measurement.

Example: Refer to the sample syringe below:

Type: <u>tuberculin</u> Volume: <u>0.3 mL</u>

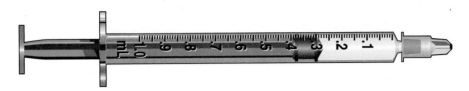

Sample

14. Refer to syringe A:

Type: _____ Volume: _____

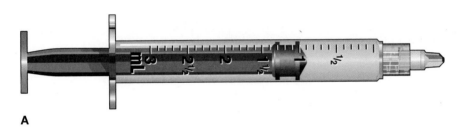

A

15. Refer to syringe B:

Type: _____ Volume: _____

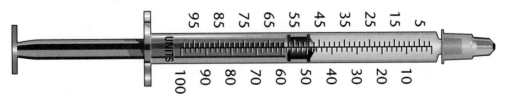

B

16. Refer to syringe C:

Type: _____ Volume: _____

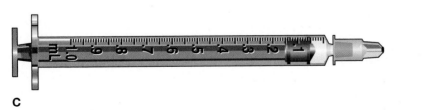

C

17. Refer to syringe D:

Type: _____ Volume: _____

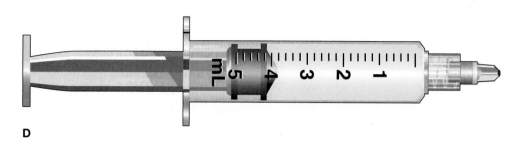

D

18. Refer to syringe E:

Type: _____ Volume: _____

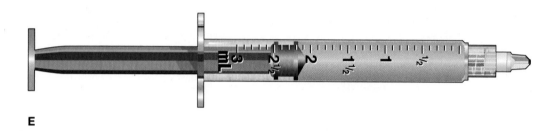

E

19. Refer to syringe F:

Type: _____ Volume: _____

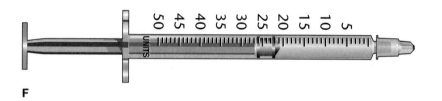

F

20. Refer to syringe G:

Type: _____ Volume: _____

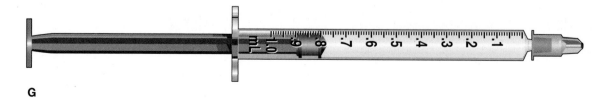

G

21. Refer to syringe H:

Type: _____ Volume: _____

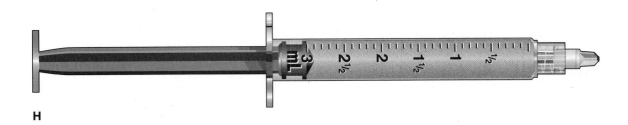

H

22. Refer to syringe I:

Type: _____ Volume: _____

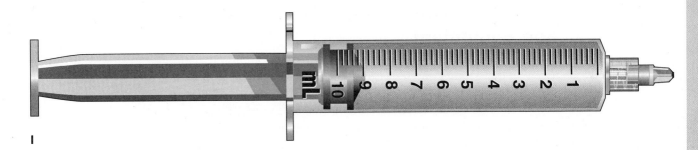

I

23. Refer to syringe J:

Type: _____ Volume: _____

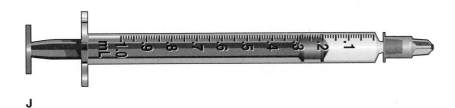

J

24. Refer to syringe K:

Type: _____ Volume: _____

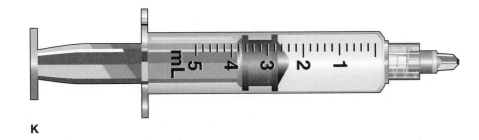

K

25. Refer to syringe L:

Type: _____ Volume: _____

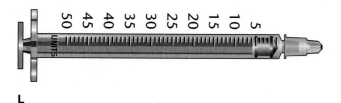

L

Other Medication Administration Forms and Equipment

Medication is given by routes other than oral and common parenteral routes. You should be aware of these routes and the equipment used for administration.

Drops, Sprays, and Mists

Different types of equipment are used to deliver medication to the nose, ears, eyes, and throat in the form of drops, sprays, and mists. Drops, also called **instillations**, deliver medication to the nose, eyes, and ears. Sprays deliver medication to the nose and throat. Drops and sprays are measured according to the dose prescribed and the manufacturer's instructions. Therefore, be sure to use the equipment that accompanies the drug when you administer these medications.

Droppers, similar to those for oral medications, are used to administer drops. Plastic squeeze bottles are used for drops and sprays. Atomizers deliver sprays by using a rubber bulb to propel the spray from a medicine container into the nose.

Another way to administer medication is to use a mist that the patient inhales. Vaporizers, or steam inhalers, use boiling water to create a mist from liquid medication. Nebulizers, often used by patients with asthma, and **metered-dose inhalers (MDIs)** also help deliver medication to the patient.

Inhalants

Inhaled medications, or **inhalants**, are administered either by metered-dose inhaler (MDI), or by nebulizer. Metered-dose inhalers provide a measured dose of medication in each puff. The physician orders the number of puffs to be given. No calculation is necessary. MDI must be primed before initial use, or if the MDI has not been used for two weeks. The plastic actuator should be cleaned weekly; the metal canister is not cleaned. See the manufacturer's instructions for priming and cleaning methods. There are three common methods for using an MDI inhaler: the closed mouth (Figure 8-22), the open mouth (Figure 8-23), and the closed mouth with a spacer (Figure 8-24). With all methods, shake the MDI, exhale fully, inhale slowly while depressing the canister, then hold the inhalation as long as possible, up to 10 seconds. If multiple doses are ordered wait 1 minute between doses, or as the manufacturer directs.

Medications given by nebulizer are supplied as liquids mixed with sterile saline solution. Single doses premixed with saline are available for most medications. A few are measured in the receptacle of the nebulizer, after which the correct amount of saline is added. Sterile saline is usually provided in 3-mL or 5-mL single-dose ampules.

Inhalant medications in multiple-dose containers are usually packaged with special droppers calibrated for the standard doses. If the dropper is not available or becomes contaminated, a sterile syringe may be used.

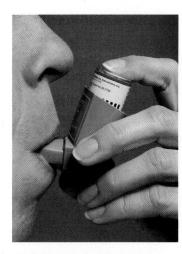

Figure 8-22 An MDI is used to deliver inhalant medications (Closed Mouth Method).

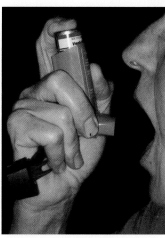

Figure 8-23 MDI Open Mouth Method.

Inhaler

Inhaler adaptor

Flow signal whistle (on some models)

Valve

Mouthpiece

Cap

Body

Figure 8-24 Spacer used for MDI.

Vaginal and Rectal Medications

Medications can be administered by the vaginal (pv) or rectal (pr) routes. Liquid vaginal medication is in the form of a douche, and solid vaginal medication is in tablet or suppository form. Liquid rectal medication is in the form of an enema, and solid rectal medication is in suppository form. Generally, suppositories cannot be accurately divided. Therefore, in most cases, only doses that are multiples of the available suppository strength may be administered.

Topical Medications

Topical medications, such as gels, creams, ointments, and pastes, are applied directly to the skin. You administer the drug with a glove, tongue blade, or cotton-tipped applicator. Topical medications are usually given for their therapeutic effect in or on the skin. Follow the instructions that accompany the product to determine how to remove the medication from its container and administer it. Avoid letting any of the medication contact your own skin.

Transdermal Systems

Transdermal medication is a form of topical medication absorbed through the skin into the bloodstream. Transdermal medications include patches, ointments, and creams. Patches usually consist of a special membrane that releases liquid medication at a constant rate. The patch has adhesive edges to hold it in place so that the membrane rests against the skin (see Figure 8-25). Before you administer a patch, be certain to remove any patches that are already in place, wipe off any residual medication, and rotate the site with each application. Patches should be applied to a reasonably hair-free site such as abdomen, shoulder, back, or hip. Be careful to avoid placing the patch on skin that is irritated or rubbed, such as under a waistband or bra strap; also avoid skin that is scarred, inflamed, or broken. Write the date, the time, and your signature on the patch when administering. Observe the patient, if he or she has a fever, since the rate of absorption may increase.

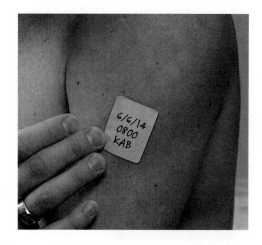

Figure 8-25 Application of a transdermal patch; date, time, and signature is written on to the patch before application.

REVIEW AND PRACTICE

8-3 Other Medication Administration Forms and Equipment

Match the medication administration forms with their descriptions. They may be used more than once.

   a. Topical

   b. Transdermal

   c. Drops

   d. Sprays

   e. Mists

   f. Vaginal

   g. Rectal

_____ **1.** Can be delivered in the form of a tablet, suppository, or douche.

_____ **2.** Applied directly to the skin.

_____ **3.** Delivered by a nebulizer, vaporizer, or metered-dose inhaler.

_____ **4.** Medication from a patch is absorbed through the skin.

_____ **5.** Can be delivered in the form of a suppository or an enema.

_____ **6.** Must be marked with your initials, date, and time of administration.

_____ **7.** Also known as instillations.

_____ **8.** An atomizer is used to deliver this medication form.

_____ **9.** Are useful when a patient has difficulty or trouble swallowing oral drugs.

_____ **10.** Are usually delivered to the nose, eyes, and ears.

LEARNING OUTCOME	KEY POINTS
8.1 Recognize medication dosage volumes in different enteral equipment. Pages 126–133	Enteral devices are for medications absorbed through the GI tract: *Medicine cup:* for liquids, measured at the bottom of the meniscus, easy administration; calibrations include mL (5 mL increments), tsp, tbs, oz ($\frac{1}{8}, \frac{1}{4}, \frac{1}{2}, \frac{3}{4}$) *Dropper:* for administering small amounts of liquids; calibrations vary; droppers may have different size openings—do not interchange droppers *Calibrated spoons:* used for small amounts of oral medication for pediatric and geriatric patients; calibrations include mL (1 mL increments) and tsp ($\frac{1}{4}$ tsp increments) *Oral syringes:* for administering small amounts of *oral* medications; calibrations include mL (in 0.1 mL increments) and tsp (in $\frac{1}{4}$ tsp increments); clean, not sterile—DO NOT USE for *parenteral* medication administration *Enteral tubes (NGT, GT, PEG, JT)* can become clogged by medications. Liquid medication is preferable; some solid medications can be crushed/opened and mixed with water. Some medications such as gel caps, enteric coated, and some capsules *should not be crushed.*
8.2 Recognize medication dosage volumes in different parenteral equipment. Pages 133–146	Parenteral devices are for medications given via the injection route: *3-mL syringe:* most commonly used for injections; calibrated to the tenths *1-mL/tuberculin syringe:* used to administer small doses; calibrated to the hundredths *Large-capacity syringes:* deliver 5, 6, 10, 12 or more mL; calibration varies *Insulin syringes:* used to administer insulin only; 1-mL standard insulin syringe is calibrated by 1 or 2 unit markings, delivers up to 100 units; 0.5-mL/low-dose syringe is calibrated by 1 unit markings, delivers up to 50 units *Prefilled syringe:* filled with single dose of medication *Syringe parts:* needle, hub, barrel, plunger, trailing ring (ring farthest from needle), leading ring (tip of plunger closest to needle), needlestick prevention safety device Safety syringes and needles include shields that cover the needles, needles that retract or have a device that cap the needle keeping the hands away from the tip to prevent needlestick injury.

LEARNING OUTCOME	KEY POINTS
	Zero calibration: edge of the barrel closest to needle *Cartridge:* prefilled container shaped like syringe barrel *Ampule:* glass, single-dose container that requires use of filtered needle to withdraw medication *Vial:* single- or multiple-dose container with rubber stopper or diaphragm through which medication is withdrawn *Needle gauge:* interior diameter of a needle; 21–25 gauge for IM injections; 23–27 gauge for subcut injections; 25–26 gauge for intradermal injections *Needle length:* 1–2 inches for IM injections; $\frac{1}{2} - \frac{5}{8}$ inches for subcut injections; $\frac{3}{8} - \frac{5}{8}$ inches for intradermal injections
8.3 Differentiate among other medication administration forms and equipment. Pages 146–148	Medications may be administered by other routes and require different equipment to administer. Topical medications, creams, gels, ointments, pastes, patches are administered on top of the skin with glove or applicator (do not let drug get on your skin). Patches usually consist of a special membrane that releases liquid medication at a constant rate. Inhalants are administered by metered-dose inhaler (MDI), which has a premeasured dose per puff, or by a nebulizer. Nebulizer medications can be premixed, or the medication may be added to sterile saline in the nebulizer. Medications in multiple-dose containers usually have a calibrated dropper to measure the dose. Vaginal/rectal medications are usually suppositories. Although never scored, some suppositories may be divided per manufacturer's direction.

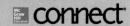

Determine if the statement is true or false. If false, explain what is incorrect about the statement.

1. Oral dosage forms are also called parenteral. (LO 8.1)

_____

2. The leading ring is closer to the needle than the trailing ring. (LO 8.2)

_____

3. Prefilled syringes can be used to give multiple injections as long as they are given to the same patient. (LO 8.2)

_____

4. Tuberculin syringes have a capacity of 3 mL. (LO 8.2)

_____

5. A vial can be used to give injections to multiple patients. (LO 8.2)

_____

6. Syringes are always calibrated in milliliters. (LO 8.2)

_____

7. Rectal medications are commonly delivered as suppositories and capsules. (LO 8.3)

_____

8. MDIs are used to administer inhalant medications. (LO 8.3)

_____

Using the accompanying illustrations of equipment for the remaining questions, mark with a line or shading where you would measure the required dose. (LO 8.1, 8.2)

9. 30 mL

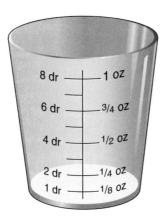

10. 0.7 mL

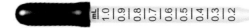

11. 2.4 mL

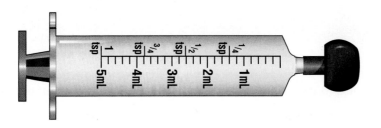

12. 2.4 mL

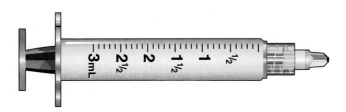

13. 18 units

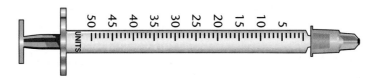

14. 0.38 mL

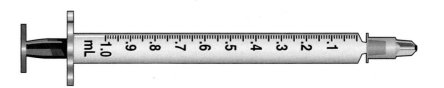

CHECK UP

For Exercises 1–10, answer the multiple-choice questions. More than one answer may be correct.

1. Which of the following equals 1 oz? (LO 8.1)

   a. 2 tbs　　　　　**b.** 20 mL　　　　　**c.** 30 mL　　　　　**d.** 22.5 mL as measured in an oral syringe

2. A patient is supposed to receive 15 mL of Mylanta. A measuring cup cannot be found. What is an equivalent dose? (LO 8.1)

   a. 1 tsp　　　　　**b.** 2 tsp　　　　　**c.** 3 tsp　　　　　**d.** 5 tsp

3. The dose of a liquid medication for oral administration is $\frac{3}{4}$ oz. Which is the correct equivalent dose? (LO 8.1)

   a. 20 mL　　　　　**b.** 25 mL　　　　　**c.** 4.5 tsp　　　　　**d.** 1.5 tbs

4. The ordered dosage of a liquid medication for oral administration is 2.5 mL. What is the appropriate method of oral administration? (LO 8.1)

   a. $\frac{1}{8}$ oz as measured in a medicine cup　　　　**b.** 1 oz as measured in a medicine cup

   c. $\frac{1}{2}$ tsp as measured in a calibrated spoon　　　**d.** 2.5 mL as measured in a calibrated dropper

5. The prescribed dosage of a medication is 5 drops. Which of the following is an appropriate method of administering the dose? (LO 8.1)

   a. 0.5 mL using only the calibrated dropper that accompanies the medicine bottle

   b. 5.0 mL using the calibrated dropper that accompanies the medicine bottle

   c. 5 drops using any calibrated dropper

   d. 5 drops using only the calibrated dropper that accompanies the medicine bottle

6. The ordered oral dosage of a medication is 5 mL. Which of the following is an appropriate method of administering the dose? (LO 8.1)

   a. 1 tsp using a calibrated spoon

   b. 5 mL using a syringe for parenteral administration with the needle removed

   c. 25 drops using a calibrated dropper

   d. 5 tsp using a calibrated spoon

7. The ordered dosage of a medication is 10 mg. The medication is mixed at a strength of 5 mg per milliliter. Using a 2.5-mL prefilled syringe, you should discard how much medication before administration? (LO 8.2)

   a. 0.2 mL　　　　　**b.** 1 mL　　　　　**c.** 0.5 mL　　　　　**d.** 2 mL

8. A tuberculin syringe is being used to administer 0.25 mL of a given medication. Which of the following is the equivalent dose? (LO 8.2)

   a. 2.5 hundredths of a milliliter　　　　**b.** 25 hundredths of a milliliter

   c. 250 hundredths of a milliliter　　　　**d.** 2.5 drops using a calibrated dropper

9. Which of the following can be used to administer a 7-mL dose via the parenteral route? (LO 8.2)

   a. A large-capacity syringe　　　　**b.** A standard syringe

   c. A tuberculin syringe　　　　　　**d.** An insulin syringe

10. Which of the following has the most precise and accurate calibrations? (LO 8.2)

    a. A 5-mL syringe attached to an established intravenous line

    b. A 3-mL syringe attached to an established intravenous line

    c. A 3-mL syringe

    d. A 1-mL tuberculin syringe

For Exercises 11–20, determine if the statement is true or false. If false, explain why it is incorrect. (LO 8.1, 8.2)

11. Based upon the calibration marks, medicine cups appear to indicate that 30 mL is equivalent to 1 oz. (LO 8.1)

_____

12. If an ordered dose calls for 3 mL, a medicine cup may be used to measure it. (LO 8.1)

_____

13. A calibrated dropper dispenses a standard drop of 3 mL. (LO 8.1)

_____

14. The standard syringe can hold more than 1 mL. (LO 8.2)

_____

15. The standard syringe is calibrated in tenths of a milliliter. (LO 8.2)

_____

16. Prefilled, single-dose syringes can be used more than once. (LO 8.2)

_____

17. The standard U-100 insulin syringe can hold up to 100 units or 1 mL. (LO 8.2)

_____

18. The tuberculin syringe is used to measure doses of drugs larger than 3 mL. (LO 8.2)

_____

19. The syringes used to deliver medication through already established intravenous systems are hypodermic syringes. (LO 8.2)

_____

20. You may administer an oral medication by injecting it parenterally. (LO 8.1)

_____

21. Vaginal suppositories are scored and can be divided per manufacturer's directions. (LO 8.3)

_____

22. You should not let the drug touch your skin when administering creams, gels, ointments, pastes, and patches. (LO 8.3)

_____

For Exercises 23–42, use the accompanying illustrations of equipment. For each question, mark with a line or with shading where you would measure the required dose:

23. 30 mL (Refer to medicine cup A.) (LO 8.1)

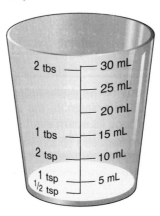

A

24. $\frac{1}{2}$ oz (Refer to medicine cup B.) (LO 8.1)

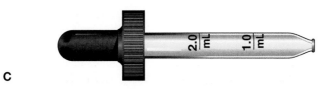

B

25. 1 mL (Refer to calibrated dropper C.) (LO 8.1)

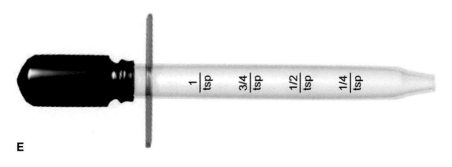

C

26. 0.6 mL (Refer to calibrated dropper D.) (LO 8.1)

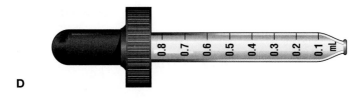

D

27. $\frac{3}{4}$ tsp (Refer to dropper E.) (LO 8.1)

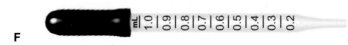

E

28. 0.5 mL (Refer to dropper F.) (LO 8.1)

F

29. $\frac{1}{4}$ tsp (Refer to dropper G.) (LO 8.1)

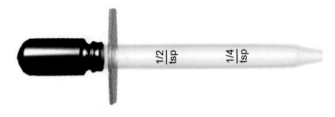

G

30. 0.32 mL (Refer to syringe H.) (LO 8.2)

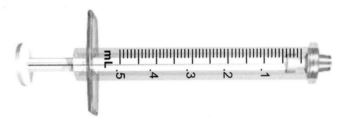

H

31. 2 mL (Refer to syringe I.) (LO 8.1)

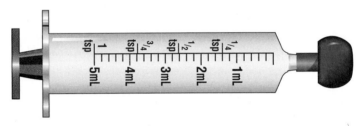

I

32. $1\frac{1}{2}$ tsp (Refer to syringe J.) (LO 8.1)

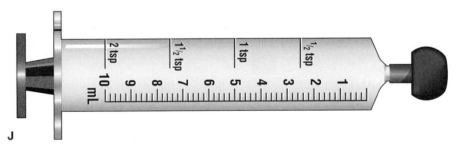

J

33. 1.5 mL (Refer to syringe K.) (LO 8.2)

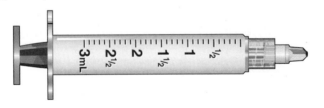

K

34. 2.3 mL (Refer to syringe L.) (LO 8.2)

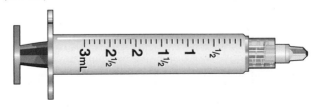

L

35. 80 units (Refer to syringe M.) (LO 8.2)

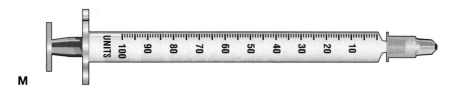

M

36. 45 units (Refer to syringe N.) (LO 8.2)

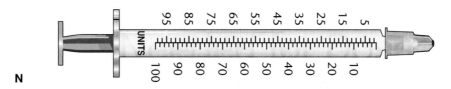

N

37. 35 units (Refer to syringe O.) (LO 8.2)

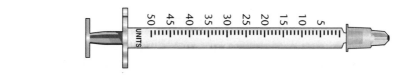

O

38. 27 units (Refer to syringe P.) (LO 8.2)

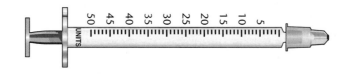

P

39. 0.5 mL (Refer to syringe Q.) (LO 8.2)

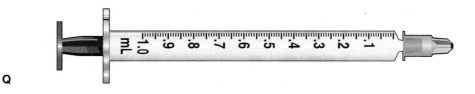

Q

40. 0.25 mL (Refer to syringe R.) (LO 8.2)

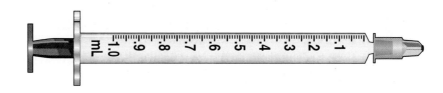

R

41. 5 mL (Refer to syringe S.) (LO 8.2)

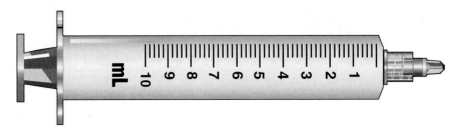

S

42. 7.2 mL (Refer to syringe T.) (LO 8.2)

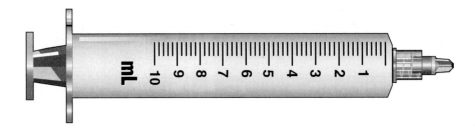

T

CRITICAL THINKING APPLICATIONS

What are the best utensils for measuring and administering the doses in each of the following situations? Choose from any of the equipment discussed in this chapter. (LO 8.1 to 8.3)

1. 1.5 mL, to be delivered parenterally

2. 39 units of insulin, to be delivered parenterally

3. 0.3 mL, to be delivered parenterally

4. Oral liquid dose of 29 mL

5. Oral liquid dose of 1 tbs

6. Parenteral dose of 1.25 mL

7. Oral liquid dose of 2 tbs

8. 8 mL, to be administered parenterally

9. 0.3 mg, to be administered transdermally

10. 0.4 mL, to be administered orally

11. $\frac{3}{4}$ tsp to be administered orally

12. An inhalant medication in a multiple-dose container

CASE STUDY

A healthcare professional must administer 10 drops of an oral medication. In attempting to administer the dose, the healthcare professional breaks the calibrated dropper. Instructions on the bottle say that 20 drops is equal to 1.5 tsp. What is the dose to be administered, and what is the best utensil for measuring it, now that the dropper is broken? (LO 8.1)

connect

Now that you have completed the materials in the chapter text, go to CONNECT and complete any chapter activities you have not yet done.

Interpreting Medication Orders

You must motivate yourself everyday!

MATTHEW STASIOR

CHAPTER 9

LEARNING OUTCOMES

When you have completed Chapter 9, you will be able to:

9.1 Interpret common medical abbreviations.

9.2 Identify components of a medication order.

9.3 Differentiate information on prescriptions and other medication orders.

9.4 Recognize the components of a medication order on the medication administration record (MAR).

KEY TERMS

Authorized prescriber (AP)

Electronic medication administration record (eMAR)

Frequency

Medication administration record (MAR)

Medication order

Prescription

Route

INTRODUCTION

To correctly calculate a medication dose, first you must be able to read and understand the medication or drug order. To do this, you must learn common medical abbreviations. You must also recognize the components of a medication order, including prescriptions. You must be motivated to read and interpret medication orders with accuracy to prevent errors and perform your job effectively.

9.1 Medical Abbreviations

To promote efficiency, **authorized prescribers** (APs) often use abbreviations on **medication orders**. APs are licensed healthcare professionals that have the authority to write medication orders, also called **prescriptions**. Table 9-1 provides a list of commonly used medical abbreviations that pertain to medication administration. Table 9-1 is organized by abbreviation type, including general abbreviations, medication form abbreviations, and abbreviations that pertain to route and frequency of medication administration. The medication **route** refers to the path by which a drug is brought into the body. For example, oral route indicates that the medication enters the body through the mouth, and the rectal route means via the rectum. **Frequency** of medication administration refers to the time(s) of day and how often a medication is to be given.

Memorize these abbreviations and have available a complete list of those accepted at your facility. Approved abbreviations vary among facilities. Abbreviations may be written in either uppercase or lowercase letters and with or without punctuation marks. APs may also put a line over general and frequency abbreviations, such as *a, ac, c, p,* and *s,* when the abbreviations are lowercase. You may also notice slight differences in the way that the abbreviations are spelled.

TABLE 9-1 Abbreviations Commonly Used in Drug Orders

General Abbreviations

ABBREVIATION	MEANING	ABBREVIATION	MEANING
aq	water	NPO, n.p.o.	nothing by mouth
$\bar{a}$	before	$\bar{p}$	after
BP	blood pressure	q, q.	every
$\bar{c}$	with	qs	quantity sufficient
d.c.*, D/C*	discontinue	$\bar{s}$	without
disp	dispense	sig, sig.	write on label
et	and	ss*, $\overline{ss}$*	one-half
iss*, $\overline{iss}$*	one and one-half	sys	systolic
NKA	no known allergies	tbsp, tbs, T	tablespoon
NKDA	no known drug allergies	tsp, t	teaspoon

Form of Medication

ABBREVIATION	MEANING	ABBREVIATION	MEANING
cap, caps	capsule	MDI	metered-dose inhaler
comp	compound	sol, soln.	solution
dil, dil.	dilute	SR	slow-release, sustained-release
EC	enteric-coated	supp, supp.	suppository
elix, elix.	elixir	susp, susp.	suspension
ext, ext.	extract	syr	syrup
fld., fl	fluid	syr	syringe
gt, gtt†	drop, drops	tab	tablet
LA	long-acting	tr, tinct, tinc.	tincture
liq	liquid	ung, oint	ointment

Route

ABBREVIATION	MEANING	ABBREVIATION	MEANING
ad*, A.D.*, AD*	right ear	NG, NGT, ng	nasogastric tube
as*, A.S.*, AS*	left ear	NJ	nasojejunal tube
au*, A.U.*, AU*	both ears	od*, O.D.*, OD*	right eye
GT	gastrostomy tube	os*, O.S.*, OS*	left eye
ID	intradermal	ou*, O.U.*, OU*	both eyes
IM, I.M.	intramuscular	per	per, by, through
IVPB	intravenous piggyback	po, p.o., PO, P.O.	by mouth; orally
IVSS	intravenous soluset	P.R., p.r., PR, pr	rectally
IV, I.V.	intravenous	subcut	subcutaneous, beneath the skin

TABLE 9-1 Continued

Route			
ABBREVIATION	**MEANING**	**ABBREVIATION**	**MEANING**
IVP	intravenous push	SL, sl	sublingual, under the tongue
KVO, TKO	keep vein open, to keep open	top, TOP	topical, applied to skin surface

Frequency			
ABBREVIATION	**MEANING**	**ABBREVIATION**	**MEANING**
a.c., ac, AC	before meals	p.r.n., prn, PRN	when necessary, when required
ad. lib., ad lib	as desired, freely	qam, q.a.m.	every morning
b.i.d., bid, BID	twice a day	qpm	every night
b.i.w.	twice a week	q.h., qh	every hour
h, hr	hour	q. _____ hrs, q_____h	every _____ hours
h.s.,* hs,* HS*	hour of sleep, at bedtime	qhs*, q.h.s.*	every night, at bedtime
LOS	length of stay	q.i.d., qid, QID	4 times a day
Min	minute	rep	repeat
non rep	do not repeat	stat	immediately
noc, noct	night	t.i.d., tid, TID	3 times a day
p.c., pc, PC	after meals	t.i.w.*	3 times a week

*Indicates an "error-prone" abbreviation as established by the ISMP.
†commonly abbreviated at gtt and gtts
Adapted from Joint Commission on Accreditation of Healthcare Organizations, 2010.

Note the abbreviations with an asterisk (*) beside them in Table 9-1. Sometimes these abbreviations are still used by APs; however, you need to remember that these abbreviations should NOT be used as they are considered error-prone. Most electronic medical records allow practitioners to select from a list of standardized abbreviations when creating medication orders. This eliminates the use of error-prone abbreviations as well as poor handwriting, thus helping to prevent medication errors. In the "Safe Medication Administration" chapter, you will learn more about error-prone abbreviations and your role in promoting safe medication administration. Be certain to check abbreviations carefully when you read drug orders.

Roman Numerals

Roman numerals are sometimes used with drug orders written in the apothecary system, although this system is used infrequently. The Institute for Safe Medication Practices (ISMP) recommends using the metric system for measuring medications. The ISMP will be discussed in more detail in the "Safe Medication Administration" chapter. Since Roman numerals are still seen in practice, you will need to understand how to change Roman numerals to Arabic numbers.

In the Roman numeral system, letters are used to represent numbers. Recall that lowercase letters are frequently used in pharmacy, especially for apothecary measurements. The Roman numerals that you are likely to encounter in a medical setting include ss ($\frac{1}{2}$), I (1), V (5), and X (10). These numerals may be written in either uppercase or lowercase, and a line is sometimes written above lowercase symbols. Thus, the number "one" can be written as I, i, or $\bar{\text{i}}$. The Roman numerals from 1 to 30 are the ones you are most likely to see in medication orders. Table 9-2 summarizes these numerals for you. Remember that "ss" could be added to the end of any of these expressions to add the value of $\frac{1}{2}$.

TABLE 9-2 Converting Roman Numerals

ROMAN NUMERAL*	ARABIC NUMBER	ROMAN NUMERAL	ARABIC NUMBER	ROMAN NUMERAL	ARABIC NUMBER
SS, $\overline{ss}$	$\frac{1}{2}$	XI, xi	11	XXII, xxii	22
I, i	1	XII, xii	12	XXIII, xxiii	23
II, ii	2	XIII, xiii	13	XXIV, xxiv	24
III, iii	3	XIV, xiv	14	XXV, xxv	25
IV, iv	4	XV, xv	15	XXVI, xxvi	26
V, v	5	XVI, xvi	16	XXVII, xxvii	27
VI, vi	6	XVII, xvii	17	XXVIII, xxviii	28
VII, vii	7	XVIII, xviii	18	XXIX, xxix	29
VIII, viii	8	XIX, xix	19	XXX, xxx	30
IX, ix	9	XX, xx	20		
X, x	10	XXI, xxi	21		

*Roman numerals written with small letters are also correctly written with a line over the top; for example, iv and $\overline{iv}$ are both correct.

COMBINING ROMAN NUMERALS   Obviously, it is often necessary to write Roman numerals other than $\frac{1}{2}$, 1, 5, or 10. To do so, the letters are combined into a single expression. The expression can be translated to an Arabic number by following two basic steps.

RULE 9-1	When you read a Roman numeral containing more than one letter, follow these two steps:
	1. If any letter with a smaller value appears *before* a letter with a larger value, subtract the smaller value from the larger.
	2. Add the values of all the letters not affected by step 1 to those that were combined.
Examples	**a.** IX = 10 − 1 = 9
	b. iv = 5 − 1 = 4
	c. XIV = 10 + (5 − 1) = 14
	d. VII = 5 + 2 = 7
	e. ivss = (5 − 1) + $\frac{1}{2}$ = $4\frac{1}{2}$
	f. VI = (5 + 1) = 6

It is important to note that there will never be more than three of the same Roman numerals in a row. If more than three need to be added to generate the new number, the convention is to subtract 1 from the larger number, rather than add four Roman numerals in a row. For

Copyright © 2016 by McGraw-Hill Education

example, the number 9 is written as ix, instead of viiii. Also, there will never be more than 1 subtracted from a larger number to generate a new number. For example, the number 8 is written as viii, instead of iix.

Understanding the Order of Roman Numerals

A medication administration record lists a drug order of gr ix. (The abbreviation "gr" stands for grains.) A healthcare professional reading the order thinks, "The Roman numeral i equals 1 and x equals 10, so I should give 11 grains of the drug."

 Think! . . . Is It Reasonable? What mistake did the healthcare professional make?

REVIEW AND PRACTICE

9-1 Medical Abbreviations

For Exercises 1–5, rewrite the medication order, interpreting the abbreviations.

1. Bactrim® (400 mg sulfamethoxazole and 80 mg trimethoprim) i tab po q 12h for 10 days.

2. Catapres® (clonidine hydrochloride, USP) 0.1 mg tablet po twice daily (morning and bedtime).

3. Lunesta® (eszopiclone) 1 mg tab i po qpm at bedtime prn insomnia.

4. Nitrostat® (Nitroglycerin) gr 1/150, tab i SL, prn chest pain; rep q 5 min prn continued pain, max 3 doses per episode.

5. Mevacor® (lovastatin) 20 mg tab ii po daily.

9.2 Components of a Medication Order

Always verify that a medication order contains all information needed to carry it out safely and accurately. Complete medication orders contain eight components: the full name of the patient, the patient's date of birth (DOB), the full name of the drug, the dose, the route, the time and frequency, the signature (electronic or written) of the authorized prescriber, and the date of the order. See Figure 9-1 and Table 9-3. A prn order must include the reason for administering the medication. If an order is unclear or incomplete, contact the AP before you carry it out.

Most facilities have a standard schedule for administering medication (see Table 9-4). To minimize errors, agencies frequently use the 24-hour clock. The person who verifies the transcription ensures that the times listed are appropriate for the medications. For example,

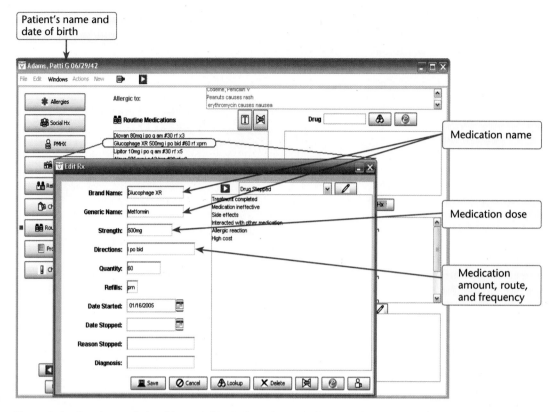

Figure 9-1 An electronic health record includes all parts of the medication order. In some cases a signature is not seen when an electronic signature is used, but will be shown on the printed or transmitted order.

some medications need to be given with food or after a meal; others, on an empty stomach. Times may need to be adjusted to accommodate a patient's meals. A patient may take two or more medications with conflicting schedules. Again, the timing may need to be adjusted.

TABLE 9-3 Components of a Medical Order	
Patient's name	Should be full name with middle name or initial.
Date	Date the order was written. The time of the order is typically included for inpatient medication orders.
Date of birth (DOB)	Patient's date of birth (Note: A medical record number or bar code may also be included on the order.)
Name of medication	Full medication or drug name
Dose	Amount of medication to be administered at one time.
Route	The path by which the drug enters the body (such as oral).
Frequency	The time of day and how often the medication is to be taken.
Authorized prescriber's (AP) signature	Handwritten or electronic signature from licensed MD (medical doctor), DO (osteopathic physician), DPM (podiatrist), DDS (dentist), PA (physician assistant), ARNP (advanced registered nurse practitioner), or other licensed healthcare professional with prescriptive authority.

TABLE 9-4 Sample Times for Medication Administration

FREQUENCY ORDERED	TIMES TO ADMINISTER
daily	0800
bid	0800, 2000
tid	0800, 1400, 2000
Qid	0800, 1200, 1600, 2000
q 12 hrs	0800, 2000
q 8 hrs	2400, 0800, 1600
q 6 hrs	2400, 0600, 1200, 1800

CRITICAL THINKING ON THE JOB

When in Doubt, Check

A healthcare practitioner is preparing medications. An entry in the MAR calls for 600 mg of Lasix® IV, higher than what she usually administers. She checks a medication reference. It indicates that doses this high may be used for congestive heart failure, the patient's diagnosis. Still, she is not comfortable with this level. She checks the original order on the medication order (see Figure 9-2).

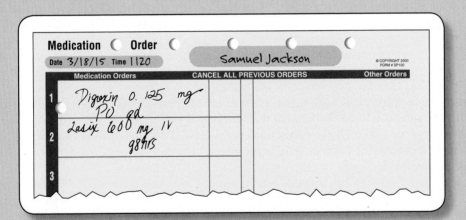

Figure 9-2 Medication order.

Think! . . . Is It Reasonable?

1. What parts of the medication order are not seen from Figure 9-2?
2. What part of the medication order is the healthcare practitioner questioning?
3. What serious error did the healthcare practitioner prevent by checking the original medication order?

9-2 Components of a Medication Order

For Exercises 1–8, match the eight components of a medication order to the corresponding order segments.

1. Patient's name   _____   a. *P. Sriker, MD*

2. Date   _____   b. Aricept (donepezil HCL)

3. Date of birth (DOB)   _____   c. 4/12/56

4. Name of medication   _____   d. daily

5. Dose   _____   e. John M. Smith

6. Route   _____   f. 2/18/14

7. Frequency   _____   g. 5 mg

8. Authorized prescriber's signature   _____   h. po

9.3 Prescription/Medication Order

The first step in the medication delivery process is a prescription. The prescription is a medication order. It can be written on a prescription tablet (pad) or transmitted through an electronic health record for medication procurement. A medication order, as discussed in the previous section, can be written or added electronically to a patient's chart for administration by healthcare practitioners in an inpatient setting.

As with all medication orders, only licensed healthcare professionals with prescriptive authority, such as medical doctors (MDs), osteopathic physicians (DOs), podiatrists (DPMs), dentists (DDSs), physician assistants (PAs), and advanced practice registered nurse practitioners (ARNPs) are permitted to write prescriptions. These are typical authorized prescribers (APs). It is important to note that those authorized to write prescriptions may differ according to state law.

Prescriptions must include all eight components of a medication order, plus the prescriber number, the quantity to be dispensed, the number of refills permitted, and instructions for the label of the container. These instructions are preceded by the word *sig* (see Figure 9-3). Sig is an abbreviation for the Latin term *signetur* which means "let it be labeled." Some APs write instructions without the use of "sig."

Note in Figure 9-3 that the patient is Arthur Simons. His date of birth (DOB) is September 29, 1949. The drug is doxycycline. The dose is 100 mg. The sig line indicates that the patient should take one capsule (1 cap) twice a day (BID) by mouth (po) after meals (pc), so the instructions on the label should read, "Take one capsule twice a day after meals." Form, number, route, frequency, and timing are all shown. The quantity, sometimes abbreviated quan, of capsules is 20. The prescription cannot be refilled. The physician's name, prescriber number, and signature are present. This order contains all the necessary components.

When medications are administered by a healthcare practitioner, the prescription will be in the form of a medication order in the patient's chart. This order will be either handwritten or entered electronically into the patient's chart. An order or group of orders will include the current *date/time* and *signature* of the AP with each order entry on an electronic or paper form marked with the *patient's name* and *date of birth (DOB)* comprising four of the eight medication

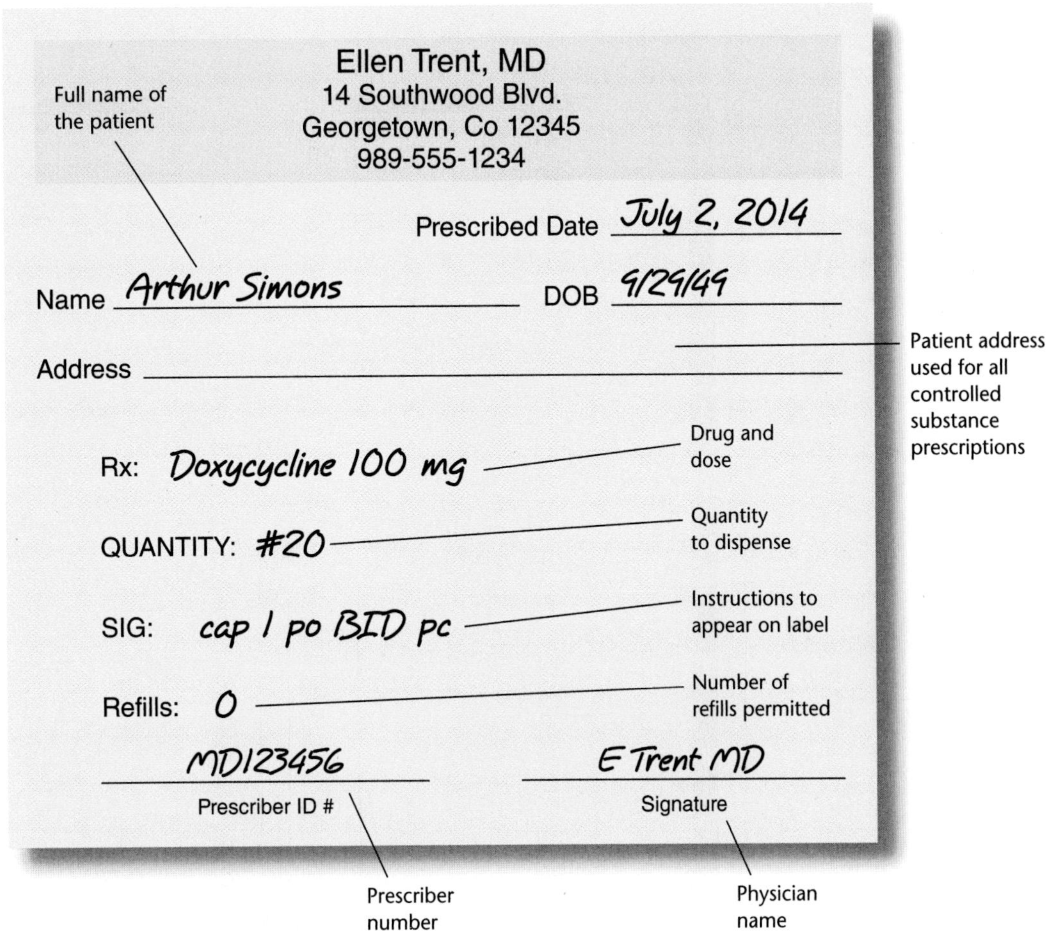

Figure 9-3 A typical outpatient prescription.

order components. The remaining four components should be identified for every medication ordered: *drug name*, *dose*, *route*, and *frequency/time*. Additional instructions are provided as needed.

The form in Figure 9-4 shows several medication orders that were written by the authorized prescriber or verbalized directly by the authorized prescriber, in person or via telephone. Review each medication order and note that some are correct and others have errors.

- Order 1 contains all necessary components. The drug is Lasix, the dose is 20 mg, the route is oral (po), and the frequency is once a day (daily).

- Order 2, for KCl (potassium chloride) elixir, is not complete. The order lists 1 tsp as the amount, but KCl elixir is available in strengths of 10, 20, 30, or 40 mEq per 15 mL. Each strength provides a different dose per teaspoon.

- Order 3 is correct. The drug is Motrin®, the dose is 200 mg, the route is oral (po), and the frequency is whenever necessary (PRN) every 4 hours (q 4 h). Motrin® may not be administered more often than every 4 h.

- Order 4 is not complete because it does not include a frequency.

- In Order 5, the physician has included instructions for "holding" (not administering) the medication. Inderal should not be given if the patient's apical pulse is below 50. However, the dose ordered includes number of tablets, but not number of milligrams, thus it is incomplete. Because Inderal is available in 10, 20, 40, 60, and 90 mg tablets, this order is unsafe.

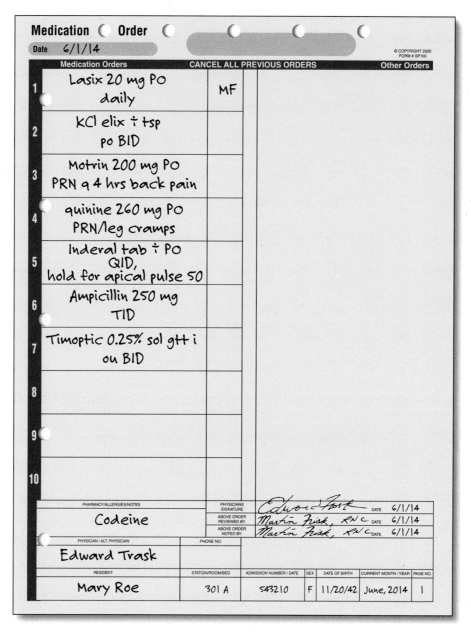

Figure 9-4 Medication order form. Do you see any errors?

- Order 6 does not specify the route for 250 mg Ampicillin, which is available in oral, intramuscular, and intravenous forms. The AP should be consulted for clarification of this order.

- Order 7 is complete. The physician specified the number of drops as well as the strength of Timoptic® desired.

9-3 Prescription/Medication Order

For Exercises 1–5, refer to prescription A.

Alan Capsella, MD
Westtown Medical Clinic
989-555-1234

Prescribed Date _July 9, 2014_

Name _Ann Pechin_   DOB _5/30/60_

Address _____

Rx: _Lopressor 50 mg_

QUANTITY: _#90_

SIG: _tab i po tid_

Refills: _5_

_MD398475_   _Alan Capsella MD_
Prescriber ID #   Signature

Prescription A

1. What components, if any, are missing from prescription A?
2. How many Lopressor® tablets should the pharmacy technician dispense?
3. How often should the patient take Lopressor®?
4. What strength tablets should be dispensed?
5. If the patient gets all the refills permitted, how long will the medication covered by this prescription last?

For Exercises 6–10, refer to prescription B.

6. What components, if any, are missing from prescription B?
7. How much Amoxil® should the pharmacy technician dispense?
8. How much Amoxil® should the patient take at one time?
9. How many times can this prescription be refilled?
10. How often should the patient take Amoxil®?

Alan Capsella, MD
Westtown Medical Clinic
989-555-1234

Prescribed Date *April 10, 2014*

Name *Mark Ward*   DOB *8/12/10*

Address _____

Rx: *Amoxil – oral susp*

QUANTITY: *100 mL*

SIG: *i tsp po q8h*

Refills: *0*

_____*MD398475*_____   *Alan Capsella MD*
Prescriber ID #   Signature

Prescription B

For Exercises 11–12, refer to Medication Order Form C.

Rhode Island Medical Center		Jane Doe DOB 3/15/55
Coventry, Rhode Island		1534 Hopkins Trail Chepachet, RI 01222
Medication Order Form		MR # 345466610

Diagnosis: *Congestive Heart Failure*   Allergies: NONE

Date	Time		
1/3/14	*8AM*	**A**	*tylenol PO q4h pm fever > 101*
		B	*furosemide 10 mg b.i.d*
		C	*valproic acid 250 mg by mouth*
		D	*10,000 units subcut q am*
			Mark Sanger, MD

Medication Order Form C

11. List the eight essential components as specified on Medication Order Form C for medication A.

12. Refer to Medication Order Form C and identify the missing component of orders A–D.

9.4 Medication Administration Records

Medication administration records (MARs) are legal documents that may be handwritten forms or electronic (see Figure 9-5). **Electronic medication administration records (eMARs)** are viewed and completed on an electronic device and the authorized prescriber's signature is protected through a unique password. MARs contain the same information as a medication order and also specify the actual times to administer the medication. Additionally the MAR provides a place to document that each medication has been given. By law, when a medication is given, it must be documented.

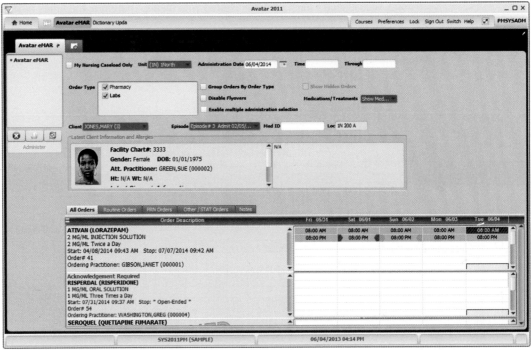

Patient identity information is fictitious.

Figure 9-5 An electronic medication administration record (eMAR) like this one allows the healthcare practitioner to document medication administration electronically.
*Netsmart Technologies (www.ntst.com)

RULE 9-2

MARs must include the following information:

1. The full name of the medication, the dose, the route, and the frequency.

2. Times that accurately reflect the frequency specified.

3. The full name and date of birth (DOB) and/or other identification number of the patient.

4. The date the order was written. If no start date is listed, then the assumption is that the date of order is the start date. Orders for narcotics and antibiotics should include end dates, according to your facility's policies.

5. Any special instructions or information as required by your facility. This includes, but is not limited to, the patient's diagnosis and weight.

Example 1

Determine whether the MAR in Figure 9-6 is complete.

In Figure 9-6 all three orders are written correctly. In order A, the drug is Nitrobid® 2% cream, the dose is $\frac{1}{2}$ inch, the route is topical, and the frequency is every 6 hr. The scheduled times are 2400 (midnight), 0600 (6:00 a.m.), 1200 (12:00 p.m.), and 1800 (6:00 p.m.).

In order B, the drug is Vasotec®, the dose is 10 mg, the route is oral, and the frequency is twice a day. This order includes a special instruction to hold the medication if the systolic blood pressure is below 100.

In order C, the drug is Glucophage®, the dose is 500 mg, the frequency is twice a day, and the route is oral. Glucophage® must be administered with meals. Therefore, the times have been adjusted to fit the facility's meal schedule.

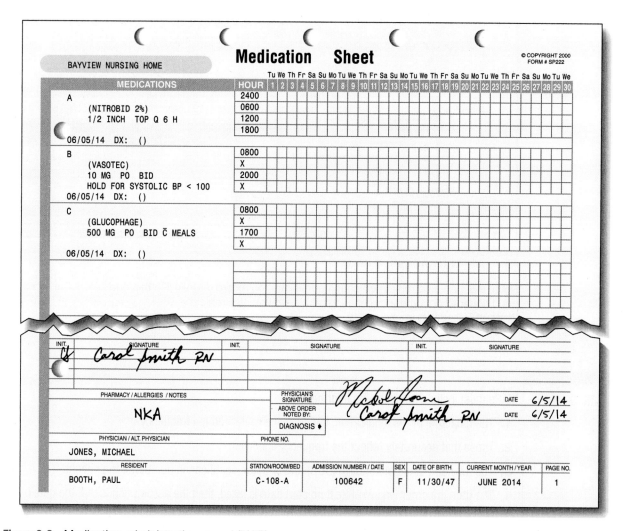

Figure 9-6 Medication administration record (MAR).

Example 2

Determine whether the MAR in Figure 9-7 is complete.

In Figure 9-7, order A is correct. The drug is Synthroid®, the dose is 50 mcg, the route is oral, and the frequency is daily.

Order B may seem to have all required information, but the dose—1 tablet—is not adequate. Erythromycin is available in several strengths. The order does not specify which dosage strength is intended. The times (0800, 2000) are for every 12 hours. Times should be listed as 0200, 0800, 1400, 2000. If the error is not corrected the patient will not receive a therapeutic level of the drug.

Order C contains an error in the times listed. Persantine® 75 mg is to be given q6h, or every 6 hours. The times (2400, 0800, 1600) are for every 8 hours. If the error is not recognized, then the patient will not receive a therapeutic level of the drug.

Order D does not include a route. Heparin can be administered either subcutaneously or intravenously. This order cannot be carried out as written.

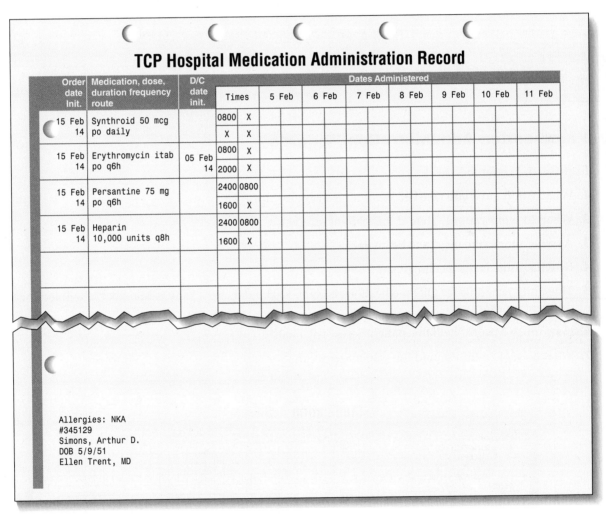

TCP Hospital Medication Administration Record

Order date Init.	Medication, dose, duration frequency route	D/C date init.	Times		5 Feb	6 Feb	7 Feb	8 Feb	9 Feb	10 Feb	11 Feb
15 Feb 14	Synthroid 50 mcg po daily		0800	X							
			X	X							
15 Feb 14	Erythromycin itab po q6h	05 Feb 14	0800	X							
			2000	X							
15 Feb 14	Persantine 75 mg po q6h		2400	0800							
			1600	X							
15 Feb 14	Heparin 10,000 units q8h		2400	0800							
			1600	X							

Allergies: NKA
#345129
Simons, Arthur D.
DOB 5/9/51
Ellen Trent, MD

Figure 9-7 Medication administration record (MAR).

When administering medications, accurate and complete information should be given to patients.

1. Explain the purpose of a medication and its side effects.

2. Review the dose, route, frequency, and time that the physician has prescribed.

3. When appropriate, be certain that the patient understands how to self-administer the medication.

4. If the patient is taking liquid oral medications at home, emphasize the importance of using calibrated spoons and measuring cups.

5. When writing instructions for patients, do not use abbreviations; write the actual unit of measurement. For example, instead of writing "2 t PO t.i.d. prn cough," write "take two teaspoons by mouth three times a day as needed for cough".

REVIEW AND PRACTICE

9-4 Medication Administration Records

For Exercises 1–7, refer to MAR 1.

1. What action must you take before administering Accupril®?

2. What dose of Accupril® should this patient receive?

3. At what time is the insulin to be given?

4. By what route is the insulin given?

5. This unit's schedule for QID medications is 0800, 1200, 1700, 2000. Why is Maalox® scheduled for different times?

6. How much Maalox® will this patient receive at 1400?

7. What dose of insulin should this patient receive?

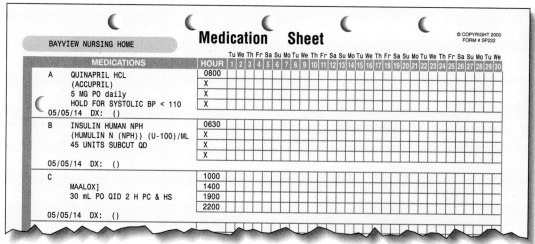

MAR 1

CHAPTER 9 SUMMARY

LEARNING OUTCOME	KEY POINTS
9.1 Interpret common medical abbreviations. Pages 159–163	See Table 9-1 for complete list. ▶ *General abbreviations:* $\overline{a}$ = before; $\overline{p}$ = after; q = every; qs = quantity sufficient; NKA = no known allergies; NKDA = no known drug allergies; NPO = nothing by mouth ▶ *Form:* cap = capsule; EC = enteric coated; gt = drop; MDI = metered-dose inhaler; tab = tablet ▶ *Route:* GT = gastrostomy tube; IM = intramuscular; IV = intravenous; IVP = intravenous push; IVPB = intravenous piggyback; KVO = keep vein open; NG = nasogastric tube; NJ = nasojejunal tube; po = by mouth; pr = per rectum; subcut = subcutaneous; SL = sublingual; top = topical ▶ *Frequency:* ac = before meals; pc = after meals; BID = twice a day; h = hour; prn = as needed; qam = every morning; qpm = every night; qh = every hour; stat = immediately; tid = 3 times a day The error-prone abbreviations identified in Table 9-1 with an asterisk should not be used. Roman numerals are used to write medication dosages in the apothecary system (see Table 9-2). The ISMP recommends using the metric system for writing medication dosages. However, if Roman numerals are used you must follow the steps in Rule 9-1 to ensure accuracy.
9.2 Identify components of a medication order. Pages 163–166	There are eight components of a medication order: **1.** Patient's name **2.** Date **3.** Date of birth (patient) **4.** Name of medication **5.** Dose **6.** Route **7.** Time and/or frequency of medication administration **8.** Authorized prescriber's signature For example, 5/11/2014 Peter Patient DOB 2/14/87 Tylenol 650 mg po q4h prn headache *A. Physician, MD*

LEARNING OUTCOME	KEY POINTS
9.3 Differentiate information on prescriptions and other medication orders. Pages 166–170	Prescriptions must include all eight components of a medication order, plus the prescriber number, the quantity to be dispensed, the number of refills permitted, and in some cases the *sig*, which is the instructions for the label of the container.
9.4 Recognize the components of a medication order on the medication administration record (MAR). Pages 171–174	Medication administration records (MARs) are transcriptions of the complete doctor's order, with an additional schedule of dates and times for the medication to be administered. A notation is made by the healthcare provider after a medication is administered. This is a legal document that can be handwritten or computer generated (eMAR). Rule 9-2 identifies what must be included on a MAR.

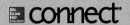
For Exercises 1–10, interpret the medical abbreviations in each order. (LO 9.1)

1. Ambien® (zolpidem tartrate) 10 mg po immediately before bedtime, prn insomnia

2. Sectral® (acebutolol hydrochloride) 400 mg po daily

3. Astelin® (azelastine hydrochloride) sprays ii each nostril BID

4. Bextra® (valdecoxib) 10 mg po daily

5. Wellbutrin XL® (bupropion hydrochloride extended-release) 300 mg po daily

6. Xigris® (drotrecogin alfa (activated)) 24 mcg/kg/hr IV for 96 hours

7. Zantac® Syrup (ranitidine hydrochloride) 150 mg/10 mL, tsp ii po BID

8. Serevent® Diskus® (salmeterol xinafoate) Inhalation Powder 50 mcg inhalation i po q 12h

9. Glucotrol® (glipizide) 5 mg tab i po daily ā breakfast

10. Lamisil® (terbinafine hydrochloride) 250 mg tab i po daily for 6 weeks

For examples 11–18, write the data that correspond with each medication order component. (LO 9.2)

RHODE ISLAND MEDICAL CENTER Coventry, Rhode Island	Jane Doe DOB 3/15/55 1534 Hopkins Trail Chepachet, RI 01222
Diagnosis: Congestive Heart Failure	**Allergies:** NONE

Date	Time	
1/3/14	8AM	tylenol 325 mg tab ii PO q4h prn fever > 101
		Mark Sanger, MD

11. Date/time _____

12. Patient's name _____

13. Patient's date of birth _____

14. Medication name _____

15. Dose _____

16. Route _____

17. Frequency _____

18. AP signature _____

For Exercises 19–21, refer to Prescription 1. (LO 9.3)

19. What instructions should be printed for the patient?

20. By what route is the medication to be administered?

21. How many refills may the patient be given?

Mark DeSantis
123 Baker Drive
Owosso, MI 48867
989-555-1234

Prescribed Date _1/23/2014_

Name _Jeannies Kucharek_   DOB _8/10/1939_

Address _____

Rx: _Synthroid 0.1 mg_

QUANTITY: _#30_

SIG: _tab i po tid_

Refills: _0_

_MD1234567_   _Mark Desantis, MD_
Prescriber ID #   Signature

Prescription 1

For Exercises 22 and 23, refer to Prescription 2. (LO 9.3)

22. What information must be obtained before this order can be filled?

23. What instructions should be printed for the patient?

Mark DeSantis
123 Baker Drive
Owosso, MI 48867
989-555-1234

Prescribed Date _1/23/2014_

Name _Jeannies Kucharek_   DOB _8/10/1939_

Address _____

Rx: _Amoxil 250 mg/5ml_

QUANTITY:

SIG: _1 tsp. p.o. q8h until gone_

Refills: _0_

_MD1234567_   _Mark Desantis, MD_
Prescriber ID #   Signature

Prescription 2

For Exercise 24, refer to Prescription 3. (LO 9.3)

24. What action must be taken before this prescription can be filled?

Mark DeSantis
123 Baker Drive
Owosso, MI 48867
989-555-1234

Prescribed Date _1/23/2014_

Name _Jeannies Kucharek_   DOB _8/10/1939_

Address _____

Rx: *Cortisporin Otic Drops*

QUANTITY: *5 ml*

SIG: *gtts. ii os quid*

Refills: *0*

_MD1234567_   _Mark Desantis, MD_
Prescriber ID #   Signature

Prescription 3

For Exercises 25–30, refer to MAR 2. (LO 9.4)

Medication Sheet

Order	Medication, dose, duration frequency route	D/C date init.	HOUR		1 Feb	2 Feb	3 Feb	4 Feb	5 Feb	6 Feb	7 Feb
A	NORMODYNE 100 MG PO BID		0800	X							
			2000	X							
B	HUMULIN N 24 UNITS before breakfast		0700	X							
			X	X							
C	DULCOLAX PR once a day PRN		X	X							
			X	X							
D	ATROVENT 2 PUFFS VIA MDI QID		0800	1200							
			1600	2000							
E	BUSPAR 15 MG PO TID		0800	1400							
			2000	X							

MAR 2

25. Why are no times marked beside the Dulcolax®?

26. Which medications should be given at 8 a.m.?

27. Which medication orders are not complete?

28. What is missing from the orders identified in the answer to question 21?

29. What is the route for the Buspar®?

30. What is the dose for the Atrovent®?

CHECK UP

For Exercises 1–10 rewrite the medication order, interpreting the abbreviations. (LO 9.1)

1. Aldactone® (spironolactone) 25 mg tab i po daily.

2. Neurontin® (gabapentin) oral solution 250 mg/5 mL, 400 mg po TID.

3. Boniva® (ibandronate sodium) 150 mg tab i taken po ā breakfast q month.

4. Paxil® (paroxetine hydrochloride) oral susp 10 mg/5 mL, 20 mg po daily in a.m.

5. Singulair® (montelukast sodium) 5 mg tab, chew i po daily.

6. Aspirin gr v, tab ii po q4h prn headache.

7. Protonix® (pantoprazole sodium) 40 mg tab i po daily.

8. Nitrong® (nitroglycerin) 1 inch top bid, remove for 8 hours at bedtime.

9. Naprosyn® (naproxen) 250 mg tab i po q8h.

10. Cozaar® (losartan potassium) 50 mg tab i po daily.

For Exercises 11–18 identify each of the components of the electronic medication order below. (LO 9.2)

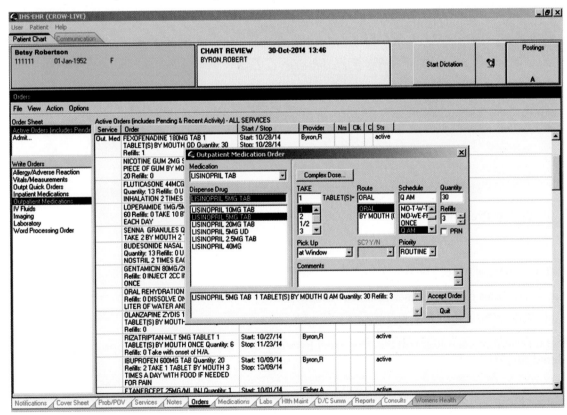

Electronic medication order

11. Date   _____

12. Medication   _____

13. Frequency   _____

14. Route   _____

15. AP   _____

16. Dose   _____

17. Patient   _____

18. DOB   _____

For Exercises 19–22, refer to Prescription 1. (LO 9.3)

Alan Capsella, MD
Westtown Medical Clinic
989-555-1234

Prescribed Date _July 8, 2014_

Name _Maria Ortiz_   DOB _____

Address _____

    Rx: _Timoptic 0.5%_

    QUANTITY: _5 mL_

    SIG: _gtts ii right eye QID_

    Refills: _2_

_____MD398475_____   _Alan Capsella MD_
Prescriber ID #   Signature

Prescription 1

19. What instructions should be printed for the patient?

20. How many times can this prescription be refilled?

21. By what route should this medication be administered?

22. What information should be on the drug label to verify that this medication is appropriate for the ordered route?

For Exercises 23–29, refer to MAR 3. (LO 9.4)

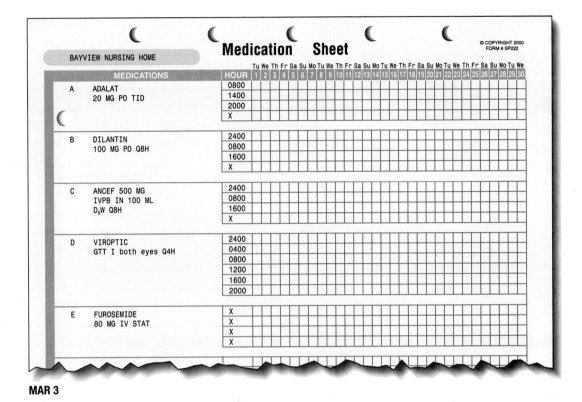

MAR 3

23. When should the furosemide be given?

24. What is the route of administration of the Viroptic®?

25. What is the route of administration of the Ancef®?

26. Which medications will be given at 4 p.m.?

27. If medications were delivered daily, how many doses of medication would be delivered for each of the medications this patient is scheduled to receive?

28. How many times a day does the patient receive Viroptic®?

29. What two medications will be administered through an IV?

For Exercises 30–34, refer to MAR 4. (LO 9.3)

TCP Hospital Medication Administration Record

Order date	Medication, dose, duration frequency route	D/C date	Times	22 Feb	23 Feb	24 Feb	25 Feb	26 Feb	27 Feb	28 Feb
5/21/14	heparin 5,000 units subcut q12h		0900							
			2100							
5/22/14	Procan SR 500 mg tab po q6h	05 Feb 14	0600 1200							
			1800 2400							
5/22/14	digoxin [Lanoxin] 125 mg tab po daily		0900							
5/22/14	furosemide [Lasix] 40 mg tab po daily		0900							

MAR 4

30. By what route will the heparin be given?

31. How many times a day will the patient receive Procan?

32. Will Lanoxin® be administered in the morning or at night?

33. How many oral medications is the patient receiving?

34. If the patient has a dose of Procan at 6 p.m., when should he receive the next dose?

CRITICAL THINKING APPLICATION

For Exercises 1–3, refer to the medication order below. (LO 9.2)

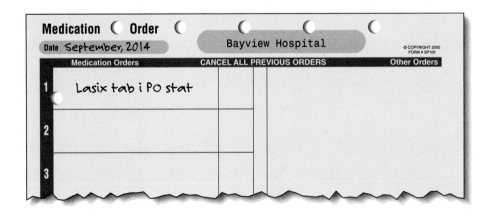

1. Interpret the medical abbreviations in this order.

2. What components of the medication order are missing?

3. Describe the importance of knowing the eight components of the medication order.

CASE STUDY

Katherine Drexel, born 20 years ago today, is complaining of pain and discomfort after the delivery of her baby. The midwife, Louise Pingree RN, APN, CNM, has ordered on this date, at this hour, eight hundred milligrams of Motrin® (ibuprofen) to be given orally every eight hours as needed for pain. Write a medication order using appropriate medical abbreviations and identify each of the eight components of the order. (LO 9.1)

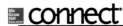

Now that you have completed the materials in the chapter text, go to CONNECT and complete any chapter activities you have not yet done.

Interpreting Medication Labels and Package Inserts

CHAPTER 10

Read in order to live.

HENRY FIELDING

LEARNING OUTCOMES

When you have completed Chapter 10, you will be able to:

10.1 Interpret information on a medication label.

10.2 Distinguish information related to administration routes for medications.

10.3 Find information on package inserts, needed for dosage calculations.

INTRODUCTION

In preparation for dosage calculations you need to know basic math, other systems of measurement, conversions, equipment, and drug orders, all of which are covered in other chapters. In this chapter you will learn about drug packaging. The drug label and package insert contain the information you need to perform dosage calculations, and they must be read carefully. Make sure you know exactly what is found on a drug label, and do not forget to read the fine print. Essential information is located there.

10.1 Information on Medication Labels

To prepare and administer drugs, you must understand information that appears on drug labels. This information includes the drug name, form, dosage strength, total amount in the container, route of administration, warnings, storage requirements, and manufacturing information.

Drug Name

Every drug has an official name—its **generic name.** By law, this name must appear on the drug's label. It is also recorded in a national listing of drugs: the *United States Pharmacopeia* (USP) and the *National Formulary* (NF). In Figures 10-1, 10-2, 10-3, and 10-4 each drug's generic name has been identified. If USP appears on the label, it indicates that this drug's name is recorded with the *United States Pharmacopeia.*

Many drug labels include the **trade name** or **brand name** used to market the drug. In Figures 10-1 and 10-2 note that the trade name is listed before the generic name. However, some drug labels list only a generic name (see Figures 10-3 and 10-4). A trade name is the property of a specific drug company. The registered mark® indicates the name has been legally registered with the U.S. Patent and Trademark Office. Several companies may manufacture a drug but market it under different trade names.

Authorized prescribers can write drug orders using either generic or trade names. Some companies produce drugs under their generic names and market them at a lower cost than the trade name equivalents. For example, ibuprofen is sold under its generic name as well as trade names such as Advil® and Motrin®.

RULE 10-1	You must know both the generic and trade names of drugs.
Example	Suppose a patient is allergic to Vicodin®, a narcotic painkiller. The generic drugs in Vicodin®—hydrocodone bitartrate and acetaminophen—are also found in the trade name drugs Anexsia®, Lortab®, and Zydone®. If you administer one of these drugs or any drug containing hydrocodone bitartrate or acetaminophen as an alternative to Vicodin®, the patient may have a similar allergic reaction. When you record a patient's drug allergy, include both the trade and generic names. Resources such as the PDR (*Physicians' Desk Reference*), drug handbook, or reliable Internet site provide information about a drug's ingredients.

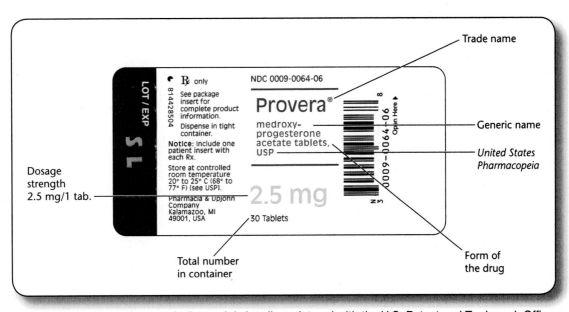

Figure 10-1 A ® beside the trade name indicates it is legally registered with the U.S. Patent and Trademark Office.

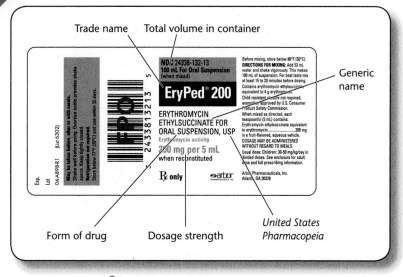

Trade name   Total volume in container   Generic name

Form of drug   Dosage strength   *United States Pharmacopeia*

Figure 10-2 E.E.S.® 200 Liquid is the trade name.

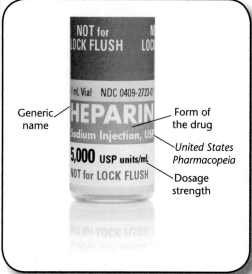

Generic name   Form of the drug   *United States Pharmacopeia*   Dosage strength

Figure 10-3 Some medications are generic only and have no trade name.

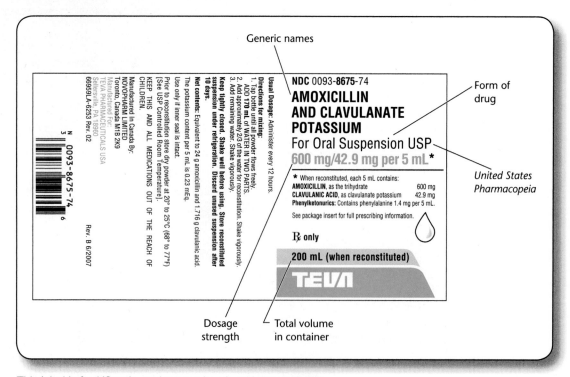

Generic names   Form of drug   *United States Pharmacopeia*   Dosage strength   Total volume in container

This label is for US only, and cannot be altered or translated.

Figure 10-4 Amoxicillin and clavulanate potassium is a combination medication.

Form of the Drug

Manufacturers may offer the same drug in different forms. For example, penicillin is available as a tablet, a capsule, a liquid for oral administration, and a liquid for injection. Every label indicates the drug's form. Solid oral medications come in the form of tablets, capsules, gelcaps, and caplets. Liquid forms include oral, injections, inhalants, drops, sprays, and mists. Other forms of medication include ointments, creams, lotions, patches, suppositories, and shampoos. See Figures 10-1, 10-2, 10-3, and 10-4.

Dosage Strength

Drug labels include information about the amount of the drug present. This amount, combined with information about the form of the drug, identifies the drug's **dosage strength** (supply dose). On the label, the dosage strength is stated as the amount of drug per dosage unit. In most cases, the amount of the drug is listed in grams (g), milligrams (mg), micrograms (mcg), or possibly grains (gr). In certain cases, such as insulin, the amount is listed in units. Certain liquid drugs, such as hydrogen peroxide and glycerin, may list the amount in milliliters (mL). Some medications are also listed as milliequivalents (mEq).

For solid medications, the dosage strength is the amount of drug present per tablet, capsule, or other form. In Figure 10-1, note the amount of Provera® (2.5 mg) present in a tablet, the form of medication. The dosage strength is 2.5 mg per tablet. *Note: For most solid medications, if the unit is not listed, assume it is one tablet, one capsule, one gelcap, and so forth.*

For liquid medications, the dosage strength is the amount of the drug present in a certain quantity of solution. For example in Figure 10-2, the dosage strength of EES is 200 mg/5 mL. In Figure 10-3 the dosage strength of heparin sodium is 5,000 units/1 mL.

Pharmaceutical companies manufacture medications with dosage strengths corresponding to commonly prescribed doses. This practice, along with the practice of packaging unit doses (discussed further in this chapter), reduces the risk of medical error by reducing the number of dosage calculations.

Combination Drugs

The generic names and dosage strengths of all components of a combination drug must appear on the label. The label in Figure 10-4 lists the components amoxicillin and clavulanate. It also provides information about the individual drugs' dosage strengths. The line 600 mg/42.9 mg per 5 mL indicates that this medication contains 600 mg of amoxicillin and 42.9 mg of clavulanate in every 5 mL. Combination drugs sometimes have a trade name, which may be used in physician orders. For example, for the drug Lortab® 5/500 (trade name), which includes 5 mg of hydrocodone bitartrate and 500 mg of acetaminophen (generic names), the order might read Lortab® 5/500 1 tab q 4-6h PRN for pain. The order would *not* read hydrocodone bitartrate 5 mg, acetaminophen 500 mg, q 4-6h PRN for pain.

Total Number or Volume in Container

Many oral medications are packaged separately in *unit doses.* These packages may contain a single dosage unit. For example a container may have a single tablet or a vial with 2 mL of solution for injection. If the container holds more than one dosage unit, the total number or volume must be listed on the label. See Figures 10-1, 10-2, and 10-4. Prescription and nonprescription medications are often packaged in multiple-dose containers. Figure 10-5 indicates that prescription-strength Ritalin® is available in containers of 100 tablets, each tablet with 5 mg of drug.

Figure 10-6 shows the label for a dose pack of Azithromycin, a prescription medication. The container has 6 tablets taken over 5 days. Two tablets are taken on the first day. Each tablet is packaged as a unit dose. In Figure 10-7, the container of generic Rocephin® has 15 mL and provides a unit dose of 1 g/15 mL in a single-use vial. The label's directions indicate that you reconstitute the drug, administer it intravenously or intramuscularly, and discard any unused portion. Single-use vials are preservative-free and should be used for one dose and then discarded.

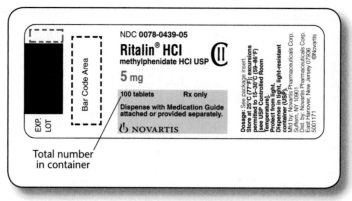

Figure 10-5 This container of Ritalin® contains 100 tablets and each tablet has 5 mg of medication.

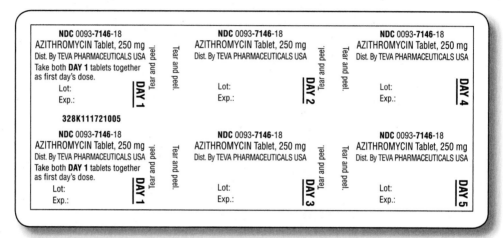

This label is for US only, and cannot be altered or translated.

Figure 10-6 A five-day dose pack of Azithromycin has one tablet in each package.

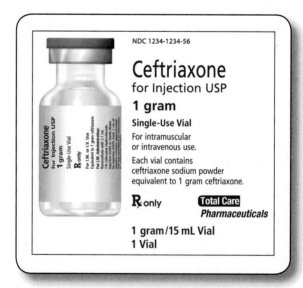

Figure 10-7 Unit-dose package of ceftriaxone (generic for Rocephin) for IV or IM administration.

RULE 10-2	Do not confuse the total amount of drug in the container with the dosage strength.
Example 1	According to Figure 10-1, the Provera® container holds 30 tablets, with a dosage strength of 2.5 mg per tablet. The entire container holds 30 × 2.5 mg, or 75 mg, of drug whereas an individual tablet holds 2.5 mg of drug.
Example 2	According to Figure 10-2, each 5 mL of E.E.S.® solution contains 200 mg of drug. The entire amount of solution is one pint or 473 mL*, not 5 mL. The entire container, therefore, holds 473 mL ÷ 5 mL = 94.6 or 94 complete doses. Even though the entire contents of the container is one pint (473 mL*), you will only administer a small portion (5 mL) of it at a time. *For practical purposes, household (pint) to metric (ml) conversions are approximate. The conversion factor 1 oz = 30 mL will yield 480 mL in 1 pint. This is an approximate conversion. When the manufacturer gives you an exact metric amount, the math is based on that number.

Route of Administration

Directions for the route of administration may be specified on the label. This information may not be included for oral medications. However, if a tablet or a capsule is not to be swallowed, additional information will be provided. For example, the label for Nitrostat® (Figure 10-8) shows it is administered sublingually, under the tongue. Chewable tablets will be labeled as such. Medications for topical use only will also be marked on the label (Figure 10-9).

Liquid medications may be given orally or injected. Labels will indicate whether an injection is given **intradermally** (ID), **intravenously** (IV), **intramuscularly** (IM), or **subcutaneously** (subcut) (see Figures 10-10 and 10-11). Labels will indicate other routes as well. For example, flunisolide (generic for Aerobid-M) is a solution for oral inhalation only (see Figure 10-12).

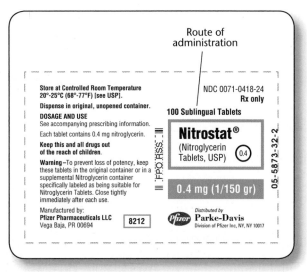

Figure 10-8 Sublingual tablets should be placed only under the tongue.

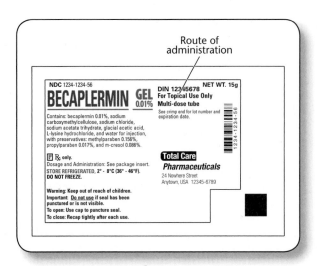

Figure 10-9 Becaplermin (generic for Regranex®) is a topical gel.

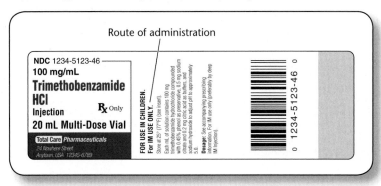

Figure 10-10 For intramuscular (IM) administration only.

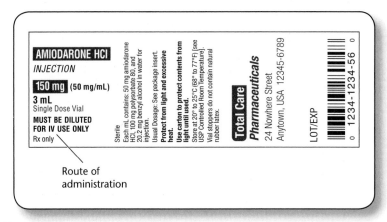

Figure 10-11 For intravenous (IV) administration only.

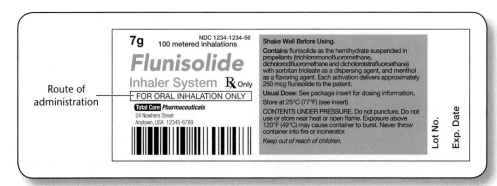

Figure 10-12 For oral inhalation only.

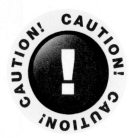

ERROR ALERT!

Read the Label Carefully!

Certain medications are available in a variety of forms, including an antibacterial suspension for otic (ear) use and an antimicrobial suspension for ophthalmic (eye) use. (See label A and B below.) The product label indicates the route. The usual dosage of the otic suspension is 4 drops instilled 3 to 4 times a day into the affected ear. The usual dosage of the ophthalmic suspension is 1 or 2 drops instilled into the affected eye every 3 or 4 h. If you were to carry out an order for the otic suspension by administering it to the patient's eye, you would not only fail to provide appropriate care for the ear, but also cause considerable irritation to the eye. *The bottom line: check labels carefully and do not administer drugs by any route other than intended, as described on the drug label and on the order.*

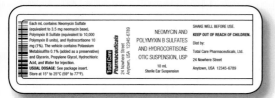

A

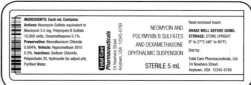

B

Warnings

Warnings on labels help healthcare workers administer drugs safely. They include statements such as "It is recommended that drug dispensing should not exceed weekly supply. Dispensing should be contingent upon the results of a WBC count." (See Figure 10-13.) Other labels indicate that the contents are poisonous. Labels may carry warnings for specific groups of patients. For example a label may caution that you should find out what medications may not be taken with the medication (see Figure 10-14) or that a medication may not be safe for pregnant women or for children. Controlled substances may contain a warning that says, "May be habit forming." Other labels describe harmful effects resulting from combinations with other products.

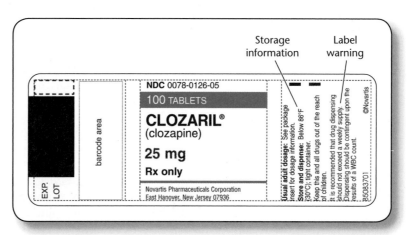

Figure 10-13 Always read label warnings. This label indicates no more than a weekly supply should be dispensed.

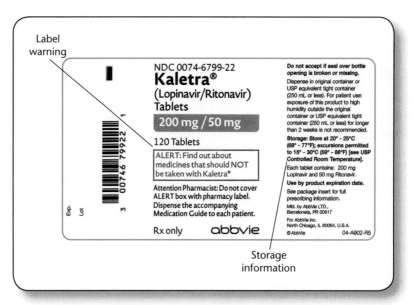

Label warning

NDC 0074-6799-22

Kaletra®

(Lopinavir/Ritonavir)
Tablets

200 mg / 50 mg

120 Tablets

ALERT: Find out about
medicines that should NOT
be taken with Kaletra®

Attention Pharmacist: Do not cover
ALERT box with pharmacy label.
Dispense the accompanying
Medication Guide to each patient.

Rx only   abbvie

Do not accept if seal over bottle
opening is broken or missing.

Dispense in original container or
USP equivalent tight container
(250 mL or less). For patient use:
exposure of this product to high
humidity outside the original
container or USP equivalent tight
container (250 mL or less) for longer
than 2 weeks is not recommended.

Storage: Store at 20° - 25°C
(68° - 77°F); excursions permitted
to 15° - 30°C (59° - 86°F) [see USP
Controlled Room Temperature].

Each tablet contains: 200 mg
Lopinavir and 50 mg Ritonavir.

Use by product expiration date.

See package insert for full
prescribing information.

Mfd. by AbbVie LTD.,
Barceloneta, PR 00617

For AbbVie Inc.
North Chicago, IL 60064, U.S.A.
© AbbVie   04-A902-R5

Storage information

Figure 10-14   Always read label storage information. Some medications may need to be refrigerated or kept in a dark location.

Every facility follows guidelines for disposing of drugs that are not used. The guidelines for medications that carry warnings are especially strict. For example, in some cases, you dispose of medications such as narcotics with a coworker as witness, then provide appropriate documentation.

Storage Information

Some drugs must be stored under specific conditions to maintain their potency and effectiveness. Storage information will appear on the drug's label. The label may have information about storage temperature, exposure to light, or the length of time the drug will remain potent after the container has been opened. Storage at the wrong temperature or exposure to light can trigger a chemical reaction that makes the drug unusable. (See Figures 10-13 and 10-14 for examples of storage information.)

Manufacturing Information

Pharmaceutical manufacturers are strictly regulated by the U.S. Food and Drug Administration (FDA). FDA regulations state that every drug label must include the name of the manufacturer; an expiration date, abbreviated EXP, after which the drug may no longer be used; and the lot number (see Figure 10-15).

Medications are produced in batches, known as *lots*. The lot number is a code that indicates when and where a drug was produced. It allows the manufacturer to trace problems linked to a particular batch. If a manufacturer has to remove an entire lot from the market because of contamination, suspected tampering, or unexpected side effects, the lot number helps identify which batch to recall.

Bar codes on medication labels are used to electronically identify the drug. This information is useful to ensure that an individual receives the correct medication. Bar coding has reduced medication administration and dispensing errors (see Figure 10-15).

Drug manufacturers assign a specific identification number to each of their drug products, called an *NDC (National Drug Code)* number. Each NDC number has 10 digits and is divided into three groups of numbers. The first group of numbers identifies the manufacturer; the second group identifies the medication, its strength, and its dosage form; and the third group

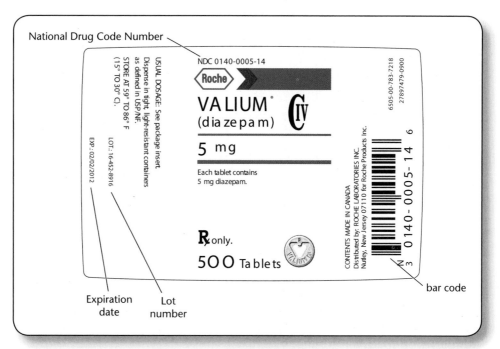

National Drug Code Number

NDC 0140-0005-14

Roche

VALIUM **C** **IV**
(dia ze pa m)

5 mg

Each tablet contains
5 mg diazepam.

R only.

500 Tablets

USUAL DOSAGE: See package insert

Dispense in tight, light-resistant containers
as defined in USP/NF.

STORE AT 59° TO 86° F
(15° TO 30° C).

LOT: 16-452-8916

EXP.: 02/02/2012

6505-00-783-7218

27897479-0900

CONTENTS MADE IN CANADA
Distributed by: ROCHE LABORATORIES INC.
Nutley, New Jersey 07110 for Roche Products Inc.

N 3 0140- 0005- 14 6

bar code

Expiration
date

Lot
number

Figure 10-15 The lot number, expiration date, and bar code are stamped on the drug label during manufacturing.

identifies the package size. If any of the three groups of numbers begin with zeros, the manufacturer may omit the zeros when printing the numbers on the product label. When ordering drugs and comparing NDC numbers on the drug label on the drug bottle, all 10 digits are used (see Figure 10-15).

RULE 10-3	Never use a drug after the expiration date has passed.
Example	Older drugs may become chemically unstable or altered. As a result, they may not provide the correct dosage strength. Worse, they could have an effect different from the intended one. Advise patients to check the expiration dates on all drug labels. If patients have not used a product by the date listed, they should dispose of it. At an inpatient setting, the medication may need to be returned to the pharmacy, depending on the facility's policy.

Information About Reconstituting Drugs

Some drugs, such as antibiotics, are packaged in powder form. You **reconstitute** the drug (add liquid to the powder) shortly before administering it. Reconstituted medications remain potent for only a short time. The label indicates the time period within which they can be safely administered (see Figures 10-16 and 10-17). Other drugs must be diluted before they are administered; they, too, must be used within a limited time. Directions for reconstituting or diluting a drug appear on the label (see Figures 10-16 and 10-17). Additional information can be found in the package insert, discussed in the next section.

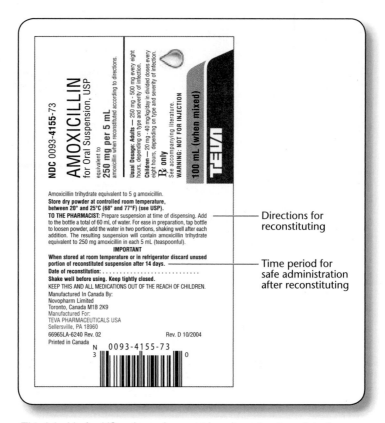

This label is for US only, and cannot be altered or translated.

Figure 10-16 To reconstitute a drug, you add liquid to a powder.

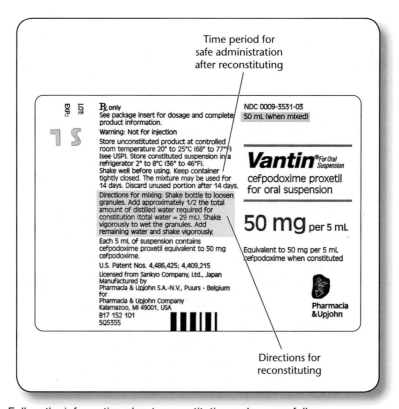

Figure 10-17 Follow the information about reconstituting a drug carefully.

Read Labels Carefully

A healthcare professional is filling the order Synthroid® 0.05 mg p.o. daily. Synthroid® is available in tablets of 11 different strengths, each in a different color. The healthcare professional has access to tablets in 0.025 mg (orange), 0.05 mg (white), 0.125 mg (brown), and 0.15 mg (blue) doses.

Looking quickly at two labels (see Figures 10-18 and 10-19), the healthcare professional sees a Synthroid® label with "5" on it. Without realizing it is for 0.15 mg, he removes a tablet. When he tries to administer it, the patient tells him that her usual pill is white, not blue.

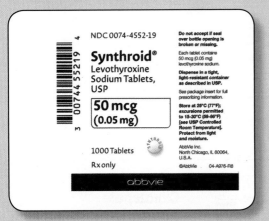

Figure 10-18 Read medication labels carefully.

Figure 10-19 Two labels may look alike but list different dosage strengths.

Think! . . . Is It Reasonable? What should the healthcare professional do? What mistake did he make?

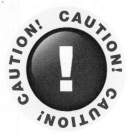

ERROR ALERT!

Consider the Age and Health Needs of Your Patient When You Administer a Drug

Suppose the drug order reads Biaxin® 250 mg po b.i.d. Biaxin®, an antibiotic, is available in 250 mg tablets and as an oral suspension with a reconstituted dosage strength of 125 mg/5 mL. (An *oral suspension* is a liquid that contains solid particles of medication. You shake the medication before administering it, suspending the particles.)

It may seem logical to fill the order with one tablet. Yet the age or health of the patient may make a liquid the better choice, especially for children or patients who have difficulty swallowing. If you see a situation in which another form of a drug may work better, consult the physician or pharmacist about changing the form of the drug.

10.1 Information on Medication Labels

For Exercises 1–6, refer to label A.

1. What is the trade name of the drug?

2. What is the generic name of the drug?

3. Does this container hold multiple doses or a unit dose? How do you know?

4. What is the name of the manufacturer?

5. What is the dosage strength?

6. What is the NDC code?

For Exercises 7–12, refer to label B.

7. What is the generic name of the drug?

8. In what type of container should this drug be dispensed?

9. What is the dosage strength?

10. What type of tablets are in this bottle?

11. What is the name of the manufacturer?

12. What are the storage requirements for this drug?

For Exercises 13–18, refer to label C.

13. What is the trade name of the drug?

14. Is this medication packaged in an ampule or a vial?

15. What is the dosage strength?

16. How would you administer this drug?

17. What is the total volume?

18. What is the total amount of medication?

For Exercises 19–24, refer to label D.

19. What is the generic name of the drug?

20. By what route is this drug administered?

21. What is the usual dose?

22. What is the dosage strength?

23. If you had a drug order for 200 mg of Zithromax®, how many teaspoons would you administer to the patient?

24. How long would two bottles last if you administered 1 dose of 10 mL daily?

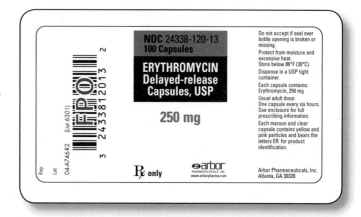

A

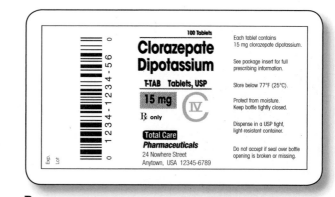

B

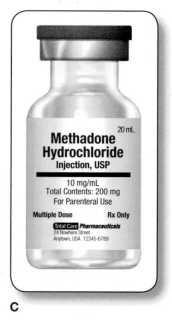

C

For Exercises 25–30, refer to label E.

25. What is the generic name of the drug?

26. By what route is this drug administered?

27. What special storage information is provided on the label?

28. How much medication is in one vial?

29. How much medication is contained in 1 mL?

30. How many doses are in one vial?

For Exercises 31–36, refer to label F.

31. When it is mixed, how many milliliters are in the bottle?

32. What is the name of the drug?

33. What is the form of the drug?

34. When it is mixed, what is the dosage strength?

35. What is the name of manufacturer?

36. If the usual dose is 5 mL, how many doses are in this container?

For Exercises 37–43, refer to label G.

37. What is the trade name of the drug?

38. What is the generic name of the drug?

39. What is the dosage strength?

40. How should this medication be stored?

41. Through what route is this drug administered?

42. How many prescriptions could be filled from this bottle if each prescription's quantity was 30 tablets?

43. What is the name of the manufacturer?

For Exercises 44–50, refer to labels A through G (labels may be used more than once).

44. Which of these drugs are tablets?

45. Which of these drugs are given orally?

FOR ORAL USE ONLY.
Store dry powder below 30°C (86°F).
PROTECT FROM FREEZING.
DOSAGE AND USE
See accompanying prescribing information.
MIXING DIRECTIONS:
Tap bottle to loosen powder.
Add 9 mL of water to the bottle.
After mixing, store suspension at
5° to 30°C (41° to 86°F).
Oversized bottle provides extra space
for shaking.
After mixing, use within 10 days.
Discard after full dosing is completed.
SHAKE WELL BEFORE USING.
Contains 600 mg azithromycin.

600 mg (15 mL when mixed)   NDC 0069-3120-19

Zithromax®
(azithromycin for
oral suspension)
CHERRY FLAVORED
200 mg* per 5 mL

Pfizer Pfizer Labs
Division of Pfizer Inc, NY, NY 10017

www.zithromax.com

6416
MADE IN USA

*When constituted as directed, each teaspoonful (5 mL) contains azithromycin dihydrate equivalent to 200 mg of azithromycin.

Rx only

05-5013-32-2

D

NDC 12345-1234-56

FUROSEMIDE

INJECTION, USP

40 mg/4 mL

(10 mg/mL)

For IM or IV Use   Rx only

4 mL Single Dose Vial

Sterile, Nonpyrogenic
Preservative Free
Discard unused portion.
Each mL contains: Furosemide 10 mg;
Water for Injection q.s. Sodium chloride to adjust isotonicity, pH adjusted with sodium hydroxide and if necessary hydrochloric acid.
Usual Dosage: See insert.
PROTECT FROM LIGHT. Do not use if discolored. Use only if solution is clear and seal intact.
Store at 20° to 25°C (68° to 77°F) [see USP Controlled Room Temperature].

Total Care Pharmaceuticals
24 Nowhere Street
Anytown, USA 12345-6789

LOT/EXP

E

NDC 0093-1075-78

CEFPROZIL
for Oral Suspension USP
125 mg/5 mL*

*Each 5 mL, when constituted according to directions, contains 125 mg anhydrous cefprozil.

℞ only

75 mL (when mixed)

TEVA

Store constituted suspension in refrigerator. Discard after 14 days.
Phenylketonurics: This product contains 10.1 mg of phenylalanine per 5 mL (approx. one teaspoonful) of suspension.
SHAKE WELL BEFORE USING.
KEEP THIS AND ALL MEDICATIONS OUT OF THE REACH OF CHILDREN.

TEVA PHARMACEUTICALS USA
Sellersville, PA 18960

LS2974
Rev. A 7/2005

To the Pharmacist: Prepare suspension at time of dispensing. Add to the bottle a total of **59 mL** water. For ease in preparation, add the water in two portions. **Shake well after each addition.** This provides 75 mL of suspension. Each 5 mL contains cefprozil equivalent to 125 mg anhydrous cefprozil.
Usual Dosage: See package insert for full prescribing information.
Store powder at 20° to 25°C (68° to 77°F) [See USP Controlled Room Temperature] prior to constitution.

F

This label is for US only, and cannot be altered or translated.

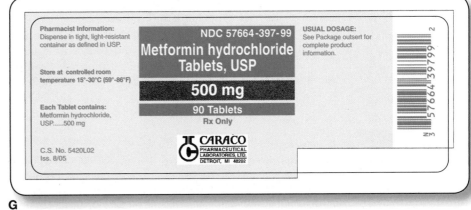

Pharmacist Information:
Dispense in tight, light-resistant container as defined in USP.

Store at controlled room temperature 15°-30°C (59°-86°F)

Each Tablet contains:
Metformin hydrochloride, USP......500 mg

C.S. No. 5420L02
Iss. 8/05

NDC 57664-397-99
Metformin hydrochloride Tablets, USP

500 mg
90 Tablets
Rx Only

USUAL DOSAGE:
See Package outsert for complete product information.

CARACO
PHARMACEUTICAL
LABORATORIES, LTD.
DETROIT, MI 48202

G

46. Which of these is a delayed release drug?

47. Which of these drugs are oral suspensions?

48. Which of these drugs would be administered parenterally?

49. Which medication(s) must be mixed before using?

50. Which medication(s) do not include a trade name?

10.2 Label Information Related to Medication Routes

Oral Medications

Medication labels contain critical information related to the route by which the medication is to be administered. You must read each label carefully and identify this information when calculating doses, or administering or dispensing medications.

Oral, also known as enteral, medications are available in either solid or liquid form. Tablets are the most common form. They may be scored, chewable, or enteric-coated. Scored tablets can be broken into equal portions so that you can administer a partial dosage, if necessary. Chewable tablets must be chewed to be effective. Enteric-coated tablets must be swallowed whole as they are covered with a substance that prevents absorption of the medication until it reaches the small intestine. Chewing them or dividing them breaks the seal provided by their coating, allowing the drug to be absorbed sooner than intended.

Capsules have a gelatin shell that contains the drug. In most cases, they should be swallowed whole. In some cases, capsules may be opened and mixed with food. *Controlled-release capsules*, also called *sustained-release* or *extended-release capsules*, release the drug over a longer time than regular release. If these capsules are not swallowed whole, they may release too much of the drug too quickly for absorption. See the chapter "Oral Dosages" for more information about solid oral medications.

RULE 10-4 You may break tablets to give a partial dose *only* when the tablets are scored. Enteric-coated, controlled-release, extended-release, and sustained-release medications should *never* be crushed or broken.

Abbreviations such as SR, CR, ER, and XL listed after the drug name indicate a special drug action. The SR following the brand name means the drug is designed for *sustained release;* CR means that a drug is *controlled release;* and ER or XL following the brand name means the drug has an *extended-release* mechanism (Figure 10-20).

Liquid oral medications are described as oral solutions, syrups, elixirs, oral suspensions, and simply liquids (see Figures 10-21 and 10-22). In liquid medications, the dosage strength corresponds to a specific volume of the solution, for example, 250 mg/5 mL.

If a medication needs to be reconstituted, the instructions are given on the label.

RULE 10-5 When you reconstitute a drug that is to be used for more than one dose, you must write your initials as well as the time and date of reconstitution on the label. Reconstituted medications are usable only for a certain length of time. The date and time you document will allow others to determine when the medication will expire. Your initials document who reconstituted the medication in case a question arises.

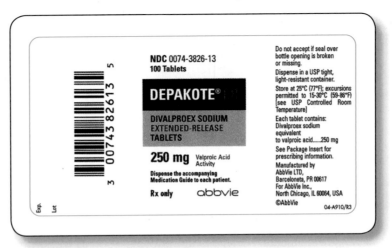

Figure 10-20 Do not break these extended-release tablets.

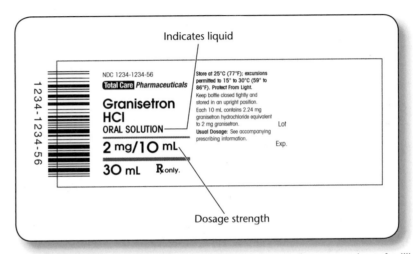

Indicates liquid

Dosage strength

Figure 10-21 For liquid medications the dosage strength corresponds to a number of milligrams per a specific volume of solution.

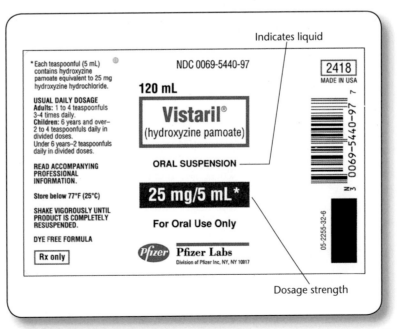

Indicates liquid

Dosage strength

Figure 10-22 The dosage strength is 25 mg per 5 mL for this oral suspension medication.

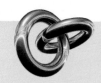

LEARNING LINK   Recall from the chapter "Equipment for Dosage Measurement" that liquids may be measured in droppers, calibrated spoons, medicine cups, or oral syringes. Calibrated cups and spoons are available at most pharmacies and sometimes come with the medication. Advise patients who take oral liquid medications at home to use a medicine cup or baking measuring spoon—not a household cup or spoon—if they do not have calibrated cups or spoons.

PATIENT EDUCATION

Healthcare workers often educate patients about the proper way to take drugs at home. This responsibility may be the duty of the pharmacy technician, the nurse, or the certified medical assistant. If you are authorized to provide patient education, you should take the following steps:

1. Ensure there is no language barrier. If a language barrier exists, obtain a healthcare interpreter.

2. Be sure the patient or caretaker can read and understand the label. Some patients cannot see the fine print on labels. Others do not have the necessary literacy skills.

3. Ask the patient about drug allergies and any medications that he or she may be taking. Check the label or the package insert for drug interactions. Also check with the patient about any over-the-counter medications and herbal remedies being taken.

4. Review the dose, frequency, and length of time the drug is to be taken. Have the patient or caretaker repeat this information to you.

5. Review any special written instructions. Have the patient or caretaker repeat this to you.

6. Describe any adverse effects of the drug that are serious enough to warrant prompt medical attention. Encourage the patient to seek help immediately if these side effects occur. Also discuss side effects that are considered normal.

7. Remind the patient to refer to the label when needed. Emphasize that the patient should call the pharmacy or physician with any questions that cannot be answered from the label or additional written instructions that are provided by the pharmacy.

Parenteral Medications

Parenteral drugs may be packaged in single-use ampules or vials, single-use prefilled syringes, or multiuse vials. These small containers have small labels that have limited space for providing comprehensive information (Figure 10-23). You must read these labels with extra care. You will often need to review the package insert to obtain complete drug information.

Parenteral drugs can be injected intradermally (ID), intramuscularly (IM), intravenously (IV), or subcutaneously (subcut). Parenteral drugs can also be inhalants and **transdermal** (through the skin) medications or any mode of administration other than through the gastrointestinal tract. For example, a medication can be administered into the vagina. The drug label specifies the appropriate route. Trimethobenzamide (generic for Tigan®) is made for IM use only (see Figure 10-10). Primaxin® is a drug that can be administered either intramuscularly or intravenously. Figure 10-24 indicates Camptosar for IV (intravenous) use only.

Recall from earlier in this chapter that on the label of medications, the dosage strength may be labeled as the amount of drug per dosage unit or in units per mL. This is also true for parenteral medication (Figure 10-24). In some cases the label is marked with milligrams and micrograms. Dosage strength may also be expressed in milliequivalents per milliliter or as a percent, which is grams per 100 mL.

Look at the labels for insulin in Figures 10-25 and 10-26. In addition to the standard components, these labels contain information about the origin of the medication and how quickly the insulin takes effect. Insulin is most commonly made from human sources known as recombinant DNA (rDNA). Different types of insulin take effect over different time periods. NPH insulin (Figure 10-25) is an intermediate-acting insulin. Regular insulin (Figure 10-26) is shorter acting. See the chapter "Parenteral Dosages" for more information about insulin.

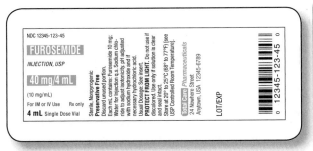

Figure 10-23 Read the label carefully and find complete information on the package insert when needed.

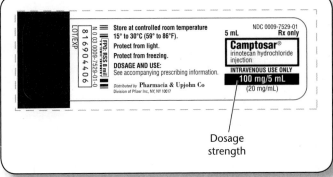

Dosage strength

Figure 10-24 This dosage strength is expressed in milligrams per milliliter: 100 mg/5 mL.

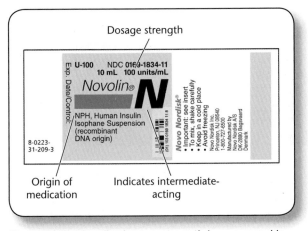

Dosage strength

Origin of medication

Indicates intermediate-acting

Figure 10-25 Insulin dosage strength is expressed in units per milliliter.

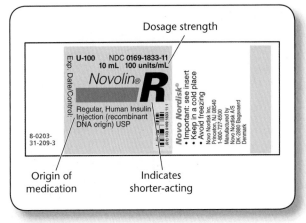

Dosage strength

Origin of medication

Indicates shorter-acting

Figure 10-26 Shorter-acting regular (R) insulin has a dosage strength of 100 units/mL.

Medications Administered by Other Routes

In addition to the oral and injection routes, there are several other routes of medication administration. They include sublingual (under the tongue), buccal (between the gums and cheek), rectal, and vaginal. Drugs may also be administered as topical ointments (used on the skin); eye or ear drops; patches applied to the skin (transdermal delivery); or nasal, oral, and throat inhalants (see Figures 10-27, 10-28, and 10-29).

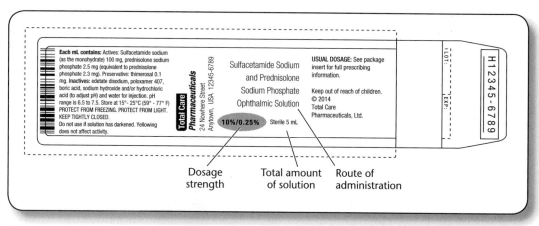

Figure 10-27 This drug is used in the eyes (opthalmic solution).

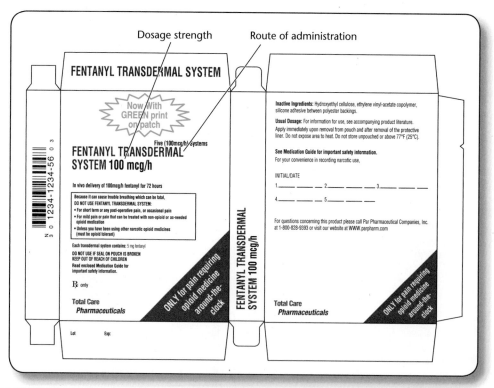

Figure 10-28 Transdermal medications deliver medication through the skin at a specified dosage rate.

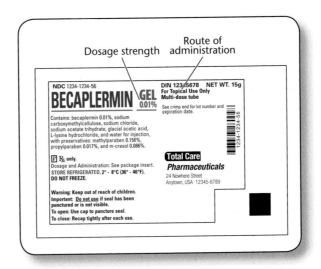

Figure 10-29 This medication is for topical use only.

The dosage strength is expressed slightly differently on these labels. In Figure 10-27, the dosage strength is the percentage of the active ingredients in the solution. Sulfacetamide 10% and prednisolone 0.25% are found in this ophthalmic medication. In Figure 10-28, the dosage rate is given as 100 mcg/h; this drug is absorbed over time through the skin. Thus the dosage rate indicates 100 mcg are delivered each hour. In Figure 10-29, the medication is measured in a percentage. Regranex® has 0.01% becaplermin in a gel base.

REVIEW AND PRACTICE

10.2 Label Information Related to Medication Routes

For Exercises 1–4, refer to label A.

1. What is the NDC number?

2. What is the dosage strength?

3. Can you store this drug on a shelf in the storeroom?

4. How many tablets are in the container?

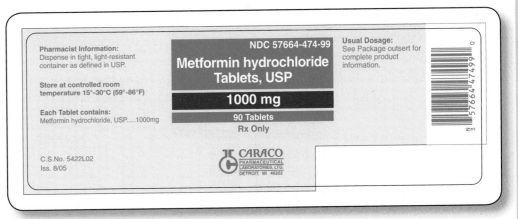

A

For Exercises 5–8, refer to label B.

5. What is the trade name of this drug?

6. Who is the manufacturer?

7. What is the dosage strength?

8. How many tablets are in the container?

For Exercises 9–12, refer to label C.

9. What is the generic name of this drug?

10. How is this medication administered?

11. What is the dosage strength?

12. How many doses are in this vial?

For Exercises 13–16, refer to label D.

13. How many milliliters of water should be used to reconstitute this drug?

14. What is the dosage strength when the drug is mixed?

15. What is the total volume in the container when the drug is mixed?

16. How long can this drug be stored after it is reconstituted?

For Exercises 17–20, refer to label E.

17. What is the generic name of this drug?

18. What is the dosage strength?

19. What is the trade name of this medication?

20. How should this drug be stored?

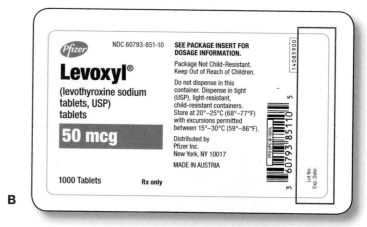

B

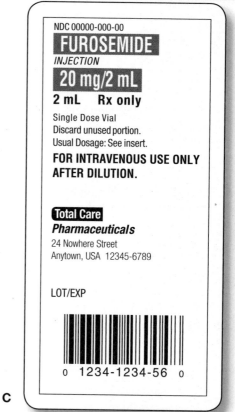

C

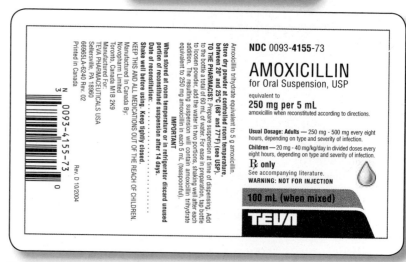

D

This label is for US only, and cannot be altered or translated.

For Exercises 21–25, refer to labels A through E.

21. Which of these medication labels indicate that there are 100 tablets in the bottle?

22. Which of these medications must be mixed before dispensing?

23. Which labels are on multiple-dose containers?

24. Which of these drugs are to be given via the oral route?

25. Which medication is to be given by injection?

For Exercises 26–29, refer to label F.

26. What is the dosage strength?

27. By what route of administration is this drug given?

28. What color is this medication?

29. What is the total volume of medication in this bottle?

For Exercises 30–33, refer to label G.

30. What is the dosage strength of this drug?

31. Who manufactures this medication?

32. What is the generic name of this medication?

33. If you were not familiar with this drug, would you be able to administer it with only the information on the label? Why?

For Exercises 34–37, refer to label H.

34. What are the storage requirements for this medication?

35. What is the dosage strength?

36. By what route of administration is this drug given?

37. If the dose is 50 mg (2 capsules), how many doses does the container hold?

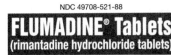

NDC 49708-521-88

FLUMADINE® Tablets
(rimantadine hydrochloride tablets)

Each tablet contains 100 mg rimantadine hydrochloride

R_x only

100 TABLETS

CARACO PHARMA, INC.

Distributed by:
Caraco Pharmaceutical Laboratories, Ltd.
Detroit, MI 48202

USUAL DOSAGE: For dosage, administration and full prescribing information, see package insert.

Dispense in a tight container as defined in the USP.

LOT NO.
EXP. DATE

Manufactured by:
Forest Pharmaceuticals, Inc., St. Louis, MO 63045

Store at 25°C (77°F); excursions permitted to 15-30°C (59-86°F) [see USP Controlled Room Temperature].

C.S. No. 7104L01
Iss. 10/09

MP 00

E

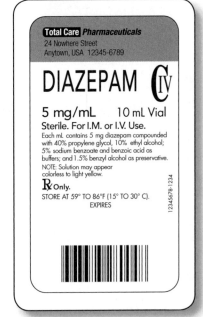

Total Care *Pharmaceuticals*
24 Nowhere Street
Anytown, USA 12345-6789

DIAZEPAM C IV

5 mg/mL   **10 mL Vial**
Sterile. For I.M. or I.V. Use.

Each mL contains 5 mg diazepam compounded with 40% propylene glycol, 10% ethyl alcohol; 5% sodium benzoate and benzoic acid as buffers; and 1.5% benzyl alcohol as preservative.
NOTE: Solution may appear colorless to light yellow.

R Only.
STORE AT 59° TO 86°F (15° TO 30° C).
EXPIRES

12345678-1234

F

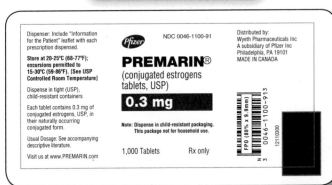

Dispenser: Include "Information for the Patient" leaflet with each prescription dispensed.

Store at 20-25°C (68-77°F); excursions permitted to 15-30°C (59-86°F). [See USP Controlled Room Temperature]

Dispense in tight (USP), child-resistant containers

Each tablet contains 0.3 mg of conjugated estrogens, USP, in their naturally occurring conjugated form.

Usual Dosage: See accompanying descriptive literature.

Visit us at www.PREMARIN.com

Pfizer   NDC 0046-1100-91

PREMARIN®
(conjugated estrogens tablets, USP)

0.3 mg

Note: Dispense in child-resistant packaging. This package not for household use.

1,000 Tablets   Rx only

Distributed by:
Wyeth Pharmaceuticals Inc
A subsidiary of Pfizer Inc
Philadelphia, PA 19101
MADE IN CANADA

FPO (80% x 9.9mm)

0046-1100-913

12110300

G

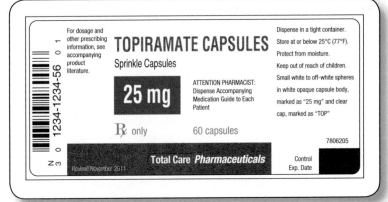

For dosage and other prescribing information, see accompanying product literature.

TOPIRAMATE CAPSULES

Sprinkle Capsules

25 mg

R only   60 capsules

Total Care *Pharmaceuticals*

ATTENTION PHARMACIST:
Dispense Accompanying Medication Guide to Each Patient

Dispense in a tight container.
Store at or below 25°C (77°F).
Protect from moisture.
Keep out of reach of children.
Small white to off-white spheres in white opaque capsule body, marked as "25 mg" and clear cap, marked as "TOP"

7806205

Control
Exp. Date

1234-1234-56   0 1

Revised November 2011

H

For Exercises 38–41, refer to label I.

38. What is the origin of this insulin?

39. What is the dosage strength of the insulin?

40. What is the generic name of this insulin?

41. What is the total volume in this container?

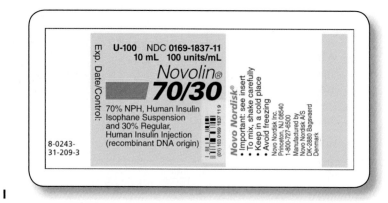

I

For Exercises 42–45, refer to label J.

42. What is the dosage strength?

43. What is the generic name of this medication?

44. How many 100 mg doses does this container hold?

45. What are the storage requirements for this drug?

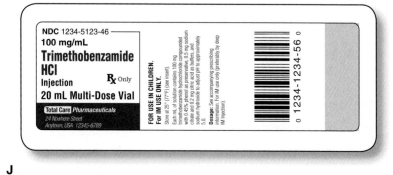

J

For Exercises 46–49, refer to label K.

46. What is the generic name?

47. What is the route of administration?

48. What instructions for administration are indicated on the label?

49. How would this medication be stored?

For Exercises 50–53, refer to label L.

50. By what route is this drug to be administered?

51. What are the drug's storage requirements?

52. What is the dosage strength?

53. What is the generic name of the drug?

K

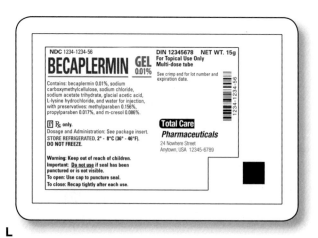

L

For Exercises 54–57, refer to label M.

54. What is the route of administration?

55. What is the generic name of the drug?

56. What is the total volume in the container?

57. What is the name of the manufacturer?

For Exercises 58–61, refer to label N.

58. By what route is this drug delivered?

59. What is the dosage strength?

60. What type of patients should use this medication?

61. How many doses are in this box?

For Exercises 62–65, refer to label O.

62. What is the generic name?

63. What is the dosage strength?

64. By what route is this drug to be administered?

65. How many doses are in this container?

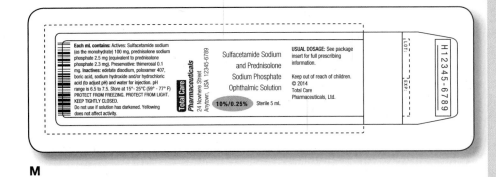

M

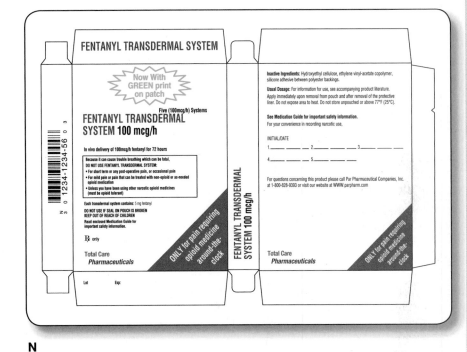

N

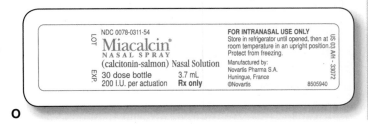

O

Package Inserts

Package inserts, **package outserts**, and **monographs** provide authoritative information about a medication. **Official package inserts** as well as package outserts and monographs provide prescribing information for a medical professional. A **patient package insert** is an easy-to-understand document provided for patients with each medication. Package inserts must be included with every medication as required by the Food and Drug Administration (FDA). Outserts and monographs are found outside the drug package, in medication

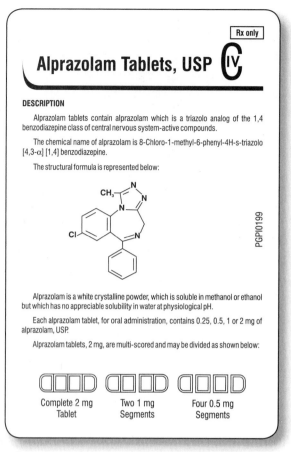

Rx only

Alprazolam Tablets, USP C IV

DESCRIPTION

Alprazolam tablets contain alprazolam which is a triazolo analog of the 1,4 benzodiazepine class of central nervous system-active compounds.

The chemical name of alprazolam is 8-Chloro-1-methyl-6-phenyl-4H-s-triazolo [4,3-α] [1,4] benzodiazepine.

The structural formula is represented below:

PGPI0199

Alprazolam is a white crystalline powder, which is soluble in methanol or ethanol but which has no appreciable solubility in water at physiological pH.

Each alprazolam tablet, for oral administration, contains 0.25, 0.5, 1 or 2 mg of alprazolam, USP.

Alprazolam tablets, 2 mg, are multi-scored and may be divided as shown below:

Complete 2 mg
Tablet

Two 1 mg
Segments

Four 0.5 mg
Segments

Figure 10-30 The top portion of a package insert. Note that this medication is scored and can be broken into two or four segments.

reference books or online at various locations including the FDA, Drug Info Net, RxList, or the *Physician's Desk Reference* (PDR).

In some cases all the information you need to perform a dosage calculation is not provided on the drug label so you must consult the complete prescribing information in order to prepare, dispense, or administer the medication. For example, when reconstituting medications you may need to review the specifics about additives and resulting dosage strengths. Figure 10-30 shows a portion of a package insert. Table 10-1 summarizes the sections of a package insert.

TABLE 10-1 Sections of a Package Insert

SECTION	DESCRIPTION	EXAMPLE INFORMATION
Description	Chemical and physical description of the drug	Alprazolam tablets contain alprazolam which is a triazolo analog of the 1,4 benzodiazepine class of central nervous system-active compounds. The chemical name of alprazolam is 8-Chloro-1-methyl-6-phenyl-4H-s-triazolo [4,3-α] [1,4] benzodiazepine. The structural formula is represented below:

TABLE 10-1 Continued

SECTION	DESCRIPTION	EXAMPLE INFORMATION
Clinical pharmacology	Description of the actions of the drug	CNS agents of the 1,4 benzodiazepine class presumably exert their effects by binding at stereo specific receptors at several sites within the central nervous system. Their exact mechanism of action is unknown. Clinically, all benzodiazepines cause a dose-related central nervous system depressant activity varying from mild impairment of task performance to hypnosis.
Indications and usage	Medical conditions in which the drug is safe and effective; instructions for use	Alprazolam tablets are indicated for the management of anxiety disorder (a condition corresponding most closely to the *APA Diagnostic and Statistical Manual* [DSM-III-R] diagnosis of generalized anxiety disorder) or the short-term relief of symptoms of anxiety. Anxiety or tension associated with the stress of everyday life usually does not require treatment with an anxiolytic.
Contraindications	Conditions and situations under which the drug should not be administered	Alprazolam tablets are contraindicated in patients with known sensitivity to this drug or other benzodiazepines. Alprazolam tablets may be used in patients with open angle glaucoma who are receiving appropriate therapy, but is contraindicated in patients with acute narrow angle glaucoma.
Warnings	Information about serious, possibly fatal, side effects	*Dependence and withdrawal reactions, including seizures.*
Precautions	Information about drug interactions and other conditions that may cause unwanted side effects	*Use with other CNS depressants:* If alprazolam tablets are to be combined with other psychotropic agents or anticonvulsant drugs, careful consideration should be given to the pharmacology of the agents to be employed, particularly with compounds that might potentiate the action of benzodiazepines.
Adverse reactions	Less serious, anticipated side effects that can be caused by the drug	Side effects to alprazolam tablets, if they occur, are generally observed at the beginning of therapy and usually disappear upon continued medication. In the usual patient, the most frequent side effects are likely to be an extension of the pharmacological activity of alprazolam, e.g., drowsiness or light-headedness.
Drug abuse and dependence	Information about potential abuse and withdrawal symptoms, if necessary	*Physical and Psychological Dependence:* Withdrawal symptoms similar in character to those noted with sedative/hypnotics and alcohol have occurred following discontinuance of benzodiazepines, including alprazolam tablets.
Highlights	Includes most important prescribing information including benefits and risks.	These highlights do not include all the information needed to use alprazolam safely and effectively. See full prescribing information for alprazolam.
Overdosage	Effects of overdoses and instructions for treatment	Manifestations of alprazolam overdosage include somnolence, confusion, impaired coordination, diminished reflexes and coma. Death has been reported in association with overdoses of alprazolam by itself, as it has with other benzodiazepines. In addition, fatalities have been reported in patients who have overdosed with a combination of a single benzodiazepine, including alprazolam, and alcohol; alcohol levels seen in some of these patients have been lower than those usually associated with alcohol-induced fatality.

(Continued)

TABLE 10-1 Continued

SECTION	DESCRIPTION	EXAMPLE INFORMATION
Dosage and administration	Recommended dosages under various conditions and recommendations for administration routes	Dosage should be individualized for maximum beneficial effect. While the usual daily dosages will meet the needs of most patients, there will be some who require doses greater than 4 mg/day. In such cases, dosage should be increased cautiously to avoid adverse effects.
Preparation for administration	Directions for reconstituting or diluting the drug, if necessary	Alprazolam tablets do not require any preparation so this section is not included. This section is essential when reconstituting medications.
Manufacturer supply	Information on dosage strengths and forms of the drug available	Alprazolam tablets are available as follows: **0.25 mg** (white, oval, biconvex, uncoated tablets, debossed with "603" on one side and breakline on the other side) Bottles of 30's with CRC.....NDC 47335-603-83

Courtesy of Caraco Pharmaceutical Laboratories.

REVIEW AND PRACTICE

10.3 Package Inserts

Match the sections of the package insert to the descriptions.

1. Description
2. Clinical pharmacology
3. Indications and usage
4. Contraindications
5. Warnings
6. Precautions
7. Adverse reactions
8. Drug abuse and dependence
9. Highlights
10. Overdosage
11. Dosage and administration
12. Preparation for administration
13. Manufacturer supply

a. Information on dosage strengths and forms of the drug available

b. Less serious, anticipated side effects that can be caused by the drug

c. Information about potential abuse and withdrawal symptoms, if necessary

d. Effects of overdoses and instructions for treatment

e. Chemical and physical description of the drug

f. Recommended dosages under various conditions and recommendations for administration routes

g. Description of the actions of the drug

h. Medical conditions in which the drug is safe and effective; instructions for use

i. Directions for reconstituting or diluting the drug, if necessary

j. Conditions and situations under which the drug should not be administered

k. Information about drug interactions and other conditions that may cause unwanted side effects

l. Includes most important prescribing information including benefits and risks.

m. Information about serious, possibly fatal, side effects

LEARNING OUTCOME	KEY POINTS
10.1 Interpret information on a medication label. Pages 186–200	Drug Name ▶ Generic—official name recorded in the *US Pharmacopeia* (USP) and *National Formulary* (NF) ▶ Trade (brand) name identified as such with registered trademark Form of Drug ▶ Solid—tablet, capsule, caplet, gelcap ▶ Liquid—oral liquid, injectable liquid, inhalant, drop, spray, mist ▶ Other—ointment, cream, lotion, patches, suppositories, shampoo Dosage Strength—amount of drug per dosage unit, e.g., 1 g/tablet or 500 mg/5 mL Combination Drugs—must list the generic name and the dosage strength of each medication in the combination, e.g., Lortab 5/500 = 5 mg of hydrocodone bitartrate with 500 mg of acetaminophen Total Volume Route of Administration Warnings Storage Information Manufacturing Information—pharmaceutical company, expiration date, lot number, bar code, and National Drug Code (NDC) Reconstitution Information—directions for mixing the medication
10.2 Distinguish information related to administration routes for medications. Pages 200–209	Oral (Enteral) Medications—medications given via the gastrointestinal (GI) tract ▶ Tablets • Scored tablets may be divided for partial dosing • Chewable tablets must be chewed to be effective • Enteric-coated (EC) tablets must be swallowed whole to protect coating that prevents absorption of medication until it reaches the small intestine • RULES: Do not break a tablet unless it is scored. Do not break or crush EC tablets.

LEARNING OUTCOME	KEY POINTS

	▶ Capsules
	   • Usually swallowed whole; some may be opened and mixed with food
	   • Controlled-release capsules, which release drug over a long period of time, are identified as sustained release (SR) or extended release (ER, XL)
	   • RULE: Do not crush or break ER, SR, XL capsules.
	▶ Liquids
	   • Available in syrups, elixirs, suspensions, solutions
	   • Reconstituted solutions should be labeled with initials as well as the date and time medication was mixed.
	   • Calibrated equipment should be used for administration.
	Parenteral Medications—medications given outside the GI tract
	▶ Injection routes—intradermal (ID), intramuscular (IM), intravenous (IV), subcutaneous (subcut)
	▶ Other routes—inhalant, transdermal, sublingual (SL), buccal (between the gum and the cheek), rectal, vaginal, topical, eye or ear drops

10.3 Find information on package inserts, needed for dosage calculations. Pages 209–212	Package insert information may need to be consulted in order to prepare, dispense, or administer medication. The package insert includes the following sections:
	   • complete chemical description
	   • indications and usage
	   • contraindications
	   • warnings
	   • precautions
	   • adverse reactions
	   • drug abuse and dependence
	   • highlights
	   • overdosage
	   • dosage and administration
	   • preparation for administration
	   • manufacturer supply

Use the identified drug labels to answer the following questions: (LO 10.1 to LO 10.3)

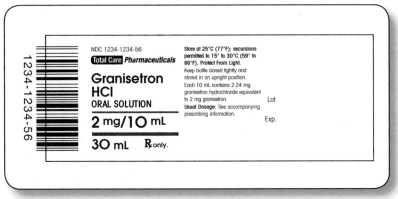

A

Label A

1. What is the generic name of this drug?

2. List three items of storage information on this label.

3. What is the total drug volume of the container?

4. 2 mg of the drug is equal to how many milliliters?

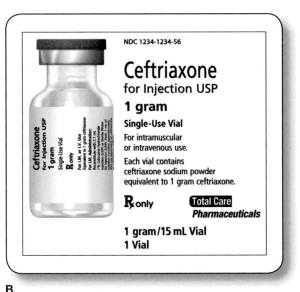

B

Ceftriaxone for Injection USP **1 gram**

Directions For Use:

For I.M. Administration: Reconstitute with 2.1 mL 1% Lidocaine Hydrochloride Injection (USP) or Sterile Water for Injection (USP). Each 1 mL of solution contains approximately 350 mg equivalent of ceftriaxone as ceftriaxone sodium.

For I.V. Administration: Reconstitute with 4.8 mL of an I.V. diluent specified in the accompanying package insert. Each 1 mL of solution contains approximately 100 mg equivalent of ceftriaxone as ceftriaxone sodium.

Withdraw entire contents and dilute to the desired concentration with the appropriate I.V. diluent.

Usual dosage: For dosage recommendations and other important prescribing information, read accompanying insert.

Storage Prior to Reconstitution: Store at 20°–25°C (68°–77°F) [see USP Controlled Room Temperature].

Protect From Light.

Storage After Reconstitution: See package insert.

Total Care *Pharmaceuticals*
24 Nowhere Street
Anytown, USA 12345-6789

N 0   1234-1234-56   0

Label B

5. What is the generic name of this drug?

6. What two routes of administration are listed on this label?

7. What are the reconstitution directions for an IM injection?

8. How many times may this vial be used?

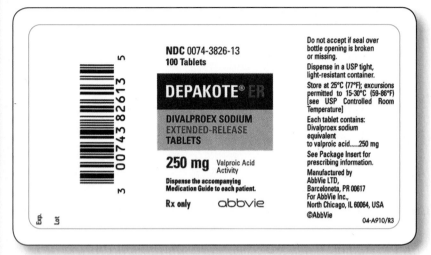

NDC 0074-3826-13
100 Tablets

DEPAKOTE® ER

DIVALPROEX SODIUM
EXTENDED-RELEASE
TABLETS

250 mg Valproic Acid Activity

Dispense the accompanying
Medication Guide to each patient.

Rx only   abbvie

Do not accept if seal over bottle opening is broken or missing.
Dispense in a USP tight, light-resistant container.
Store at 25°C (77°F); excursions permitted to 15-30°C (59-86°F) [see USP Controlled Room Temperature]
Each tablet contains: Divalproex sodium equivalent to valproic acid......250 mg
See Package Insert for prescribing information.
Manufactured by AbbVie LTD, Barceloneta, PR 00617
For AbbVie Inc., North Chicago, IL 60064, USA
©AbbVie
04-A910/R3

C

Label C

9. What is the brand name of this drug?

10. What does ER after the drug name mean?

11. How many tablets are in the container?

12. What is the name of the manufacturer?

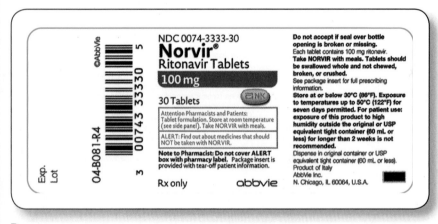

NDC 0074-3333-30
Norvir®
Ritonavir Tablets
100 mg

30 Tablets   NK

Attention Pharmacists and Patients:
Tablet formulation. Store at room temperature (see side panel). Take NORVIR with meals.

ALERT: Find out about medicines that should NOT be taken with NORVIR.

Note to Pharmacist: Do not cover ALERT box with pharmacy label. Package insert is provided with tear-off patient information.

Rx only   abbvie

Do not accept if seal over bottle opening is broken or missing.
Each tablet contains 100 mg ritonavir.
Take NORVIR with meals. Tablets should be swallowed whole and not chewed, broken, or crushed.
See package insert for full prescribing information.
Store at or below 30°C (86°F). Exposure to temperatures up to 50°C (122°F) for seven days permitted. For patient use: exposure of this product to high humidity outside the original or USP equivalent tight container (60 mL or less) for longer than 2 weeks is not recommended.
Dispense in original container or USP equivalent tight container (60 mL or less).
Product of Italy
AbbVie Inc.
N. Chicago, IL 60064, U.S.A.

D

Label D

13. What is the generic name of this drug?

14. If the usual dose is one tablet, how many doses are available in this container?

15. Can this medication be crushed?

16. At what temperature should this medication be stored?

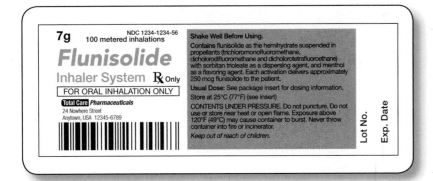

Label E

17. What is the route of administration for this drug?

18. Approximately how much medication is delivered with each inhalation?

19. How many inhalations are in this container?

20. What are the before-use instructions for this drug?

21. What section of the package insert would be used to determine how to reconstitute a medication?

CHECK UP

1. Distinguish a drug's trade name from its generic name. (LO 10.1)

2. Which name, generic or trade name, is followed by the symbol ®? (LO 10.1)

3. Explain the difference between IM and IV. (LO 10.2)

4. List the types of tablets that cannot be divided, broken, or crushed for administration, and explain why. (LO 10.2)

5. Describe when you would use a package insert. (LO 10.1)

6. Explain the importance of a lot number. (LO 10.1)

In Exercises 7–10, refer to label A. (LO 10.1)

7. What is the dosage strength of the drug?

8. How many tablets of medication are in this container?

9. What is the name of the manufacturer of the drug?

10. How is it administered?

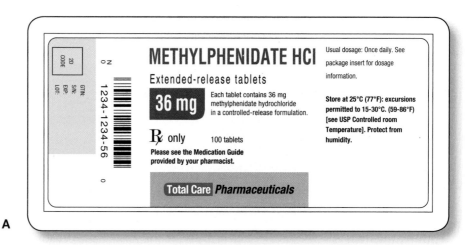

A

In Exercises 11–14, refer to label B. (LO 10.1)

11. What is the generic name of this drug?

12. How is this drug administered?

13. What is the dosage strength?

14. How many doses are in the container?

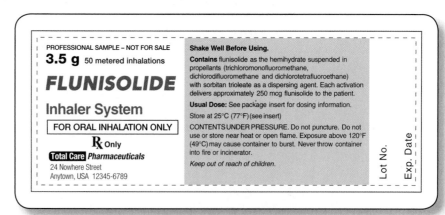

B

In Exercises 15–18, refer to label C. (LO 10.1)

15. How is this drug administered?

16. What is the dosage strength?

17. What is the drug name?

18. How many capsules are in the container?

In Exercises 19–22, refer to label D. (LO 10.1)

19. What is the origin of this insulin?

20. What word on the label describes the time frame in which this insulin acts?

21. How is this drug administered?

22. What is the dosage strength?

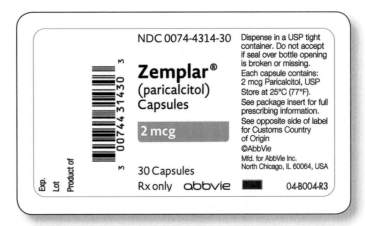

C

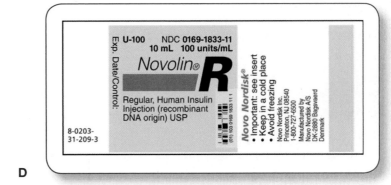

D

CRITICAL THINKING APPLICATION

You are working in a clinic that serves many adult homeless people. Two forms of erythromycin are available (see labels below). If the patient needs to take erythromycin for 5 days, which form of the medication would be better and why? (LO 10.2)

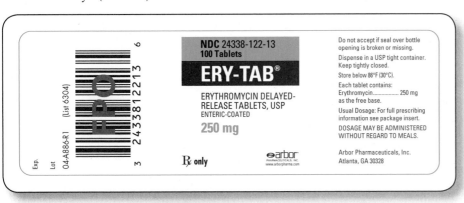

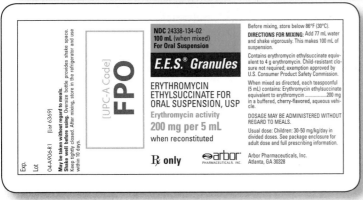

CASE STUDY

A drug order reads Gentamicin 5 mg IV now. (LO 10.2)

You have available a drug with the following label:

1. What would you do to prepare for administering this drug?

2. How would you administer the drug?

3. What would you do with the vial after administering a dose of the drug?

4. Where would you look to see what other forms of this medication are supplied by the manufacturer?

Gentamicin
Pediatric INJECTION, USP
equivalent to 10 mg/mL

20 mg/2 mL

For IM or IV Use.
Must be diluted for IV use.
2 mL Single Dose Vial
Preservative Free   Rx Only
Sterile, Nonpyrogenic

Total Care *Pharmaceuticals*
24 Nowhere Street
Anytown, USA 12345-6789

LOT/EXP

0 1234-1234-56 0

connect

Now that you have completed the materials in the chapter text, go to CONNECT and complete any chapter activities you have not yet done.

Safe Medication Administration

"It is better to be safe than sorry."

AMERICAN PROVERB

LEARNING OUTCOMES

When you have completed Chapter 11, you will be able to:

11.1 Apply The Joint Commission steps to receiving and writing a verbal order.

11.2 Execute safe transcription practices.

11.3 Identify error-prone abbreviations and symbols.

11.4 Identify the three checks in the medication administration procedure.

11.5 Implement the "rights" of medication administration.

11.6 Recognize the importance of observation in safe medication administration.

11.7 Describe the appropriate use of patient teaching as it relates to safe drug administration.

INTRODUCTION

Medication errors are mistakes in prescribing, dispensing, and administering medications. According to Mayo Clinic, medication errors injure more than 1 million people a year in the United States. The importance of safe medication administration cannot be overstated. Medication administration is a complex process that may involve several individuals (the authorized prescriber, the pharmacist, and the healthcare practitioner who administers the medication), often from several departments. The elements of safe medication administration include prescription, transcription, three "checks" of medication administration, "rights of medication administration," observation, and patient teaching. This chapter will focus on the vital role of the healthcare professional in preventing medication errors by attending to the elements of safe medication administration.

The first step in the medication delivery process is the medication order or prescription. The prescription is one type of medication order. You already know that a medication order can be written on a prescription tablet (pad) or printed through an electronic health record. Healthcare practitioners must verify the parts of a medication order to dispense or administer medications safely.

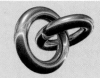

LEARNING LINK Recall the components of a medication order addressed in the chapter "Interpreting Medication Orders": name of patient, patient's date of birth, date and time the order is written, drug name, drug dose, route, time and/or frequency of medication administration, and signature of authorized prescriber (AP).

11.1 Verbal Orders

Usually, orders must be written and/or personally signed by hand or electronically by the licensed prescribing practitioner. However, if the authorized prescriber is not able to write an order that must be carried out quickly, verbal orders may be permitted. This may occur, for example, when a physician is performing a sterile procedure on the patient, and verbally orders that the patient receive a sedative, to facilitate the safe completion of the procedure.

Verbal orders are orders from an authorized prescriber stated directly, in person or via the telephone, to a nurse or other practitioner whose scope of practice includes the authorization to receive and document such orders. State laws govern which personnel may accept such orders and how soon the prescriber must countersign them. Accepting verbal orders is a serious task, since it can readily lead to medication errors. Most healthcare agencies limit the use of verbal orders, so learn the agency's policy before accepting a verbal order. To minimize errors when receiving verbal orders, **The Joint Commission (TJC)**, the accrediting body for healthcare organizations, has identified three guidelines for verbal orders:

1. **Write the order.** If you are legally permitted to accept a telephone order, write it carefully and legibly *as* you receive it, *not after* the call. In some cases, you may write the order on the physician's order form, identifying it as a verbal order. Verify that all components of the medication order are included. For example, if the AP forgets to include the route, ask: "By what route would you like that medication administered?"

2. **Read the order.** Read the order back to the prescribing practitioner to verify that you have transcribed it correctly. If you are not certain of the spelling of the drug name, ask the prescriber to spell it. Many drugs have names that are pronounced or spelled similarly.

3. **Confirm the order.** Get confirmation from the prescriber that the order is correct.

ERROR ALERT!

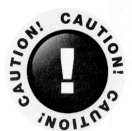

Always Be Certain That You Are Administering

and/or Dispensing the Correct Medication

Many drugs have names that are very similar. Read the order carefully and, when in doubt, contact the authorized prescriber. The following list gives just a few examples of how similar the names of different drugs can look and sound. It is especially easy to confuse them when they are written rather than printed.

Accupril—Aciphex	Dioval—Diovan	Neurontin—Motrin
Benadryl—Benazepril	Epinephrine—Ephedrine	Novolin—Humulin
Cozaar—Zocor	Heparin—Hespan	Oxycontin—Oxycodone
Clozaril—Colazal	Inderal—Adderall	Quinidine—Quinine
Darvon—Diovan	Iodine—Lodine	Regranex—Granulex
Diamox—Diabinese	Neulasta—Lunesta	Topomax—Toprol-XL

For example, Nurse Jones is receiving a telephone order from Dr. Smith for patient Robert Brown. After physician and nurse have identified themselves, and then identified the patient by double identifier, the order would proceed as follows:

Step 1: The *authorized prescriber* states the order:

"Acetaminophen every four hours as needed for fever greater than 101."

The *receiver* writes the order as stated:

Acetaminophen   q4h prn fever greater than 101

The *receiver* asks:

"How much acetaminophen and by what route should it be administered?"

The *authorized prescriber* states:

"650 mg po"

The *receiver* fills in the blanks as the order is stated:

Acetaminophen 650 mg po q4h prn fever greater than 101

Step 2: The *receiver* reads the order back to the prescriber, as written:

"OK, that is: acetaminophen 650 mg po q4h prn fever greater than 101."

Step 3: The *receiver* continues on to confirm the order:

"Is that correct?"

The *authorized prescriber* answers "yes."

The order would have the date and time recorded, and the signature would begin: T.O. (for telephone order), and have the AP's name and license printed, followed by the receiver's professional signature.

Date/time   Acetaminophen 650 mg po q4h prn fever greater than 101

T.O. S. Smith, MD/J. Jones, RN

Note that once the verbal order is included on the patient medical record, the authorized prescriber must go back into the medical record and provide a signature, usually within 24 hours. So if you take a verbal order, you should verify at a later date that the order is signed by the authorized prescriber.

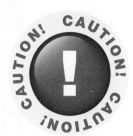

ERROR ALERT!

Never Guess What the Prescriber Meant

If an order is not legible, always contact the authorized prescriber to clarify the order.

In Figure 11-1, the physician intended to order Zyrtec® 10 mg po qd. However, the order is illegible, and you could read Zantac®. The loop on the m in mg could be an extra zero, or 100 mg. A small extra loop in qd makes it hard to tell if the order is *qd* (once every day) or qod (every other day).

Note: The abbreviations qd and qod are on the "Do not use" list by TJC. The physician should not use them, but instead write *daily*.

Because you bear the responsibility of administering the correct dose at the correct frequency, you must contact the physician to clarify the order. Also contact the physician if any part of the order is missing.

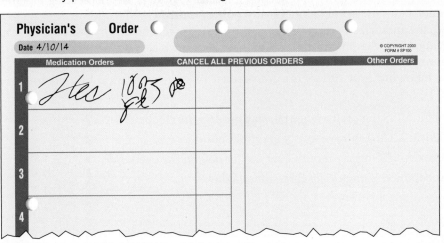

Figure 11-1 Handwritten physician's orders can be difficult to read.

11.1 Verbal Orders

Complete the steps the receiver will take during a verbal order:
The nurse is receiving a telephone order from the physician. The physician and nurse have identified themselves, and then identified the patient by double identifier.

Step 1: The *authorized prescriber* states the order: "cefixime 200 mg every 12 hours for 10 days"

   The receiver writes: _____

   The receiver asks: _____

   The *authorized prescriber* states: "by mouth"

   The receiver fills in the blanks as the order is stated: cefixime 200 mg po q12h for 10 days

Step 2: *The receiver* states: _____

Step 3: *The receiver* continues on to confirm the order: _____

11.2 Safe Medication Order Transcription

Transcription of a medication order is the process of taking the information from the prescribing practitioner's order (prescription) and transferring it to the prescription label for outpatient settings (done by a pharmacist) or to the medication administration record (MAR) (done by a nurse or pharmacist) for inpatient settings. *Incorrect transcription is one of the main causes of medication errors.* Although the transcription process may not be the responsibility of the person who is administering medications, it is the duty of the registered nurse in the inpatient setting to ensure that a transcribed order is accurate and complete before signing off an order for implementation. It is important that the transcriber be familiar with medical terminology and abbreviations. If the medication order is not written neatly and is difficult to interpret, the nurse must contact the authorized prescriber for clarification. An entry on the order sheet should be written, reflecting the clarification. If the medicating practitioner does not understand an abbreviation, or any part of a medication order as it is written or transcribed, the authorized prescriber or pharmacist, or registered nurse, should be contacted for clarification. Transcribing identifying information, such as the patient name, is also necessary to ensure a safe medication order transcription.

The following four orders are transcribed on the medication administration record in Figure 11-2.

- Dilantin 125 mg orally twice per day around the clock
- Cleocin 225 mg intravenously every six hours
- Digoxin 0.125 mg by mouth every other day on the even days
- Probanthine 15 mg orally three times a day

Medication Administration Record (MAR)

MO/YR: 2/2014 Start/Stop Date		Facility Name: RIMC																																
Medication		Hour	1	2	3	4	5	6	7	8	9	10	11	12	13	14	15	16	17	18	19	20	21	22	23	24	25	26	27	28	29	30	31
Dilantin 125 mg PO q12h	Start	0800																																
		2000																																
	Stop																																	
Cleocin 225 mg IV q6h	Start	0600																																
		1200																																
		1800																																
		2400																																
	Stop																																	
Digoxin 0.125 mg PO every other day; even days	Start	0800	X		X		X		X		X		X		X		X		X		X		X		X		X		X		X		X
	Stop																																	
Probanthine 15 mg PO tid	Start	0600																																
		1400																																
		2200																																
	Stop																																	
	Start																																		
	Start																																		
	Start																																		
	Stop																																	

Diagnosis: angina

Allergies: NKA

DIET (Special instructions. e.g. Texture, Bite Size, Position, etc.)
NPO

Physician Name: **Jack Buckwalter, DO**

Phone Number

Comments

A. Put initials in appropriate box when medication is given.
B. Circle initials when not given.
C. State reason for refusal / omission on back of form.
D. PRN Medications: Reason given and results must be noted on back of form.
E. Legend: S = School; H = Home visit; W = Work; P = Program.

NAME: **Kaylyn Renee White**

Record #

Date of Birth: **6/26/54** Sex: **F**

VITAL SIGNS	1	2	3	4	5	6	7	8	9	10	11	12	13	14	15	16	17	18	19	20	21	22	23	24	25	26	27	28	29	30	31
TEMPERATURE																															
PULSE																															
RESPIRATION																															
WEIGHT																															

PRN AND MEDICATIONS NOT ADMINSTERED								Initials	Staff Signature
Date	Hour	Initials	Medication	Reason		Result			
							1		
							2		
							3		
							4		
							5		

Figure 11-2 Medication administration record sample.

11.2 Safe Medication Order Transcription

Use the information below to complete Exercises 1–3 on the medication administration record. Transcribe orders E, F, and G on the medication order form to the MAR.

- t.i.d. = 6 a.m.–2 p.m.–10 p.m.
- daily = 10 a.m.
- bedtime = 10 p.m.

Rhode Island Medical Center
Coventry, Rhode Island
Medication Order Form

Jane Doe   DOB 9/22/50
1534 Hopkins Trail Chepachet, RI 01222
MR# 123456789

Diagnosis: Urinary Retention

Allergies: NONE

Date	Time	
1/3/14	8AM	E probanthine 15 mg po t.i.d
		F heparin 10,000 units subout daily
		G diphenhydramine 50 mg PO at bedtime
		Mark Sanger, MD

Medication Administration Record (MAR)

MO/YR: Start/Stop Date		Facility Name:																															
Medication		Hour	1	2	3	4	5	6	7	8	9	10	11	12	13	14	15	16	17	18	19	20	21	22	23	24	25	26	27	28	29	30	31
Exercise 1: Order E	Start																																	
	Stop																																	
Exercise 2: Order F	Start																																	
	Stop																																	
Exercise 3: Order G	Start																																	
	Stop																																	

Diagnosis:	DIET (Special instructions. e.g. Texture, Bite Size, Position, etc.)	Comments
Allergies:	Physician Name	A. Put initials in appropriate box when medication is given.
		B. Circle initials when not given.
	Phone Number	C. State reason for refusal / omission on back of form.
		D. PRN Medications: Reason given and results must be noted on back of from.
		E. Legend: S = School; H = Home visit; W = Work; P = Program.
NAME:	Record #	Date of Birth:	Sex:

11.3 Error-Prone Abbreviations and Symbols

The Joint Commission (TJC) and the **Institute for Safe Medication Practice (ISMP)** are two healthcare organizations whose mission includes promotion of patient safety. These organizations have identified frequently misinterpreted abbreviations and symbols that have contributed to harmful medication errors. To reduce transcription errors, TJC, in 2005, published the *Official "Do Not Use" List,* a standardized list of abbreviations, acronyms, and symbols (U, IU, QD, QOD, trailing zero, lack of leading zero, MS, MSO_4, $MgSO_4$) that are not to be used on prescriptions and medication orders. The ISMP publishes a more comprehensive *ISMP's List of Error-Prone Abbreviations, Symbols, and Dose Designations* which is updated periodically. This list includes all of the abbreviations on TJC's "Do Not Use" list, denoting them with a double asterisk (**). The ISMP, through its Medication Errors Reporting Program, has compiled this table of error-prone abbreviations that should *not* be used in the processes of prescription and transcription. It is found at http://www.ismp.org/tools/errorproneabbreviations.pdf and in Table 11-1. Although you may see these on preprinted order sheets, *do not use* the error-prone abbreviations when transcribing an order.

TABLE 11-1 ISMP's List of Error-Prone Abbreviations, Symbols, and Dose Designations*

ABBREVIATIONS	INTENDED MEANING	MISINTERPRETATION	CORRECTION
μg	Microgram	Mistaken as "mg"	Use "mcg"
AD, AS, AU	Right ear, left ear, each ear	Mistaken as OD, OS, OU (right eye, left eye, each eye)	Use "right ear," "left ear," or "each ear"
OD, OS, OU	Right eye, left eye, each eye	Mistaken as AD, AS, AU (right ear, left ear, each ear)	Use "right eye," "left eye," or "each eye"
BT	Bedtime	Mistaken as "BID" (twice daily)	Use "bedtime"
cc	Cubic centimeters	Mistaken as "u" (units)	Use "mL"
D/C	Discharge or discontinue	Premature discontinuation of medications if D/C (intended to mean "discharge") has been misinterpreted as "discontinued" when followed by a list of discharge medications	Use "discharge" and "discontinue"
IJ	Injection	Mistaken as "IV" or "intrajugular"	Use "injection"
IN	Intranasal	Mistaken as "IM" or "IV"	Use "intranasal" or "NAS"
HS hs	Half-strength At bedtime, hours of sleep	Mistaken as bedtime Mistaken as half-strength	Use "half-strength" or "bedtime"
IU**	International unit	Mistaken as IV (intravenous) or 10 (ten)	Use "units"
o.d. or OD	Once daily	Mistaken as "right eye" (OD-oculus dexter), leading to oral liquid medications administered in the eye	Use "daily"
OJ	Orange juice	Mistaken as OD or OS (right or left eye); drugs meant to be diluted in orange juice may be given in the eye	Use "orange juice"
Per os	By mouth, orally	The "os" can be mistaken as "left eye" (OS-oculus sinister)	Use "PO," "by mouth," or "orally"

(Continued)

TABLE 11-1 Continued

ABBREVIATIONS	INTENDED MEANING	MISINTERPRETATION	CORRECTION
q.d. or QD**	Every day	Mistaken as q.i.d., especially if the period after the "q" or the tail of the "q" is misunderstood as an "i"	Use "daily"
qhs	Nightly at bedtime	Mistaken as "qhr" or every hour	Use "nightly"
qn	Nightly or at bedtime	Mistaken as "qh" (every hour)	Use "nightly" or "at bedtime"
q.o.d. or QOD**	Every other day	Mistaken as "q.d." (daily) or "q.i.d." (four times daily) if the "o" is poorly written	Use "every other day"
q1d	Daily	Mistaken as q.i.d. (four times daily)	Use "daily"
q6PM, etc.	Every evening at 6 PM	Mistaken as every 6 hours	Use "daily at 6 PM" or "6 PM daily"
SC, SQ, sub q	Subcutaneous	SC mistaken as SL (sublingual); SQ mistaken as "5 every"; the "q" in "sub q" has been mistaken as "every" (e.g., a heparin dose ordered "sub q 2 hours before surgery" misunderstood as every 2 hours before surgery)	Use "subcut" or "subcutaneously"
ss	Sliding scale (insulin) or $\frac{1}{2}$ (apothecary)	Mistaken as "55"	Spell out "sliding scale"; use "one-half" or "$\frac{1}{2}$"
SSRI	Sliding scale regular insulin	Mistaken as selective-serotonin reuptake inhibitor	Spell out "sliding scale (insulin)"
SSI	Sliding scale insulin	Mistaken as Strong Solution of Iodine (Lugol's)	
i/d	One daily	Mistaken as "tid"	Use "1 daily"
TIW or tiw	TIW: 3 times a week BIW: 2 times a week	TIW mistaken as "3 times a day"	Use "3 times weekly"
U or u**	Unit	Mistaken as the number 0 or 4, causing a 10-fold overdose or greater (e.g., 4U seen as "40" or 4u seen as "44"); mistaken as "cc" so dose given in volume instead of units (e.g., 4u seen as 4cc)	Use "unit"
UD	As directed ("ut dictum")	Mistaken as unit dose (e.g., diltiazem 125 mg IV infusion "UD" misinterpreted as meaning to give the entire infusion as a unit [bolus] dose)	Use "as directed"

DOSE DESIGNATIONS AND OTHER INFORMATION	INTENDED MEANING	MISINTERPRETATION	CORRECTION
Trailing zero after decimal point (e.g., 1.0 mg)**	1 mg	Mistaken as 10 mg if the decimal point is not seen	Do not use trailing zeros for doses expressed in whole numbers
"Naked" decimal point (e.g., .5 mg)**	0.5 mg	Mistaken as 5 mg if the decimal point is not seen	Use zero before a decimal point when the dose is less than a whole unit

TABLE 11-1 Continued

ABBREVIATIONS	INTENDED MEANING	MISINTERPRETATION	CORRECTION
Abbreviations such as mg. or mL. with a period following the abbreviation	mg mL	The period is unnecessary and could be mistaken as the number 1 if written poorly	Use mg, mL, etc. without a terminal period
Drug name and dose run together (especially problematic for drug names that end in "l" such as Inderal 40 mg; Tegretol 300 mg)	Inderal 40 mg Tegretol 300 mg	Mistaken as Inderal 140 mg Mistaken as Tegretol 1,300 mg	Place adequate space between the drug name, dose, and unit of measure
Numerical dose and unit of measure run together (e.g., 10mg, 100mL)	10 mg 100 mL	The "m" is sometimes mistaken as a zero or two zeros, risking a 10- to 100-fold overdose	Place adequate space between the dose and unit of measure
Large doses without properly placed commas (e.g., 100000 units; 1000000 units)	100,000 units 1,000,000 units	100000 has been mistaken as 10,000 or 1,000,000; 1000000 has been mistaken as 100,000	Use commas for dosing units at or above 1,000, or use words such as 100 "thousand" or 1 "million" to improve readability

DRUG NAME ABBREVIATIONS	INTENDED MEANING	MISINTERPRETATION	CORRECTION
APAP	acetaminophen	Not recognized as acetaminophen	Use complete drug name
ARA A	vidarabine	Mistaken as cytarabine (ARA C)	Use complete drug name
AZT	zidovudine (Retrovir)	Mistaken as azathioprine or aztreonam	Use complete drug name
CPZ	Compazine (prochlorperazine)	Mistaken as chlorpromazine	Use complete drug name
DPT	Demerol-Phenergan-Thorazine	Mistaken as diphtheria-pertussis-tetanus (vaccine)	Use complete drug name
DTO	Diluted tincture of opium, or deodorized tincture of opium (Paregoric)	Mistaken as tincture of opium	Use complete drug name
HCl	hydrochloric acid or hydrochloride	Mistaken as potassium chloride (the "H" is misinterpreted as "K")	Use complete drug name unless expressed as a salt of a drug
HCT	hydrocortisone	Mistaken as hydrochlorothiazide	Use complete drug name
HCTZ	hydrochlorothiazide	Mistaken as hydrocortisone (seen as HCT 250 mg)	Use complete drug name
$MgSO_4$**	magnesium sulfate	Mistaken as morphine sulfate	Use complete drug name
MS, MSO_4**	morphine sulfate	Mistaken as magnesium sulfate	Use complete drug name
MTX	methotrexate	Mistaken as mitoxantrone	Use complete drug name
PCA	procainamide	Mistaken as patient controlled analgesia	Use complete drug name

(Continued)

TABLE 11-1 Continued

ABBREVIATIONS	INTENDED MEANING	MISINTERPRETATION	CORRECTION
PTU	propylthiouracil	Mistaken as mercaptopurine	Use complete drug name
T3	Tylenol with codeine No. 3	Mistaken as liothyronine	Use complete drug name
TAC	triamcinolone	Mistaken as tetracaine, adrenalin, cocaine	Use complete drug name
TNK	TNKase	Mistaken as "TPA"	Use complete drug name
$ZnSO_4$	zinc sulfate	Mistaken as morphine sulfate	Use complete drug name

STEMMED DRUG NAMES	INTENDED MEANING	MISINTERPRETATION	CORRECTION
"Nitro" drip	nitroglycerin infusion	Mistaken as sodium nitroprusside infusion	Use complete drug name
"Norflox"	norfloxacin	Mistaken as Norflex	Use complete drug name
"IV Vanc"	intravenous vancomycin	Mistaken as Invanz	Use complete drug name

SYMBOLS	INTENDED MEANING	MISINTERPRETATION	CORRECTION
ℨ	Dram	Symbol for dram mistaken as "3"	Use the metric system
ℳ	Minim	Symbol for minim mistaken as "mL"	Use the metric system
x3d	For three days	Mistaken as "3 doses"	Use "for three days"
> and <,	Greater than and less than	Mistaken as opposite of intended; mistakenly use incorrect symbol; "< 10" mistaken as "40"	Use "greater than" or "less than"
/ (slash mark)	Separates two doses or indicates "per"	Mistaken as the number 1 (e.g., "25 units/10 units" misread as "25 units and 110 units")	Use "per" rather than a slash mark to separate doses
@	At	Mistaken as "2"	Use "at"
&	And	Mistaken as "2"	Use "and"
+	Plus or and	Mistaken as "4"	Use "and"
°	Hour	Mistaken as a zero (e.g., q2° seen as q 20)	Use "hr," "h," or "hour"
Ø	zero, null sign	Mistaken as the numerals 4, 6, or 9	Use the number "0" or the word "zero"

*ISMP's List of Error-Prone Abbreviations, Symbols, and Dose Designation, copyright 2010, Institute for Safe Medication Practices, Horsham, PA. Reprinted with permission.

**These abbreviations are included on The Joint Commission's "minimum list" of dangerous abbreviations, acronyms, and symbols that must be included on an organization's "Do Not Use" list, effective January 1, 2004. Visit www.jointcommission.org for more information about this Joint Commission requirement.

11.3 Error-Prone Abbreviations and Symbols

For Exercise 1, refer to the following medication order.

1. Identify the error-prone abbreviations transcribed on this medication order form.

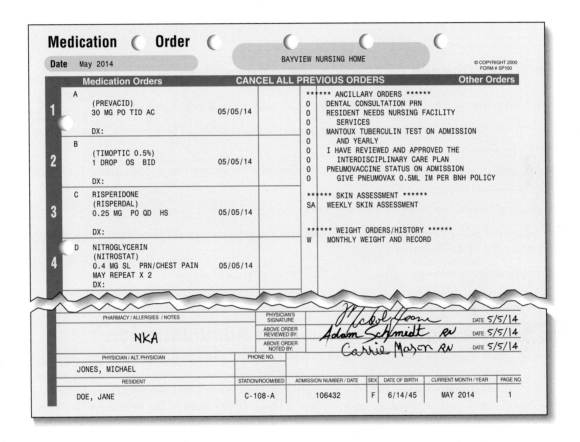

For Exercises 2–5, correct the medication orders, using the published list from the ISMP (Table 11-1). Hint: See items marked with a double asterisk.

2. Give Coumadin® 5.0 mg p.o. QD

3. MS 4 mg sc q4h prn pain

4. Vitamin D 1000 IU QOD

5. Digoxin 0.125 mg (125 µg) p.o. q.d.

11.4 The Three Checks of Medication Administration

To promote accuracy and safety with medication administration, the drug label should be checked three times (see Rule 11-1).

RULE 11-1	Check medication three times:
	1st check—when you take it from the storage container and match it to the MAR
	2nd check—when you prepare it
	3rd check—before you close the storage container or just before you administer the medication to the patient
	Check the medication three times even if the dose is prepackaged, labeled, and ready to be administered.

REVIEW AND PRACTICE

11.4 The Three Checks of Medication Administration

In Scenarios 1–5, identify which check (1, 2, or 3) the healthcare practitioner demonstrates.

1. The certified medication technician is at the patient's bedside about to administer acetaminophen tablets. _____

2. The licensed practical nurse draws up 4 units Humalog® insulin to be administered via subcutaneous route. _____

3. The medical technician takes the influenza vaccine out of the refrigerator. _____

4. The registered nurse reads the medication label on the intravenous (IV) medication bag before connecting the IV to the patient. _____

5. The physician retrieves epinephrine from the emergency cart. _____

11.5 The Rights of Medication Administration

The rights of medication administration are a set of safety checks the practitioner follows to prevent a medication administration error. When administering medications, the healthcare practitioner should observe the rights of medication administration (see Table 11-2) to reduce errors and help ensure patient safety. These rights include the original five rights, which are right patient, right drug, right dose, right route, and right time. Additional rights include right documentation, right reason, right to know, right to refuse, and right technique. Medication rights are desired outcomes of safe medication practices. Individuals administering medications should follow the procedures needed to ensure that these desired outcomes are achieved, not just memorize the rights.

TABLE 11-2 The Rights of Medication Administration	
1. Right patient	6. Right documentation
2. Right drug	7. Right reason
3. Right dose	8. Right to know
4. Right route	9. Right to refuse
5. Right time	10. Right technique

RIGHT PATIENT Before you give a medication to a patient you must check two identifiers: the full name and another identifier such as the patient's date of birth, social security number, or medical record number. Check that the name on the medication order is exactly the same as the name of the patient. Two patients with the same last name may have the same first initials, or even the same first names. Ask the patient to state his or her full name and date of birth or other identifying information. If the patient is unable to do so, ask the parent or caregiver to state the patient's full name. In outpatient settings, you may be required to ask for photographic identification, such as a driver's license. In an inpatient setting, check the patient's name and date of birth. In many facilities you may be required to scan the bar code on the patient's identification bracelet as well as the medication you will be administering. Remember, you are not only identifying that you have the right patient, you are also identifying that you are using the *right patient's MAR*. This is why recognizing the patient is not good enough, but a comparison of double identifiers from the patient to the MAR must be completed before medication administration.

RIGHT DRUG Be certain that a patient receives the *right drug*. Administer only drugs you have prepared yourself or that are clearly and completely labeled. Carefully check the medication label at least three times (see Rule 11-1) before administering the medication. Check that the medication and the drug order have not expired. (See Chapter 10 for more details on drug labels.) If a patient questions a medication, recheck the original order. Patients are often familiar with their medications. Listening to them may prevent an error.

CRITICAL THINKING ON THE JOB

The Importance of the Right Drug

A patient is brought to the hospital with a severe thumb laceration. The attending physician verbally orders lidocaine 1% solution 2 mL as a local anesthetic. The healthcare professional picks up a vial labeled lidocaine 1% with epinephrine and draws up 2 mL. He then says, "This is lidocaine 1% solution 2 mL," but neither mentions the epinephrine nor shows the physician the label.

A while later, the patient expresses concern about continuing numbness in his thumb. After locating the vial, the staff member realized that the patient received epinephrine, a vasoconstricting drug, in addition to the lidocaine. The patient is reassured that feeling will return to his thumb, although not quite as quickly as was first anticipated.

 Think! . . . Is It Reasonable? What could have been done to prevent the patient from losing feeling in his thumb?

RIGHT DOSE The patient must be given the *right dose* of medication. In later chapters, you will learn to calculate the amount to administer to a patient, factoring in the strength of the medication and the equipment you are using. Use extreme caution with dosage calculations. Pay special attention to decimal points. They can easily be placed in the wrong location or missed altogether when an order is copied. If you misread a decimal point, the patient could receive a dose significantly different from the one ordered.

RIGHT ROUTE You must give patients drugs by the *right route*. A drug intended for one route is often not safe if administered via another route. For example, only drugs labeled *for ophthalmic use* should be instilled (applied with a dropper) into the eye. Some medications are produced in different versions for different routes. The drug label (see Chapter 10) indicates the intended route. For example, Compazine® is available as a suppository, a tablet, and an injection. Always check that the route listed on the drug label matches the route ordered.

The Importance of the Right Dose

A medication order reads Compazine® supp i pr q4h PRN/nausea. The healthcare professional interprets this order as "administer 1 Compazine® suppository rectally every four hours as necessary for nausea."

He assumes that the patient is an adult and dispenses 25 mg suppositories, the normal adult dose. In turn another healthcare professional, who does not notice that the dose is not specified in the order, administers the 25 mg suppository to the patient, a 6-year-old boy.

The usual dose of Compazine® for children is a 2.5 mg suppository. The pediatrician who wrote the order did not include the dose, assuming the staff would know this information. The child receives 10 times the normal dose of Compazine®. He has a seizure and develops fever, respiratory distress, severe hypotension, and tachycardia because of drug toxicity. He is admitted to the intensive care unit for treatment.

Think! . . . Is It Reasonable? What could have been done to prevent this problem?

RIGHT TIME   Give medications at the *right time.* In most cases, to be "on time," you must administer medications within 30 minutes of the scheduled time. The right time may refer to an absolute time, such as 6:00 p.m., or to a relative time, such as "before breakfast." Some medications, such as insulin, antibiotics, and antidysrhythmic drugs, must be given at specific times because of how they interact with food or the patient's body. Other medications may be spaced over waking hours without changing their effectiveness. The drug order must identify special timing considerations to be followed. If a medication is ordered PRN (whenever necessary), a time interval and/or condition should be specified (e.g., q4h for temperature greater than or equal to 101). Before you administer a PRN drug, check that enough time has passed since the previous dose was given. Otherwise, the patient could receive the medication too soon, leading to severe consequences.

RIGHT DOCUMENTATION   Medication administration should be followed by the *right documentation* on the patient's medication administration record (MAR). Recall that the MAR is a paper form or electronic record that tracks the medication that a patient receives. Users of electronic systems must log in to the computer, entering their names and secure passwords. With some electronic medication administration systems, both the medication bar code and the patient's identification band are scanned. This information is documented directly into the patient's eMAR. This system allows medication administration to be tracked electronically to help reduce errors. (See Figure 11-3.) If medication administration is not documented, then the documentation is not considered complete. If the patient declines the medication, consumes only part of the dose, or vomits shortly after taking the medication, this information must be documented, as well.

RIGHT REASON   The healthcare professional who administers the medication should know the reason the drug is ordered and ensure that it is given for the right reason. Knowing why a medication is ordered also helps the practitioner know when not to give (hold) a medication. For example, if a medication is ordered to slow down a rapid heart rate and the patient's heart rate is slower than normal (less than 60 beats/minute), the drug should be held until the prescriber is notified of the situation.

RIGHT TO KNOW   All patients have the right to be educated about the medications they are receiving. Information that patients should receive includes dose, schedule, reason, and the intended effect and side effects of medications.

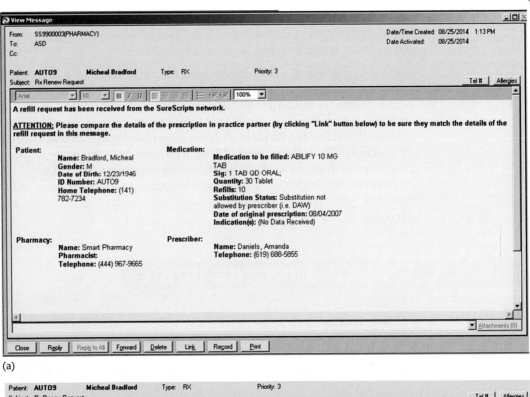

(a)

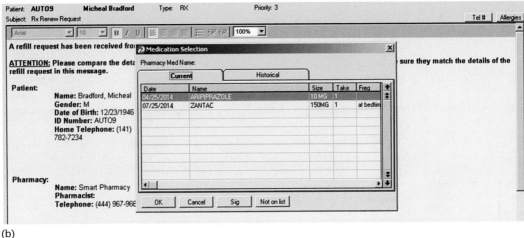

(b)

Figure 11-3 With electronic health records, the nurse in an outpatient practice can verify that the medication refill requested electronically by the pharmacy through SureScripts is the same medication as the original medication ordered on the patient chart. (a) An order for Abilify is received and viewed and then the Link button is selected; (b) Once the Link button is selected, the patient's medication record with the original order is viewed and compared to the refill request. In this case the order is for aripiprazole, the generic equivalent of Abilify.

PATIENT EDUCATION

Patient education, although not one of the five basic rights of medication administration, is critical to the patient's right to know. Patients should always be provided with basic information regarding their medications.

1. Explain the purpose of a medication and its side effects.
2. Review the dose, route, frequency, and time that the physician has prescribed.
3. When appropriate, be certain that the patient understands how to self-administer the medication.
4. If the patient is taking liquid oral medications at home, emphasize the importance of using calibrated spoons and measuring cups.

RIGHT TO REFUSE   Every patient has the *right to refuse* a medication. If a patient refuses a medication, the physician should be notified and this information should be documented in the patient's medical record.

RIGHT TECHNIQUE   Be familiar with the *right technique* to administer a medication. For example, both buccal and sublingual medications are applied to the mucous membranes of the mouth. A buccal medication, such as fentanyl tablets, is placed between the cheek and the gum, whereas a sublingual medication, such as nitroglycerin, is placed under the tongue. If you are not familiar with the correct technique to use, check resources such as the **Physicians' Desk Reference (PDR)**, a current drug reference book, the facility policy and procedure manual, or a valid Internet resource for more information.

   Following the "rights" of medication administration needs to become automatic, just like looking both ways before crossing the street. Following the "rights" of medication administration will avert dangerous medication errors.

CRITICAL THINKING ON THE JOB

The Importance of the Right Drug and Right Reason

Over the course of several days, a staff nurse administered quinidine to a patient whose order was for quinine. Quinine is usually ordered to treat malaria, while quinidine is typically ordered to treat altered heart rhythms. The patient had no documented heart problems. The nurse assumed that the order writer must have intended to order quinidine as it was a typical medication ordered for many patients on this particular medical unit. The nurse also rationalized that quinine must be an alternate name or brand name for quinidine. The consequence to the patient was a critical drop in blood pressure, a side effect of quinidine.

 Think! . . . Is It Reasonable? What went wrong?

REVIEW AND PRACTICE

11.5 The Rights of Medication Administration

Match the rights of drug administration with an example of how that right can be violated.

   a. Right patient

   b. Right drug

   c. Right dose

   d. Right route

   e. Right time

   f. Right documentation

g. Right reason

h. Right to know

i. Right to refuse

j. Right technique

_____ **1.** The medication bottle said *for optic use,* and the medication was instilled into the patient's ears.

_____ **2.** A patient with a bleeding disorder is scheduled to be given an anticoagulant (blood thinner).

_____ **3.** James F. Jones received James E. Jones's medication.

_____ **4.** The nurse charted a medication on the medication record before the patient had taken the medication.

_____ **5.** A patient asks why she is getting a medication and although the nurse knows why, she does not answer and administers the medication anyway.

_____ **6.** The dose to be administered was ½ tsp, and the patient received 5 mL.

_____ **7.** The medication was ordered at bedtime, and the patient took it at 9 a.m.

_____ **8.** The physician ordered Uracel, and the patient received uracil.

_____ **9.** The medication was to be given under the tongue, and the patient was told to swallow it.

_____ **10.** The nurse is giving a patient medication and the patient states, "I am not going to take that now. I want to talk to my doctor."

11.6 Observation

Observation refers to observing that the medication is safely received. Observation is an essential part of medication administration. Observation takes place before, during, and after medication administration. Before preparing medications to be administered, the healthcare practitioner should assess the patient's allergy status, condition, and ability to take medications via the prescribed route, which might include checking the intravenous site and available equipment. Before administering the medication, the healthcare professional observes the patient to determine if it is safe or appropriate to administer the medication: Has the patient's condition changed so that the route or the medication itself is no longer indicated? Is there sufficient access to administer the medication: Is the IV functional? Is the nasogastric tube (NGT) in place? If the authorized prescriber (AP) is present, such as in a doctor's office or a clinic, the AP, who just ordered the medication, will perform this observation. If the AP has not just examined the patient, the practitioner should inform the RN or question the AP as to whether the medication should be given as ordered.

During medication administration the practitioner observes that the medication is received and retained. Did the patient swallow the medication? Was the suppository retained? Did the infusion enter the vein, or did the IV infiltrate? The practitioner also observes for any untoward reactions that may occur during administration.

After medication administration the practitioner observes for any untoward reactions. The AP and the nurse also observe to see if the medication has had the desired effect.

11.6 Observation

For Questions 1–5 write the observation that would occur during this phase of medication administration.

1. The patient is scheduled to receive an IV antibiotic.

2. The patient is receiving eye drops.

3. The patient has just received an IM injection.

4. The patient is about to receive an oral medication.

5. The patient is about to receive a medication through a nasogastric tube.

11.7 Patient Teaching

Patient teaching refers to teaching the patient and/or caregiver how to procure the medication, administer the medication, and what to look for when administering a medication outside of the healthcare setting. If the patient/family will be administering the medication, the patient must be informed of all the steps in medication administration, including observation. Additionally, patients have the right to know about the medications they receive as well as the right to refuse medications. This basic right to know is an essential right of all patients' rights. The medicating practitioner, after assessing the patient's knowledge and literacy level, should ensure that all patients have this basic information regarding their drugs:

1. Name of the medication, including generic and brand name
2. Purpose of the medication
3. Dose and use of calibrated equipment for liquid medications
4. Route and self-administration guidelines, as needed
5. Medication schedule, related to food intake
6. Drug-drug interactions
7. Side effects and other reportable concerns
8. Where to procure the medication
9. Additional instructions, as needed

Proper patient education promotes accuracy and compliance with the medication regime. Patients should maintain a complete and up-to-date list of medications to provide for any AP they encounter.

Medication Reference Materials

In order to provide patient teaching when you dispense or administer medications, you are responsible for knowing their effects. Hundreds of drugs exist. New ones are produced and approved all the time. You cannot memorize all the information you might need to know. Therefore, you need to be familiar with drug information sources.

The PDR is an authoritative, current drug reference containing comprehensive information from the drug manufacturer regarding prescription drugs. Some versions feature non-prescription medications and herbal medications. A new volume is produced each year. Many physicians' offices, pharmacies, and healthcare facilities have the PDR available for employee use.

Many other guides are available for healthcare professionals, including the *United States Pharmacopeia/National Formulary*, found in most pharmacies. Most are updated every year or two. Other books have titles suggesting they are for nurses, but they are useful to all healthcare professionals. Their information is similar to that of the PDR, but they often have easy-to-understand language.

Internet users can access information about the 200 most commonly prescribed drugs at www.rxlist.com. This site provides information about the most frequently prescribed drugs. For each drug listed, the site lists appropriate doses of the drug for specific indications, available dosages and dosage forms, descriptions of the pills or liquids, and the drug's effects. Another Internet site, www.druginfonet.com, lists drug information, allows searches by brand or generic names, and provides many other useful features.

Also available are software programs that can run on a handheld computer or smartphone. One such program is called Epocrates. This program is updated regularly and is a handy resource for any healthcare professional needing the latest medication information. When an electronic health record (EHR) system is used, medication database software programs are frequently linked and can be accessed easily while working within the EHR programs.

REVIEW AND PRACTICE

11.7 Patient Teaching

For Exercises 1–5 match each patient teaching with the situation that requires it.

Patient Teaching:

a. Procedure for administering an injection

b. Use of calibrated equipment

c. Medication schedule, related to food intake

d. Drug-drug interactions

e. Side effects and reportable concerns

Situation:

_____ 1. If the patient develops a nonproductive cough related to this medication, the AP will discontinue the medication.

_____ 2. The patient has been newly prescribed subcutaneous insulin.

_____ 3. The patient has been prescribed a medication that interacts with several over-the-counter medications.

_____ 4. The patient has been prescribed a medication to take before meals.

_____ 5. The patient has been prescribed a liquid cough syrup.

LEARNING OUTCOME	KEY POINTS
11.1 Apply The Joint Commission steps to receiving and writing a verbal order. Pages 222–224	Step 1: Write the order Step 2: Read the order Step 3: Confirm the order
11.2 Execute safe transcription practices. Pages 224–226	▶ Transfer information from the AP's order to the prescription label or to the medication administration record (MAR) ▶ Accurate ▶ Legible ▶ Contact AP if order is not clear

11.3 Identify error-prone abbreviations and symbols. Pages 227–231	▶ Result in death or injury when misinterpreted
	▶ TJC's Do Not Use List:
	  • U (write unit)
	  • IU (write international unit)
	  • qd, QD, OD, or q1d (write daily)
	  • QOD (write every other day)
	  • MS or MSO$_4$ (write morphine sulfate)
	  • MgSO$_4$ (write magnesium sulfate)
	▶ Include leading zeros (write 0.4 mg not .4 mg)
	▶ Omit trailing zeros (write 4 mg not 4.0 mg)
	▶ Common ISMP's Error-Prone Abbreviations:
	  • µg (write mcg)
	  • AD, AS, AU (write right ear, left ear, both ears)
	  • OD, OS, OU (write right eye, left eye, both eyes)
	  • cc (write mL)
	  • d/c (write discontinue or discharge)
	  • HS (write half-strength or hour of sleep/bedtime)
	  • qhs (write nightly or bedtime)
	  • SC or sq (write subcut)
	  • ss (write sliding scale or one-half)

LEARNING OUTCOME	KEY POINTS
11.4 Identify the three checks in the medication administration procedure. Pages 231–232	**1:** When you take it from the storage container and match it to the MAR **2:** When you prepare it **3:** Before closing the storage container or just before you administer the medication to the patient
11.5 Implement the "rights" of medication administration. Pages 232–237	▶ Right patient ▶ Right drug ▶ Right dose ▶ Right route ▶ Right time/frequency ▶ Right documentation ▶ Also right reason, right to know, right to refuse, and right technique
11.6 Recognize the importance of observation in safe medication administration. Pages 237–238	Observe that the medication is safely received ▶ Before medication administration ▶ During medication administration ▶ After medication administration
11.7 Describe the appropriate use of patient teaching as it relates to safe drug administration. Pages 238–240	Teach patient or caregiver: ▶ How to procure the medication ▶ How to administer the medication ▶ Reportable side effects and concerns

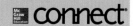
For Exercise 1, apply The Joint Commission steps to receiving and writing a verbal order. (LO 11.1)

1. The nurse is receiving a telephone order from the physician. The physician and nurse have identified themselves, and then identified the patient by double identifier.

   Step 1: The *authorized prescriber* states the order: "fentanyl 100 mcg now, may repeat once after 30 minutes if pain is not relieved."

   The receiver writes: _____

   The receiver asks: _____

   The *authorized prescriber* states: "buccal"

   The receiver fills in the blanks as the order is stated:

   Step 2: *The receiver* states: _____

   Step 3: *The receiver* continues on to confirm the order: _____

For Exercises 2–3, transcribe the following orders onto MAR 1. (LO 11.2)

2. Keflex 250 mg p.o. every six hours starting at midnight

3. Docusate sodium 100 mg p.o. twice a day in the morning and at bedtime

Medication Administration Record (MAR)

MO/YR:	Start/Stop Date		Hour	Facility Name:

Medication			Hour	1	2	3	4	5	6	7	8	9	10	11	12	13	14	15	16	17	18	19	20	21	22	23	24	25	26	27	28	29	30	31
		Start																																
		Stop																																
		Start																																
		Stop																																

Diagnosis:	DIET (Special instructions. e.g. Texture, Bite Size, Position, etc.)	Comments
Allergies: NKA	Physician Name **Harleigh Haddix**	A. Put initials in appropriate box when medication is given. B. Circle initials when not given. C. State reason for refusal / omission on back of form. D. PRN Medications: Reason given and results must be noted on back of from. E. Legend: S = School; H = Home visit; W = Work; P = Program.
	Phone Number **888-888-8888**	
NAME: **Jim Wiley**	Record # **234-885-123**	Date of Birth: **04/30/57** Sex: **M**

MAR 1

For Exercises 4–5, rewrite the orders, correcting the error-prone abbreviations. (LO 11.3)

4. MS 4.0 mg sc QD prn pain

5. Tylenol with codeine 5 cc p.o. QHS

For Exercise 6, name which check in the three-check medication administration procedure is described. (LO 11.4)

6. The RN withdraws the narcotic from the vial.

For Exercises 7–8, identify which "right" of medication administration is violated. (LO 11.5)

7. The 6 p.m. dose of propanol is given at 1930.

8. "Hydromorphone 2 mg subcut now" is ordered. Hydromorphone 2 mg is administered intramuscularly from a pre-filled syringe with a 1.5 inch pre-attached needle.

For Exercises 9–10, describe which observation should be made to promote safe medication administration. (LO 11.6)

9. The patient is about to receive the first dose of a newly prescribed medication.

10. The patient has received a medication.

For Exercise 11, indicate the appropriate patient teaching to be provided. (LO 11.7)

11. The patient has just been ordered an Epi-Pen® for subcutaneous injection.

CHAPTER 11 REVIEW

CHECK UP

1. What action should you take when you receive this drug order? Dilaudid® tab 2 mg po PRN for pain q4h. (LO 11.4, 11.5)

2. What action should you take when you receive this drug order? Codeine tab 30 mg po qid. (LO 11.4, 11.5)

For Exercises 3–8, refer to medication order form 1. (LO 11.2)

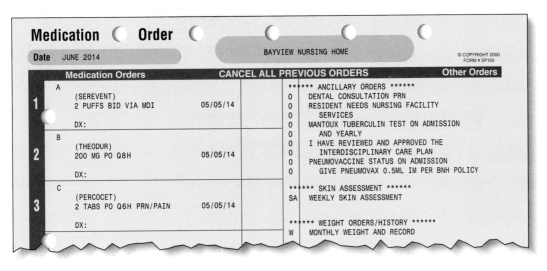

Medication Order Form 1

3. How often should Theodur® be given?

4. By what route is Serevent® administered?

5. If the patient receives Percocet® for pain at 4:00 a.m., when can the next dose be given?

6. If medications are delivered to this unit once daily, how many Percocet® tablets should be dispensed at one time?

7. What dose of Theodur® should be given?

8. How often should Serevent® be given?

For Exercises 9–15, refer to MAR 2 for Arthur Simmons. (LO 11.2, 11.3, 11.5)

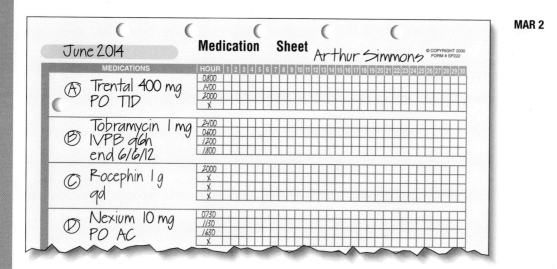

MAR 2

9. By what route is the tobramycin to be given?

10. What dose of Nexium® does Arthur Simmons receive?

11. What medications does Arthur Simmons receive at 8:00 p.m.?

12. How frequently does Arthur Simmons receive Trental®?

13. Should Arthur Simmons be served breakfast at 7:00 a.m., 7:30 a.m., or 8:00 a.m.? Why?

14. Which orders do *not* have all the essential elements for a MAR order? State what is missing from each.

15. Identify and correct the error-prone abbreviation in order C.

For Exercises 16–26, refer to MAR 3 for Carrie Kay Smith. (LO 11.2, 11.3, 11.5)

MAR 3

TCP Hospital Medication Administration Record

Carrie Kay Smith

Order date	Medication, dose, duration frequency route	D/C date	Times		Dates Administered						
					5 Feb	6 Feb	7 Feb	8 Feb	9 Feb	10 Feb	11 Feb
5 Feb 14	heparin 5000 units subcut on MAR 4 q8h		2400	0800							
			1600	X							
5 Feb 14	Bleph-10 OD q6h	05 Feb 14	0800	1400							
			2000	0200							
5 Feb 14	Premarin 1.25 mg daily		0800								
5 Feb 14	Proventil 2 mg PO bid		0800	X							
			1600	X							
5 Feb 14	Sinemet 25/100 tab i PO tid		0800	1400							
			2000								
5 Feb 14	Benadryl 25 mg PO q4h PRN/ITCH										

16. By what route will the heparin be given?

17. What dose of Premarin® will be given to Carrie Kay Smith?

18. At what times should Carrie Smith receive her Sinemet®?

19. Which medications will be administered at 1600?

20. If Carrie Smith has a dose of Benadryl® at 0200, when can she have her next dose?

21. How often should Carrie Smith receive heparin?

22. If the Proventil® were to be given TID instead of BID, how would the MAR be changed?

23. Which two medication orders are not complete, and what elements are missing?

24. Identify and correct the error-prone abbreviation in the Bleph-10 order.

25. At 1:30 p.m., you are preparing medications for patients who have just returned from lunch. Describe some precautions you might take to ensure that you administer the right dose.

26. You have just started your shift on a unit with geriatric and pediatric patients. You are scheduled to administer drugs to several elderly patients with Alzheimer's as well as to several children. What steps should you take to ensure that you administer the right drugs to the right patients?

For Exercise 27, apply The Joint Commission steps to receiving and writing a verbal order. (LO 11.1)

27. The nurse is receiving a telephone order from the physician. The physician and nurse have identified themselves, and then identified the patient by double identifier.
    Step 1: The *authorized prescriber* states the order:
    "Tylenol 650 mg pr"
    The receiver writes: _____
    The receiver asks: _____
    The *authorized prescriber* states:
    "every 4 hours as needed for headache."
    The receiver fills in the blanks as the order is stated:
    Tylenol 650 mg pr *q4h prn headache*
    Step 2: *The receiver* states: _____
    Step 3: *The receiver* continues on to confirm the order: _____

For Exercises 28–29, identify which of the three checks in the medication administration procedure is indicated. (LO 11.4)

28. The medication technician is about to hand the medication to the patient.

29. The medical assistant takes the bronchodilator out of the cabinet.

For Exercises 30–31, identify what observation should be made to promote safe medication administration. (LO 11.6)

30. The nurse is about to administer a subcutaneous injection.

31. The patient has received a medication.

32. If "yellow vision" is a sign of toxicity due to the drug digoxin, describe the appropriate patient teaching for this medication. (LO 11.7)

For Exercises 33–35, using international time and the following information, transcribe the orders to the blank MAR 4. (LO 11.2)
    • Daily refers to 8 a.m.
    • Three times per day refers to 0600, 1400, 2200.
    • Every six hours should be initiated at midnight.

Medication Administration Record (MAR)

MO/YR:	Start/Stop Date		Facility Name:	1	2	3	4	5	6	7	8	9	10	11	12	13	14	15	16	17	18	19	20	21	22	23	24	25	26	27	28	29	30	31
Medication		Hour																																
	Start																																	
	Stop																																	
	Start																																	
	Stop																																	
	Start																																	
	Stop																																	
	Start																																	
	Stop																																	
	Start																																	
	Stop																																	
	Start																																	
	Stop																																	

Diagnosis:	DIET (Special instructions. e.g. Texture, Bite Size, Position, etc.)	Comments
Allergies: **Levaquin**	Physician Name **Hunter Glaspell**	A. Put initials in appropriate box when medication is given. B. Circle initials when not given. C. State reason for refusal / omission on back of form.
	Phone Number **777-777-7777**	D. PRN Medications: Reason given and results must be noted on back of from. E. Legend: *S* = School; *H* = Home visit; *W* = Work; *P* = Program.
NAME: **Isaiah Shaw**	Record # **876-898-432**	Date of Birth: **12/28/64** Sex: **M**

MAR 4

33. Give Lasix 40 mg orally every day.

34. Give nifedipine 10 mg orally three times each day.

35. Give ampicillin 1 g intravenously every six hours.

CRITICAL THINKING APPLICATIONS

The medications on the following drug order need to be administered. What items should be observed when administering these medications? (LO 11.6)

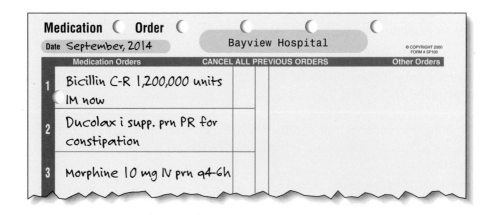

CASE STUDY

A physician gives a patient the following prescription. (LO 11.7)

Alan Capsella, MD
Westtown Medical Clinic
989-555-1234

Prescribed Date _January 6, 2014_

Name _Martin Burke_   DOB _2/22/57_

Address _105 North Main, Bolivia, KS 88807_

Rx: _Xanax 0.5 mg_

QUANTITY: _120_

SIG: _tab i po tid with meals_

Refills: _1_

_MD398475_   _Alan Capsella MD_
Prescriber ID #   Signature

1. One of your jobs is to instruct patients on how to take prescription drugs. What should you tell Martin Burke?

2. If you are filling the prescription, how many tablets will you dispense to the patient? Will you refill the prescription?

connect

Now that you have completed the materials in the chapter text, go to CONNECT and complete any chapter activities you have not yet done.

For examples 1 and 2, rewrite the medication order, interpreting the abbreviations.

1. Montelukast 10 mg tab i po q evening

2. Morphine sulfate 10 mg supp pr q4h prn pain

For Examples 3 and 4, identify which component of the medication order is missing.

3.

> Paul Mayor, DOB 8/27/53
>
> 5/4/2014 Paroxetine 25 mg po
>
> T. Holmes, MD

4.

> Carolyn Flynn, DOB 2/28/80
>
> 9/14/2014 Rifaximin po TID for 3 days.
>
> Y Xong, MD

5. Which medications will be administered at 9:00 a.m. on 6/2, according to the following MAR?

Robert Reams, DOB 4/12/48		Allergies : iodine		Room 412				
Order	Time	6/1	6/2	6/3	6/4	6/5	6/6	6/7
Rosuvastatin 10 mg PO daily	0900	GF						
Cefuroxime Sodium 500 mg IV q12h	0900	GF						
	2100	SS						
Phenytoin 100 mg Po TID	0800	GF						
	1400	GF						
	2200	SS						

6. 30 milliliters (mL) equals how many cubic centimeters?

7. An order calls for 2 teaspoons of a liquid oral medication. The only available medicine cup is calibrated in mL. How many mL will you pour into the medicine cup?

8. What is the volume of medicine in the cup?

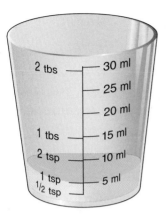

9. What is the volume of medicine in the dropper?

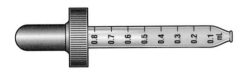

10. What is the volume of medicine in the following syringe?

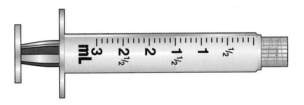

11. Answer the following questions about medication label A.

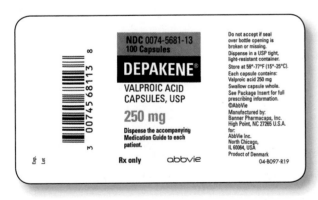

    a. Differentiate the brand name and the generic name of the drug.
    b. What is the dosage strength?
    c. What are the special adminstration instructions for this medicaton?
    d. If the patient is ordered to take 1 capsule tid, how long would this bottle last?
    e. How should this medication be stored?

12. Explain the following medication administration routes.
    a. PO
    b. IM
    c. IV
    d. Subcut
    e. SL

13. Describe three types of information found on a medication package insert.

14. List eight components of a medication order and identify each component that is also considered a "right of medication administration."

15. How does the medication technician ensure that the "right patient" is given the "right medication"?

16. Give an example of patient teaching that might accompany medication administration.

17. What important observation should the nurse make after administration of ibuprofen for pain?

18. Correct the following error-prone abbreviations and indicate why the abbreviation is no longer used.
    a. OD
    b. qhs
    c. QD
    d. SC
    e. U

19. What potential transcription error may occur from the following order? Coumadin 5.0 mg PO daily. How can this error be avoided?

20. Identify three guidelines from The Joint Commission (TJC) regarding verbal orders.

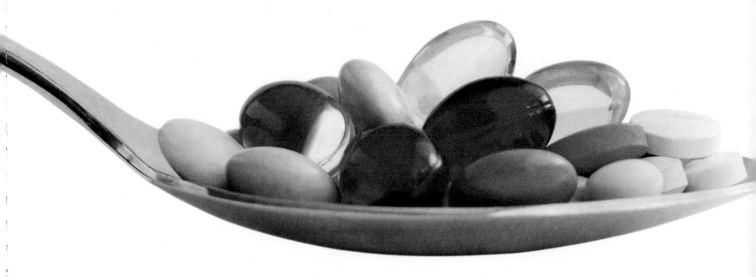

UNIT 4

Calculating Dosages

12

CHAPTER

Methods of Dosage Calculations

Each problem that I solved became a rule, which served afterwards to solve other problems.

RENÉ DESCARTES

LEARNING OUTCOMES

When you have completed Chapter 12, you will be able to:

12.1 Determine information needed to perform dosage calculations.

12.2 Utilize three methods of dosage calculations.

INTRODUCTION

It is time to bring together all the information you have learned in previous chapters to calculate the amount of medication to be administered to a patient. You will bring together basic math, information from the physician's order and drug labels, and methods of converting quantities from one unit of measurement to another.

12.1 Information Needed to Perform Dosage Calculations

The purpose of dosage calculations is to determine the amount of a drug to give to a patient, or **amount to administer (A)**. The dosage calculation process includes three steps:

Step A: Gather information and convert (if necessary)
Step B: Calculate the dosage
Step C: Think!...Is It Reasonable?

Gathering the Information

To perform Step A, you need to know certain basic facts and understand the terminology used (see Table 12-1). First, you need to know the **dosage ordered**—how much of the medication the patient is to receive. You can find this information on the medication order or prescription.

Then determine the **dosage unit (Q)**. This is the form of the medication that is available to you, such as tablets or capsules, and you can get this information from the drug label. For example, the label in Figure 12-1 states that the dosage unit is capsules. Next, find the **dose on hand (H),** which is the amount of the drug in each dosage unit of the medication. This information is also on the drug label. The label in Figure 12-1 states that each capsule contains 10 mg, so 10 mg is the dose on hand. The **desired dose (D)** is the dosage ordered, stated in the same unit of measurement as the dose on hand.

Converting the Dosage Ordered

If the dosage ordered is already in the same units as the dose on hand, then the dosage ordered is the same as the desired dose. In some cases, however, you may discover that the

TABLE 12-1 The Language of Dosage Calculations

TERM	ABBREVIATION	DEFINITION	EXAMPLE (REFER TO FIGURE 12-1)
Dosage ordered	O	The amount of drug to be given to the patient and how often it is to be given. *Obtain this value from the drug order or prescription.*	20 mg daily
Dosage unit	Q	The quantity of solid or liquid in which the dose is supplied. *Obtain this value from the drug label.*	Capsules
Dose on hand	H	The amount of drug contained in each dosage unit. *Obtain this value from the drug label.*	10 mg
Desired dose	D	The amount of drug to be given at a single time, stated in the same unit of measurement as the dose on hand. *This is the same amount as the dosage ordered, converted if necessary to the same unit of measurement as the dose on hand.*	20 mg
Dosage strength (supply dose)	$\dfrac{H}{Q}$	The dose on hand per dosage unit. *Obtain this value from the drug label.*	10 mg per capsule
Amount to administer	A	The volume of a liquid or the number of solid dosage units that contains the desired dose. *Find this value by performing a dosage calculation.*	2 capsules

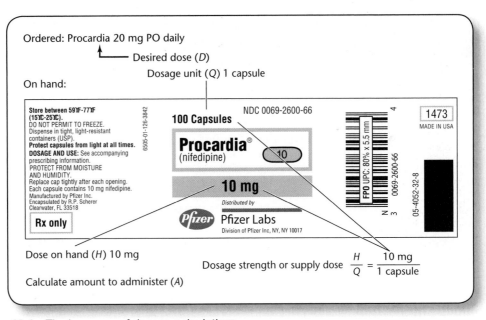

Figure 12-1 The language of dosage calculations.

dosage ordered is not in the same unit of measurement as the dose on hand. For example, the dosage ordered might be 0.2 mg once a day, and the medication you have on hand might have a dosage strength of 100 mcg per tablet. The dose on hand would therefore be 100 mcg. If the units of measurement are different, you must convert the dosage ordered to the same units of measurement as the dose on hand before you continue with the dosage calculations.

Recall from the chapter "Converting Units" that there are several ways to perform unit conversions. The proportion method and dimensional analysis are reviewed here to show how these methods apply to converting dosages.

RULE 12-1	Converting the Dosage Ordered to Like Units of Measurement Convert the unit of measure of the desired dose to the unit of measure of the dose on hand.
EXAMPLE	The physician has ordered the patient to receive 0.2 mg of medication. This is the dosage ordered.
	The dosage strength (supply dose) is 100 mcg/tablet, so the unit of measure of the dose on hand is micrograms (mcg). *Recall that the dosage strength is the dose on hand per dosage unit,* or *H/Q.*
	Since the bottle of medication comes in micrograms and the order is for milligrams, you must change the units of measure of the dosage ordered (0.2 mg) to the same unit of measurement as the dose on hand (micrograms) to obtain the desired dose.

PROPORTION METHOD

In the proportion method, you first write a conversion factor. Then set up the proportion as described in the "Converting Units" chapter. The proportion can be written as a ratio ($A{:}B = C{:}D$) or as a fraction $\left(\dfrac{A}{B} = \dfrac{C}{D}\right)$. In both cases, the proportion is read as "A is to B as C is to D." If you set up a ratio, multiply the means to equal the extremes ($B \times C = A \times D$). If you set up a fraction, cross-multiply the numerators with the denominators ($A \times D = B \times C$).

 LEARNING LINK Recall the chapter "Converting Units," Procedure Checklist 6-1: Writing Conversion Factors as Fractions, and 6-2: Writing Conversion Factors as Ratios.

Procedure Checklist 6-3
Converting by the Proportion Method Using Fractions

1. Write a conversion factor with the units needed in the answer in the numerator and the units you are converting from in the denominator. *The units needed in the answer are the units of the dose on hand. The units you are converting from are the units of the dosage ordered.*

2. Write a proportion with the unknown x in the numerator and the quantity that you are converting from in the denominator. The unknown is the desired dose (D) and the quantity that you are converting from is the dose ordered (O).

3. Set the two fractions as a proportion.

4. Cancel units.

5. Cross-multiply and solve for the unknown value.

EXAMPLE 1   Ordered: Nitrostat® 800 mcg sublingually PRN chest pain

On hand: See Figure 12-2.

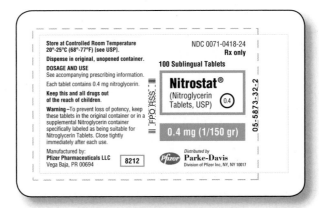

Figure 12-2

In this case, the drug is measured in micrograms on the drug order and in milligrams on the drug label. The units for the *desired dose* must match those found on the drug label, which means that we will convert 800 mcg to milligrams.

Follow the steps of Procedure Checklist 6-3.

1. The first fraction should have mg in the numerator since this is the units of the dose on hand and mcg in the denominator since this is the units of the dose ordered.

$$\frac{1 \text{ mg}}{1{,}000 \text{ mcg}}$$

2. The second fraction should have the unknown D in the numerator and the dose ordered in the denominator.

$$\frac{D}{800 \text{ mcg}}$$

3. Set up the fractions.

$$\frac{D}{800 \text{ mcg}} = \frac{1 \text{ mg}}{1{,}000 \text{ mcg}}$$

4. Cancel units.

$$\frac{D}{800 \text{ mcg}} = \frac{1 \text{ mg}}{1{,}000 \text{ mcg}}$$

5. Cross-multiply and then solve for the unknown.

$$D \times 1{,}000 = 800 \times 1 \text{ mg}$$

$$D \times \frac{1{,}000}{1{,}000} = \frac{800}{1{,}000} \times 1 \text{ mg}$$

$$D = \frac{800}{1{,}000} = 0.8 \text{ mg} = \text{desired dose}$$

EXAMPLE 2

Ordered: 500 mg PO q6h

Dosage strength available: 250 mg per tablet
Find the desired dose.
In this case the unit for the dose ordered is the same as that for the dose on hand. No calculation is needed. The drug is measured in milligrams on both the order and the drug label, so the desired dose $D = 500$ mg.

DIMENSIONAL ANALYSIS

Recall from the chapter "Converting Units" that the dimensional analysis (DA) method is similar to the proportion method, but starts with the unknown value x standing alone on one side of the equation.

Procedure Checklist 6-5
Converting by Dimensional Analysis

1. Write a conversion factor with the units you are converting to in the numerator and the units you are converting from in the denominator. *The units you are converting to are the units of the dose on hand. The units you are converting from are the units of the dosage ordered.*

2. Write an equation with the unknown value x on one side and the quantity being converted multiplied by the conversion factor on the other side. *The unknown value x is the desired dose (D). The quantity being converted is the dosage ordered (O).*

3. Cancel units.

4. Solve the equation.

EXAMPLE 1

The dosage ordered is 0.2 mg once a day.

The dosage strength is 100 mcg per tablet.

Find the desired dose.

The drug is measured in milligrams on the drug order and in micrograms on the drug label. The units for the desired dose must match the units of the dose on hand. We must determine how many micrograms is equivalent to 0.2 mg.

Follow the steps of Procedure Checklist 6-5.

1. Write a conversion factor with mcg in the numerator and mg in the denominator. Mcg is the units of the dose on hand, which is what you are converting to. Mg is the units of the dosage ordered and what you are converting from. Our conversion factor is $\dfrac{1{,}000 \text{ mcg}}{1 \text{ mg}}$.

2. Write the equation with the unknown value D on one side and the quantity being converted, which is the dosage ordered, multiplied by the conversion factor $\dfrac{1{,}000 \text{ mcg}}{1 \text{ mg}}$.

$$D = 0.2 \text{ mg} \times \frac{1{,}000 \text{ mcg}}{1 \text{ mg}}$$

3. Cancel units

$$D = 0.2 \text{ \sout{mg}} \times \frac{1{,}000 \text{ \sout{mcg}}}{1 \text{ \sout{mg}}}$$

4. Solve the equation.

$$D = 0.2 \times 1{,}000 \text{ mcg}$$

$$D = 200 \text{ mcg} = \text{desired dose}$$

| EXAMPLE 2 | Ordered: 10 mg PO daily |

Dosage strength available: 5 mg per tablet

Find the desired dose.

In this case the unit for the dose ordered is the same as that for the dose on hand. No calculation is needed. The drug is measured in milligrams on both the order and the drug label, so the desired dose $D = 10$ mg.

ERROR ALERT!

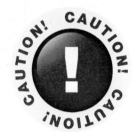

Canceling Units in Dimensional Analysis

In an earlier example, the dosage ordered was in milligrams and the dosage strength was measured in micrograms. Suppose that you had used the conversion factor $\frac{1 \text{ mg}}{1,000 \text{ mcg}}$ instead of $\frac{1,000 \text{ mcg}}{1 \text{ mg}}$. Your equation would then have been:

$$D = \frac{1 \text{ mg}}{1,000 \text{ mcg}} \times 0.2 \text{ mcg}$$

You may cancel units within a fraction only when they are found in both the numerator and the denominator. Here, the common unit (milligrams) is found in the numerator only and cannot be canceled. You should immediately realize that the conversion factor is incorrect because the units cannot be canceled. If you had not included the units when setting up the equation, the error might have gone unnoticed. *Always include the units when you are performing calculations.*

REVIEW AND PRACTICE

12.1 Information Needed to Perform Dosage Calculations

For Exercises 1–20, for each order: identify the dose on hand, dosage unit, desired dose, and if necessary identify the conversion factor and convert to like units of measurement. Use conversion tables from the chapter "Converting Units" as needed. For Exercises 8–20, use Labels A–M located following the table.

medication order	dose on hand	dosage unit	conversion factor	desired dose
1. Ordered: Amoxicillin 0.25 g PO QID On hand: Amoxicillin 125 mg capsules				
2. Ordered: Erythromycin 0.5 g PO q6h On hand: Erythromycin 500 mg tablets				
3. Ordered: Phenobarbital 30 mg PO TID On hand: Phenobarbital 15 mg tablets				

(Continued)

medication order	dose on hand	dosage unit	conversion factor	desired dose
4. Ordered: Penicillin VK 0.25 g PO now On hand: Penicillin VK 500 mg scored tablet				
5. Ordered: Levoxyl 0.075 mg PO daily On hand: Levoxyl 150 mcg tablets				
6. Ordered: Docusate 100 mg PO daily On hand: Docusate sodium elixir 150 mg/15 mL Available measuring device is marked in teaspoons				
7. Ordered: 2 tsp Robitussin 5 mg/5 mL PO q4h for cough On hand: Robitussin 5 mg/5 mL syrup Available measuring device is marked in mL				
8. Ordered: Biaxin 1 g PO daily On hand: Refer to label A.				
9. Ordered: Tricor 145 mg PO daily On hand: Refer to label B.				
10. Ordered: Synthroid 0.05 mg PO daily On hand: Refer to label C.				
11. Ordered: Synthroid 0.088 mg PO daily On hand: Refer to label D.				
12. Ordered: Depakote 0.25 g PO BID On hand: Refer to label E.				
13. Ordered: Synthroid 250 mcg PO daily On hand: Refer to label F.				
14. Ordered: $1\frac{1}{2}$ teaspoon Zinthromax 200 mg/5 mL PO q6h On hand: Refer to label G. (Only available measuring device is marked in mL.)				
15. Ordered: 7.5 mL of Amoxicillin 250 mg/5 mL PO q4h On hand: Refer to label H. (Available measuring device is a teaspoon.)				
16. Ordered: Levothroid 0.137 mg PO daily On hand: Refer to label I.				
17. Ordered: Levothroid 0.112 mg PO daily On hand: Refer to label J.				
18. Ordered: Risperidone 500 mcg PO daily On hand: Refer to label K.				
19. Ordered: Prandin 750 mcg PO before meals On hand: Refer to label L.				
20. Ordered: Metformin 1 g PO BID On hand: Refer to label M.				

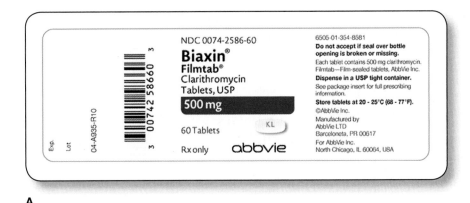

A

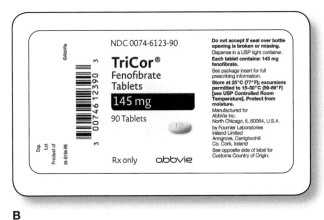

B

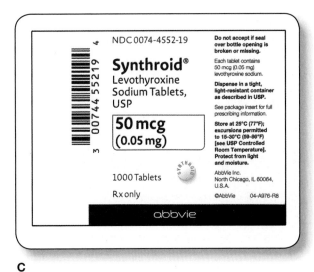

C

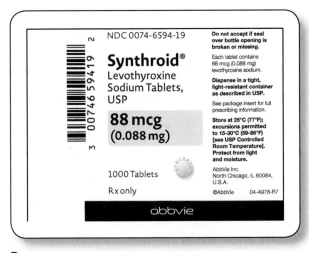

D

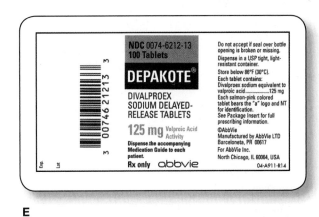

E

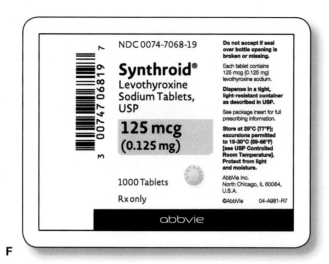

F

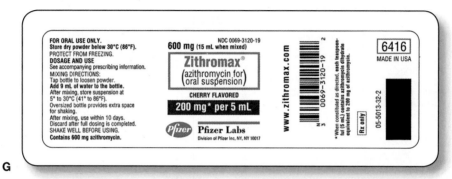

G

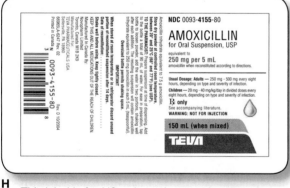

H

This label is for US only, and cannot be altered or translated.

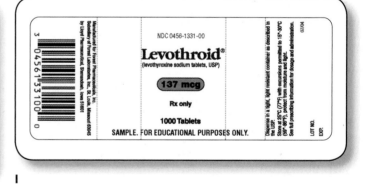

I

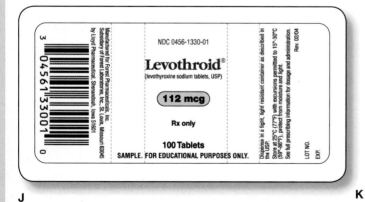

J

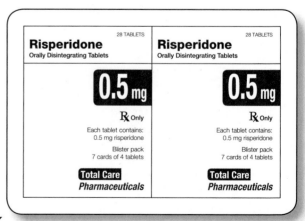

K

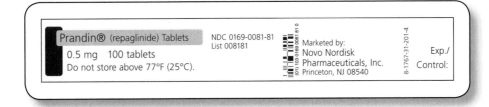

Prandin® (repaglinide) Tablets

NDC 0169-0081-81
List 008181

0.5 mg   100 tablets

Do not store above 77°F (25°C).

Marketed by:
Novo Nordisk
Pharmaceuticals, Inc.
Princeton, NJ 08540

Exp./
Control:

L

Pharmacist Information:
Dispense in tight, light-resistant
container as defined in USP

**Store at controlled room
temperature 15°-30°C (59°-86°F)**

Each Tablet contains:
Metformin hydrochloride, USP.......500mg

NDC 57664-397-18

**Metformin hydrochloride
Tablets, USP**

500 mg

1000 Tablets
Rx Only

USUAL DOSAGE:
See Package outsert
for complete product
information.

CARACO
PHARMACEUTICAL
LABORATORIES, LTD.
DETROIT, MI 48202

C.S.No. 5274L04
Iss. 4/05

M

12.2 Methods of Dosage Calculation

Once you have completed Step A, including converting the desired dose if necessary, you are ready to move on to Step B: Calculate the dosage. There are several methods for calculating the dosage. In this section, three methods are presented: proportion method, dimensional analysis method, and formula method. You are already familiar with using the proportion and dimensional analysis method for unit conversions. Now you will discover how to use these methods, as well as the formula method, for dosage calculation.

Regardless of the method you choose to use, always follow the steps of dosage calculation. These were presented at the beginning of the chapter, but are repeated here as Rule 12-2.

RULE 12-2

Calculating the Amount to Administer
Step A: Gather Information and Convert
Gather the information needed for the dosage calculation: the dosage ordered, dose on hand, dosage unit, and desired dose. If necessary, convert the desired dose to the same unit of measurement as the dose on hand. NOTE: When using the dimensional analysis method introduced later in this chapter, step A will include determining the conversion factor.

(Continued)

Step B: Calculate

Perform the dosage calculation using the method of your choice: proportion method, dimensional analysis, or formula method.

Step C: Think! . . . Is It Reasonable?

Think about your answer. Is it reasonable? Apply common sense and rules of dosage calculation.

For example, suppose the physician has ordered erythromycin 0.5 g PO twice daily. You have on hand the medication shown in the label in Figure 12-3. Begin by performing Step A. First, gather the information you will need. The dosage ordered is 0.5 g, the dose on hand is 250 mg, and the dosage unit is 1 capsule. Since the dosage ordered is in a different unit of measurement from the dose on hand, you will need to perform a unit conversion calculation. In this case, you will convert 0.5 g to milligrams to find the desired dose of 500 mg.

Now you are ready to proceed to Step B, the actual dosage calculation, and Step C, checking to be sure the answer is reasonable. Study each method of dosage calculation and the examples provided in this section. Remember that each of these methods will give you the same result, and the method you use is a matter of personal preference. Once you identify the method you prefer, follow the color coding for that method:

- Proportion method: orange
- Dimensional analysis: green
- Formula method: red

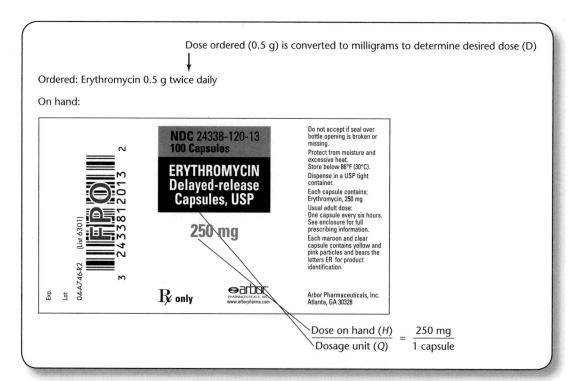

Figure 12-3 Information necessary to calculate the amount to administer. In this case the dose ordered must be converted to milligrams to obtain the desired dose.

Procedure Checklist 12-1

Calculating the Amount to Administer by Proportion Method Using Fractions

1. Set up the proportion as follows:

$$\frac{\text{Dose on hand}}{\text{Dosage unit}} = \frac{\text{Desired dose}}{\text{Amount to administer}} \quad \text{or} \quad \frac{H}{Q} = \frac{D}{A} \quad \text{or} \quad H{:}Q = D{:}A$$

2. Cancel units.

3. Cross-multiply, and then solve for the unknown value.

EXAMPLE 1

Find the amount to administer.

Ordered: Famvir® 1,000 mg PO BID

On hand: See label in Figure 12-4.

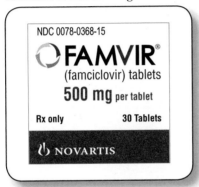

Figure 12-4

STEP A: GATHER INFORMATION AND CONVERT

The drug is ordered in milligrams, which is the same unit used on the label. Therefore, the dosage ordered is the same as the desired dose (1,000 mg), so no conversion is needed. By reading the label, we find that the dosage unit is 1 tablet and the dose on hand is 500 mg. Therefore,

$$D = 1{,}000 \text{ mg}$$
$$Q = 1 \text{ tablet}$$
$$H = 500 \text{ mg}$$

STEP B: CALCULATE

Follow Procedure Checklist 12-1.

1. Set up the proportion.

$$\frac{500 \text{ mg}}{1 \text{ tablet}} = \frac{1{,}000 \text{ mg}}{A}$$

2. Cancel units.

$$\frac{500 \text{ m\cancel{g}}}{1 \text{ tablet}} = \frac{1{,}000 \text{ m\cancel{g}}}{A}$$

3. Cross-multiply and solve for the unknown.

$$500 \times A = 1 \text{ tablet} \times 1{,}000$$

$$A = \frac{1{,}000}{500} \text{ tablets}$$

$$A = 2 \text{ tablets} = \text{amount to administer}$$

STEP C: THINK! . . . IS IT REASONABLE?

If 1 tablet equals 500 mg, then how many tablets equal 1,000 mg? Do I need more or less than the dose on hand? (*1,000 is greater than 500; therefore, more than 1 tablet is administered.*)

What is the relationship between the dose on hand and the ordered dose? (*The ordered dose is twice a large as the dose on hand and 2 tablets is twice as many as 1 tablet, so it is reasonable.*)

EXAMPLE 2

Find the amount to administer.

Ordered: Norvir® 200 mg PO now

On hand: See label in Figure 12-5.

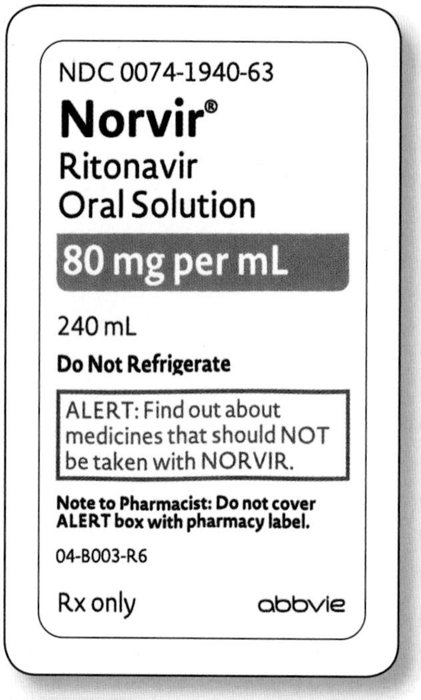
NDC 0074-1940-63
Norvir®
Ritonavir
Oral Solution
80 mg per mL
240 mL
Do Not Refrigerate
ALERT: Find out about medicines that should NOT be taken with NORVIR.
Note to Pharmacist: Do not cover ALERT box with pharmacy label.
04-B003-R6
Rx only
abbvie

Figure 12-5

STEP A: GATHER INFORMATION AND CONVERT

Again, the drug order and the drug label use the same units, so no conversion is necessary. Our desired dose is 200 mg. Reading the label tells us that the dosage unit is 1 mL and the dose on hand is 80 mg. Therefore,

$D = 200 \text{ mg}$

$Q = 1 \text{ mL}$

$H = 80 \text{ mg}$

STEP B: CALCULATE

Follow the Procedure Checklist 12-1.

1. Set up the proportion.

$$\frac{80 \text{ mg}}{1 \text{ mL}} = \frac{200 \text{ mg}}{A}$$

2. Cancel units.

$$\frac{80 \cancel{\text{mg}}}{1 \text{ mL}} = \frac{200 \cancel{\text{mg}}}{A}$$

3. Solve for the unknown.

$$80 \times A = 1 \text{ mL} \times 200$$

$$A = \frac{200}{80} = 2.5 \text{ mL} = \text{amount to administer}$$

STEP C: THINK! . . . IS IT REASONABLE?

If 80 mg is in 1 mL, is it reasonable that 40 mg would be in 0.5 mL? *(80 is two times 40 and 1 is two times 0.5, so it is reasonable.)* Eighty times 2.5 equals 200, the number of mg ordered. *(So 2.5 mL is reasonable.)*

EXAMPLE 3 | **Find the amount to administer.**

Ordered: ampicillin 250 mg IM now

On hand: ampicillin 0.5 g/mL

STEP A: GATHER INFORMATION AND CONVERT

The label tells us that the dose on hand (*H*) is 0.5 g and the dosage unit (*Q*) is 1 mL. However, in this case, the order is written in milligrams and the drug is labeled in grams. Before we can determine the amount to administer, we must calculate the desired dose in grams.
Follow the Procedure Checklist 6-3.

1. Recall that 1 g = 1,000 mg. Since we are converting to grams, our conversion factor is
$$\frac{1\ g}{1,000\ mg}.$$

2. The other fraction for our proportion is $\frac{D}{250\ mg}$.

3. Setting the two fractions into a proportion gives us the following equation:
$$\frac{D}{250\ mg} = \frac{1\ g}{1,000\ mg}$$

4. Cancel units.
$$\frac{D}{250\ \cancel{mg}} = \frac{1\ g}{1,000\ \cancel{mg}}$$

5. Solve for the unknown.
$$1,000 \times D = 250 \times 1\ g$$
$$D = \frac{250}{1,000} = 0.25\ g = \text{desired dose}$$

STEP B: CALCULATE

Follow the Procedure Checklist 12-1.

1. Set up the proportion. (Recall $\frac{H}{Q} = \frac{D}{A}$)
$$\frac{0.5\ g}{1\ mL} = \frac{0.25\ g}{A}$$

2. Cancel units.
$$\frac{0.5\ \cancel{g}}{1\ mL} = \frac{0.25\ \cancel{g}}{A}$$

3. Cross-multiply and solve for the unknown.
$$0.5 \times A = 1\ mL \times 0.25$$
$$A = \frac{0.25}{0.5} = 0.5\ mL = \text{amount to administer}$$

STEP C: THINK! . . . IS IT REASONABLE?

If 0.5 g is in 1 mL, is it reasonable that there is 0.25 g in 0.5 mL? *(Yes, it is reasonable; 0.25 is one half of 0.5 and 0.5 is one half of 1.)*

EXAMPLE 4 | **Find the amount to administer.**

Ordered: Metformin 2 g PO daily

On hand: See label in Figure 12-6.

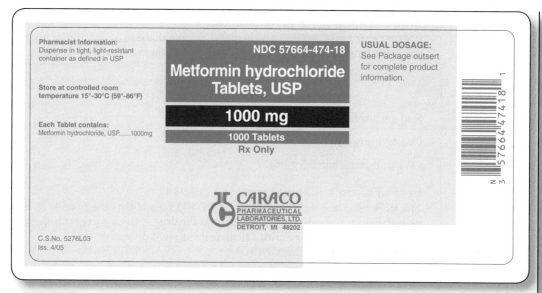

Figure 12-6

STEP A: GATHER INFORMATION AND CONVERT

In this case, we see from the label that the dosage unit (Q) is 1 tablet and the dose on hand (H) is 1,000 mg. Since the ordered dose is written in grams, we must calculate a desired dose that is in milligrams. Follow Procedure Checklist 6-3.

1. Recall that 1 g = 1,000 mg. Since we are converting to milligrams, our conversion factor is $\dfrac{1{,}000 \text{ mg}}{1 \text{ g}}$.

2. The other fraction for our proportion is $\dfrac{D}{2 \text{ g}}$.

3. Set up the proportion.

$$\frac{D}{2 \text{ g}} = \frac{1{,}000 \text{ mg}}{1 \text{ g}}$$

4. Cancel units.

$$\frac{D}{2 \cancel{\text{ g}}} = \frac{1{,}000 \text{ mg}}{1 \cancel{\text{ g}}}$$

5. Solve for the unknown.

$$1 \times D = 1{,}000 \text{ mg} \times 2$$

$$D = 2{,}000 \text{ mg} = \text{desired dose}$$

STEP B: CALCULATE

Follow the Procedure Checklist 12-1.

1. Set up the proportion. (Recall $\dfrac{H}{Q} = \dfrac{D}{A}$)

$$\frac{1{,}000 \text{ mg}}{1 \text{ tablet}} = \frac{2{,}000 \text{ mg}}{A}$$

2. Cancel units.

$$\frac{1{,}000 \cancel{\text{ mg}}}{1 \text{ tablet}} = \frac{2{,}000 \cancel{\text{ mg}}}{A}$$

3. Cross-multiply and solve for the unknown.

$$1{,}000 \times A = 1 \text{ tablet} \times 2{,}000$$

$$A = \frac{2{,}000}{1{,}000} = 2 \text{ tablets} = \text{amount to administer}$$

STEP C: THINK! . . . IS IT REASONABLE?

If 1,000 mg is in 1 tablet, is it reasonable that there is 2,000 mg in 2 tablets? (*Yes it is reasonable, 1,000 is one-half of 2,000 and 1 is half of 2.*)

LEARNING LINK Recall from the chapter "Converting Units," Procedure Checklist 6-4 that the proportion method can also be performed using ratios. When calculating the amount to administer using ratios, you would fill in the proportion *H:Q = D:A* and then multiply the means and extremes and solve for the unknown.

DIMENSIONAL ANALYSIS

Procedure Checklist 12-2

Calculating the Amount to Administer by Dimensional Analysis

With dimensional analysis you will not need to calculate the desired dose and amount to administer separately. You will place your unknown (amount to administer) on one side of the equation and then multiply a series of factors on the right side of the equation. Canceling units will help you determine that the equation has been set up correctly.

1. Determine the unit of measure for the answer, and place it as the unknown on one side of the equation. (In this case the answer would be the amount to administer. The unit of measure will be the same unit of measure as that of the dosage unit.)

2. If the desired dose (dose ordered) is a different unit of measure than the dose on hand, use a conversion factor as your first factor. The conversion factor should have the same unit of measure as the dose on hand on top and the same unit of measure as the dose ordered on the bottom.

3. Multiply the conversion factor by a second factor—the dosage unit over the dose on hand.

4. Multiply by a third factor—dosage ordered over the number 1.

5. Cancel units on the right side of the equation. The remaining unit of measure on the right side of the equation should match the unknown unit of measure on the left side of the equation.

6. Solve the equation.

EXAMPLE 1

Find the amount to administer.

Ordered: Famvir® 500 mg PO q8h

On hand: Famvir® 250 mg per tablet.

STEP A: GATHER INFORMATION AND CONVERT
The dose on hand is 250 mg, the dosage unit is 1 tablet, and the dosage ordered is 500 mg. The unit of measurement for the dosage ordered and the dose on hand are both milligrams. No conversion factor is needed.

STEP B: CALCULATE
Follow Procedure Checklist 12-2.

1. The unit of measure for the amount to administer will be tablets. This is the dosage unit.

   A tablets =

2. No conversion factor needed.

3. The dosage unit is 1 tablet. The dose on hand is 250 mg. This is our first factor.

$$A \text{ tablets} = \frac{1 \text{ tablet}}{250 \text{ mg}}$$

4. The dosage ordered is 500 mg. Place this quantity over the number 1 for the next factor.

$$A \text{ tablets} = \frac{1 \text{ tablet}}{250 \text{ mg}} \times \frac{500 \text{ mg}}{1}$$

5. Cancel the units.

$$A \text{ tablets} = \frac{1 \text{ tab}}{250 \text{ \cancel{mg}}} \times \frac{500 \text{ \cancel{mg}}}{1}$$

Since the remaining unit is tablets, and the unit of measure for the amount to administer is also tablets, the equation is set up correctly.

6. Solve the equation.

$$A \text{ tablets} = \frac{1 \text{ tablet}}{250 \text{ \cancel{mg}}} \times \frac{500 \text{ \cancel{mg}}}{1}$$

$$A = \frac{500}{250} = 2 \text{ tablets} = \text{amount to administer}$$

STEP C: THINK! . . . IS IT REASONABLE?

If 1 tablet equals 250 mg, then how many tablets equal 500 mg? Do I need more or less than the dose on hand? (*500 is greater than 250; therefore, more than 1 tablet is administered.*)

Consider the relationship between the dose on hand and the ordered dose. (*The ordered dose is twice a large as the dose on hand and 2 tablets is twice as many as 1 tablet, so it is reasonable.*)

EXAMPLE 2 | **Find the amount to administer.**

Ordered: Norvir® liquid 40 mg PO daily

On hand: Norvir® 80 mg/1 mL. See Figure 12-5 on page 264.

STEP A: GATHER INFORMATION AND CONVERT

The dose on hand is 80 mg, the dosage unit is 1 mL, and the dosage ordered is 40 mg. The unit of measurement for the dosage ordered and the dose on hand are both milligrams. No conversion factor needed.

STEP B: CALCULATE

Follow Procedure Checklist 12-2.

1. The amount to administer will be in milliliters. This is the dosage unit or how the medication is supplied.

$$A \text{ mL} =$$

2. No conversion factor needed.

3. The dosage unit is 1 mL. The dose on hand is 80 mg. This is our first factor.

$$A \text{ mL} = \frac{1 \text{ mL}}{80 \text{ mg}}$$

4. The dosage ordered is 40 mg. Place this over 1.

$$A \text{ mL} = \frac{1 \text{ mL}}{80 \text{ mg}} \times \frac{40 \text{ mg}}{1}$$

5. Cancel units on the right side of the equation.

$$A \text{ mL} = \frac{1 \text{ mL}}{80 \text{ \cancel{mg}}} \times \frac{40 \text{ \cancel{mg}}}{1}$$

6. Solve the equation.

$$A = \frac{40}{80} = 0.5 \text{ mL} = \text{amount to administer}$$

STEP C: THINK! . . . IS IT REASONABLE?

If 80 mg is in 1 mL, is it reasonable that 40 mg would be in half a mL? (*80 is two times greater than 40, so it is reasonable.*) Eighty times 2.5 equals 200, the number of mg ordered. (*So 2.5 mL is reasonable.*)

EXAMPLE 3	**Find the amount to administer.**

Ordered: ampicillin 250 mg IM now

On hand: ampicillin 0.5 g/mL

STEP A: GATHER INFORMATION AND CONVERT
The dosage ordered is 250 mg, the dose on hand is 0.5 g, and the dosage unit is 1 mL. Because the dose on hand is stated in grams and the dosage ordered is stated in milligrams, you will need to determine the conversion factor for grams to milligrams. In this case, the conversion factor is 1 g/1,000 mg. Grams (g) is the same unit of measure as the dose on hand and mg is the same unit of measure as the dosage ordered.

STEP B: CALCULATE
Follow Procedure Checklist 12-2.

   1. The unit of measure for the amount to administer will be milliliters.

     $A \text{ mL} =$

   2. Use the conversion factor.

     $A = \dfrac{1 \text{ g}}{1,000 \text{ mg}}$

   3. The dosage unit is 1 mL, and the dose on hand is 0.5 g. This is our second factor.

     $A \text{ mL} = \dfrac{1 \text{ g}}{1,000 \text{ mg}} \times \dfrac{1 \text{ mL}}{0.5 \text{ g}}$

   4. The dosage ordered is 250 mg. Place this over 1.

     $A \text{ mL} = \dfrac{1 \text{ g}}{1,000 \text{ mg}} \times \dfrac{1 \text{ mL}}{0.5 \text{ g}} \times \dfrac{250 \text{ mg}}{1}$

   5. Cancel units to check your equation.

     $A \text{ mL} = \dfrac{1 \cancel{g}}{1,000 \cancel{mg}} \times \dfrac{1 \text{ mL}}{0.5 \cancel{g}} \times \dfrac{250 \cancel{mg}}{1}$

   6. Solve the equation.

     $A \text{ mL} = \dfrac{250 \text{ mL}}{500}$ (Reduce the fraction to its lowest terms.)

     $A = \dfrac{1}{2} \text{ mL} = 0.5 \text{ mL} = \text{amount to administer}$

STEP C: THINK! . . . IS IT REASONABLE?
If 0.5 g is in 1 mL, is it reasonable that there is 0.25 g in 0.5 mL? (*Yes, it is reasonable; 0.25 is one half of 0.5 and 0.5 is one half of 1.*) |
| **EXAMPLE 4** | **Find the amount to administer.**

Ordered: Metformin 2 g PO daily

On hand: Metformin hydrochloride 1,000 mg. See Figure 12-6 on page 266.

STEP A: GATHER INFORMATION AND CONVERT
The dosage ordered is 2 g, the dose on hand is 1,000 mg, and the dosage unit is 1 tablet. Because the dose on hand is stated in milligrams and the dosage ordered is stated in grams, you will need to determine the conversion factor for milligrams to grams. In this case, the conversion factor is 1,000 mg/1 g.

STEP B: CALCULATE
Follow Procedure Checklist 12-2.

   1. The unit of measure for the amount to administer will be tablets.

     $A \text{ tablets} =$

   2. Use the conversion factor.

     $A \text{ tablets} = \dfrac{1,000 \text{ mg}}{1 \text{ g}}$

   3. The dosage unit is 1 tablet, and the dose on hand is 1,000 mg. This is our second factor.

     $A \text{ tablets} = \dfrac{1,000 \text{ mg}}{1 \text{ g}} \times \dfrac{1 \text{ tablet}}{1,000 \text{ mg}}$ |

4. The dosage ordered is 2 g. Place this over 1.

$$A \text{ tablets} = \frac{1{,}000 \text{ mg}}{1 \text{ g}} \times \frac{1 \text{ tablet}}{1{,}000 \text{ mg}} \times \frac{2 \text{ g}}{1}$$

5. Cancel units.

$$A \text{ tablets} = \frac{1{,}000 \cancel{\text{mg}}}{1 \cancel{\text{g}}} \times \frac{1 \text{ tablet}}{1{,}000 \cancel{\text{mg}}} \times \frac{2 \cancel{\text{g}}}{1}$$

6. Solve the equation.

$$A \text{ tablets} = \frac{2{,}000}{1{,}000} \quad \text{(Reduce the fraction to its lowest terms.)}$$

$$A = 2 \text{ tablets} = \text{amount to administer}$$

STEP C: THINK! . . . IS IT REASONABLE?
If 1,000 mg are in 1 tablet, is it reasonable that there are 2,000 mg in 2 tablets? (*Yes it is reasonable, 1,000 is one half of 2,000 and 1 is half of 2.*)

FORMULA METHOD

Procedure Checklist 12-3
Calculating the Amount to Administer by the Formula Method

1. Determine the components of the formula method, *D*, *H*, and *Q*, and fill in the formula:

$$\frac{D}{H} \times Q = A$$

where *D* = desired dose—the dose ordered changed to the same unit of measure as the dose on hand.
   H = dose on hand—the amount of drug contained in each unit.
   Q = dosage unit—how the drug will be administered, such as tablets or milliliters.
   A = unknown or amount to administer.

2. Cancel the units.

3. Solve for the unknown.

EXAMPLE 1

Find the amount to administer.

Ordered: Famvir® 500 mg PO q8h

On hand: Famvir® 250 mg per tablet.

STEP A: GATHER INFORMATION AND CONVERT
The dosage ordered is 500 mg, the dose on hand is 250 mg, and the dosage unit is 1 tablet. The drug is ordered in milligrams, which is the same unit used on the label, so no conversion is needed. So the desired dose *D* is the same as the dosage ordered.

STEP B: CALCULATE
Follow Procedure Checklist 12-3.

1. Determine the values of *D*, *H*, and *Q*, and fill in the formula.

D (desired dose) = 500 mg
Q (dosage unit) = 1 tablet
H (dose on hand) = 250 mg

$$\frac{500 \text{ mg}}{250 \text{ mg}} \times 1 \text{ tablet} = A$$

2. Cancel units.

$$\frac{500 \text{ m\cancel{g}}}{250 \text{ m\cancel{g}}} \times 1 \text{ tablet} = A$$

3. Solve for the unknown.

A = 2 tablets = amount to administer

STEP C: THINK! . . . IS IT REASONABLE?

If 1 tablet equals 250 mg, then how many tablets equal 500 mg? Do I need more or less than the dose on hand? (*500 is greater than 250, therefore, more than 1 tablet is administered.*)

What is the relationship between the dose on hand and the ordered dose? (*The ordered dose is twice as large as the dose on hand and 2 tablets are twice as many as 1 tablet, so it is reasonable.*)

| EXAMPLE 2 | **Calculate the amount to administer.** |

Ordered: Norvir® liquid 40 mg PO daily

On hand: Norvir® 8 mg/1 mL. See Figure 12-5 on page 264.

STEP A: GATHER INFORMATION AND CONVERT
The dosage ordered is 40 mg, the dose on hand is 8 mg, and the dosage unit is 1 mL. The drug order and the drug label use the same units, so no conversion is necessary. So the desired dose is the same as the dosage ordered.

STEP B: CALCULATE
Follow Procedure Checklist 12-3.

1. Determine the values of *D*, *H*, and *Q* and insert them into the formula.

D (desired dose) = 40 mg

Q (dosage unit) = 1 mL

H (dose on hand) = 80 mg

$$\frac{40 \text{ mg}}{80 \text{ mg}} \times 1 \text{ mL} = A$$

2. Cancel units.

$$\frac{40 \text{ m\cancel{g}}}{80 \text{ m\cancel{g}}} \times 1 \text{ mL} = A$$

3. Solve for the unknown.

0.5 mL = A = amount to administer

STEP C: THINK! . . . IS IT REASONABLE?
If 80 mg is in 1 mL, is it reasonable that 40 mg would be in 0.5 mL? (*80 is two times greater than 40 and 1 is two times greater than 0.5, so it is reasonable.*)

| EXAMPLE 3 | **Find the amount to administer.** |

Ordered: ampicillin 250 mg IM now

On hand: ampicillin 0.5 g/mL

STEP A: GATHER INFORMATION AND CONVERT
The dosage ordered is 250 mg, the dose on hand is 0.5 g, and the dosage unit is 1 mL. In this case, the order is written in milligrams, and the drug is labeled in grams. Before we can determine the amount to administer, we must calculate a desired dose that is in grams. In this example we will use the proportion method, Procedure Checklist 6-3.

1. Recall that 1 g = 1,000 mg. Since we are converting to grams, our conversion factor is:

$$\frac{1 \text{ g}}{1,000 \text{ mg}}$$

2. The other fraction for our proportion is $\frac{D}{250 \text{ mg}}$.

3. Setting the two fractions into a proportion gives us the following equation:

$$\frac{D}{250 \text{ mg}} = \frac{1 \text{ g}}{1,000 \text{ mg}}$$

4. Cancel units.

$$\frac{D}{250 \text{ m\cancel{g}}} = \frac{1 \text{ g}}{1,000 \text{ m\cancel{g}}}$$

5. Solve for the unknown.

$$1,000 \times D = 250 \times 1 \text{ g}$$
$$D = 0.25 \text{ g} = \text{desired dose}$$

STEP B: CALCULATE

Follow Procedure Checklist 12-3.

1. Determine the values of D, H, and Q and insert them into the formula.

   D (desired dose) = 0.25 g

   Q (dosage unit) = 1 mL

   H (dose on hand) = 0.5 g

   $$\frac{0.25 \text{ g}}{0.5 \text{ g}} \times 1 \text{ mL} = A$$

2. Cancel units.

   $$\frac{0.25 \text{ \cancel{g}}}{0.5 \text{ \cancel{g}}} \times 1 \text{ mL} = A$$

3. Solve for the unknown.

   0.5 mL = A = amount to administer

STEP C: THINK! . . . IS IT REASONABLE?

If 0.5 g is in 1 mL, is it reasonable that there is 0.25 g in 0.5 mL? (*Yes, it is reasonable; 0.25 is one half of 0.5 and 0.5 is one half of 1.*) Eighty times 2.5 equals 200, the number of mg ordered. (*So 2.5 mL is reasonable.*)

EXAMPLE 4	Calculate the amount to administer.

Ordered: Metformin 2 g PO daily

On hand: Metformin hydrochloride 1,000 mg. See Figure 12-6 on page 266.

STEP A: GATHER INFORMATION AND CONVERT

The dosage ordered is 2 g, the dose on hand is 1,000 mg, and the dosage unit is 1 tablet. In this case, the order is written in grams, and the drug is labeled in milligrams. Before we can determine the amount to administer, we must calculate a desired dose that is in milligrams. In this example we will use the proportion method, Procedure Checklist 6-3.

1. Recall that 1 g = 1,000 mg. Since we are converting to milligrams, our conversion factor is:

   1,000 mg : 1 g

2. The other ratio in our proportion is:

   $D : 2 \text{ g}$

3. Set up the ratio proportion equation.

   1,000 mg:1 g = D:2 g

4. Cancel units.

$$1{,}000 \text{ mg}{:}1\,\cancel{g} = D{:}2\,\cancel{g}$$

5. Multiply the means and extremes and solve the equation.

$$1 \times D = 1{,}000 \text{ mg} \times 2$$
$$D = 2{,}000 \text{ mg} = \text{desired dose}$$

STEP B: CALCULATE
Follow Procedure Checklist 12-3.

1. Determine the values of D, H, and Q and insert them into the formula.
   D (desired dose) = 2,000 mg
   Q (dosage unit) = 1 tablet
   H (dose on hand) = 1,000 mg

$$\frac{2{,}000 \text{ g}}{1{,}000 \text{ g}} \times 1 \text{ tablet} = A$$

2. Cancel units.

$$\frac{2{,}000 \,\cancel{g}}{1{,}000 \,\cancel{g}} \times 1 \text{ tablet} = A$$

3. Solve for the unknown.

$$2 \text{ tablets} = A = \text{amount to administer}$$

STEP C: THINK! . . . IS IT REASONABLE?
If 1,000 mg are in 1 tablet, is it reasonable that there are 2,000 mg in 2 tablets? (*Yes it is reasonable, 1,000 is half of 2,000 and 1 is half of 2.*)

CRITICAL THINKING ON THE JOB

When in Doubt, Check

Jorge was working in the emergency room when a patient arrived with life-threatening internal bleeding. The physician in charge told Jorge, "Aminocaproic acid 5 grams STAT! You'd better give him liquid, I don't think he's able to swallow pills." Jorge repeated the order, "Aminocaproic acid liquid 5 grams STAT."

On hand, Jorge had Amicar Syrup (aminocaproic acid) 0.25 g/mL (see Figure 12-7). Jorge determined the amount to administer by using the ratio proportion method.

$$\frac{0.25 \text{ g}}{1 \text{ mL}} = \frac{5 \text{ g}}{A}$$

$$\frac{0.25 \,\cancel{g}}{1 \text{ mL}} = \frac{5 \,\cancel{g}}{A}$$

$$0.25 \times A = 5 \text{ mL} \times 1$$

$$A = \frac{5 \text{ mL}}{0.25}$$

$$A = 20 \text{ mL} = 4 \text{ tsp}$$

(Continued)

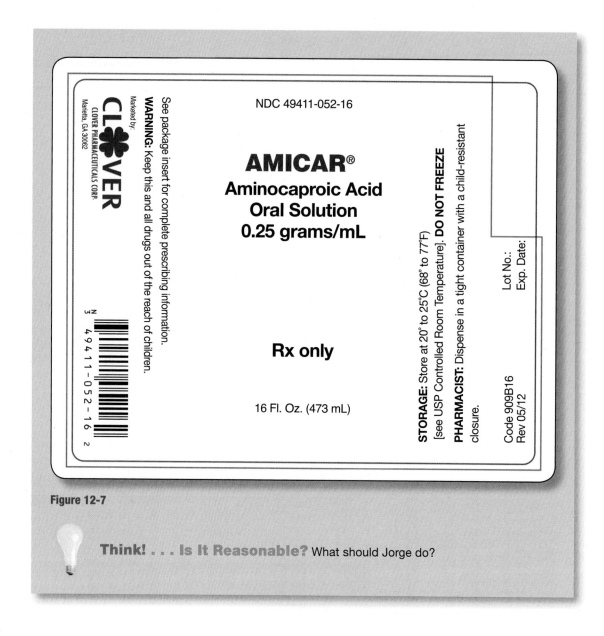

Figure 12-7

Think! . . . Is It Reasonable? What should Jorge do?

REVIEW AND PRACTICE

12.2 Methods of Dosage Calculation

In Exercises 1–20, calculate the amount to administer.

1. Ordered: Thorazine® 20 mg PO tid
On hand: Thorazine® 10 mg tablets

2. Ordered: Ranitidine hydrochloride 150 mg PO bid
On hand: Zantac® syrup 15 mg ranitidine hydrochloride per mL

3. Ordered: Ceclor® 0.375 g PO bid
On hand: Ceclor® Oral Suspension 187 mg per 5 mL

4. Ordered: Nitroglycerin gr $\frac{1}{100}$ SL stat
   On hand: Nitroglycerin 0.3 mg tablets

5. Ordered: Amoxicillin 250 mg PO tid
   On hand: Refer to label A.

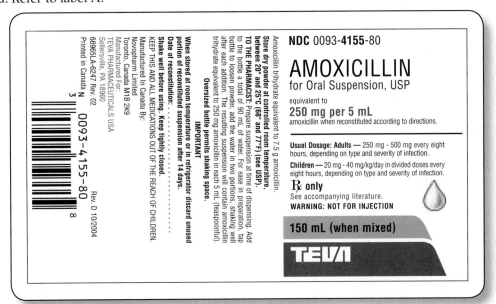

A

This label is for US only, and cannot be altered or translated.

6. Ordered: Tricor® 48 mg PO daily
   On hand: Refer to label B.

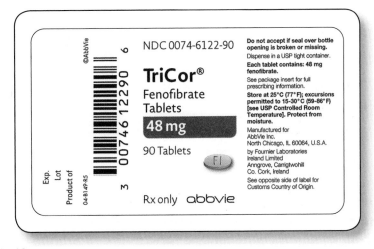

B

7. Ordered: Procardia 10 mg
   On hand: Refer to label C.

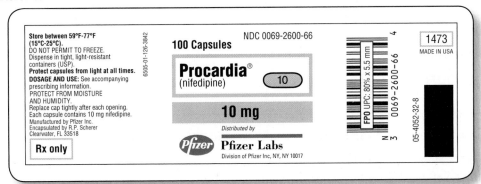

C

8. Ordered: Kaletra 400 mg/100 mg PO BID
   On hand: Refer to label D.

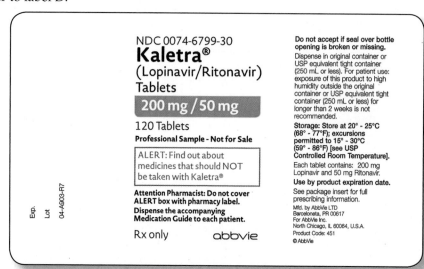

9. Ordered: Synthroid® 0.3 mg PO daily
   On hand: Refer to label E.

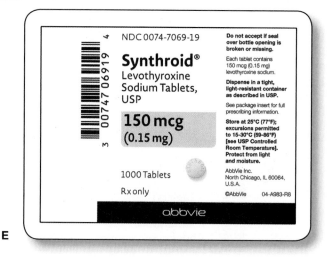

10. Ordered: Atomoxetine HCl 0.1 g PO bid
   On hand: Refer to label F.

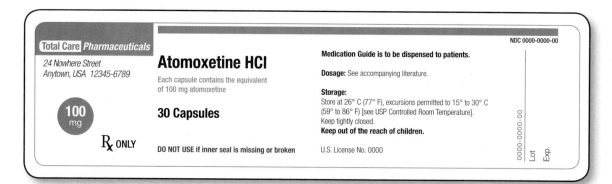

11. Ordered: Keflex® 500 mg PO q12h
   On hand: Keflex® 250 mg per 5 mL

12. Ordered: Decadron® 6 mg IM q.i.d.
   On hand: Decadron® 4 mg per mL

13. Ordered: Ketoconazole® 100 mg PO daily.
   On hand: Ketoconazole® 200 mg scored tablets

14. Ordered: Dilaudid® 2 mg IM prn for pain q6h
   On hand: Dilaudid® for injection, 4 mg per mL

15. Ordered: Erythromycin Oral Suspension 150 mg PO bid
   On hand: Refer to label G.

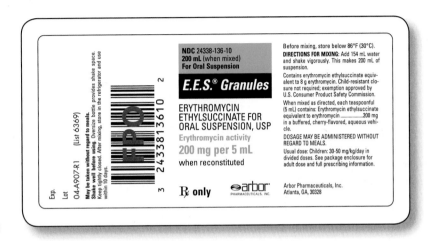

G

16. Ordered: Provera 5 mg PO daily
   On hand: Refer to label H.

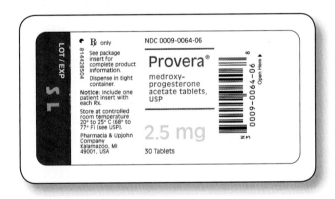

H

17. Ordered: Vistaril 35 mg PO now.
   On hand: Refer to label I.

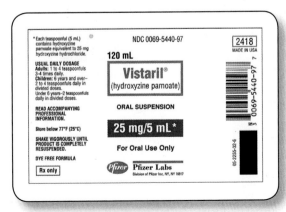

I

18. Ordered: Insulix-R 28 units subcut stat
   On hand: Refer to label J.

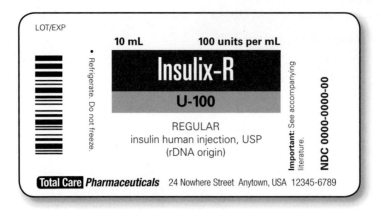

J

19. Ordered: Ritalin® 15 mg PO bid ac
   On hand: Refer to label K.

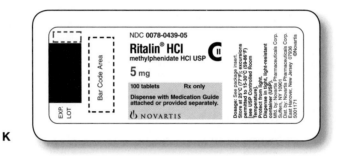

K

20. Ordered: Camptosar 250 mg IV now
   On hand: Refer to label L.

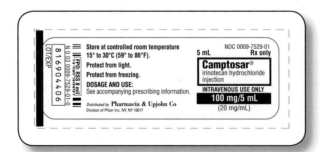

L

LEARNING OUTCOME	KEY POINTS
12.1 Determine information needed to perform dosage calculations. Pages 252–261	*Dose ordered:* found on order, prescription, MAR, or eMAR *Dosage strength:* found on medication label as dosage unit (Q) per dose on hand (H) If the dose ordered is in a different unit of measurement from the dose on hand, convert the dose ordered to the same unit of measurement as the dose on hand. For example, if the dose ordered is 500 mg and the dose on hand is 1 g, convert 500 mg to grams using the calculation method of your choice.

12.2 Utilize three methods of dosage calculations. Pages 261–283	Follow three steps to perform dosage calculations:
	
	  A. Gather information and convert
	
	  B. Calculate
	
	  C. Think! Is it reasonable?
	
	Remember, D = desired dose, H = dose on hand, Q = dosage unit, A = amount to administer, Conversion factor = Units of measurement on hand/units of measurement ordered
	
	Proportion Method:
	
	The proportion of the units you have to the units you desire can be written two ways:
	
	Fraction $\dfrac{H}{Q} = \dfrac{D}{A}$
	
	As a fraction, cross-multiply the numerators with the denominators ($H \times A = Q \times D$).
	
	Ratio $H : Q = D : A$
	
	As a ratio multiply the means to equal the extremes ($Q \times D = H \times A$)
	
	Use the Procedure Checklist 12-1 to calculate the amount to administer using a fraction or a ratio.

	Dimensional Analysis Method: **Step A: Gather Information and Convert** Determine if a conversion factor is needed **Step B: Calculate** Amount to administer = conversion factor $\times \dfrac{Q}{H} \times \dfrac{D}{1}$

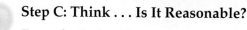

LEARNING OUTCOME	KEY POINTS

Step C: Think . . . Is It Reasonable?

Example: Ordered: Metformin 2 g po daily On hand: Metformin hydrochloride 1,000 mg per 1 tablet.

Step A: Gather Information and Convert A conversion factor is needed since the tablet strength is measured in mg, and the order calls for g.

Step B: Calculate

$$A = \frac{1,000 \text{ mg}}{1 \text{ g}} \times \frac{1 \text{ tablet}}{1,000 \text{ mg}} \times \frac{2 \text{ g}}{1}$$

Cancel and reduce

2 tablets = 1 tablet × 2

Step C: Think! . . . Is It Reasonable? We know we will need more than 1 tablet since 2 g is more than the amount in 1 tablet (1 tablet is 1 g) and 1,000 mg = 1 g.

We also know that we need twice the amount found in 1 tablet, since 2 g is twice as much as 1 g. 2 tablets is twice as much as 1 tablet, so the answer is reasonable

---

Formula Method:

$$\frac{D}{H} \times Q = A$$

Example: Ordered: Metformin 2 g po daily

On hand: Metformin hydrochloride 1,000 mg per 1 tablet

Step A: Gather Information and Convert

$$\frac{1,000 \text{ mg}}{1 \text{ g}} \times 2 \text{ g} = 2,000 \text{ mg}$$

Step B: Calculate

$$\frac{2,000 \text{ mg}}{1,000 \text{ mg}} \times 1 \text{ tablet} = A$$

Cancel units and reduce

2 × 1 tablet = 2 tablets

Step C: Think! . . . Is It Reasonable? We know we will need more than 1 tablet since 2 g is more than the amount in 1 tablet (1 tablet is 1 g) and 1,000 mg = 1 g.

We also know that we need twice the amount found in 1 tablet, since 2 g is twice as much as 1 g. 2 tablets is twice as much as 1 tablet, so the answer is reasonable

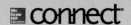
Answer the following questions. (LO 12.1)

1. Define the term *desired dose.*

2. Define the term *dosage unit.*

3. Define the term *dose on hand.*

4. Define the term *amount to administer.*

5. Define the term *conversion factor* and tell when it is used.

For Exercises 6–10, for each order: identify the dose on hand, dosage unit, desired dose, and if necessary identify the conversion factor and convert to like units of measurement. Use conversion tables from the "Converting Units" chapter as needed. (LO 12.1)

medication order	dose on hand	dosage unit	conversion factor	desired dose
6. Ordered: Flagyl 0.50 g po tid On hand: Flagyl 500 mg tablets				
7. Ordered: Synthroid 0.05 mg po daily On hand: Synthroid 25 mcg tablets				
8. Ordered: Tolbutamide 250 mg po tid On hand: Tolbutamide 0.5 g scored tablets				
9. Ordered: Dexamethasone 1,000 mcg po now On hand: Dexamethasone 1 mg tablets				
10. Ordered: Erythromycin 0.5 g po q6h On hand: Erythromycin 250 mg tablets				

Select the appropriate label (pp. 282–283) for the following drug orders and indicate the number of tablets/capsules/milliliters that will be required to administer the dosage ordered. Labels may be used for more than one example. (LO 12.2)

Notice that both generic and brand names are used for the orders.

11. Ordered: amoxicillin 2 grams liquid

    Label _____

    Amount to administer: _____

12. Ordered: Zemplar® 1 mcg

    Label _____

    Amount to administer: _____

13. Ordered: Gleevec® 300 mg

Label _____

Amount to administer: _____

14. Ordered: nifedipine 10 mg

Label _____

Amount to administer: _____

15. Ordered: cefprozil 500 mg liquid

Label _____

Amount to administer: _____

16. Ordered: valproic acid 250 mg

Label _____

Amount to administer: _____

17. Ordered: sertraline HCL 100 mg

Label _____

Amount to administer: _____

18. Ordered: Trileptal 450 mg

Label _____

Amount to administer: _____

19. Ordered: amoxicillin 300 mg liquid

Label _____

Amount to administer: _____

20. Ordered: risperidone 1 mg

Label _____

Amount to administer: _____

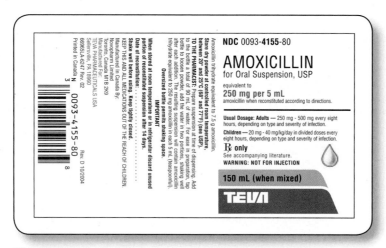

This label is for US only, and cannot be altered or translated.

Label A

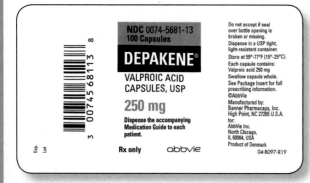

Label B

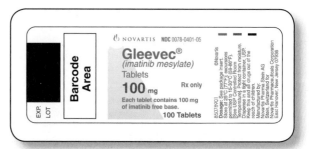

Label C

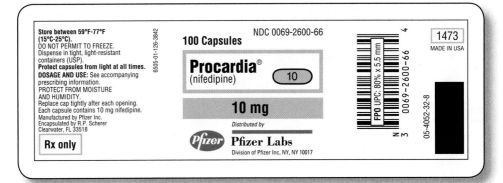

Label D

Store between 59°F-77°F
(15°C-25°C).
DO NOT PERMIT TO FREEZE.
Dispense in tight, light-resistant
containers (USP).
Protect capsules from light at all times.
DOSAGE AND USE: See accompanying
prescribing information.
PROTECT FROM MOISTURE
AND HUMIDITY.
Replace cap tightly after each opening.
Each capsule contains 10 mg nifedipine.
Manufactured by Pfizer Inc.
Encapsulated by R.P. Scherer
Clearwater, FL 33518

Rx only

6505-01-126-3842

100 Capsules   NDC 0069-2600-66

Procardia®   ⬭ 10
(nifedipine)

10 mg

Distributed by

Pfizer **Pfizer Labs**
Division of Pfizer Inc, NY, NY 10017

FPO UPC: 80% x 5.5 mm   0069-2600-66   N 3

1473
MADE IN USA

05-4052-32-8

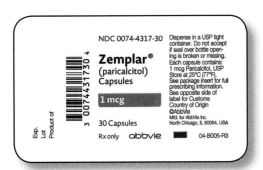

Label E

NDC 0074-4317-30

Zemplar®
(paricalcitol)
Capsules

1 mcg

30 Capsules

Rx only   abbvie

3 0074431730 4

Exp.
Lot
Product of

Dispense in a USP tight
container. Do not accept
if seal over bottle open-
ing is broken or missing.
Each capsule contains:
1 mcg Paricalcitol, USP
Store at 25°C (77°F).
See package insert for full
prescribing information.
See opposite side of
label for Customs
Country of Origin
©AbbVie
Mfd. for AbbVie Inc.
North Chicago, IL 60064, USA

04-B005-R3

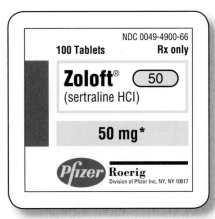

Label F

NDC 0049-4900-66

100 Tablets   **Rx only**

Zoloft®   ⬭ 50
(sertraline HCl)

50 mg*

Pfizer Roerig
Division of Pfizer Inc, NY, NY 10017

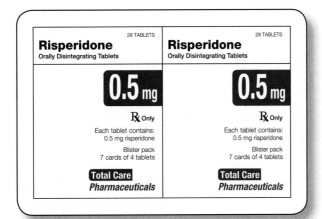

Label G

28 TABLETS	28 TABLETS
Risperidone Orally Disintegrating Tablets	**Risperidone** Orally Disintegrating Tablets
0.5 mg	**0.5 mg**
Rx Only	**Rx Only**
Each tablet contains: 0.5 mg risperidone	Each tablet contains: 0.5 mg risperidone
Blister pack 7 cards of 4 tablets	Blister pack 7 cards of 4 tablets
Total Care *Pharmaceuticals*	**Total Care** *Pharmaceuticals*

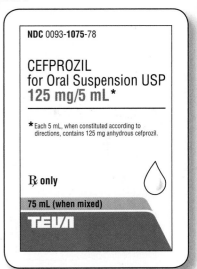

Label H   *This label is for US
only, and cannot be
altered or translated.*

NDC 0093-1075-78

CEFPROZIL
for Oral Suspension USP
125 mg/5 mL*

* Each 5 mL, when constituted according to
directions, contains 125 mg anhydrous cefprozil.

Rx only

75 mL (when mixed)

TEVA

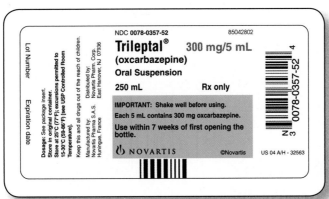

Label I

NDC 0078-0357-52   85042802

Trileptal®   **300 mg/5 mL**
(oxcarbazepine)
Oral Suspension

250 mL   **Rx only**

IMPORTANT: Shake well before using.
Each 5 mL contains 300 mg oxcarbazepine.
Use within 7 weeks of first opening the
bottle.

☊ NOVARTIS   ©Novartis   US 04 A/H - 32563

Lot Number   Expiration date

Dosage: See package insert.
Store in original container.
Store at 25°C (77°F); excursions permitted to
15-30°C (59-86°F) [see USP Controlled Room
Temperature].
Keep this and all drugs out of the reach of children.

Distributed by:
Novartis Pharm. Corp.
East Hanover, NJ 07936

Manufactured by:
Novartis Pharma S.A.S.
Huningue, France

N 3 0078-0357-52 4

CHAPTER 12 REVIEW

CHECK UP

For Exercises 1–23, calculate the desired dose. Then calculate the amount to administer. (LO 12.1, 12.2)

1. Ordered: Valium® 5 mg PO tid
   On hand: Valium® 2 mg scored tablets
   Desired dose: _____   Amount to administer: _____

2. Ordered: Atacand® 16 mg PO bid
   On hand: Atacand® 8 mg tablets
   Desired dose: _____   Amount to administer: _____

3. Ordered: Cimetidine 400 mg PO qid
   On hand: Cimetidine 200 mg tablets
   Desired dose: _____   Amount to administer: _____

4. Ordered: Noroxin® 800 mg PO daily ac $\bar{c}$ H_2O
   On hand: Noroxin® 400 mg tablets
   Desired dose: _____   Amount to administer: _____

5. Ordered: Tenex® 2 mg PO nightly at bedtime
   On hand: Tenex® 1 mg tablets
   Desired dose: _____   Amount to administer: _____

6. Ordered: Tranxene® 7.5 mg PO nightly at bedtime
   On hand: Tranxene® 3.75 mg tablets
   Desired dose: _____   Amount to administer: _____

7. Ordered: Pergolide mesylate 100 mcg PO tid
   On hand: Pergolide mesylate 0.05 mg tablets
   Desired dose: _____   Amount to administer: _____

8. Ordered: Zyloprim® 0.25 g PO bid
   On hand: Zyloprim® 100 mg scored tablets
   Desired dose: _____   Amount to administer: _____

9. Ordered: Zaroxolyn® 7.5 mg PO daily
   On hand: Zaroxolyn® 2.5 mg tablets
   Desired dose: _____   Amount to administer: _____

10. Ordered: Depakote ER 500 mg PO q12h

On hand: Refer to label A.

Desired dose: _____   Amount to administer: _____

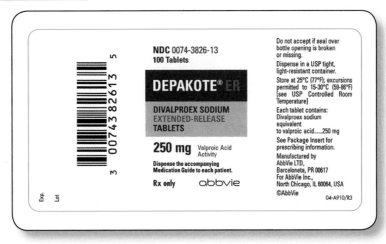

A

11. Ordered: Lexapro® 20 mg PO daily

On hand: Refer to label B.

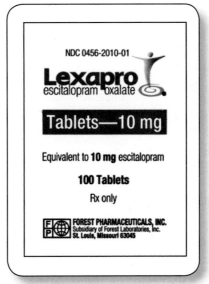

B

12. Ordered: Erythromycin 500 mg PO BID

On hand: Refer to label C.

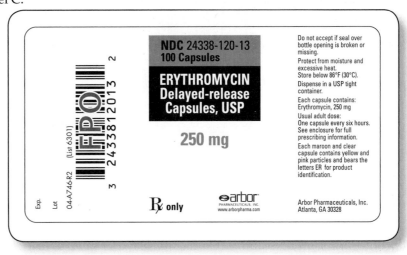

C

13. Ordered: Depakene® 250 mg PO bid
   On hand: Refer to label D.

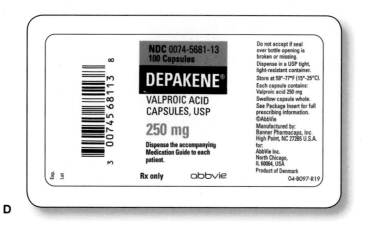

D

14. Ordered: Dilantin® 60 mg PO daily
   On hand: Refer to label E.

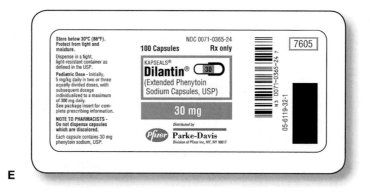

E

15. Ordered: Lisinopril 40 mg PO daily
   On hand: Refer to label F.

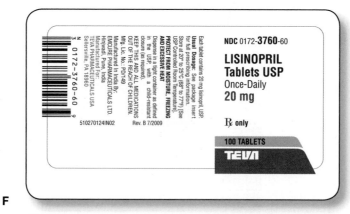

F

This label is for US only, and cannot be altered or translated.

16. Ordered: EES Granules® 100 mg PO tid

On hand: Refer to label G.

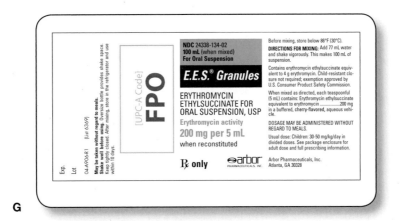

G

17. Ordered: amoxicillin 1 gram PO bid

On hand: Refer to label H.

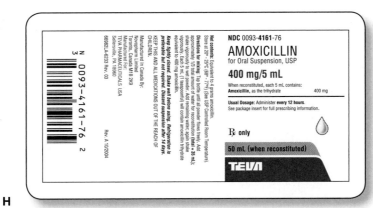

H

This label is for US only, and cannot be altered or translated.

18. Ordered: Metformin 1 g daily

On hand: Refer to label I.

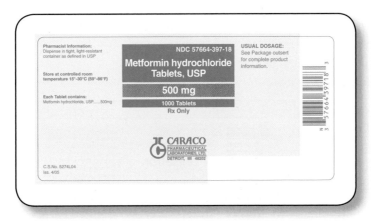

I

19. Ordered Cefprozil 200 mg PO q8h
   On hand: Refer to label J.

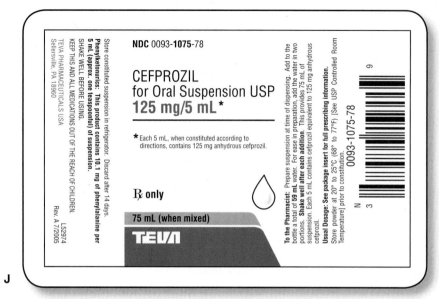

This label is for US only, and cannot be altered or translated.

20. Ordered: Sandostatin 150 mcg subcut BID
   On hand: Refer to label K.

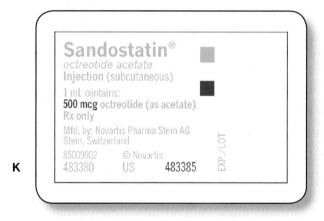

21. Ordered: Granisetron HCL Oral Solution 4 mg PO tid
   On hand: Refer to label L.

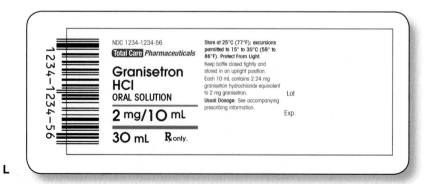

22. Ordered: Furosemide 100 mg IM now
   On hand: Refer to label M.

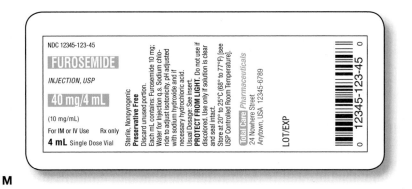

M

23. Ordered: Lipitor® 20 mg PO daily
   On hand: Refer to label N.

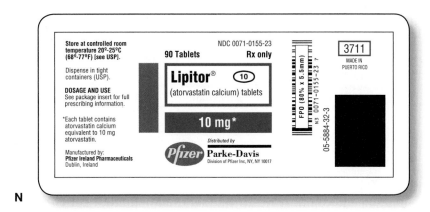

N

CRITICAL THINKING APPLICATIONS

Use the following label to answer questions 1 through 4. (LO 12.1, 12.2)

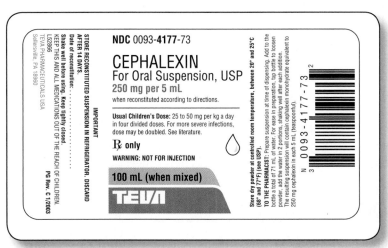

This label is for US only, and cannot be altered or translated.

1. A physician's order reads Cephalexin 250 mg PO q6h for 1 week. Calculate the amount to administer.

2. The physician changes the dose to Cephalexin 375 mg PO q6h for 2 weeks. Calculate the amount to administer for this dose.

3. After two weeks, the physician orders Cephalexin 250 PO TID for 30 days. Calculate the amount to administer for 1 dose.

4. In each of the cases above, determine the total amount of medication the patient will need.

CASE STUDY

You are working in a pharmacy when the following prescription comes in: diazepam 7 mg PO tid for 7 days. The drug labels below represent what you have on hand for filling this prescription. (LO 12.2)

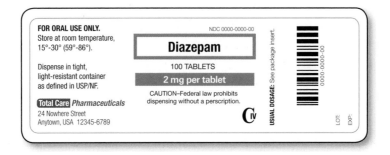

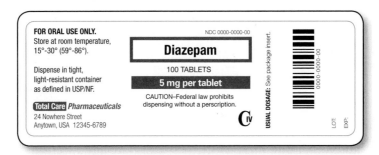

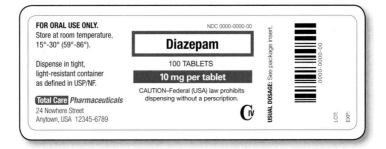

1. What is the amount to administer for 1 dose?

2. How many total tablets will the patient need?

3. What changes would you make in filling the order if the prescription read diazepam 15 mg PO tid for 7 days? How many tablets will the patient need for this new order?

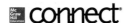

Now that you have completed the materials in the chapter text, go to CONNECT and complete any chapter activities you have not yet done.

Oral Dosages

*If you want to achieve excellence, you can get there today.
As of this second, quit doing less-than-excellent work.*

THOMAS JOHN WATSON, JR.

LEARNING OUTCOMES

When you have completed Chapter 13, you will be able to:

13.1 Calculate dosages for solid oral medications and explain principles related to their administration.

13.2 Calculate dosages for liquid oral medications, and explain principles related to their administration.

KEY TERMS

Caplet

Capsule

Enteric coated

Gelcap

Reconstitution

Scored

Spansules

Sustained release

Tablet

INTRODUCTION

You have learned the proportion, formula, and dimensional analysis methods for basic dosage calculations. In this chapter you will apply these methods to oral dosages, including solids and liquids. By now you may have chosen one method with which you are most comfortable. If so, follow that method throughout this chapter, using the corresponding color coding in the examples given; then complete the practice problems, using your method of choice. In this chapter you will also apply the principles of label reading learned in the chapter "Interpreting Medication Labels and Package Inserts." Many practice problems in this chapter will require you to carefully read medication labels. While you are practicing these problems, remember that excellence is a *must* with dosage calculations.

13.1 Solid Oral Medications

Solid oral medications come in several forms, including tablets, caplets, capsules, and gelcaps (see Figure 13-1). The **tablet** is the most common form of solid oral medication. It combines a specific amount of drug with inactive ingredients such as starch or talc to form a solid disk or cylinder that is convenient for swallowing. Certain tablets are specially designed to be administered sublingually (under the tongue) or buccally (between the cheek and gum). Sublingual and buccal tablets release medication into an area rich in blood vessels, where it can be quickly absorbed for rapid action. Some tablets are designed to be chewed; others dissolve in water to make a liquid that the patient can drink. Always check the drug label to determine how a tablet is meant to be administered.

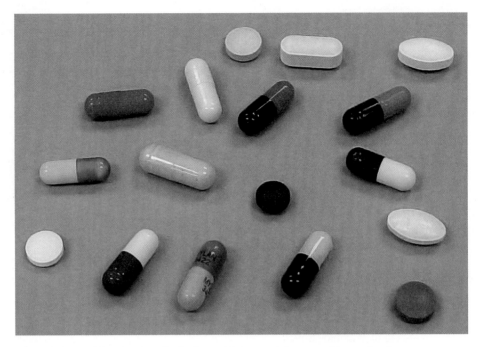

Figure 13-1 Solid oral medications including tablets, caplets, capsules, and gelcaps.

Caplets are similar to tablets. Oval-shaped, they have a special coating that makes them easy to swallow. **Capsules** are usually oval-shaped gelatin shells that contain medication in powder or granule form. The gelatin shell usually has two pieces that fit together. These pieces may sometimes be separated to remove the medication when the patient cannot swallow a pill. **Gelcaps** consist of medication, usually liquid, in gelatin shells that are not designed to be opened.

Calculating Dosages for Solid Oral Medications

Tablets are sometimes **scored** so that they can be divided when smaller doses are ordered. Most often, scored tablets divide into halves (see Figure 13-2), but some are scored to divide

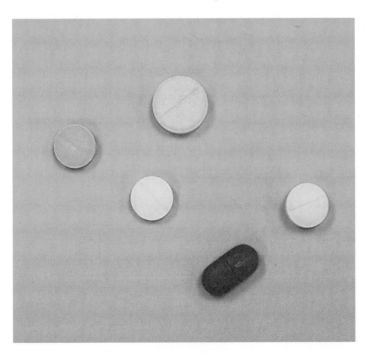

Figure 13-2 Scored tablets.

into thirds or quarters. The medication in scored tablets is evenly distributed throughout the tablet, allowing the dose to be divided evenly when the tablet is broken. Tablets may be broken into parts *only if they are scored*, and they must be broken only along the line of the scoring. Gloves must be worn when handling medication to prevent absorption of medication through the skin. Unscored tablets *must not* be broken into parts. Remember, breaking scored tablets to administer an ordered dosage is permitted but not optimal. Determine whether another dosage strength is available before you break scored tablets.

RULE 13-1	Always question and verify any calculation that indicates you should give a portion of a tablet when the tablet is not scored.

- Do not administer $\frac{1}{2}$ of an unscored tablet.
- Do not administer $\frac{1}{3}$ or $\frac{1}{4}$ of a tablet scored for division in two.

RULE 13-2	Question and recheck any calculation that indicates that you should administer more than 3 tablets or capsules.

If the situations in Rules 13-1 and 13-2 arise, recheck your calculations. If you are confident that your calculations are correct, then check with the physician or pharmacist, or your drug reference book, to be sure there is no error in the order or the dosage strength you are using.

 LEARNING LINK   Recall from the "Methods of Dosage Calculations" chapter that to calculate the amount to administer, you must know the desired dose and the dosage strength. The dosage strength is the amount of medication (dose on hand, or *H*) per unit dose (dosage unit, or *Q*). This information should be clearly marked on the medication label. The desired dose and the dose on hand must be in the same unit of measurement.

RULE 13-3	Follow these steps when you are determining the amount of oral medication to administer to a patient.

Step A: Gather Information and Convert
Read the physician's order and the drug label to find the information necessary to calculate the amount to administer. If necessary, convert the dosage ordered *O* to the desired dose *D* that has the same unit of measure as the dose on hand *H*.

Step B: Calculate
Perform the dosage calculation using the method of your choice and round the volume for liquid medications according to the calibration of the equipment used for administration.

- The proportion method (using Procedure Checklist 12-1)
- Dimensional analysis (using Procedure Checklist 12-2)
- The formula method (using Procedure Checklist 12-3)

(Continued)

Step C: Think! . . . Is It Reasonable?
Apply critical thinking skills to determine whether the amount you have calculated is reasonable, keeping in mind both Rules 13-1 and 13-2. Recheck your calculation, if necessary.

PROPORTION METHOD

EXAMPLE 1

The order is to give the patient 15 mg codeine PO now. You have 30 mg scored tablets available.

STEP A: GATHER INFORMATION AND CONVERT

The dosage ordered is 15 mg. The dose on hand H is 30 mg, and the dosage unit Q is 1 tablet. Because the dosage ordered and the dose on hand have the same units, no conversion is needed and the dosage ordered is the desired dose D.

STEP B: CALCULATE
Follow Procedure Checklist 12-1.

1. Set up the proportion.

$$\frac{H}{Q} = \frac{D}{A} \quad \text{or} \quad \frac{\text{Dose on hand}}{\text{Dosage unit}} = \frac{\text{Desired dose}}{\text{Amount to administer}}$$

$$\frac{30 \text{ mg}}{1 \text{ tablet}} = \frac{15 \text{ mg}}{A}$$

2. Cancel units.
$$\frac{30 \cancel{\text{ mg}}}{1 \text{ tablet}} = \frac{15 \cancel{\text{ mg}}}{A}$$

3. Cross-multiply and solve for the unknown.

$$30 \times A = 1 \text{ tablet} \times 15$$

$$A = 1 \text{ tablet} \times \frac{15}{30}$$

$$A = 0.5 \text{ tablet}$$

STEP C: THINK! . . . IS IT REASONABLE?

Because 15 mg is one-half of 30 mg, $\frac{1}{2}$ tablet is a reasonable answer since the tablets are scored.

EXAMPLE 2

The order is Inderal 80 mg PO qid. You have 40 mg tablets available.

STEP A: GATHER INFORMATION AND CONVERT

The dose on hand H is 40 mg, and the dosage unit Q is 1 tablet. Because the dosage ordered and the dose on hand have the same units, no conversion is needed. The desired dose D is 80 mg.

STEP B: CALCULATE
Follow Procedure Checklist 12-1.

1. Set up in the proportion.
$$\frac{40 \text{ mg}}{1 \text{ tablet}} = \frac{80 \text{ mg}}{A}$$

2. Cancel units.

$$\frac{40 \text{ mg}}{1 \text{ tablet}} = \frac{80 \text{ mg}}{A}$$

3. Cross-multiply and solve for the unknown.

$$40 \times A = 1 \text{ tablet} \times 80$$

$$A = 1 \text{ tablet} \times \frac{80}{40}$$

$$A = 2 \text{ tablets}$$

STEP C: THINK! . . . IS IT REASONABLE?

80 is twice 40 so this dose requires twice 1 tablet. The calculated dosage does not call for more than 3 tablets, so this answer seems reasonable.

EXAMPLE 3 | Refer to Figures 13-3 and 13-4.

STEP A: GATHER INFORMATION AND CONVERT

The dose on hand H is 250 mg, and the dosage unit Q is 1 tablet. Because the dosage ordered and the dose on hand are in different units, you need to convert the dosage ordered to milligrams.

Convert the dosage ordered to the same unit of measurement as the dose on hand to obtain the desired dose (D) of 0.5 g.

1. Set up the proportion, recalling that 1 g = 1,000 mg and you are converting to mg.

$$\frac{1,000 \text{ mg}}{1 \text{ g}} = \frac{x}{0.5 \text{ g}}$$

2. Cancel units.

$$\frac{1,000 \text{ mg}}{1 \text{ g}} = \frac{x}{0.5 \text{ g}}$$

3. Cross-multiply and solve for the unknown.

$$1 \times x = 0.5 \times 1,000 \text{ mg}$$

$$x = 500 \text{ mg}$$

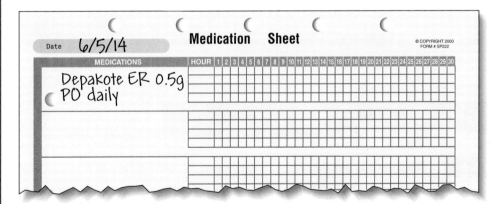

Figure 13-3 Medication ordered.

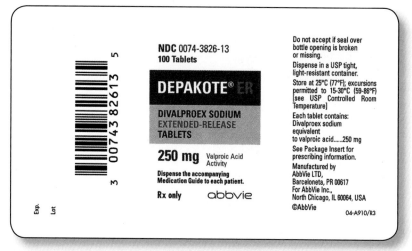

Figure 13-4 Medication on hand.

STEP B: CALCULATE

Follow Procedure Checklist 12-1.

1. Set up the proportion. *Note that ratios are also shown for this example.*

$$\frac{250 \text{ mg}}{1 \text{ tablet}} = \frac{500 \text{ mg}}{A} \qquad \text{or} \qquad 250 \text{ mg} : 1 \text{ tablet} = 500 \text{ mg} : A$$

2. Cancel units.

$$\frac{250 \text{ mg}}{1 \text{ tablet}} = \frac{500 \text{ mg}}{A} \qquad \text{or} \qquad 250 \text{ mg} : 1 \text{ tablet} = 500 \text{ mg} : A$$

3. Cross-multiply or multiply the means and extremes and solve for the unknown.

$$250 \times A = 1 \text{ tablet} \times 500$$

$$A = 1 \text{ tablet} \times \frac{500}{250}$$

$$A = 2 \text{ tablets}$$

STEP C: THINK! . . . IS IT REASONABLE?

500 mg is twice as large as 250 mg. It is logical to give more than 1 tablet. The calculation does not call for more than 3 tablets. The answer of 2 tablets is reasonable.

DIMENSIONAL ANALYSIS

| EXAMPLE 1 | The order is to give the patient 15 mg codeine PO now. You have 30 mg scored tablets available. |

STEP A: GATHER INFORMATION AND CONVERT

The dosage ordered is 15 mg, the dose on hand is 30 mg, and the dosage unit is scored tablets. The unit of measurement for the desired dose and the dose on hand is milligrams. No conversion factor is needed.

STEP B: CALCULATE

Follow Procedure Checklist 12-2.

1. The unit of measure for the amount to administer will be tablets.

   A tablets $=$

2. No conversion factor is needed.

3. The dosage unit is 1 tablet. The dose on hand is 30 mg.

   A tablets $= \dfrac{1 \text{ tablet}}{30 \text{ mg}}$

4. The dosage ordered is 15 mg.

   A tablets $= \dfrac{1 \text{ tablet}}{30 \text{ mg}} \times \dfrac{15 \text{ mg}}{1}$

5. Cancel units.

   A tablets $= \dfrac{1 \text{ tablet}}{30 \text{ m\cancel{g}}} \times \dfrac{15 \text{ m\cancel{g}}}{1}$

   Since the remaining unit is tablets on both sides of the equation, it is set up correctly.

6. Solve the equation.

   A tablets $= \dfrac{1 \text{ tablet}}{30} \times \dfrac{15}{1}$

   $A = 0.5 \text{ tablet} = \dfrac{1}{2} \text{ tablet}$

STEP C: THINK! . . . IS IT REASONABLE?

Because 15 mg is one-half of 30 mg, $\frac{1}{2}$ tablet is an appropriate answer since the tablets are scored.

| EXAMPLE 2 | The order is Inderal® 80 mg PO qid. You have 40 mg tablets available. |

STEP A: GATHER INFORMATION AND CONVERT

The dosage ordered is 80 mg, the dose on hand is 40 mg, and the dosage unit is tablets. The unit of measurement for the desired dose and the dose on hand is milligrams. No conversion factor is needed.

STEP B: CALCULATE

Follow Procedure Checklist 12-2.

1. The unit of measure for the amount to administer will be tablets.

   A tablets $=$

2. No conversion factor needed.

3. The dosage unit is 1 tablet. The dose on hand is 40 mg.

   A tablets $= \dfrac{1 \text{ tablet}}{40 \text{ mg}}$

4. The dosage ordered is 80 mg.

   A tablets $= \dfrac{1 \text{ tablet}}{40 \text{ mg}} \times \dfrac{80 \text{ mg}}{1}$

5. Cancel units.

   A tablets $= \dfrac{1 \text{ tablet}}{40 \text{ m\cancel{g}}} \times \dfrac{80 \text{ m\cancel{g}}}{1}$

6. Solve the equation.

$$A \text{ tablets} = \frac{1 \text{ tablet}}{40 \text{ mg}} \times \frac{80}{1}$$

$$A = 2 \text{ tablets}$$

STEP C: THINK! . . . IS IT REASONABLE?

80 is 40 × 2, so this dose requires twice 1 tablet. The calculated dosage does not call for more than 3 tablets, so the dosage is reasonable.

EXAMPLE 3 — Refer to Figures 13-3 and 13-4 on pages 295–296

STEP A: GATHER INFORMATION AND CONVERT

The dosage ordered is 0.5 g, the dose on hand is 250 mg, and the dosage unit is 1 tablet. Because the units of measurement are different in the dosage ordered and the dose on hand, you will need to determine the conversion factor for converting milligrams to grams. Recall that 1 g = 1,000 mg.

STEP B: CALCULATE

Follow Procedure Checklist 12-2.

1. The unit of measure for the amount to administer will be tablets.

$$A \text{ tablets} =$$

2. Insert the conversion factor you determined in Step A. Because we wish to convert to milligrams (the units of the dose on hand), our first factor must have milligrams on top.

$$A \text{ tablets} = \frac{1,000 \text{ mg}}{1 \text{ g}}$$

3. The dosage unit is 1 tablet. The dose on hand is 250 mg. This is the second factor.

$$A \text{ tablets} = \frac{1,000 \text{ mg}}{1 \text{ g}} \times \frac{1 \text{ tablet}}{250 \text{ mg}}$$

4. The dosage ordered is 0.5 g. Place this over 1 to complete the equation.

$$A \text{ tablets} = \frac{1,000 \text{ mg}}{1 \text{ g}} \times \frac{1 \text{ tablet}}{250 \text{ mg}} \times \frac{0.5 \text{ g}}{1}$$

5. Cancel units.

$$A \text{ tablets} = \frac{1,000 \, \cancel{\text{mg}}}{1 \, \cancel{\text{g}}} \times \frac{1 \text{ tablet}}{250 \, \cancel{\text{mg}}} \times \frac{0.5 \, \cancel{\text{g}}}{1}$$

6. Solve the equation.

$$A \text{ tablets} = \frac{1,000}{1} \times \frac{1 \text{ tablet}}{250} \times \frac{0.5}{1}$$

$$A = 2 \text{ tablets}$$

STEP C: THINK! . . . IS IT REASONABLE?

500 mg is larger than 250 mg. It is logical to give more than 1 tablet. The calculation does not call for more than 3 tablets. The answer of 2 tablets is reasonable.

FORMULA METHOD

EXAMPLE 1

The order is to give the patient 15 mg codeine PO now. You have 30 mg scored tablets available.

STEP A: GATHER INFORMATION AND CONVERT

The dosage ordered is 15 mg, the dose on hand is 30 mg, and the dosage unit is scored tablets. The drug is ordered in milligrams, which is the same unit of measure as that for the dose on hand. No conversion is needed.

STEP B: CALCULATE

Follow Procedure Checklist 12-3.

1. Determine the components of the formula method and fill in the formula.

$D = 15$ mg

$Q = 1$ tablet

$H = 30$ mg

$$\frac{D}{H} \times Q = A$$

$$\frac{15 \text{ mg}}{30 \text{ mg}} \times 1 \text{ tablet} = A$$

2. Cancel units.

$$\frac{15 \text{ mg}}{30 \text{ mg}} \times 1 \text{ tablet} = A$$

3. Solve for the unknown.

$$\frac{1}{2} \times 1 \text{ tablet} = A$$

$$A = 0.5 \text{ tablet} = \frac{1}{2} \text{ tablet}$$

STEP C: THINK! . . . IS IT REASONABLE?

Because 15 mg is one-half of 30 mg, $\frac{1}{2}$ tablet is a reasonable answer since the tablets are scored.

EXAMPLE 2

The order is Inderal® 80 mg PO qid. You have 40 mg tablets available.

STEP A: GATHER INFORMATION AND CONVERT

The dosage ordered is 80 mg, the dose on hand is 40 mg, and the dosage unit is tablets. The drug is ordered in milligrams, which is the same unit of measure as that for the dose on hand. No conversion is needed.

STEP B: CALCULATE

Follow Procedure Checklist 12-3.

1. Determine the components of the formula method and fill in the formula.

$D = 80$ mg

$Q = 1$ tablet

$H = 40$ mg

$$\frac{80 \text{ mg}}{40 \text{ mg}} \times 1 \text{ tablet} = A$$

2. Cancel units.

$$\frac{80 \text{ mg}}{40 \text{ mg}} \times 1 \text{ tablet} = A$$

3. Solve for the unknown.

$2 \times 1 \text{ tablet} = A$

$A = 2 \text{ tablets}$

STEP C: THINK! . . . IS IT REASONABLE?
80 is 40 × 2, so this dose requires twice 1 tablet. The calculated dosage does not call for more than 3 tablets so the answer is reasonable.

EXAMPLE 3   Refer to Figures 13-3 and 13-4 on pages 295–296.

STEP A: GATHER INFORMATION AND CONVERT
The dosage ordered is 0.5 g, the dose on hand is 250 mg, and the dosage unit is 1 tablet. Because the units of measurement are different in the dosage ordered and dose on hand, you will need to convert the dosage ordered, 0.5 g, to the same unit of measurement as the dose on hand, milligrams. Recall that 1 g = 1,000 mg, therefore, convert by setting up the proportion:

$$\frac{1,000 \text{ mg}}{1 \text{ g}} = \frac{D}{0.5 \text{ g}}$$
$D = 500 \text{ mg}$

STEP B: CALCULATE
Follow Procedure Checklist 12-3.

1. Determine the components of the formula method and fill in the formula.

$D = 500 \text{ mg}$

$Q = 1 \text{ tablet}$

$H = 250 \text{ mg}$

$$\frac{500 \text{ mg}}{250 \text{ mg}} \times 1 \text{ tablet} = A$$

2. Cancel units.

$$\frac{500 \text{ mg}}{250 \text{ mg}} \times 1 \text{ tablet} = A$$

3. Solve for the unknown.

$2 \times 1 \text{ tablet} = A$

$2 \text{ tablets} = A$

STEP C: THINK! . . . IS IT REASONABLE?
500 mg is larger than 250 mg. It is logical to give more than 1 tablet. The calculation does not call for more than 3 tablets. The answer of 2 tablets is reasonable.

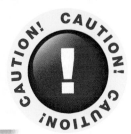

Observe Patients as They Take Their Medications

Medications left at the bedside lead to errors because patients may:
- Forget to take the medication or may consume it at an incorrect time.
- Inadvertently spill or drop medication.
- Encounter difficulty when swallowing, leading to potential aspiration.

Crushing Tablets or Opening Capsules

For patients who have difficulty swallowing pills, you may crush certain tablets and open certain capsules. However, in many settings, such as nursing homes, you must first get a physician's order. Check with your facility about these policies before you crush tablets. See Figure 13-5.

Sometimes you can mix a crushed tablet or an opened capsule with soft food or liquid. First check for interactions between the medication and the food or fluid being mixed with it or other medications that are being administered (Table 13-1). For example, tetracycline is inactivated by milk. It must not be dissolved in foods that contain milk. In addition, it should not be given with either antacids or vitamin and mineral supplements. Grapefruit juice can increase the effects and side effects of many medications so avoid using it.

Oral forms of medication are also ordered for patients with nasogastric, gastrostomy, or jejunostomy tubes. Review the figure in the chapter "Equipment for Dosage Measurement." Before administering medication through the tube, you first dissolve the contents from a crushed tablet or opened capsule in a small amount of warm water.

Some medications cannot be crushed. If these medications are ordered for a patient with a feeding tube or one who cannot swallow pills, determine whether an alternative form of the medication exists. Consult a drug reference or pharmacist for information, then ask the physician if the medication could be ordered in one of these forms. Always follow the policy of the facility where you are employed regarding substituting forms of medications.

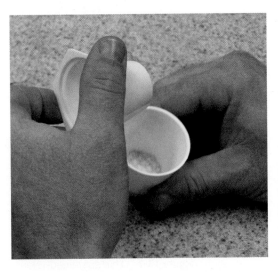
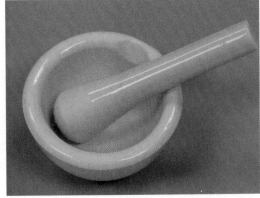

Figure 13-5   A pill crusher or mortar and pestle may be used to crush tablets when necessary.

TABLE 13-1 Examples of Food and Drug Interactions

DRUG	FOOD	INTERACTION
Antipsychotics	Coffee and tea	Reduced effectiveness of drug
Bronchodilators	Caffeine	Stimulation of the nervous system
Central nervous system (CNS) depressants	Black cohosh, ginseng kava kava, St. John's wort, valerian, ETOH	Intensified sedative effects of CNS depressant
Erythromycin	Acidic fruits or juices, carbonated beverages	Decreased antimicrobial activity
Ferrous sulfate	Tea	Decreased absorption
Haloperidol	Coffee and tea	Decreased absorption
Insulin	Coffee	Stimulated excretion
Monoamine oxidase inhibitors	Foods containing tyramine, such as hard cheeses, chocolate, red wine, and beef or chicken liver	Headache, nosebleed, chest pain, severe hypertension
Tetracyclines	Dairy products, antacids, vitamin and mineral supplements	Reduced effectiveness of drug
Antihistamines, cholesterol lowering agents, calcium channel blockers	Grapefruit and grapefruit juice	Increased effects and side effects

Enteric-coated tablets have a coating that dissolves only in an alkaline environment, such as the small intestine. These tablets deliver medication that would be destroyed by stomach acid or that could injure the stomach lining. Enteric-coated tablets often look like candies that have a soft center and a hard shell. Some aspirins are enteric-coated, as are certain iron tablets such as ferrous gluconate. Enteric-coated tablets must *never* be crushed, broken, or chewed. A patient must swallow them with their coating intact (see Figure 13-6).

Some medications are available in **sustained-release** forms. (See Figure 13-7.) They allow the drug to be released slowly into the bloodstream over a period of several hours. If the medication is scored, you may break it at the scored line. Otherwise you must not break it. Crushing or dissolving sustained-release tablets would allow more than the intended amount of medication to be absorbed at one time, causing overdose or toxicity of the drug.

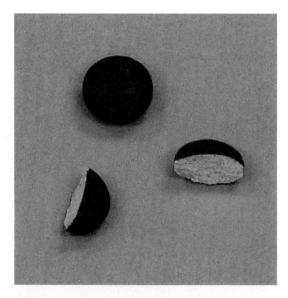

Figure 13-6 Enteric-coated tablet. One tablet has been split for visualization only. Enteric-coated tablets should never be split when given to patients.

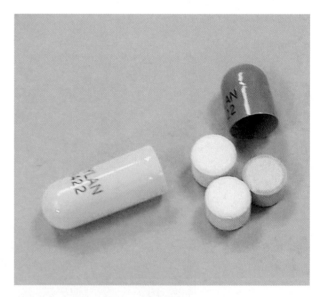

Figure 13-7 This sustained-release capsule has three smaller tablets inside that release medication into the bloodstream over a period of several hours.

Special capsules, often called **spansules**, contain granules of medication with different coatings that delay release of some of the medication. You may open spansules and gently mix the granules in soft food, but you must not crush or dissolve the granules.

RULE 13-4	To prevent an incorrect dose of medication, do not crush or otherwise alter any of the following: • Enteric-coated tablets • Sustained-release forms of medication • Any tablet with a hard shell or coating • Any tablet with layers or speckles of different colors • Tablets for sublingual or buccal use • Capsules with seals that prevent separating the two parts
Example	The following lists indicate some medications that should not be crushed or altered. Crushing or altering these medications could cause an inaccurate dose of the medication to be administered. • Names that indicate sustained release, such as:

-Bid	LA	Tempule
-Dur	CR	Chronotab
Plateau cap	XL	Repetab
Span	Sequel	Tembid
SA	Spansule	
SR	Extentab	

• Names that indicate enteric coated, such as:

EC
Enseal

PATIENT EDUCATION

Perform all necessary calculations, so that you can tell patients how many pills to take.

Review with patients the following guidelines for taking tablets and capsules:

1. Tell patients whether they need to take a medication with food. Encourage them to drink at least 8 oz of water with any medication.

2. Tell patients who need to divide tablets that pharmacists can provide this service on request. If the patients will be dividing the tablets, demonstrate and advise them as follows:

   a. Wash hands before you handle tablets.

   b. Grasp the tablet with the scored line between your fingers. Exert pressure in the same direction—downward or upward—with both hands, until the tablet breaks along the scored line.

> **c.** You may use a knife or pill cutter to break the tablet. Place the tablet on a clean surface, place the blade in the scored line, and press directly downward until the tablet breaks.
>
> **3.** For patients who have difficulty swallowing, offer the following suggestions:
>
> **a.** Drink water before taking pills, so your mouth is moist.
>
> **b.** Place whole tablets or capsules in a small amount of food, such as applesauce or pudding. The pill will go down when the food is swallowed. *Note:* Also tell patients which foods should **not** be used.
>
> **c.** Crush tablets by placing them on a spoon and pressing another spoon down on top of them or use a pill crusher. **Note:** Warn patients not to crush any medication without first checking with the pharmacist or physician.

REVIEW AND PRACTICE

13.1 Solid Oral Medications

For Exercises 1–20, calculate the amount to administer. Unless otherwise noted, all scored tablets are scored in half.

1. Ordered: Tegretol® 400 mg PO bid   Administer: _____
   On hand: Tegretol® 200 mg unscored tablets

2. Ordered: Seroquel® 75 mg PO tid   Administer: _____
   On hand: Seroquel® 25 mg unscored tablets

3. Ordered: Tolectin® 300 mg PO tid   Administer: _____
   On hand: Tolectin® 200 mg scored tablets

4. Ordered: Isordil® Titradose 15 mg PO now   Administer: _____
   On hand: Isordil® Titradose 10 mg deep-scored tablets

5. Ordered: Felbatol® 600 mg PO qid   Administer: _____
   On hand: Felbatol® 400 mg scored tablets

6. Ordered: Decadron® 1.5 mg PO daily   Administer: _____
   On hand: Decadron® 0.75 mg unscored tablets

7. Ordered: Coumadin® 8 mg PO daily   Administer: _____
   On hand: Coumadin® 2 mg scored tablets

8. Ordered: Cardizem® 90 mg PO tid   Administer: _____
   On hand: Cardizem® 60 mg scored tablets

9. Ordered: Tambocor® 150 mg PO q12h   Administer: _____
   On hand: Tambocor® 100 mg scored tablets

10. Ordered: Clozaril® 50 mg PO daily   Administer: _____

On hand: Refer to label A. Tablets are unscored.

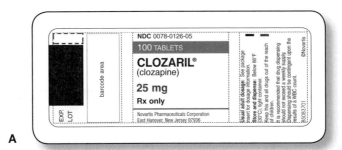

A

11. Ordered: Alprazolam 0.5 mg PO tid   Administer: _____

On hand: Refer to label B. Tablets are scored into fourths.

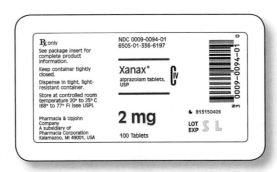

B

12. Ordered: Diazepam 10 mg PO q12h   Administer: _____

On hand: Refer to label C.

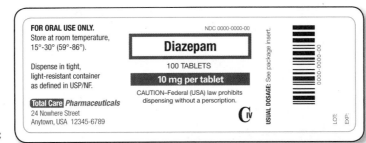

C

13. Ordered: Famvir® 250 mg PO bid   Administer: _____

On hand: Refer to label D. Tablets are unscored.

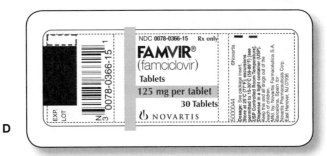

D

14. Ordered: Aricept® 10 mg PO daily

On hand: Refer to label E. Tablets are unscored.

Administer: _____

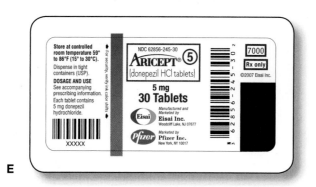

E

15. Ordered: Prandin 1 mg PO bid

On hand: Refer to labels F and G. Tablets are unscored.
Determine dosage strength to use.

Administer: _____

Dosage strength: _____

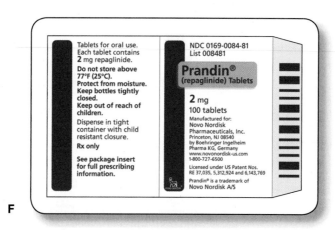

F

G

16. Ordered: Synthroid 0.132 mg PO daily   Administer: _____

On hand: Refer to label H. Tablets are scored in half.

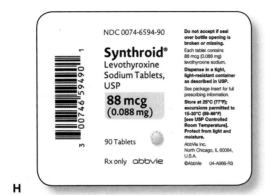

NDC 0074-6594-90

Synthroid®
Levothyroxine
Sodium Tablets,
USP

88 mcg
(0.088 mg)

90 Tablets

Rx only abbvie

Do not accept if seal
over bottle opening is
broken or missing.

Each tablet contains
88 mcg (0.088 mg)
levothyroxine sodium.

Dispense in a tight,
light-resistant container
as described in USP.

See package insert for full
prescribing information.

Store at 25°C (77°F);
excursions permitted to
15-30°C (59-86°F)
[see USP Controlled
Room Temperature].
Protect from light and
moisture.

AbbVie Inc.
North Chicago, IL 60064,
U.S.A.
©AbbVie   04-A966-R3

H

17. Ordered: Lipitor® 30 mg PO daily   Administer: _____

On hand: Refer to label I. Tablets are unscored.

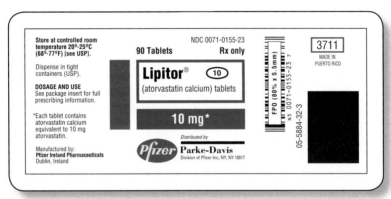

Store at controlled room
temperature 20°-25°C
(68°-77°F) [see USP].

Dispense in tight
containers (USP).

DOSAGE AND USE
See package insert for full
prescribing information.

*Each tablet contains
atorvastatin calcium
equivalent to 10 mg
atorvastatin.

Manufactured by:
Pfizer Ireland Pharmaceuticals
Dublin, Ireland

NDC 0071-0155-23

90 Tablets   Rx only

Lipitor®   10
(atorvastatin calcium) tablets

10 mg*

Pfizer *Distributed by*
Parke-Davis
Division of Pfizer Inc, NY, NY 10017

3711
MADE IN
PUERTO RICO

FPO (80% x 5.5mm)

I

18. Ordered: Zoloft® 50 mg PO daily   Administer: _____

On hand: Refer to label J. Tablets are scored.

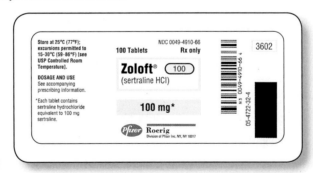

Store at 25°C (77°F);
excursions permitted to
15-30°C (59-86°F) [see
USP Controlled Room
Temperature].

DOSAGE AND USE
See accompanying
prescribing information.

*Each tablet contains
sertraline hydrochloride
equivalent to 100 mg
sertraline.

NDC 0049-4910-66

100 Tablets   Rx only

Zoloft®   100
(sertraline HCl)

100 mg*

Pfizer **Roerig**
Division of Pfizer Inc, NY, NY 10017

3602

J

19. Ordered: Gleevec® 200 mg PO daily   Administer: _____

On hand: Refer to label K. Tablets are not scored.

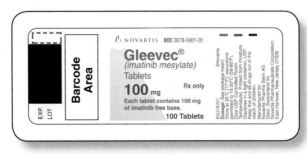

Barcode
Area

EXP.
LOT

ᚼ NOVARTIS   NDC 0078-0401-05

Gleevec®
(imatinib mesylate)
Tablets
100 mg   Rx only
Each tablet contains 100 mg
of imatinib free base.

100 Tablets

K

20. Ordered: Clonazepam 1 mg PO tid   Administer: _____

On hand: Clonazepam 2 mg scored tablets

For Exercises 21–24, match the term to the description:

   a. tablet   **b.** spansule   **c.** gelcap   **d.** enteric coating   **e.** capsule

21. Contains granules that delay the release of the medication   _____

22. Hard shell that is absorbed in the small intestine, not the stomach   _____

23. Most common form of oral medication   _____

24. Liquid medication in a gelatin shell   _____

25. Under what circumstances can pills be split or crushed?   _____

13.2 Liquid Oral Medications

Many medications are available in liquid form. Liquids can be measured in small units of volume; thus, a greater range of dosages can be ordered and administered. Because they are easier to swallow than tablets and capsules, they are often used for children, elderly, and other patients who have difficulty swallowing. Liquids can also be administered easily through feeding tubes.

Liquids may be less stable than solid forms of drugs. Many medications that are intended to be administered as liquids are provided as powders because they rapidly lose their power once they are mixed into a solution. These drugs will then have to be **reconstituted,** or mixed with a liquid, before they can be administered. Many liquids, especially antibiotics, require refrigeration.

The directions for reconstitution are located on the medication label (or package insert). If clarification of reconstitution information is needed, contact the pharmacist who dispensed the medication.

 LEARNING LINK Recall from the chapter "Interpreting Medication Labels and Package Inserts" that directions for reconstituting or diluting a drug appear on the label or in the package insert.

RULE 13-5

When reconstituting liquid medications:

- Use only the liquid specified on the drug label.

- Use the exact amount of liquid specified on the drug label.

- Check the label to determine whether the medication should be shaken before administering.

- Check the label to determine whether the reconstituted medication must be refrigerated.

- Write on the label the date and time you reconstitute the medication. Also, write your initials. Check the label to determine how long the reconstituted medication may be stored. Discard any medication left after this time period has passed.

- When medication can be reconstituted in different strengths, write on the label the strength that you choose.

- When medication can be reconstituted in different strengths, select the strength that will allow the desired dose to be administered in the smallest volume.

- Read the order carefully when you calculate the amount to administer. The physician usually orders the dose in units of drug, not volume of liquid. The person administering the medication calculates the volume needed to administer the desired dose.

Small volumes are given in oral syringes and amounts are rounded according to the calibration on the syringe:

- Amounts less than 1 mL should be rounded to the hundredths.

- Amounts greater than 1 mL should be rounded to the tenths.

Example 1

How would you reconstitute the following medication? Find the amount to administer.

Ordered: granisetron 5 mg PO now

On hand: Refer to Figure 13-8.

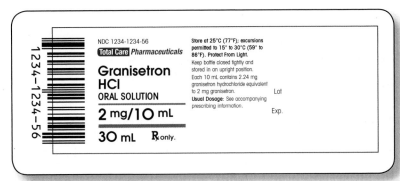

Figure 13-8

According to the label, this medication is already in liquid form as a solution, so no reconstitution is necessary.

Calculate the amount to administer. The dosage ordered is 5 mg. The dosage strength is 2 mg/10 mL, which makes the dose on hand 2 mg and the dosage unit 10 mL.

PROPORTION METHOD

EXAMPLE 1

Calculate the amount of granisetron to administer (refer to Figure 13-8).

STEP A: GATHER INFORMATION AND CONVERT

Ordered: granisetron 5 mg PO now
Dosage strength: 2 mg/10 mL
The dose on hand is the same unit of measure as the dose ordered. No conversion is needed.

STEP B: CALCULATE

Follow Procedure Checklist 12-1.

1. Set up the proportion.

$$\frac{H}{Q} = \frac{D}{A} \quad \text{or} \quad \frac{\text{Dose on hand}}{\text{Dosage unit}} = \frac{\text{Desired dose}}{\text{Amount to administer}}$$

$$\frac{2\text{ mg}}{10\text{ mL}} = \frac{5\text{ mg}}{A}$$

2. Cancel units.

$$\frac{2 \cancel{mg}}{10 \text{ mL}} = \frac{5 \cancel{mg}}{A}$$

3. Cross-multiply and solve for the unknown.

$$2 \times A = 10 \text{ mL} \times 5$$

$$A = \frac{10 \text{ mL} \times 5}{2}$$

$$A = \frac{50 \text{ mL}}{2}$$

$$A = 25 \text{ mL}$$

STEP C: THINK! . . . IS IT REASONABLE?
Since 2 mg of medication is in 10 mL of liquid, it is reasonable that 5 mg of medication would be in 25 mL of liquid.

DIMENSIONAL ANALYSIS

EXAMPLE 1

Calculate the amount of granisetron to administer (refer to Figure 13-8 on page 309).

STEP A: GATHER INFORMATION AND CONVERT
Ordered: granisetron 5 mg PO now
Dosage strength: 2 mg/10 mL
The unit of measurement for the desired dose and the dose on hand is milligrams. No conversion factor is needed.

STEP B: CALCULATE
Follow Procedure Checklist 12-2.

1. The unit of measure for the amount to administer will be milliliters.

$$A \text{ mL} =$$

2. No conversion factor is needed.

3. The dosage unit is 10 mL. The dose on hand is 2 mg. This is the first factor.

$$A \text{ mL} = \frac{10 \text{ mL}}{2 \text{ mg}}$$

4. The dosage ordered is 5 mg. Place this over 1 for the second factor.

$$A \text{ mL} = \frac{10 \text{ mL}}{2 \text{ mg}} \times \frac{5 \text{ mg}}{1}$$

5. Cancel units.

$$A \text{ mL} = \frac{10 \text{ mL}}{2 \cancel{mg}} \times \frac{5 \cancel{mg}}{1}$$

6. Solve the equation.

$$A \text{ mL} = \frac{50 \text{ mL}}{2}$$

$$A = 25 \text{ mL}$$

STEP C: THINK! . . . IS IT REASONABLE?
Since 2 mg of medication is in 10 mL of liquid, it is reasonable that 5 mg of medication would be in 25 mL of liquid.

FORMULA METHOD

EXAMPLE 1

Calculate the amount of granisetron to administer (refer to Figure 13-8 on page 309).

STEP A: GATHER INFORMATION AND CONVERT

Ordered: granisetron 5 mg PO now
Dosage strength: 2 mg/10 mL
The dose on hand is the same unit of measure as the dose ordered. No conversion is needed.

STEP B: CALCULATE

Follow Procedure Checklist 12-3.

1. Determine the components of the formula method and fill in the formula.

   $D = 5$ mg

   $Q = 10$ mL

   $H = 2$ mg

   $$\frac{D}{H} \times Q = A$$

   $$\frac{5 \text{ mg}}{2 \text{ mg}} \times 10 \text{ mL} = A$$

2. Cancel units.

   $$\frac{5 \text{ mg}}{2 \text{ mg}} \times 10 \text{ mL} = A$$

3. Solve for the unknown.

   $$\frac{50 \text{ mL}}{2} = A$$

   $$A = 25 \text{ mL}$$

STEP C: THINK ABOUT IT! . . . IS IT REASONABLE?

Since 2 mg of medication is in 10 mL of liquid, it is reasonable that 5 mg of medication would be in 25 mL of liquid.

Example 2

How would you reconstitute the following medication? Calculate the amount to administer.

Ordered: E.E.S.® susp 400 mg PO q6h
On hand: Refer to Figure 13-9.

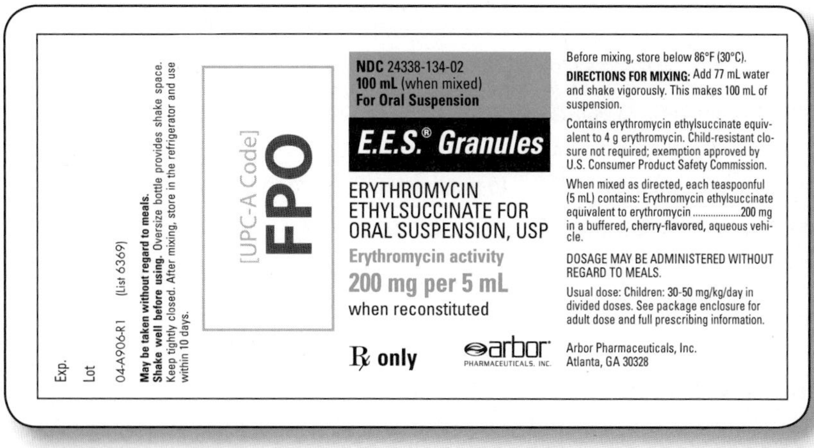

[UPC-A Code]
FPO

May be taken without regard to meals.
Shake well before using. Oversize bottle provides shake space.
Keep tightly closed. After mixing, store in the refrigerator and use within 10 days.

Exp.
Lot
04-A906-R1   (List 6369)

NDC 24338-134-02
100 mL (when mixed)
For Oral Suspension

E.E.S.® Granules

ERYTHROMYCIN
ETHYLSUCCINATE FOR
ORAL SUSPENSION, USP

Erythromycin activity
200 mg per 5 mL
when reconstituted

℞ **only**

⬤arbor
PHARMACEUTICALS, INC.

Before mixing, store below 86°F (30°C).
DIRECTIONS FOR MIXING: Add 77 mL water and shake vigorously. This makes 100 mL of suspension.

Contains erythromycin ethylsuccinate equivalent to 4 g erythromycin. Child-resistant closure not required; exemption approved by U.S. Consumer Product Safety Commission.

When mixed as directed, each teaspoonful (5 mL) contains: Erythromycin ethylsuccinate equivalent to erythromycin ....200 mg in a buffered, cherry-flavored, aqueous vehicle.

DOSAGE MAY BE ADMINISTERED WITHOUT REGARD TO MEALS.

Usual dose: Children: 30-50 mg/kg/day in divided doses. See package enclosure for adult dose and full prescribing information.

Arbor Pharmaceuticals, Inc.
Atlanta, GA 30328

Figure 13-9

According to the label, you add 77 mL of water to the bottle of granules and shake vigorously. You then have a total of 100 mL of oral suspension that must be stored in the refrigerator for up to 10 days.

Calculate the amount to administer. The dosage ordered is 400 mg. The dosage strength is 200 mg/5 mL, which makes the dose on hand 200 mg and the dosage unit 5 mL.

PROPORTION METHOD

EXAMPLE 2 Calculate the amount of E.E.S.® to administer. Refer to the label in Figure 13-9.

STEP A: GATHER INFORMATION AND CONVERT
Ordered: E.E.S.® susp 400 mg PO q6h
Dosage strength: 200 mg per 5 mL
The dose on hand is the same unit of measure as the dose ordered. No conversion is needed.

STEP B: CALCULATE
Follow Procedure Checklist 12-1.

1. Set up the proportion.

$$\frac{H}{Q} = \frac{D}{A} \quad \text{or} \quad \frac{\text{Dose on hand}}{\text{Dosage unit}} = \frac{\text{Desired dose}}{\text{Amount to administer}}$$

$$\frac{200 \text{ mg}}{5 \text{ mL}} = \frac{400 \text{ mg}}{A}$$

2. Cancel units.

$$\frac{200 \text{ mg}}{5 \text{ mL}} = \frac{400 \text{ mg}}{A}$$

3. Cross-multiply and solve for the unknown.

$$200 \times A = 5 \text{ mL} \times 400$$

$$A = 5 \text{ mL} \times \frac{400}{200}$$

$$A = 5 \text{ mL} \times 2$$

$$A = 10 \text{ mL}$$

STEP C: THINK! . . . IS IT REASONABLE?
If 5 mL of liquid contain 200 mg of medication, it is reasonable that 10 mL of liquid contains 400 mg of medication.

DIMENSIONAL ANALYSIS

EXAMPLE 2 Calculate the amount of E.E.S.® to administer. Refer to the label in Figure 13-9.

STEP A: GATHER INFORMATION AND CONVERT
Ordered: E.E.S.® susp 400 mg PO q6h
Dosage strength: 200 mg per 5 mL
The unit of measurement for the desired dose and the dose on hand is milligrams. No conversion factor is needed.

STEP B: CALCULATE
Follow Procedure Checklist 12-2.

1. The unit of measure for the amount to administer will be milliliters.

$$A \text{ mL} =$$

2. No conversion factor is needed.

3. The dosage unit is 5 mL. The dose on hand is 200 mg. This is your first factor.

$$A \text{ mL} = \frac{5 \text{ mL}}{200 \text{ mg}}$$

4. The dosage ordered is 400 mg. Place this over 1 for the second factor.

$$A \text{ mL} = \frac{5 \text{ mL}}{200 \text{ mg}} \times \frac{400 \text{ mg}}{1}$$

5. Cancel units.

$$A \text{ mL} = \frac{5 \text{ mL}}{200 \text{ \cancel{mg}}} \times \frac{400 \text{ \cancel{mg}}}{1}$$

6. Solve the equation.

$$A \text{ mL} = \frac{2,000 \text{ mL}}{200}$$

$$A = 10 \text{ mL}$$

STEP C: THINK! . . . IS IT REASONABLE?

If 5 mL of liquid contain 200 mg of medication, it is reasonable that 10 mL of liquid contains 400 mg of medication.

FORMULA METHOD

EXAMPLE 2   Calculate the amount of E.E.S.® to administer. Refer to the label in Figure 13-9.

STEP A: GATHER INFORMATION AND CONVERT

Ordered: E.E.S.® susp 400 mg PO q6h
Dosage strength: 200 mg per 5 mL
The dose on hand is the same unit of measure as the dose ordered. No conversion is needed.

STEP B: CALCULATE

Follow Procedure Checklist 12-3.

1. Determine the components of the formula and fill in the formula.

$D = 400 \text{ mg}$

$Q = 5 \text{ mL}$

$H = 200 \text{ mg}$

$$\frac{D}{H} \times Q = A$$

$$\frac{400 \text{ mg}}{200 \text{ mg}} \times 5 \text{ mL} = A$$

2. Cancel units.

$$\frac{400 \text{ \cancel{mg}}}{200 \text{ \cancel{mg}}} \times 5 \text{ mL} = A$$

3. Solve for the unknown.

$$\frac{2,000 \text{ mL}}{200} = A$$

$$A = 10 \text{ mL}$$

STEP C: THINK! . . . IS IT REASONABLE?

If 5 mL of liquid contains 200 mg of medication, it is reasonable that 10 mL of liquid contains 400 mg of medication.

Example 3	How would you reconstitute the following medication? Find the amount to administer.

Ordered: Amoxicillin 500 mg PO q8h
On hand: Refer to Figure 13-10.

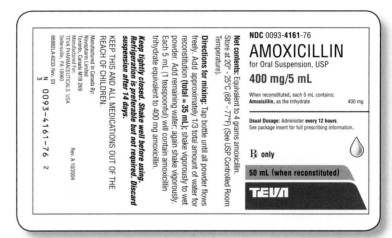

This label is for US only, and cannot be altered or translated.

Figure 13-10

To reconstitute, tap the bottle until all powder flows freely. Add approximately $\frac{1}{3}$ the total amount of water for reconstitution. Shake vigorously to wet the powder. Add the remaining water, and again shake vigorously. The total amount of water to add is 35 mL.

When it is reconstituted, you will have a total of 50 mL of oral suspension.

Calculate the amount to administer. The dosage ordered is 500 mg. The dosage strength is 400 mg/5 mL, which makes the dose on hand 400 mg and the dosage unit 5 mL.

PROPORTION METHOD

EXAMPLE 3	Calculate the amount of amoxicillin to administer. Refer to the label in Figure 13-10.

STEP A: GATHER INFORMATION AND CONVERT
Ordered: amoxicillin 500 mg PO q8h
Dosage strength: 400 mg per 5 mL
The dose on hand is the same unit of measure as the dose ordered. No conversion is needed.

STEP B: CALCULATE
Follow Procedure Checklist 12-1.

1. Set up the proportion.

$$\frac{H}{Q} = \frac{A}{D} \quad \text{or} \quad \frac{\text{Dose on hand}}{\text{Dosage unit}} = \frac{\text{Desired dose}}{\text{Amount to administer}}$$

$$\frac{400 \text{ mg}}{5 \text{ mL}} = \frac{500 \text{ mg}}{A}$$

2. Cancel units.

$$\frac{400 \text{ mg}}{5 \text{ mL}} = \frac{500 \text{ mg}}{A}$$

3. Cross-multiply and solve for the unknown.

$$400 \times A = 5 \text{ mL} \times 500$$

$$A = 5 \text{ mL} \times \frac{500}{400}$$

$$A = 6.25 \text{ rounded to } 6.3 \text{ mL}$$

STEP C: THINK! . . . IS IT REASONABLE?
If there is 400 mg in 5 mL of liquid, it is reasonable that 500 mg would be a little more than 5 mL or 6.25 mL rounded to 6.3 according to Rule 13-5.

DIMENSIONAL ANALYSIS

EXAMPLE 3

Find the amount of amoxicillin to administer. Refer to the label in Figure 13-10.

STEP A: GATHER INFORMATION AND CONVERT
Ordered: Amoxicillin 500 mg PO q8h
Dosage strength: 400 mg per 5 mL
The unit of measurement for the desired dose and the dose on hand are both milligrams. No conversion factor is needed.

STEP B: CALCULATE
Follow Procedure Checklist 12-2.

1. The unit of measure for the amount to administer will be milliliters.

$A \text{ mL} =$

2. No conversion factor is needed.

3. The dosage unit is 5 mL. The dose on hand is 400 mg.

$$A \text{ mL} = \frac{5 \text{ mL}}{400 \text{ mg}}$$

4. The dosage ordered is 500 mg.

$$A \text{ mL} = \frac{5 \text{ mL}}{400 \text{ mg}} \times \frac{500 \text{ mg}}{1}$$

5. Cancel units.

$$A \text{ mL} = \frac{5 \text{ mL}}{400 \text{ mg}} \times \frac{500 \text{ mg}}{1}$$

6. Solve the equation.

$$A \text{ mL} = \frac{2,500 \text{ mL}}{400}$$

$$A = 6.25 \text{ rounded to } 6.3 \text{ mL}$$

STEP C: THINK! . . . IS IT REASONABLE?
If there is 400 mg in 5 mL of liquid, it is reasonable that 500 mg would be a little more than 5 mL or 6.25 mL rounded to 6.3 according to Rule 13-5.

FORMULA METHOD

EXAMPLE 3   Calculate the amount of amoxicillin to administer. Refer to the label in Figure 13-10.

STEP A: GATHER INFORMATION AND CONVERT
Ordered: Amoxicillin 500 mg PO q8h
Dosage strength: 400 mg per 5 mL
The dose on hand has the same unit of measure as the dose ordered. No conversion is needed.

STEP B: CALCULATE
Follow Procedure Checklist 12-3.

1. Determine the components of the formula and fill in the formula.

   $D = 500$ mg

   $Q = 5$ mL

   $H = 400$ mg

   $\dfrac{D}{H} \times Q = A$

   $\dfrac{500 \text{ mg}}{400 \text{ mg}} \times 5 \text{ mL} = A$

2. Cancel units.

   $\dfrac{500 \text{ m\cancel{g}}}{400 \text{ m\cancel{g}}} \times 5 \text{ mL} = A$

3. Solve for the unknown.

   $\dfrac{2{,}500 \text{ mL}}{400} = A$

   $A = 6.25$ rounded to 6.3 mL

STEP C: THINK! . . . IS IT REASONABLE?
If there is 400 mg in 5 mL of liquid, it is reasonable that 500 mg would be a little more than 5 mL or 6.25 mL rounded to 6.3 according to Rule 13-5.

PATIENT EDUCATION

Review information with patients who are taking liquid medications in a home environment. If the medication is to be reconstituted at home, copy Rule 13-5 for the patient and discuss the steps. If you are dispensing medications, give the patients the same information that the pharmacist would, if you are allowed to do so. Review with patients the following information about handling liquid medication:

1. Read the label to learn how to store the medication.
2. Use the measuring device provided or a device purchased specifically to measure medications. Household teaspoons and tablespoons do not measure liquid accurately.
3. Do not store medication longer than the label indicates. Medication used after its expiration date may have lost potency, or its chemical composition may have changed.

4. Wash the measuring device with hot water and a dishwashing detergent after each use. Dry it thoroughly. Store it in a clean container such as a plastic sandwich bag.

5. Keep liquid medication in its original container. Do not transfer it to other containers.

CRITICAL THINKING ON THE JOB

Reconstituting Powders

A healthcare professional is preparing a bottle of amoxicillin suspension for this order: amoxicillin 500 mg PO q8h × 5 days. The pharmacy has available 100 mL bottles and 150 mL bottles containing 250 mg/5 mL (see Figures 13-11 and 13-12). After calculating as follows:

$$\frac{500 \text{ mg}}{250 \text{ mg}} \times 5 \text{ mL} = A$$

$$\frac{500 \text{ mg}}{250 \text{ mg}} \times 5 \text{ mL} = A$$

$$2 \times 5 \text{ mL} = 10 \text{ mL}$$

the healthcare professional determines that the patient will receive 10 mL for each dose and 3 doses each day. This will require 30 mL of suspension each day for 5 days, or a total of 150 mL. The reconstituted medication can be refrigerated for 14 days.

The healthcare professional selects the 150 mL bottle and adds 150 mL of water to it. However, the liquid overflows from the bottle.

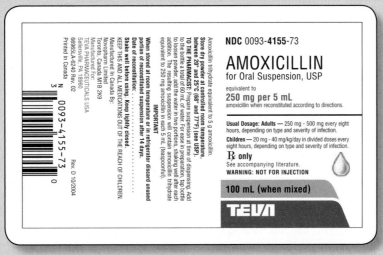

This label is for US only, and cannot be altered or translated.

Figure 13-11

(Continued)

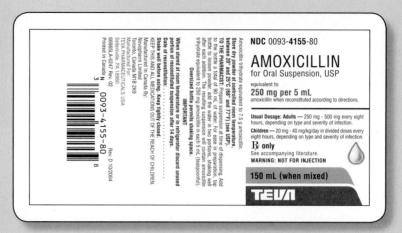

NDC 0093-4155-80

AMOXICILLIN
for Oral Suspension, USP
equivalent to
250 mg per 5 mL
amoxicillin when reconstituted according to directions.

Usual Dosage: Adults — 250 mg - 500 mg every eight hours, depending on type and severity of infection.
Children — 20 mg - 40 mg/kg/day in divided doses every eight hours, depending on type and severity of infection.

℞ only
See accompanying literature.
WARNING: NOT FOR INJECTION

150 mL (when mixed)

TEVA

This label is for US only, and cannot be altered or translated.

Figure 13-12

Think! . . . Is It Reasonable? What went wrong? How will this problem affect the patient's care?

REVIEW AND PRACTICE

13.2 Liquid Oral Medications

For Exercises 1–20, calculate the amount to administer. Provide answers in milliliters.

1. Ordered: Trilisate® 400 mg PO tid   Administer: _____
   On hand: Trilisate® liquid labeled 500 mg/5 mL

2. Ordered: MSIR sol 15 mg PO q4h   Administer: _____
   On hand: MSIR solution labeled 10 mg/5 mL

3. Ordered: Megace® 200 mg PO qid   Administer: _____
   On hand: Megace® solution labeled 40 mg/mL

4. Ordered: Norvir® 60 mg PO bid   Administer: _____
   On hand: Norvir® solution labeled 80 mg/mL

5. Ordered: Zofran® 8 mg PO q12h   Administer: _____
   On hand: Zofran® liquid labeled 4 mg/5 mL

6. Ordered: Motrin® 600 mg PO tid   Administer: _____
   On hand: Motrin® liquid labeled 100 mg/5 mL

7. Ordered: E.E.S.® 500 mg via NGT bid

Administer: _____

On hand: Refer to label A.

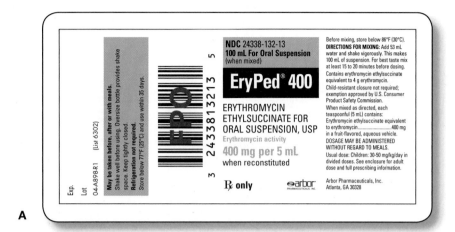

A

8. Ordered: Amoxicillin 270 mg PO q8h

Administer: _____

On hand: Refer to label B.

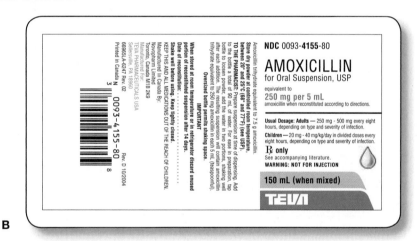

B

This label is for US only, and cannot be altered or translated.

9. Ordered: Zithromax® 250 mg PO daily

Administer: _____

On hand: Refer to label C.

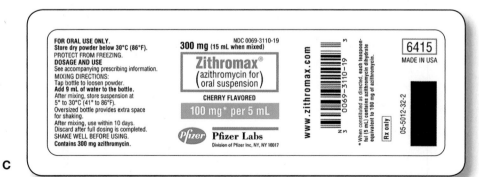

C

10. Ordered: Vistaril® 12.5 mg via NGT bid   Administer: _____
On hand: Refer to label D.

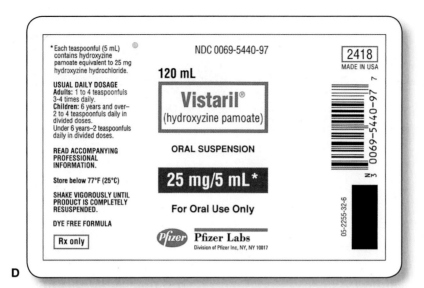

D

11. Ordered: Granisetron 1 mg PO bid   Administer: _____
On hand: Refer to label E.

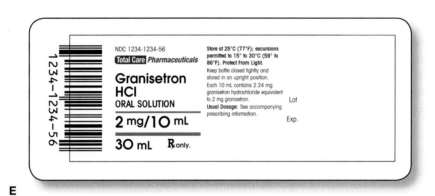

E

12. Ordered: CellCept® 500 mg PO bid   Administer: _____
On hand: Refer to label F.

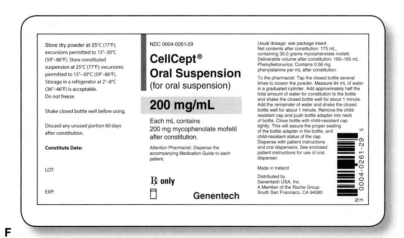

F

13. Ordered: EES Granules® 250 mg PO q12h   Administer: _____
On hand: Refer to label G.

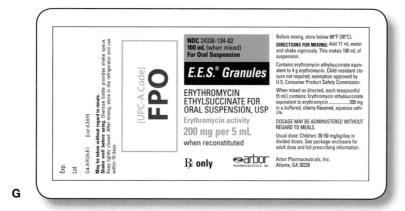

G

14. Ordered: Cefzil® 500 mg PO q24h   Administer: _____
On hand: Cefzil® 125 mg/5 mL oral suspension

15. Ordered: Augmentin® 300 mg via NGT bid   Administer: _____
On hand: Refer to label H.

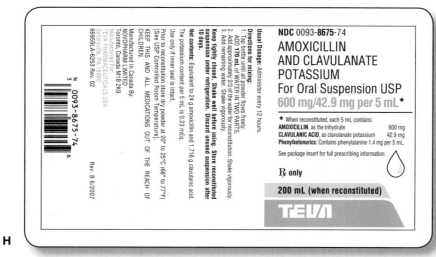

H

This label is for US only, and cannot be altered or translated.

16. Ordered: Zithromax® 500 mg PO daily   Administer: _____
On hand: Refer to label I.

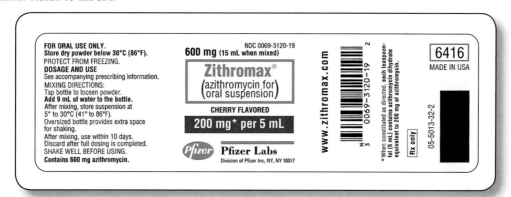

I

17. Ordered: Griseofulvin 500 mg PO daily   Administer: _____
On hand: Griseofulvin 125 mg/5 mL suspension

18. Ordered: Cefprozil® 75 mg PO q12h
On hand: Refer to label J.

Administer: _____

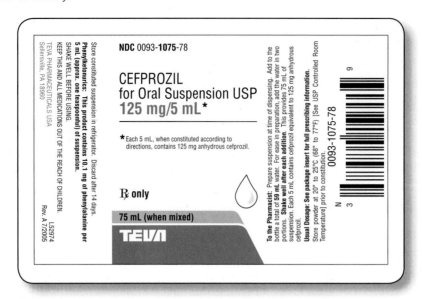

J

This label is for US only, and cannot be altered or translated.

19. Ordered: Trileptal® 75 mg PO q6h
On hand: Refer to label K.

Administer: _____

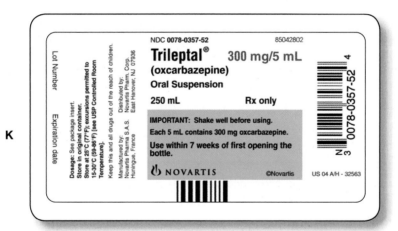

K

20. Ordered: Prozac® 60 mg PO daily
On hand: Prozac® 20 mg/5 mL oral solution

Administer: _____

LEARNING OUTCOME	KEY POINTS
13.1 Calculate dosages for solid oral medications, and explain principles related to their administration. Pages 291–308	Calculate the amount to administer using these steps: **A.** Gather information and convert the desired dose to the same unit of measurement as the dose on hand, if needed. **B.** Calculate using the proportion method, dimensional analysis, or the formula method. **C.** Think!. . .Is it reasonable? Use the guidelines for administering oral medications to decide. Tablet—most common form of solid oral medication; may be scored allowing for splitting in half, if needed; unscored tablets must not be divided Caplets—similar to tablets; oval-shaped with a special coating to make them easy to swallow Capsules—oval-shaped gelatin shells that contain medication in powder or granule form NOTE: For patients with difficulty swallowing, some tablets and caplets may be crushed and capsules may be opened and mixed with food (or dissolved in liquid and given via NGT); to determine which medications can be crushed, consult a drug reference or pharmacist. Gelcaps—liquid medication in gelatin shells that are not designed to be opened Enteric-coated tablets—have a coating that dissolves in the small intestine (not the stomach); these tablets should never be split or crushed Spansules—capsules with granules that delay the release of the medication
13.2 Calculate dosages for liquid oral medications, and explain principles related to their administration. Pages 308–322	Like dosages for solid oral medications, calculate dosages for liquid oral medications following these steps: **A.** Gather information and convert. **B.** Calculate using your method of choice. **C.** Think!. . .Is it reasonable? Liquids—can be measured in small units of volume; thus, a greater range of dosages can be ordered and administered; may be less stable than solid forms of drugs because they rapidly lose their power once they are mixed into a solution—these drugs will then have to be reconstituted, or mixed with a liquid, before they can be administered.

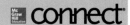
Answer the following questions.

1. Define each of the following terms: scored tablet, sublingual, buccal, capsule, spansule. (LO 13.1)

2. List four solid forms of medications that may not be crushed and explain why. (LO 13.1)

3. Explain one technique for preparing a solid medication for administration through a nasogastric, gastrostomy, or jejunostomy tube. (LO 13.1, 13.2)

4. List three techniques that may be suggested to a patient who complains of difficulty swallowing a tablet. (LO 13.1, 13.2)

5. Children or elderly patients who require medication that is easily swallowed are often prescribed what form of medication? (LO 13.2)

6. Define the term *reconstitution*. (LO 13.2)

7. List four things to be written on the label of a reconstituted medication. (LO 13.2)

Use the identified drug labels to answer the following questions:

8. In Label A, what are the generic name and the form of this drug? (LO 13.1)

9. The order is for 50 mg of the drug in Label A. What amount would you administer? (LO 13.1)

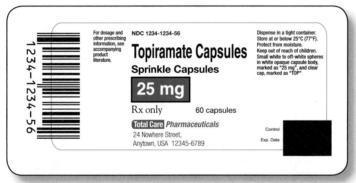

Label A

10. In Label B, what are the generic name and the form of this drug? (LO 13.1)

11. Is it acceptable to crush this drug? (LO 13.1)

12. The order is for 40 mg of the drug in Label B. What amount would you administer? (LO 13.1)

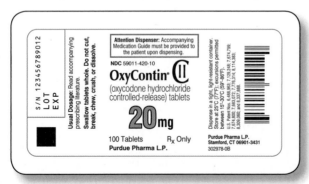

Label B

13. In Label C, what are the generic name and the form of this drug? (LO 13.1)

14. The order is for 1 mcg of the drug in Label C. What action would you take? (LO 13.1)

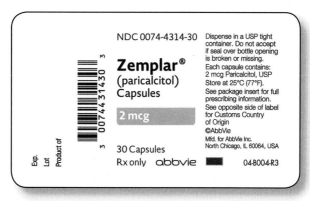

NDC 0074-4314-30

Zemplar®
(paricalcitol)
Capsules

2 mcg

30 Capsules

Rx only abbvie 04-B004-R3

Dispense in a USP tight container. Do not accept if seal over bottle opening is broken or missing.
Each capsule contains: 2 mcg Paricalcitol, USP
Store at 25°C (77°F).
See package insert for full prescribing information.
See opposite side of label for Customs Country of Origin
©AbbVie
Mfd. for AbbVie Inc.
North Chicago, IL 60064, USA

Exp. Lot Product of

Label C

15. In Label D, what are the generic name and the form of this drug? (LO 13.2)

16. The order is for 15 mg of the drug in Label D. What amount would you administer? (LO 13.2)

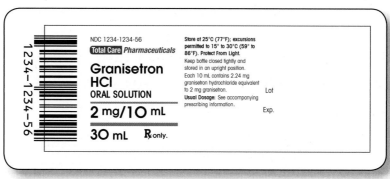

NDC 1234-1234-56

Total Care *Pharmaceuticals*

Granisetron HCl
ORAL SOLUTION

2 mg/10 mL

30 mL ℞ only.

Store at 25°C (77°F); excursions permitted to 15° to 30°C (59° to 86°F). Protect From Light.
Keep bottle closed tightly and stored in an upright position.
Each 10 mL contains 2.24 mg granisetron hydrochloride equivalent to 2 mg granisetron.
Usual Dosage: See accompanying prescribing information.

Lot

Exp.

Label D

17. In Label E, how many milliliters of water would you add to reconstitute this drug to a 75 mL suspension? (LO 13.2)

18. How are you instructed to reconstitute this drug? (LO 13.2)

19. What is the warning on the label? (LO 13.2)

20. The order is for 200 mg of the drug in Label E. What amount would you administer? (LO 13.2)

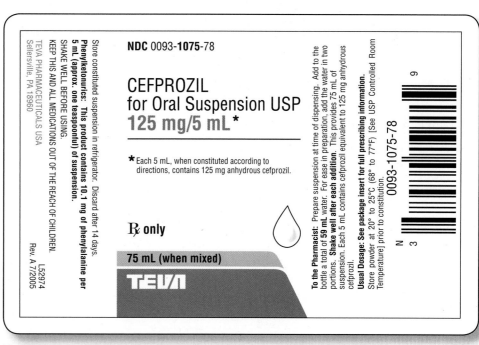

Store constituted suspension in refrigerator. Discard after 14 days.
Phenylketonurics: This product contains 10.1 mg of phenylalanine per 5 mL (approx. one teaspoonful) of suspension.
SHAKE WELL BEFORE USING.
KEEP THIS AND ALL MEDICATIONS OUT OF THE REACH OF CHILDREN.

TEVA PHARMACEUTICALS USA
Sellersville, PA 18960

L52974
Rev. A 7/2005

NDC 0093-1075-78

CEFPROZIL
for Oral Suspension USP
125 mg/5 mL *

* Each 5 mL, when constituted according to directions, contains 125 mg anhydrous cefprozil.

℞ only

75 mL (when mixed)

TEVA

To the Pharmacist: Prepare suspension at time of dispensing. Add to the bottle a total of **59 mL** water. For ease in preparation, add the water in two portions. **Shake well after each addition.** This provides 75 mL of suspension. Each 5 mL contains cefprozil equivalent to 125 mg anhydrous cefprozil.
Usual Dosage: See package insert for full prescribing information.
Store powder at 20° to 25°C (68° to 77°F) [See USP Controlled Room Temperature] prior to constitution.

0093-1075-78

N 3

This label is for US only, and cannot be altered or translated.

Label E

CHECK UP

For Exercises 1–17, calculate the amount to administer. Unless otherwise noted, tablets are scored in half.

1. Ordered: Dilaudid® 4 mg PO q6h   Administer: _____ (LO 13.1)

   On hand: Dilaudid® 8 mg scored tablets

2. Ordered: DiaBeta® 2.5 mg PO qam ac   Administer: _____ (LO 13.1)

   On hand: DiaBeta® 1.25 mg scored tablets

3. Ordered: Biltricide 450 mg PO q8h   Administer: _____ (LO 13.1)

   On hand: Biltricide 600 mg tablets scored in quarters

4. Ordered: Amoxicillin 300 mg PO q12h   Administer: _____ (LO 13.2)

   On hand: Amoxicillin suspension labeled 50 mg/mL

5. Ordered: Artane® 3 mg PO daily   Administer: _____ (LO 13.2)

   On hand: Artane® solution labeled 2 mg/5 mL

6. Ordered: Fosamax® 10 mg PO qam 30 min ac with water   Administer: _____ (LO 13.1)

   On hand: Fosamax® 5 mg unscored tablets

7. Ordered: Biaxin® liquid 62.5 mg via NGT q12h   Administer: _____ (LO 13.2)

   On hand: Biaxin® liquid labeled 125 mg/5 mL

8. Ordered: Isoptin® 270 mg PO qam   Administer: _____ (LO 13.1)

   On hand: Isoptin® 180 mg scored tablets

9. Ordered: Duricef® 0.5 g PO bid   Administer: _____ (LO 13.2)

   On hand: Duricef® suspension labeled 250 mg/5 mL

10. Ordered: Levoxyl® 0.45 mg PO daily   Administer: _____ (LO 13.1)

    On hand: Levoxyl® 300 mcg scored tablets

11. Ordered: Hivid 750 mcg PO q8h   Administer: _____ (LO 13.1)

    On hand: Hivid 0.375 mg unscored tablets

12. Ordered: Duricef® 500 mg PO bid   Administer: _____ (LO 13.1)

    On hand: Duricef® 1 g scored tablets

13. Ordered: Famvir 750 mg PO q12h   Administer: _____ (LO 13.1)

    On hand: Famvir 250 tablets

14. Ordered: Felbatol® 400 mg via NGT tid   Administer: _____ (LO 13.2)

    On hand: Felbatol® liquid labeled 600 mg/5 mL

15. Ordered: Synthroid® 0.175 mg PO daily

Administer: _____ (LO 13.1)

On hand: Refer to label A. Tablets are unscored.

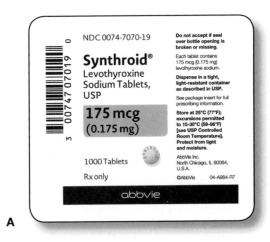

A

16. Ordered: Metformin 0.5 g po daily

On hand: Refer to label B. Tablets are scored.

Administer: _____ (LO 13.1)

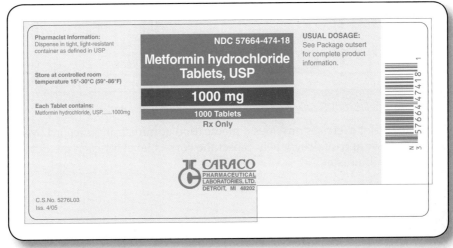

B

17. Ordered: Cefprozil 125 mg via NGT tid

On hand: Refer to label C.

Administer: _____ (LO 13.2)

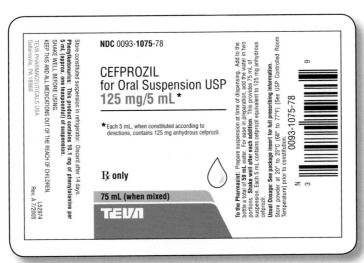

C

This label is for US only, and cannot be altered or translated.

18. What combination will provide the desired dose with the fewest tablets? (LO 13.1)
Ordered: Hytrin® 5 mg PO qpm
On hand: Hytrin® 1 mg unscored tablets and Hytrin® 2 mg unscored tablets

19. A patient receives 15 mL of Lortab® elixir every 6 h. Lortab® elixir contains 7.5 mg hydrocodone and 500 mg acetaminophen in each 15 mL. How much acetaminophen will this patient receive in 24 h? (LO 13.1)

20. How would you reconstitute the following medication? Find the amount to administer. (LO 13.2)
Ordered: Cephalexin 375 mg PO bid
On hand: Refer to label D.

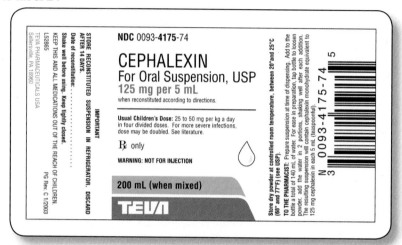

D

This label is for US only, and cannot be altered or translated.

Each of the following sets of exercises provides a medication administration record (MAR) listing several medication orders and a variety of drug labels. Select the correct label for each medication order. Then calculate the amount to administer.

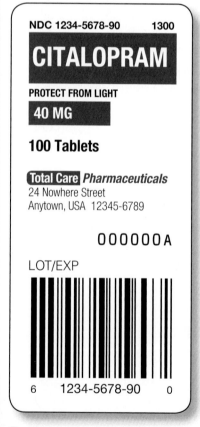

E Tablets are scored in half.

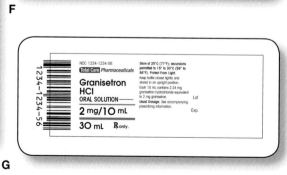

F

G

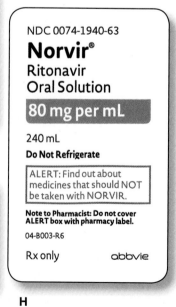

H

Medication Sheet

Date: 6/1/14

MEDICATIONS	HOUR	1	2	3	4	5	6	7	8	9	10	11	12	13	14	15	16	17	18	19	20	21	22	23	24	25	26	27	28	29	30
21. Ritonavir liquid 600 mg PO BID	0800 X																														
	2000 X																														
22. Citalopram 20 mg PO daily	0800 X X X																														
23. Granisetron 2 mg PO Daily	0800 X X X																														
24. Vistaril 20 mg PO TID	0800 1600 2400 X																														
	0800 X 2000 X																														

INIT.	SIGNATURE	INIT.	SIGNATURE	INIT.	SIGNATURE
C	Carol Smith				

PHARMACY / ALLERGIES / NOTES	PHYSICIAN'S SIGNATURE	Mary Jones	DATE 6/1/14
NKA	ABOVE ORDER NOTED BY:	Carol Smith	DATE 6/1/14
	DIAGNOSIS ◆		

PHYSICIAN / ALT. PHYSICIAN	PHONE NO.					
RESIDENT	STATION/ROOM/BED	ADMISSION NUMBER / DATE	SEX	DATE OF BIRTH	CURRENT MONTH / YEAR	PAGE NO.
Ridge, Jason	512 B	2468102	M	6/9/35	June 2014	1

Figure 13-13   MAR 1

Refer to Figure 13-13 MAR 1 above and labels E to H on the previous page.

21. Use: _____   Administer: _____ (LO 13.2)

22. Use: _____   Administer: _____ (LO 13.1)

23. Use: _____   Administer: _____ (LO 13.1)

24. Use: _____   Administer: _____ (LO 13.2)

Refer to Figure 13-14 MAR 2 and labels I to O on the next page.

25. Use: _____   Administer: _____ (LO 13.1)

26. Use: _____   Administer: _____ (LO 13.1)

27. Use: _____   Administer: _____ (LO 13.2)

28. Use: _____   Administer: _____ (LO 13.1)

29. Use: _____   Administer: _____ (LO 13.1)

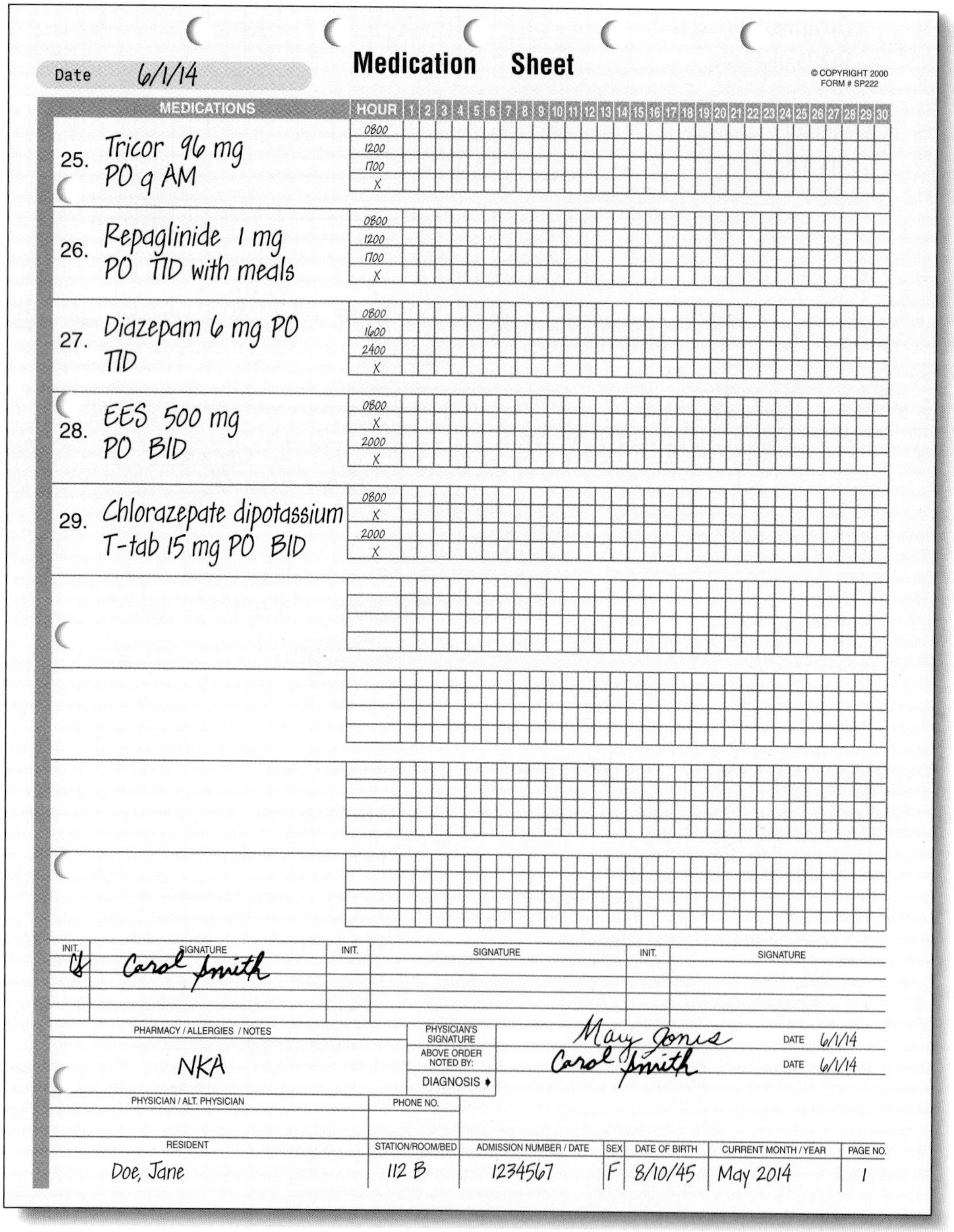

Figure 13-14   MAR 2

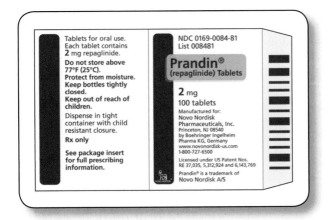

I

Tablets for oral use. Each tablet contains **2 mg** repaglinide.

Do not store above 77°F (25°C). Protect from moisture. Keep bottles tightly closed. Keep out of reach of children.

Dispense in tight container with child resistant closure.

Rx only

See package insert for full prescribing information.

NDC 0169-0084-81
List 008481

Prandin®
(repaglinide) Tablets

2 mg
100 tablets

Manufactured for:
Novo Nordisk
Pharmaceuticals, Inc.
Princeton, NJ 08540
by Boehringer Ingelheim
Pharma KG, Germany
www.novonordisk-us.com
1-800-727-6500

Licensed under US Patent Nos.
RE 37,035, 5,312,924 and 6,143,769

Prandin® is a trademark of
Novo Nordisk A/S

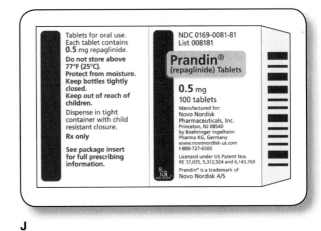

J

Tablets for oral use. Each tablet contains **0.5 mg** repaglinide.

Do not store above 77°F (25°C). Protect from moisture. Keep bottles tightly closed. Keep out of reach of children.

Dispense in tight container with child resistant closure.

Rx only

See package insert for full prescribing information.

NDC 0169-0081-81
List 008181

Prandin®
(repaglinide) Tablets

0.5 mg
100 tablets

Manufactured for:
Novo Nordisk
Pharmaceuticals, Inc.
Princeton, NJ 08540
by Boehringer Ingelheim
Pharma KG, Germany
www.novonordisk-us.com
1-800-727-6500

Licensed under US Patent Nos.
RE 37,035, 5,312,924 and 6,143,769

Prandin® is a trademark of
Novo Nordisk A/S

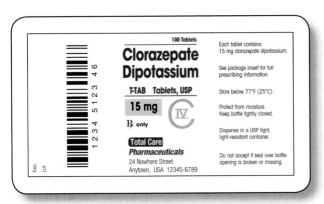

K

100 Tablets

Clorazepate Dipotassium

T-TAB   Tablets, USP

15 mg   C IV

℞ only

Total Care
Pharmaceuticals
24 Nowhere Street
Anytown, USA 12345-6789

Each tablet contains 15 mg clorazepate dipotassium.

See package insert for full prescribing information.

Store below 77°F (25°C).

Protect from moisture. Keep bottle tightly closed.

Dispense in a USP tight, light-resistant container.

Do not accept if seal over bottle opening is broken or missing.

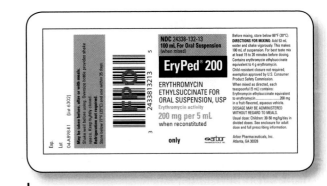

L

NDC 24338-132-13
100 mL For Oral Suspension
(when mixed)

EryPed® 200

ERYTHROMYCIN
ETHYLSUCCINATE FOR
ORAL SUSPENSION, USP

Erythromycin activity

200 mg per 5 mL
when reconstituted

only   ◆arbor

Before mixing, store below 86°F (30°C).
DIRECTIONS FOR MIXING: Add 53 mL water and shake vigorously. This makes 100 mL of suspension. For best taste mix at least 15 to 20 minutes before dosing. Contains erythromycin ethylsuccinate equivalent to 4 g erythromycin. Child-resistant closure not required; exemption approved by U.S. Consumer Product Safety Commission.
When mixed as directed, each teaspoonful (5 mL) contains: Erythromycin ethylsuccinate equivalent to erythromycin.................200 mg in a fruit-flavored, aqueous vehicle. DOSAGE MAY BE ADMINISTERED WITHOUT REGARD TO MEALS.
Usual dose: Children: 30-50 mg/kg/day in divided doses. See enclosure for adult dose and full prescribing information.

Arbor Pharmaceuticals, Inc.
Atlanta, GA 30328

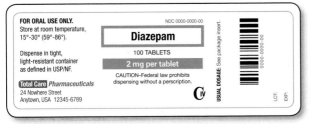

M

FOR ORAL USE ONLY.
Store at room temperature, 15°-30° (59°-86°).

Dispense in tight, light-resistant container as defined in USP/NF.

Total Care *Pharmaceuticals*
24 Nowhere Street
Anytown, USA 12345-6789

NDC 0000-0000-00

Diazepam

100 TABLETS

2 mg per tablet

CAUTION—Federal law prohibits dispensing without a perscription.

C IV

USUAL DOSAGE: See package insert.

0000-0000-00

LOT: EXP:

N

FOR ORAL USE ONLY.
Store at room temperature, 15°-30° (59°-86°).

Dispense in tight, light-resistant container as defined in USP/NF.

Total Care *Pharmaceuticals*
24 Nowhere Street
Anytown, USA 12345-6789

NDC 0000-0000-00

Diazepam

100 TABLETS

5 mg per tablet

CAUTION—Federal law prohibits dispensing without a perscription.

C IV

USUAL DOSAGE: See package insert.

0000-0000-00

LOT: EXP:

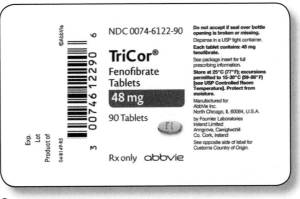

O

©AbbVie

NDC 0074-6122-90

TriCor®
Fenofibrate
Tablets

48 mg

90 Tablets

F ∞

Rx only   abbvie

Do not accept if seal over bottle opening is broken or missing.
Dispense in a USP tight container.
Each tablet contains: 48 mg fenofibrate.
See package insert for full prescribing information.
Store at 25°C (77°F); excursions permitted to 15-30°C (59-86°F) [see USP Controlled Room Temperature]. Protect from moisture.
Manufactured for AbbVie Inc.
North Chicago, IL 60064, U.S.A.
by Fournier Laboratories Ireland Limited
Anngrove, Carrigtwohill
Co. Cork, Ireland
See opposite side of label for Customs Country of Origin.

Exp.
Lot
Product of
04-B149-R5

CRITICAL THINKING APPLICATIONS

The following medications are ordered for a patient with a gastrostomy tube who cannot swallow and must receive all medications through the tube.

   a. Depakote® ER 250 mg daily

   b. Valium® 4 mg qid

   c. Hydroxyzine pamoate 50 mg PO prn for anxiety

   d. Cephalexin 500 mg

On hand: Refer to labels P, Q, R, and S.

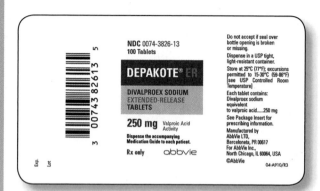

P

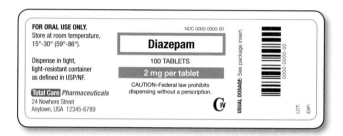

Q

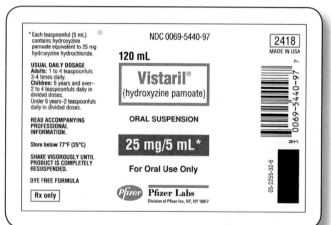

R

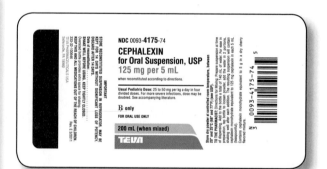

S This label is for US only, and cannot be altered or translated.

   1. For each medication, calculate the amount to administer. (LO 13.1, 13.2)

   2. Are there any medications on the list that cannot be given as ordered? (LO 13.1)

   3. How would you administer these medications? (LO 13.1, 13.2)

   4. What action would you take if you could not give a medication as ordered? (LO 13.1)

CASE STUDY

Ordered: Cefprozil® liquid 187.5 mg PO qid

On hand: Refer to label T.

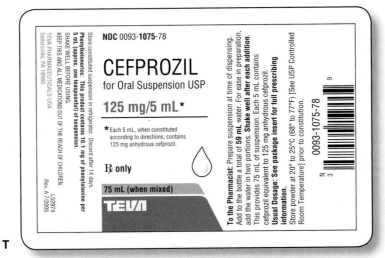

T

This label is for US only, and cannot be altered or translated.

1. Describe how you would reconstitute this medication. (LO 13.2)

2. Calculate the amount to administer. (LO 13.2)

3. What measuring device would you use to give this dose? (LO 13.2)

4. Calculate the daily dose. (LO 13.2)

connect

Now that you have completed the materials in the chapter text, go to CONNECT and complete any chapter activities you have not yet done.

14

CHAPTER

Parenteral Dosages

The best way to escape from a problem is to solve it.

ALAN SAPORTA

LEARNING OUTCOMES

When you have completed Chapter 14, you will be able to:

14.1 Calculate dosages of parenteral medication in solution and select a syringe based on the dosage calculation.

14.2 Calculate dosages of medications expressed in percent or ratio format.

14.3 Calculate dosages of reconstituted parenteral medications.

14.4 Calculate dosages for other administration forms.

14.5 Calculate subcutaneous dosages of the high-alert medication insulin.

14.6 Calculate subcutaneous dosages of the high-alert medication heparin.

INTRODUCTION

Parenteral medications are *not* taken by mouth, so they bypass the digestive tract. They include medications that are administered by injection and other medications, such as inhalants and rectal and transdermal drugs. Injection routes include intravenous (IV), intramuscular (IM), subcutaneous (subcut), and intradermal (ID). These routes have different absorption rates, which is the rate at which the medication is absorbed and dispersed into the bloodstream. Because of this, dosages may vary if the same medication is administered via different routes. See Figure 14.1

- Intravenous (IV; into a vein)—fastest absorption rate of 30 to 60 seconds
- Intramuscular (IM; into a muscle)—absorption rate varies: 10 minutes or longer
- Subcutaneous (subcut; under the skin, into fatty tissue)—absorption rate varies: 15 minutes or longer
- Intradermal (ID; between layers of skin)—sustained absorption rate because medication is absorbed through the capillaries of skin

This chapter will focus on dosage calculations for parenteral medications with the exception of intravenous medications, which will be covered in the "Intravenous Calculations" chapter. So get ready to solve some problems.

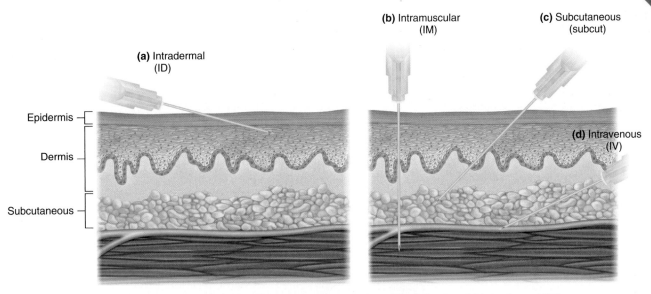

Figure 14-1 Absorption rates of medications vary based on the location of the injection: (a) intradermal (ID), (b) intramuscular (IM), (c) subcutaneous (subcut), and (d) intravenous (IV).

14.1 Calculating Parenteral Dosages in Solution

Injections are mixtures that contain the drug dissolved in an appropriate liquid. The dosage or solution strength on an injectable medication's label indicates the amount of drug contained within a volume of solution (see Table 14-1). Dosage strength may be expressed in milligrams per milliliter, as a percent, or as a ratio.

TABLE 14-1 Sample Solution Strengths

LABEL DESCRIPTION	INTERPRETATION
Compazine 5 mg/mL	1 mL contains 5 mg of Compazine
Epogen 3,000 units/mL	1 mL contains 3,000 units of Epogen
Lidocaine 1%	100 mL contains 1 g of lidocaine
Epinephrine 1:1,000	1,000 mL contains 1 g of epinephrine

Physicians' orders for injections usually specify the amount of medication to be administered to the patient. Before the injection can be administered, it is necessary to calculate how many milliliters of the solution contain the desired dose of the medication.

As with oral medications, follow the ABCs of dosage calculation. Start with Step A: gather the information regarding dosage ordered, dose on hand, and dosage unit. If the dosage ordered and dose on hand have different units, then you must convert the units of the dosage ordered to the units of the dose on hand to find the desired dose. Then follow Step B: calculate the amount to administer, using any of the three methods of dosage calculations: the proportion method, dimensional analysis, or the formula method. Then verify your calculation with Step C: Think! . . . Is it reasonable?

Syringe Sizes

Once you have determined the amount to administer, you must select the appropriate syringe and needle. Rule 14-1 provides guidelines for selecting the syringe. See the chapter "Equipment for Dosage Measurement" for a discussion of needles.

RULE 14-1	Select the proper syringe.
	1. If the amount of injection to administer is 1 mL or more, round the amount to the tenths and use a standard 3 mL syringe.
	2. If the amount of injection to administer is less than 1 mL but greater than or equal to 0.5 mL and calculates evenly to the tenths, use a 1 mL tuberculin syringe or a standard 3 mL syringe.
	3. If the amount of injection to administer is less than 1 mL, round to the hundredths and use a 1 mL tuberculin syringe. For amounts less than 0.5 mL use a 0.5-mL tuberculin syringe, if available.
Example 1	The amount to administer intramuscularly is calculated at 2.4 mL. Since this is greater than 1 mL, a standard syringe should be used. See Figure 14-2.

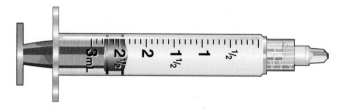

Figure 14-2   Standard syringe with 2.4 mL.

Example 2	The amount to administer subcutaneously is calculated at 0.6 mL. Since this amount is greater than 0.5 mL and calculates evenly to the tenths, either a 1 mL tuberculin syringe or a 3 mL syringe can be used. See Figures 14-3a and 14-3b.

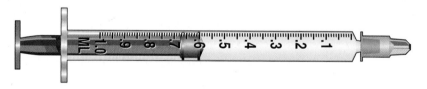

Figure 14-3a   A 1 mL tuberculin syringe with 0.6 mL.

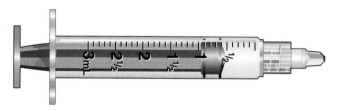

Figure 14-3b   A standard 3 mL syringe with 0.6 mL.

Example 3	The amount to administer is calculated at 0.34 mL. Since this is less than 1 mL, a 1 mL tuberculin syringe or a 0.5 mL tuberculin syringe should be used. See Figure 14-4.

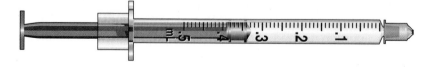

Figure 14-4   A 0.5 mL tuberculin syringe with 0.34 mL.

The amount to administer will not always be in whole milliliters, and it will sometimes be necessary to round your answer.

RULE 14-2	Correctly round the amount of an injection to administer.
	1. Round volumes greater than 1 mL to the nearest tenth because the 3 mL syringe is calibrated in tenths.
	2. Round volumes less than 1 mL to the nearest hundredth because tuberculin syringes are calibrated in hundredths.
Example 1	The amount to administer is calculated at 1.66 mL. Since the volume is greater than 1 mL, you round 1.66 mL to the nearest tenth, which is 1.7 mL.
Example 2	The amount to administer is calculated at 0.532 mL. Since the volume is less than 1 mL, you round 0.532 mL to the nearest hundredth, which is 0.53 mL.

 LEARNING LINK   Recall from the chapter "Decimals" the rule about rounding decimals.

Once you determine the proper syringe, you must also decide whether the amount to be administered can be safely injected in a single site. When the amount to administer exceeds the amount that can be safely given in one site, divide the amount into equal (or nearly equal) parts. Then administer them in separate sites.

RULE 14-3	Do not exceed maximum volume for an injection in a single site.
	Intramuscular injections:
	• Adult, excluding deltoid 3 mL
	• Adult deltoid (arm) 1 mL
	• Child 6 to 12 years 2 mL
	• Child 0 to 5 years 1 mL
	• Premature infant 0.5 mL
	Subcutaneous injections: 1 mL

Example

The amount to administer intramuscularly to an adult is 4.5 mL. After checking and verifying the amount, you draw up 2 mL into one syringe and 2.5 mL into another. Inject the contents of each syringe into a different site. See Figure 14-5.

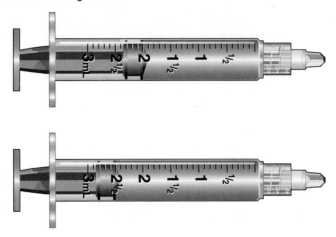

Figure 14-5 Two standard syringes would be used for a dose greater than the maximum volume for an injection, such as 4.5 mL.

When calculating the amount to administer for injectable medications, you must determine how many milliliters contain the desired dose of medication and then apply Rules 14-1 to 14-3.

PROPORTION METHOD

EXAMPLE 1

Find the amount to administer and select the proper syringe. Refer to Figure 14-6.

STEP A: GATHER INFORMATION AND CONVERT

Ordered: Diazepam 7.5 mg IM now

Dosage strength: 5 mg per mL

Patient: A 175-lb, 45-year-old male

The dosage ordered O and the dose on hand H are already expressed in the same units, so the desired dose D is 7.5 mg.

STEP B: CALCULATE
Follow Procedure Checklist 12-1.

1. Set up the proportion.

    $$\frac{H}{Q} = \frac{D}{A}$$

    Using Fractions:

    $$\frac{5 \text{ mg}}{1 \text{ mL}} = \frac{7.5 \text{ mg}}{A}$$

2. Cancel units.

    $$\frac{5 \text{ m\!g}}{1 \text{ mL}} = \frac{7.5 \text{ m\!g}}{A}$$

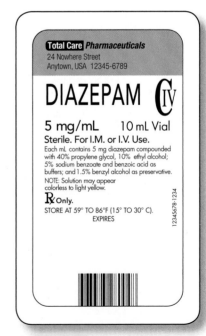

Total Care *Pharmaceuticals*
24 Nowhere Street
Anytown, USA 12345-6789

DIAZEPAM C IV

5 mg/mL   10 mL Vial
Sterile. For I.M. or I.V. Use.
Each mL contains 5 mg diazepam compounded with 40% propylene glycol, 10% ethyl alcohol; 5% sodium benzoate and benzoic acid as buffers; and 1.5% benzyl alcohol as preservative.
NOTE: Solution may appear colorless to light yellow.
℞ Only.
STORE AT 59° TO 86°F (15° TO 30° C).
          EXPIRES

12345678-1234

Figure 14-6

3. Cross-multiply and solve.

$$5 \times A = 1 \text{ mL} \times 7.5$$

$$A = \frac{1 \text{ mL} \times 7.5}{5}$$

$$A = 1.5 \text{ mL}$$

STEP C: THINK! . . . IS IT REASONABLE?

Since 7.5 mg is $1\frac{1}{2}$ times larger than 5 mg, the volume to administer should be $1\frac{1}{2}$ times larger than the volume on hand. 1.5 mL is $1\frac{1}{2}$ times larger than 1 mL, so the answer is reasonable.

The amount to administer is 1.5 mL.

- Referring to Rule 14-1, a standard 3 mL syringe would be used.
- Referring to Rule 14-2, we find that it is not necessary to round in this example.
- Referring to Rule 14-3, the total volume may be given as a single injection.

EXAMPLE 2   Find the amount to administer and select the proper syringe. Refer to Figure 14-7.

STEP A: GATHER INFORMATION AND CONVERT

Ordered: Lorazepam 800 mcg IM now

Dosage strength: 2 mg per mL

Patient: An 85-lb, 12-year-old female

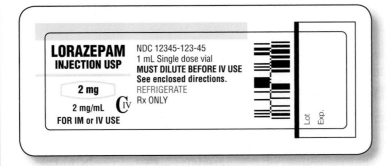

Figure 14-7

The dosage ordered O is in micrograms, and the dose on hand H is in milligrams, so the desired dose D, in milligrams, must be calculated.

1. Fill in the proportion, recalling that 1 mg = 1,000 mcg.

$$\frac{1 \text{ mg}}{1,000 \text{ mcg}} = \frac{D}{800 \text{ mcg}}$$

2. Cancel units.

$$\frac{1 \text{ mg}}{1,000 \text{ mcg}} = \frac{D}{800 \text{ mcg}}$$

3. Cross-multiply and solve for the unknown.

$$1,000 \times D = 1 \times 800 \text{ mg}$$

$$D = 0.8 \text{ mg}$$

We now have the necessary pieces of information: $D = 0.8$ mg, $Q = 1$ mL, and $H = 2$ mg.

STEP B: CALCULATE

Follow Procedure Checklist 12-1, using fractions.

1. Set up the proportion.

$$\frac{2\text{ mg}}{1\text{ mL}} = \frac{0.8\text{ mg}}{A}$$

2. Cancel units.

$$\frac{2\text{ mg}}{1\text{ mL}} = \frac{0.8\text{ mg}}{A}$$

3. Cross-multiply and solve for the unknown.

$$2 \times A = 1\text{ mL} \times 0.8$$

$$A = 1\text{ mL} \times \frac{0.8}{2}$$

$$A = 0.4\text{ mL}$$

STEP C: THINK! . . . IS IT REASONABLE?

Since 1 is half of 2, then A should be half of 0.8. The answer is reasonable because 0.4 is half of 0.8.

The amount to administer is 0.4 mL.

- Referring to Rule 14-1, a 1 mL or 0.5 mL tuberculin syringe would be used.
- Referring to Rule 14-2, we find that it is not necessary to round in this example.
- Referring to Rule 14-3, the total volume may be given as a single injection.

DIMENSIONAL ANALYSIS

EXAMPLE 1

Find the amount to administer and select the proper syringe. Refer to Figure 14-6 on page 338.

STEP A: GATHER INFORMATION AND CONVERT

Ordered: Diazepam 7.5 mg IM now

Dosage strength: 5 mg per mL

Patient: A 175-lb, 45-year-old male

Because the dosage ordered and the dose on hand have the same units, no conversion is needed to find the desired dose D, which is 7.5 mg.

STEP B: CALCULATE

Follow Procedure Checklist 12-2.

1. The unit of measure for the amount to administer is milliliters.

A mL =

2. No conversion factor is needed.

3. The dosage unit is 1 mL. The dose on hand is 5 mg. This is your first factor.

$$\frac{1\text{ mL}}{5\text{ mg}}$$

4. The dosage ordered is 7.5 mg. Set up the equation.

$$A\text{ mL} = \frac{1\text{ mL}}{5\text{ mg}} \times \frac{7.5\text{ mg}}{1}$$

5. Cancel units.

$$A \text{ mL} = \frac{1 \text{ mL}}{5 \text{ mg}} \times \frac{7.5 \text{ mg}}{1}$$

6. Solve the equation.

$$A \text{ mL} = \frac{1 \text{ mL}}{5} \times \frac{7.5}{1}$$

$$A = 1.5 \text{ mL}$$

STEP C: THINK! . . . IS IT REASONABLE?

Since 7.5 is $1\frac{1}{2}$ times larger than 5, the volume to be administered should be $1\frac{1}{2}$ times larger than 1. The amount to administer, 1.5, is $1\frac{1}{2}$ times larger than 1, so the answer is reasonable.

The amount to administer is 1.5 mL.

- Referring to Rule 14-1, a standard 3 mL syringe would be used.
- Referring to Rule 14-2, we find that it is not necessary to round in this example.
- Referring to Rule 14-3, the total volume may be given as a single injection.

EXAMPLE 2

Find the amount to administer and select the proper syringe. Refer to Figure 14-7 on page 339.

STEP A: GATHER INFORMATION AND CONVERT

Ordered: Lorazepam 800 mcg IM now

Dosage strength: 2 mg per mL

Patient: An 85-lb, 12-year-old female

The unit of measure for the dose on hand is milligrams. The unit of measure for the dose ordered is micrograms. Determine the conversion factor for milligrams to micrograms. The conversion factor is 1 mg/1,000 mcg.

STEP B: CALCULATE

Follow Procedure Checklist 12-2.

1. The unit of measure for the amount to administer will be milliliters.

$$A \text{ mL} =$$

2. The conversion factor is the first factor of the equation.

$$A \text{ mL} = \frac{1 \text{ mg}}{1,000 \text{ mcg}}$$

3. The dosage unit is 1 mL. The dose on hand is 2 mg. This is our second factor.

$$A \text{ mL} = \frac{1 \text{ mg}}{1,000 \text{ mcg}} \times \frac{1 \text{ mL}}{2 \text{ mg}}$$

4. The dosage ordered is 800 mcg. Complete the equation.

$$A \text{ mL} = \frac{1 \text{ mg}}{1,000 \text{ mcg}} \times \frac{1 \text{ mL}}{2 \text{ mg}} \times \frac{800 \text{ mcg}}{1}$$

5. Cancel units.

$$A \text{ mL} = \frac{1 \text{ mg}}{1,000 \text{ mcg}} \times \frac{1 \text{ mL}}{2 \text{ mg}} \times \frac{800 \text{ mcg}}{1}$$

6. Solve the equation.

$$A \text{ mL} = \frac{1}{1,000} \times \frac{1 \text{ mL}}{2} \times \frac{800}{1}$$

$$A = 0.4 \text{ mL}$$

The concentration is 2 mg per 1 mL, so the volume to be administered will be half the dose (in milligrams). It is reasonable because 0.4 is half of 0.8.

The amount to administer is 0.4 mL.

- Referring to Rule 14-1, a 1 mL or 0.5 mL tuberculin syringe would be used.
- Referring to Rule 14-2, we find that it is not necessary to round in this example.
- Referring to Rule 14-3, the total volume may be given as a single injection.

FORMULA METHOD

EXAMPLE 1 | Find the amount to administer and select the proper syringe. Refer to Figure 14-6 on page 338.

STEP A: GATHER INFORMATION AND CONVERT

Ordered: Diazepam 7.5 mg IM now

Dosage strength: 5 mg per mL

Patient: A 175-lb, 45-year-old male

The drug is ordered in milligrams, which is the same unit of measure as that of the dose on hand. No conversion is necessary.

STEP B: CALCULATE
Follow Procedure Checklist 12-3.

1. Desired dose $D = 7.5$ mg

Dose on hand $H = 5$ mg

Quantity to be administered $Q = 1$ mL

$$\frac{D}{H} \times Q = A$$

$$\frac{7.5 \text{ mg}}{5 \text{ mg}} \times 1 \text{ mL} = A$$

2. Cancel units.

$$\frac{7.5 \cancel{\text{ mg}}}{5 \cancel{\text{ mg}}} \times 1 \text{ mL} = A$$

3. Solve for the unknown.

$$\frac{7.5}{5} \times 1 \text{ mL} = A$$

$$1.5 \text{ mL} = A$$

STEP C: THINK! . . . IS IT REASONABLE?
Since the desired dose is $1\frac{1}{2}$ times larger than the dose in 1 mL, the volume to be administered should be $1\frac{1}{2}$ times larger than 1 mL. The amount to administer, 1.5 mL, is $1\frac{1}{2}$ times larger than 1 mL, so it is reasonable.

The amount to administer is 1.5 mL.

- Referring to Rule 14-1, a standard 3 mL syringe would be used.
- Referring to Rule 14-2, we find that it is not necessary to round in this example.
- Referring to Rule 14-3, the total volume may be given as a single injection.

EXAMPLE 2

Find the amount to administer and select the proper syringe. Refer to Figure 14-7 on page 339.

STEP A: GATHER INFORMATION AND CONVERT

Ordered: Lorazepam 800 mcg IM now

Dosage strength: 2 mg per mL

Patient: An 85-lb, 12-year-old female

The dosage ordered Q is in micrograms, and the dose on hand H is in milligrams, so the desired dose D, in milligrams, must be calculated.

1. Set up the proportion, recalling that 1 mg = 1,000 mcg.

$$\frac{1 \text{ mg}}{1,000 \text{ mcg}} = \frac{D}{800} \text{ mcg}$$

2. Cancel units.

$$\frac{1 \text{ mg}}{1,000 \text{ mcg}} = \frac{D}{800} \text{ mcg}$$

3. Cross-multiply and solve for the unknown.

$$1,000 \times D = 1 \times 800 \text{ mg}$$

$$D = 0.8 \text{ mg}$$

We now have the necessary pieces of information: $D = 0.8$ mg, $Q = 1$ mL, and $H = 2$ mg.

STEP B: CALCULATE
Follow Procedure Checklist 12-3.

1. Fill in the formula.

$$\frac{0.8 \text{ mg}}{2 \text{ mg}} \times 1 \text{ mL} = A$$

2. Cancel units.

$$\frac{0.8 \text{ mg}}{2 \text{ mg}} \times 1 \text{ mL} = A$$

3. Solve for the unknown.

$$\frac{0.8}{2} \times 1 \text{ mL} = A$$

$$0.4 \text{ mL} = A$$

STEP C: THINK! . . . IS IT REASONABLE?
The concentration is 2 mg per 1 mL, so the volume to administer will be half as large as the desired dose. 0.4 is half as large as 0.8, so it is reasonable.

The amount to administer is 0.4 mL.

- Referring to Rule 14-1, a 1 mL or 0.5 mL tuberculin syringe would be used.
- Referring to Rule 14-2, we find that it is not necessary to round in this example.
- Referring to Rule 14-3, the total volume may be given as a single injection.

Confirming the Physician's Order

A patient in an agitated state is brought to the emergency department. The physician verbally orders 2 mL IM of Vistaril. The healthcare professional draws up 2 mL from a vial labeled 50 mg/mL. She then notices another vial labeled 25 mg/mL.

Think! . . . Is It Reasonable? What should she do? How is the patient's care affected if she does not take action?

REVIEW AND PRACTICE

14.1 Calculating Parenteral Dosages in Solution

For Exercises 1–16, find the amount to administer, and then determine the proper syringe and write it in the space provided.

1. Ordered: Thiamine 100 mg IM now

On hand: Refer to label A.

Administer: _____   Syringe: _____

NDC 0073-3811-09   1300

THIAMINE HYDROCHLORIDE

PROTECT FROM LIGHT

100 mg/mL

2 mL Multiple Use Vial
For I.M or I.V. Use.

Total Care *Pharmaceuticals*
24 Nowhere Street
Anytown, USA 12345-6789

000000A

LOT/EXP

6   0073-3811-09   0

A

2. Ordered: Heparin 700 units subcut daily

   On hand: Refer to label B.

   Administer: _____   Syringe: _____

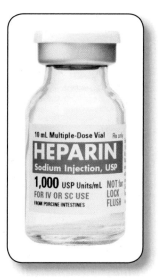

B

3. Ordered: Trimethobenzamide 200 mg IM TID

   On hand: Refer to label C.

   Administer: _____   Syringe: _____

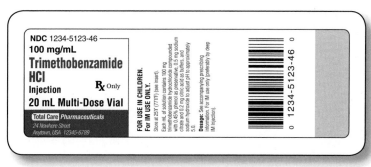

C

4. Ordered: Sandostatin® 200 mcg subcut q12h

   On hand: Refer to label D.

   Administer: _____   Syringe: _____

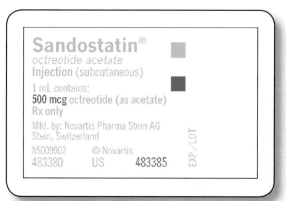

D

5. Ordered: Filgrastim® 180 mcg subcut daily

On hand: Refer to label E.

Administer: _____   Syringe: _____

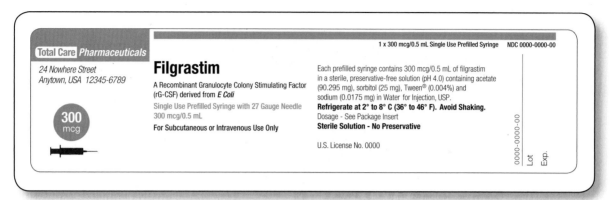

Total Care *Pharmaceuticals*

24 Nowhere Street
Anytown, USA 12345-6789

300 mcg

1 x 300 mcg/0.5 mL Single Use Prefilled Syringe   NDC 0000-0000-00

Filgrastim

A Recombinant Granulocyte Colony Stimulating Factor
(rG-CSF) derived from *E Coli*

Single Use Prefilled Syringe with 27 Gauge Needle
300 mcg/0.5 mL

For Subcutaneous or Intravenous Use Only

Each prefilled syringe contains 300 mcg/0.5 mL of filgrastim
in a sterile, preservative-free solution (pH 4.0) containing acetate
(90.295 mg), sorbitol (25 mg), Tween® (0.004%) and
sodium (0.0175 mg) in Water for Injection, USP.
Refrigerate at 2° to 8° C (36° to 46° F). Avoid Shaking.
Dosage - See Package Insert
Sterile Solution - No Preservative

U.S. License No. 0000

0000-0000-00   Lot   Exp.

E

6. Ordered: Filgrastim® 240 mcg subcut daily

On hand: Refer to label F.

Administer: _____   Syringe: _____

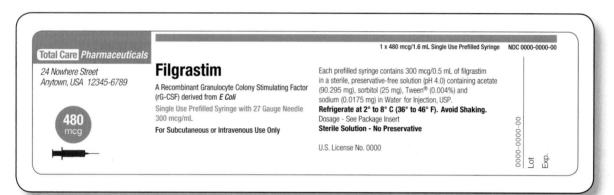

Total Care *Pharmaceuticals*

24 Nowhere Street
Anytown, USA 12345-6789

480 mcg

1 x 480 mcg/1.6 mL Single Use Prefilled Syringe   NDC 0000-0000-00

Filgrastim

A Recombinant Granulocyte Colony Stimulating Factor
(rG-CSF) derived from *E Coli*

Single Use Prefilled Syringe with 27 Gauge Needle
300 mcg/mL

For Subcutaneous or Intravenous Use Only

Each prefilled syringe contains 300 mcg/0.5 mL of filgrastim
in a sterile, preservative-free solution (pH 4.0) containing acetate
(90.295 mg), sorbitol (25 mg), Tween® (0.004%) and
sodium (0.0175 mg) in Water for Injection, USP.
Refrigerate at 2° to 8° C (36° to 46° F). Avoid Shaking.
Dosage - See Package Insert
Sterile Solution - No Preservative

U.S. License No. 0000

0000-0000-00   Lot   Exp.

F

7. Ordered: Heparin 4,000 units subcut
daily

On hand: Refer to label G.

Administer: _____

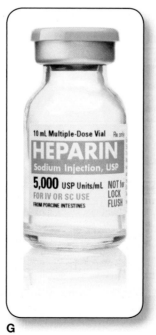

10 mL Multiple-Dose Vial   Rx only

HEPARIN
Sodium Injection, USP

5,000 USP Units/mL   NOT for
FOR IV OR SC USE   LOCK
FROM PORCINE INTESTINES   FLUSH

Syringe: _____

G

8. Ordered: Haloperidol 12 mg deep IM now
   On hand: Refer to label H.
   Administer: _____   Syringe: _____

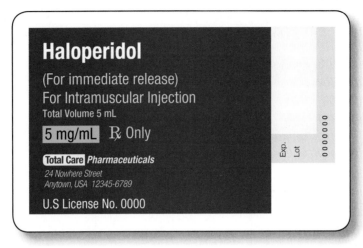

Haloperidol

(For immediate release)
For Intramuscular Injection
Total Volume 5 mL

5 mg/mL ℞ Only

Total Care *Pharmaceuticals*
24 Nowhere Street
Anytown, USA 12345-6789

U.S License No. 0000

Exp. Lot 0000000

H

9. Ordered: Zemplar™ 3 mcg IM daily
   On hand: Refer to label I.
   Administer: _____   Syringe: _____

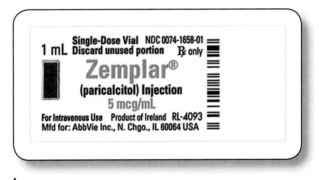

1 mL Single-Dose Vial NDC 0074-1658-01
Discard unused portion ℞ only

Zemplar®
(paricalcitol) Injection
5 mcg/mL

For Intravenous Use Product of Ireland RL-4093
Mfd for: AbbVie Inc., N. Chgo., IL 60064 USA

I

10. Ordered: Oxytocin 8 units IM now.
    On hand: Refer to label J.
    Administer: _____   Syringe: _____

NDC 00000-000-00

OXYTOCIN

INJECTION, USP (SYNTHETIC)

10 USP Units/mL

For IV Infusion or IM Use

10 mL Multiple Dose Vial
Rx only

Sterile
Each mL contains: Oxytocic activity equivalent to 10 USP Oxytocin Units; chlorobutanol anhydrous (chloral derivative) 0.5%; Water for Injection q.s. Acetic acid may have been added for pH adjustment. Usual Dosage: See Insert. Store at 20° to 25°C (68° to 77°F) [see USP Controlled Room Temperature]. Do not permit to freeze.

Total Care
Pharmaceuticals
24 Nowhere Street
Anytown, USA 12345-6789

LOT/EXP

0 1234-1234-56 0

J

11. Ordered: Clindamycin 600 mg IM pre-op

On hand: Refer to label K.

Administer: _____   Syringe: _____

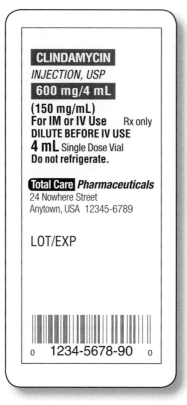

K

12. Ordered: ceftriaxone 160 mg IM now

On hand: Refer to label L.

Administer: _____   Syringe: _____

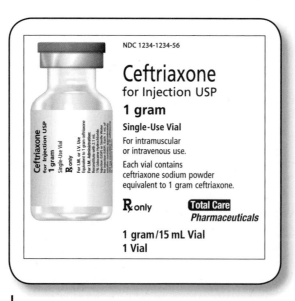

L

13. Ordered: Oxytocin 15 units IM q 12h prn

On hand: Refer to label M.

Administer: _____   Syringe: _____

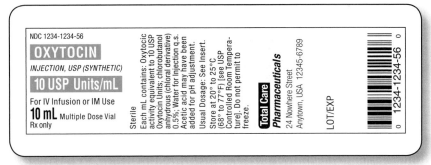

M

14. Ordered: Furosemide 20 mg IM at 0800

On hand: Refer to label N.

Administer: _____   Syringe: _____

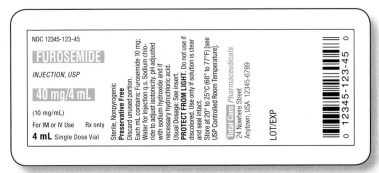

N

15. Ordered: Darbepoetin Alfa 25 mcg subcut now

On hand: Refer to label O.

Administer: _____   Syringe: _____

NDC 1076-5467-12   1300

DARBEPOETIN ALFA

Single Use Vial

40 mcg/1 mL

2 mL Multiple Use Vial
Usual Dosage: See Insert
For Subcutaneous Use

Total Care *Pharmaceuticals*
24 Nowhere Street
Anytown, USA 12345-6789

000000A

LOT/EXP

6   1076-5467-12   0

O

16. Ordered: Diazepam® 10 mg IM stat

On hand: Refer to label P.

Administer: _____   Syringe: _____

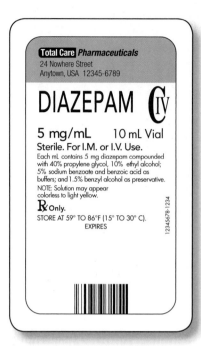

Total Care *Pharmaceuticals*
24 Nowhere Street
Anytown, USA 12345-6789

DIAZEPAM C IV

5 mg/mL   10 mL Vial
Sterile. For I.M. or I.V. Use.
Each mL contains 5 mg diazepam compounded
with 40% propylene glycol, 10% ethyl alcohol;
5% sodium benzoate and benzoic acid as
buffers; and 1.5% benzyl alcohol as preservative.
NOTE: Solution may appear
colorless to light yellow.
℞ Only.
STORE AT 59° TO 86°F (15° TO 30° C).
EXPIRES

P

14.2 Medications Expressed in Percent or Ratio Format

When the dosage strength is expressed as a percent or a ratio, convert it to the appropriate concentration fraction before calculating the amount to administer. For example, to administer 1% lidocaine, rewrite the strength as 1 g (dose on hand) per 100 mL (dosage unit) then calculate. If the labeled strength were 1:2,000, rewrite it as 1 g (dose on hand) per 2,000 mL (dosage unit). Some drugs, such as heparin, are measured in units and may have their solution strength expressed in ratio format. The ratio indicates the number of units contained in 1 mL. For example, heparin sodium 10,000:1 contains 10,000 units in 1 mL.

RULE 14-4	When a solution strength is expressed as a percent or ratio:
	1. Convert the percent or ratio to the dosage strength, such as grams per milliliter, milligrams per milliliter, or units per milliliter.
	2. Calculate the amount to administer, then apply Rules 14-1 to 14-3.

PROPORTION METHOD

EXAMPLE 1

Find the amount to administer and select the proper syringe.

STEP A: GATHER INFORMATION AND CONVERT

Ordered: Magnesium sulfate 300 mg IM now

On hand: Magnesium sulfate 10% solution

Patient: A 75-lb, 8-year-old female

The dosage strength of a 10% solution is 10 g (H) per 100 mL (Q).

The dose on hand H is now in grams, and the dosage ordered O is in milligrams. To calculate the desired dose D, we must convert the dosage ordered—300 mg—to the same unit of measure as that of the dose on hand, grams.

1. Set up the proportion, recalling that 1 g = 1,000 mg.

$$\frac{1\text{ g}}{1{,}000\text{ mg}} = \frac{D}{300\text{ mg}}$$

2. Cancel units.

$$\frac{1\text{ g}}{1{,}000\text{ mg}} = \frac{D}{300\text{ mg}}$$

3. Cross-multiply and solve for the unknown.

$$1{,}000 \times D = 300 \times 1\text{ g}$$
$$D = \frac{300 \times 1\text{ g}}{1{,}000}$$
$$D = 0.3\text{ g}$$

We now have the necessary pieces of information: $D = 0.3$ g, $Q = 100$ mL, and $H = 10$ g.

STEP B: CALCULATE
Follow Procedure Checklist 12-1.

1. Fill in the proportion.

$$\frac{10\text{ g}}{100\text{ mL}} = \frac{0.3\text{ g}}{A}$$

2. Cancel units.

$$\frac{10\text{ g}}{100\text{ mL}} = \frac{0.3\text{ g}}{A}$$

3. Cross-multiply and solve for the unknown.

$$10 \times A = 100\text{ mL} \times 0.3$$
$$A = \frac{100\text{ mL} \times 0.3}{10}$$
$$A = 3\text{ mL}$$

STEP C: THINK! . . . IS IT REASONABLE?
Since the concentration of the medication is 1 to 10, the volume to be administered should be 10 times larger than the desired dose. 3 is 10 times larger than 0.3, so it is reasonable.

The amount to administer is 3 mL.

- Referring to Rule 14-1, a standard 3 mL syringe would be used.
- Referring to Rule 14-2, we find that it is not necessary to round in this example.
- Referring to Rule 14-3, the dose would need to be divided into two parts because of the age of the patient. Draw 1.5 mL into each of two syringes and administer them into different sites.

EXAMPLE 2 Find the amount to administer and select the proper syringe.

STEP A: GATHER INFORMATION AND CONVERT

Ordered: Epinephrine 0.2 mg subcut stat

On hand: Vial of epinephrine 1:2,000 solution for injection

Patient: A 150-lb, 35-year-old adult

The dosage strength of a 1:2,000 solution is 1 g (*H*) per 2,000 mL (*Q*).

The dose on hand *H* is now in grams, and the dosage ordered *O* is in milligrams. To calculate the desired dose *D*, we must convert the dosage ordered—0.2 mg—to the same unit of measure as that of the dose on hand, grams.

1. Set up the proportion, recalling that 1 g = 1,000 mg.

$$\frac{1 \text{ g}}{1{,}000 \text{ mg}} = \frac{D}{0.2 \text{ mg}}$$

2. Cancel units.

$$\frac{1 \text{ g}}{1{,}000 \text{ mg}} = \frac{D}{0.2 \text{ mg}}$$

3. Cross-multiply and solve for the unknown.

$$1{,}000 \times D = 0.2 \times 1 \text{ g}$$

$$D = \frac{0.2 \times 1 \text{ g}}{1{,}000}$$

$$D = 0.0002 \text{ g}$$

We now have the necessary pieces of information: *D* = 0.0002 g, *Q* = 2,000 mL, and *H* = 1 g.

STEP B: CALCULATE
Follow Procedure Checklist 12-1 using fractions.

1. Fill in the proportion.

$$\frac{1 \text{ g}}{2{,}000 \text{ mL}} = \frac{0.0002 \text{ g}}{A}$$

2. Cancel units.

$$\frac{1 \text{ g}}{2{,}000 \text{ mL}} = \frac{0.0002 \text{ g}}{A}$$

3. Cross-multiply and solve for the unknown.

$$1 \times A = 2{,}000 \text{ mL} \times 0.0002$$

$$A = \frac{2{,}000 \text{ mL} \times 0.0002}{1}$$

$$A = 0.4 \text{ mL}$$

STEP C: THINK! . . . IS IT REASONABLE?
The medication concentration is 1 mg/2 mL. Since 0.4 is twice as much as 0.2, it is reasonable.

The amount to administer is 0.4 mL.

- Referring to Rule 14-1, a 1 mL or 0.5 mL tuberculin syringe would be used.
- Referring to Rule 14-2, we find that it is not necessary to round in this example.
- Referring to Rule 14-3, the dose would not need to be divided into two because the amount is less than 0.5 mL.

| EXAMPLE 3 | **Find the amount to administer and select the proper syringe.** |

STEP A: GATHER INFORMATION AND CONVERT

Ordered: Heparin sodium 5,000 units subcut q8h

On hand: Heparin 10,000:1 for injection

Patient: A 145-lb, 60-year-old male

The dosage strength of heparin 10,000:1 is 10,000 units (H) per 1 mL (Q).

The dosage ordered O and the dose on hand H are both expressed as units, so no conversion is necessary to find the desired dose, which is 5,000 units.

STEP B: CALCULATE
Follow Procedure Checklist 12-1

1. Set up the proportion.

$$\frac{10{,}000 \text{ units}}{1 \text{ mL}} = \frac{5{,}000 \text{ units}}{A}$$

2. Cancel units.

$$\frac{10{,}000 \text{ \sout{units}}}{1 \text{ mL}} = \frac{5{,}000 \text{ \sout{units}}}{A}$$

3. Cross-multiply and solve for the unknown.

$$10{,}000 \times A = 1 \text{ mL} \times 5{,}000$$

$$A = 1 \text{ mL} \times \frac{5{,}000}{10{,}000}$$

$$A = 0.5 \text{ mL}$$

STEP C: THINK! . . . IS IT REASONABLE?
5,000 units is half as much as 10,000 units, so the volume to administer should be half of 1 mL. 0.5 is one-half of 1, so the answer is reasonable.

The amount to administer is 0.5 mL.

- Referring to Rule 14-1, a 1 mL tuberculin syringe would be used.
- Referring to Rule 14-2, we find that it is not necessary to round in this example.
- Referring to Rule 14-3, the total volume may be given as a single injection.

DIMENSIONAL ANALYSIS

| EXAMPLE 1 | **Find the amount to administer and select the proper syringe.** |

STEP A: GATHER INFORMATION AND CONVERT

Ordered: Magnesium sulfate 300 mg IM now

On hand: Magnesium sulfate 10% solution

Patient: A 75-lb, 8-year-old female

The dosage strength of a 10% solution is 10 g (*H*) per 100 mL (*Q*).

The unit of measure for the dosage ordered is milligrams. The unit of measure for the dose on hand is grams. Recall that 1 g equals 1,000 mg. Because we wish to convert to grams (the units of the dose on hand), our first factor must have grams on top.

STEP B: CALCULATE

Follow Procedure Checklist 12-2.

1. The unit of measure for the amount to administer is milliliters.

$$A \text{ mL} =$$

2. The conversion factor is the first factor in the equation.

$$A \text{ mL} = \frac{1 \text{ g}}{1,000 \text{ mg}}$$

3. The dosage unit is 100 mL. The dose on hand is 10 g. This is our second factor.

$$A \text{ mL} = \frac{1 \text{ g}}{1,000 \text{ mg}} \times \frac{100 \text{ mL}}{10 \text{ g}}$$

4. The dosage ordered is 300 mg. Place this over 1 to complete the equation.

$$A \text{ mL} = \frac{1 \text{ g}}{1,000 \text{ mg}} \times \frac{100 \text{ mL}}{10 \text{ g}} \times \frac{300 \text{ mg}}{1}$$

5. Cancel units.

$$A \text{ mL} = \frac{1 \text{ \cancel{g}}}{1,000 \text{ \cancel{mg}}} \times \frac{100 \text{ mL}}{10 \text{ \cancel{g}}} \times \frac{300 \text{ \cancel{mg}}}{1}$$

6. Solve the equation.

$$A \text{ mL} = \frac{1}{1,000} \times \frac{100 \text{ mL}}{10} \times \frac{300}{1}$$

$$A = 3 \text{ mL}$$

STEP C: THINK! . . . IS IT REASONABLE?

The medication is in a 1 to 10 solution. 3 is 10 times larger than 0.3, so it is reasonable.

The amount to administer is 3 mL.

- Referring to Rule 14-1, a standard 3 mL syringe would be used.
- Referring to Rule 14-2, we find that it is not necessary to round in this example.
- Referring to Rule 14-3, the dose would need to be divided into two parts because of the age of the patient. Draw 1.5 mL into each of two syringes, and administer them into different sites.

EXAMPLE 2 | Find the amount to administer and select the proper syringe.

STEP A: GATHER INFORMATION AND CONVERT

Ordered: Epinephrine 0.2 mg subcut stat

On hand: Vial of epinephrine 1:2,000 solution for injection

Patient: A 150-lb, 35-year-old adult

The dosage strength of a 1:2,000 solution is 1 g (*H*) per 2,000 mL (*Q*).

The dose on hand *H* is now in grams, and the dosage ordered *O* is in milligrams. To calculate the desired dose *D*, we must determine the conversion factor to first change the dosage ordered—0.2 mg—to the same unit of measure as that of the dose on hand, grams. We wish to convert to grams, so our conversion factor must have grams on top. The conversion factor is 1 g/1,000 mg.

STEP B: CALCULATE

Follow Procedure Checklist 12-2.

1. The unit of measure for the amount to administer is milliliters.

$$A \text{ mL} =$$

2. The conversion factor is the first factor in the equation.

$$A \text{ mL} = \frac{1 \text{ g}}{1,000 \text{ mg}}$$

3. The dosage unit is 2,000 mL. The dose on hand is 1 g. This is our next factor.

$$A \text{ mL} = \frac{1 \text{ g}}{1,000 \text{ mg}} \times \frac{2,000 \text{ mL}}{1 \text{ g}}$$

4. The dosage ordered is 0.2 mg. Place this over 1 to complete the equation.

$$A \text{ mL} = \frac{1 \text{ g}}{1,000 \text{ mg}} \times \frac{2,000 \text{ mL}}{1 \text{ g}} \times \frac{0.2 \text{ mg}}{1}$$

5. Cancel units.

$$A \text{ mL} = \frac{1 \text{ \cancel{g}}}{1,000 \text{ \cancel{mg}}} \times \frac{2,000 \text{ mL}}{1 \text{ \cancel{g}}} \times \frac{0.2 \text{ \cancel{mg}}}{1}$$

6. Solve the equation.

$$A \text{ mL} = \frac{2,000 \text{ mL} \times 0.2 \text{ \cancel{mg}}}{1,000 \text{ \cancel{mg}}}$$

$$A = 0.4 \text{ mL}$$

STEP C: THINK! . . . IS IT REASONABLE?

The medication concentration is 1 mg/2 mL. Since 0.4 is twice as much as 0.2, it is reasonable.

The amount to administer is 0.4 mL.

- Referring to Rule 14-1, a 1-mL or 0.5 mL tuberculin syringe would be used.
- Referring to Rule 14-2, we find that it is not necessary to round in this example.
- Referring to Rule 14-3, the dose would not need to be divided into two because the amount is less than 0.5 mL.

EXAMPLE 3

Find the amount to administer and select the proper syringe.

STEP A: GATHER INFORMATION AND CONVERT

Ordered: Heparin sodium 5,000 units subcut q8h

On hand: Heparin 10,000:1 for injection

Patient: A 145-lb, 60-year-old male

The dosage strength of heparin 10,000:1 is 10,000 units (H) per 1 mL (Q).

The dosage ordered O and the dose on hand H are both expressed as units, so no conversion is necessary to find the desired dose, which is 5,000 units.

STEP B: CALCULATE
Follow Procedure Checklist 12-2.

1. The unit of measure for the amount to administer is milliliters.

$$A \text{ mL} =$$

2. No conversion factor is required.

3. The dosage unit is 1 mL. The dose on hand is 10,000 units. This is the first factor.

$$A \text{ mL} = \frac{1 \text{ mL}}{10,000 \text{ units}}$$

4. The dosage ordered is 5,000 units. Set 5,000 units over 1 to complete the equation.

$$A \text{ mL} = \frac{1 \text{ mL}}{10,000 \text{ units}} \times \frac{5,000 \text{ units}}{1}$$

5. Cancel units.

$$A \text{ mL} = \frac{1 \text{ mL}}{10,000 \text{ units}} \times \frac{5,000 \text{ units}}{1}$$

6. Solve the equation.

$$A \text{ mL} = \frac{1 \text{ mL}}{10,000} \times \frac{5,000}{1}$$

$$A = 0.5 \text{ mL}$$

STEP C: THINK! . . . IS IT REASONABLE?

5,000 units is half as much as 10,000 units, so the volume to administer should be half of 1 mL. It is reasonable since 0.5 is one-half of 1.

The amount to administer is 0.5 mL.

- Referring to Rule 14-1, a 1 mL tuberculin syringe would be used.
- Referring to Rule 14-2, we find that it is not necessary to round in this example.
- Referring to Rule 14-3, the total volume may be given as a single injection.

FORMULA METHOD

EXAMPLE 1

Find the amount to administer and select the proper syringe.

STEP A: GATHER INFORMATION AND CONVERT

Ordered: Magnesium sulfate 300 mg IM now

On hand: Magnesium sulfate 10% solution

Patient: A 75-lb, 8-year-old female

The dosage strength of a 10% solution is 10 g (*H*) per 100 mL (*Q*).

The dosage ordered *O* is in milligrams, and the dose on hand *H* is in grams, so the desired dose *D*, in grams, must be calculated.

1. Set up the proportion, recalling that 1 g = 1,000 mg.

$$\frac{1 \text{ g}}{1,000 \text{ mg}} = \frac{D}{300 \text{ mg}}$$

2. Cancel units.

$$\frac{1 \text{ g}}{1,000 \text{ mg}} = \frac{D}{300 \text{ mg}}$$

3. Cross-multiply and solve for the unknown.

$$1,000 \times D = 300 \times 1\text{g}$$

$$D = \frac{300 \times 1 \text{ g}}{1,000}$$

$$D = 0.3 \text{ g}$$

We now have the necessary pieces of information: *D* = 0.3 g, *Q* = 100 mL, and *H* = 10 g.

STEP B: CALCULATE

Follow Procedure Checklist 12-3.

1. Fill in the formula.

$$\frac{0.3 \text{ g}}{10 \text{ g}} \times 100 \text{ mL} = A$$

2. Cancel units.

$$\frac{0.3 \cancel{\text{g}}}{10 \cancel{\text{g}}} \times 100 \text{ mL} = A$$

3. Solve for the unknown.

$$\frac{0.3}{10} \times 100 = A$$

$$3 \text{ mL} = A$$

STEP C: THINK! . . . IS IT REASONABLE?

The medication is in a 10 to 1 solution. 3 is 10 times larger than 0.3, so it is reasonable.

The amount to administer is 3 mL.

- Referring to Rule 14-1, a standard 3 mL syringe would be used.
- Referring to Rule 14-2, we find that it is not necessary to round in this example.
- Referring to Rule 14-3, the dose would need to be divided into two parts because of the age of the patient. Draw 1.5 mL into each of two syringes, and administer them into different sites.

EXAMPLE 2   Find the amount to administer and select the proper syringe.

STEP A: GATHER INFORMATION AND CONVERT

Ordered: Epinephrine 0.2 mg subcut stat

On hand: Vial of epinephrine 1:2,000 solution for injection

Patient: A 150-lb, 35-year-old adult

The dosage strength of a 1:2,000 solution is 1 g (H) per 2,000 mL (Q).

The dose on hand H is now in grams, and the dosage ordered O is in milligrams. To calculate the desired dose D, we must convert the dosage ordered—0.2 mg—to the same unit of measure as that of the dose on hand, grams.

1. Set up the proportion, recalling that 1 g = 1,000 mg.

$$\frac{1 \text{ g}}{1,000 \text{ mg}} = \frac{D}{0.2 \text{ mg}}$$

2. Cancel units.

$$\frac{1 \text{ g}}{1,000 \cancel{\text{mg}}} = \frac{D}{0.2 \cancel{\text{mg}}}$$

3. Cross-multiply and solve for the unknown.

$$1,000 \times D = 0.2 \times 1 \text{ g}$$

$$D = \frac{0.2 \times 1 \text{ g}}{1,000}$$

$$D = 0.0002 \text{ g}$$

We now have the necessary pieces of information: $D = 0.0002$ g, $Q = 2,000$ mL, and $H = 1$ g.

STEP B: CALCULATE
Follow Procedure Checklist 12-3.

1. Fill in the formula.

$$\frac{0.0002 \text{ g}}{1 \text{ g}} \times 2,000 \text{ mL} = A$$

2. Cancel units.

$$\frac{0.0002 \cancel{\text{ g}}}{1 \cancel{\text{ g}}} \times 2,000 \text{ mL} = A$$

3. Solve for the unknown.

$$\frac{0.0002}{1} \times 2,000 \text{ mL} = A$$
$$0.4 \text{ mL} = A$$

STEP C: THINK! . . . IS IT REASONABLE?
The medication concentration is 1 mg/2 mL. Since 0.4 is twice as much as 0.2, it is reasonable.

The amount to administer is 0.4 mL.

- Referring to Rule 14-1, a 1 mL or 0.5 mL tuberculin syringe would be used.
- Referring to Rule 14-2, we find that it is not necessary to round in this example.
- Referring to Rule 14-3, the dose would not need to be divided into two because the amount is less than 0.5 mL.

EXAMPLE 3 | **Find the amount to administer and select the proper syringe.**

STEP A: GATHER INFORMATION AND CONVERT

Ordered: Heparin sodium 5,000 units subcut q8h

On hand: Heparin 10,000:1 for injection

Patient: A 145-lb, 60-year-old male

The dosage strength of heparin 10,000:1 is 10,000 units (H) per 1 mL (Q).

The dosage ordered O and the dose on hand H are both expressed as units, so no conversion is necessary to find the desired dose, which is 5,000 units.

STEP B: CALCULATE
Follow Procedure Checklist 12-3.

1. Fill in the formula.

$$\frac{5,000 \text{ units}}{10,000 \text{ units}} \times 1 \text{ mL} = A$$

2. Cancel units.

$$\frac{5,000 \cancel{\text{ units}}}{10,000 \cancel{\text{ units}}} \times 1 \text{ mL} = A$$

3. Solve for the unknown.

$$\frac{5,000 \text{ mL}}{10,000} = A$$
$$0.5 \text{ mL} = A$$

STEP C: THINK! . . . IS IT REASONABLE?
5,000 units is half as much as 10,000 units, so the volume to administer should be half of 1 mL. 0.5 is half of 1, so the answer is reasonable.

The amount to administer is 0.5 mL.

- Referring to Rule 14-1, a 1 mL tuberculin syringe would be used.
- Referring to Rule 14-2, we find that it is not necessary to round in this example.
- Referring to Rule 14-3, the total volume may be given as a single injection.

Confusing the Amount of Solution with the Dosage Unit

A patient is brought to the physician's office with severe vomiting. The physician orders Compazine™ 5 mg IM stat. The healthcare professional obtains a vial labeled 5 mg/mL. The label also lists the total quantity of medication as 5 mL. The healthcare professional misinterprets the solution strength as 5 mg/5 mL and injects a total of 5 mL of Compazine™.

Think! . . . **Is It Reasonable?** What mistake was made? How could the healthcare professional have avoided this mistake?

REVIEW AND PRACTICE

14.2 Medication Expressed in Percent or Ratio Format

In Exercises 1–9, find the amount to administer for each order. Then mark the syringe with the correct amount to administer.

1. Ordered: Magnesium sulfate 750 mg stat
   On hand: Magnesium sulfate 20% solution

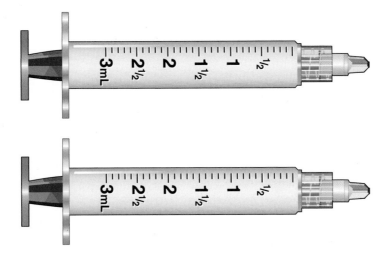

2. Ordered: Lidocaine 200 mg IM stat
   On hand: Lidocaine 10% solution

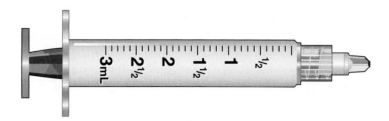

3. Ordered: Epinephrine 0.3 mg subcut stat
   On hand: Epinephrine 1:1,000 solution

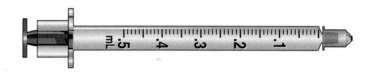

4. Ordered: Adrenalin 0.5 mg subcut stat
   On hand: Adrenalin 1:1,000 solution

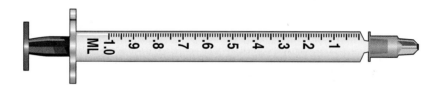

5. Ordered: Prostigmin 0.2 mg IM post-op q6h
   On hand: Prostigmin 1:4,000 solution

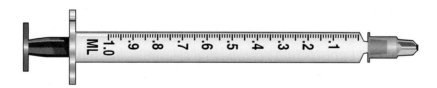

6. Ordered: Prostigmin 0.5 mg IM stat
   On hand: Prostigmin 1:2,000 solution

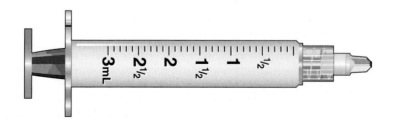

7. Ordered: Heparin sodium 8,000 units subcut q8h

On hand: Heparin sodium 5,000:1 solution

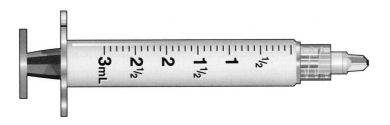

8. Ordered: Heparin sodium 5,000 units subcut q12h × 7 days

On hand: Heparin sodium 10,000:1 solution

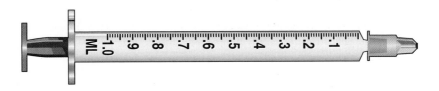

9. Ordered: Lidocaine 25 mg subcut now

On hand: Lidocaine 5% solution

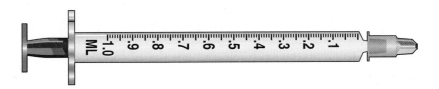

14.3 Preparing Parenteral Medications for Administration

Medications that lose potency quickly in **solution** or **suspension** may be supplied in powdered form. When in a solution, the solute or powdered medication does not settle out of the solution and the mixture is usually clear. In a suspension, the solute or powdered medication does not completely dissolve and is suspended in the solvent. Suspension medications always need to be shaken or swirled before administration. When needed, powdered medications are reconstituted by dissolving them in an appropriate solvent (or diluent). The drug label, package insert, and PDR provide instructions for reconstituting a medication. Be sure to use the directions specific to the medication you plan to administer.

First, determine what solvent should be used to dilute the medication. Common solvents include sterile water, saline, or a bacteriostatic solution containing a preservative that prevents the growth of microorganisms. Some medications are packaged with a separate container of the appropriate solvent.

Many medications, especially antibiotics, can cause burning and pain when injected. They may be mixed with lidocaine, a local anesthetic, to reduce this pain. The label or package insert indicates when lidocaine can be used. *Because lidocaine is itself a medication, you need a physician's order to use it.* Therefore, check whether the physician has ordered lidocaine. Be careful to use only lidocaine and *not* a combination of lidocaine and epinephrine in solution, because epinephrine causes vasoconstriction, a tightening of the blood vessels, which delays medication absorption.

The label or package insert lists how much solvent to combine with the medication. Read the directions carefully. Sometimes different amounts of solvent are used, based on the concentration needed to administer the least amount possible or whether the medication is for IM or IV use.

RULE 14-5

To reconstitute a powdered medication:

1. Find the directions on the medication label or package insert.

2. Use a sterile syringe and aseptic (germ-free) technique to draw up the correct amount of the appropriate diluent.

3. Inject the diluent into the medication vial.

4. Agitate the mixture by rolling, inverting, or shaking the vial. Check the directions on the label or package insert for which of these methods to use.

5. Make sure that the powdered medication is completely dissolved or suspended. A solution should be free of visible particles before you use it. For a suspension, the particles may not dissolve completely, but your goal is to distribute them evenly by shaking or swirling.

Use the exact amount of solvent indicated in the directions to produce a solution or suspension with the correct dosage strength. Powder takes up volume even when dissolved. The volume of the reconstituted medication includes the volume of the solvent and the volume of the powder.

If less than the recommended amount of solvent is used, the powder may not dissolve completely, making the solution unsafe to administer. If too much solvent is used, then the patient will not receive the desired dose. When preparing a suspension, remember that the particles will not dissolve completely. Your goal is to distribute them evenly.

Some vials contain a single dose of medication. Many must be reconstituted immediately before administering them, because they quickly lose potency. Other medications can be stored for a short time after reconstitution. In some facilities, medications are reconstituted in the pharmacy and delivered ready to use.

RULE 14-6

When you store a medication after reconstituting it record the:

- Date and time the medication was reconstituted

- Date and time of expiration

- Your name or initials

- The solution strength of the mixture for medications that can be reconstituted to different strengths

Check the drug label or package insert for the length of time a reconstituted medication may be stored. Storage time may depend on whether the medication is refrigerated.

Example 1	How would you reconstitute and label the following medication? Ordered: Glucagon 1 mg IM stat On hand: Refer to the labels in Figure 14-8.

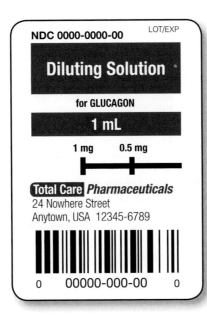
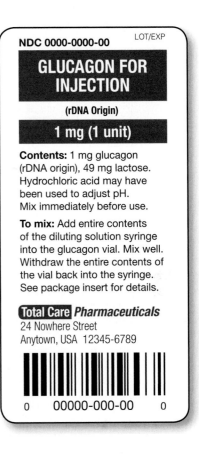

Figure 14-8

A 1 mL vial of diluting solution is provided. Once mixed, the solution must either be used immediately or be discarded. Because the mixed solution will not be stored, you do not need to label the vial.

Example 2	How would you reconstitute and label the following medication? Find the amount to administer. Ordered: Zyprexa® 5 mg IM now On hand: Refer to the label and portion of package insert shown in Figures 14-9 and 14-10.

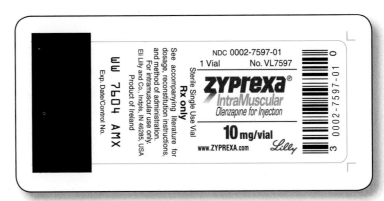

Figure 14-9

ZYPREXA® IntraMuscular (olanzapine for injection) Dosing
ZYPREXA IntraMuscular is approved for the treatment of agitation associated with schizophrenia and bipolar mania.

Dose (mg)	Injection volume (mL)
10.0 mg	Withdraw total contents of vial
7.5 mg	1.5 mL
5.0 mg	1.0 mL
2.5 mg	0.5 mL

10 mg is the recommended dose for agitation associated with bipolar mania and schizophrenia.

Follow the steps below to reconstitute and use ZYPREXA IntraMuscular:

1. Inject 2.1 mL of Sterile Water for Injection into single-packaged vial for up to 10-mg dose.
2. Dissolve contents of vial completely; resulting solution should be clear and yellow.
3. Use solution within 1 hour; discard any unused portion.
4. Refer to table for injection volumes and corresponding doses of ZYPREXA IntraMuscular.
5. Immediately after use, dispose of syringe in approved sharps box.

Figure 14-10 Package insert.

The diluent used to reconstitute this medication is 2.1 mL of sterile water for doses up to 10 mg. Contents must be dissolved completely, and fluid will be clear and yellow. The solution can only be used for 1 h. When it is prepared, you will administer 1 mL to deliver 5 mg of medication.

Example 3

How would you reconstitute and label the following medication? Find the amount to administer.

Ordered: Methylprednisolone 30 mg IM at 0930

On hand: Refer to the label (Figure 14-11) and package insert (Figure 14-12).

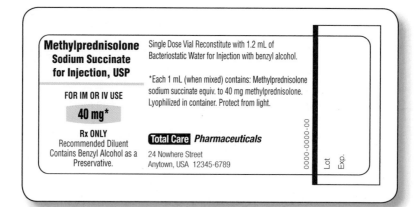

Methylprednisolone Sodium Succinate for Injection, USP

FOR IM OR IV USE

40 mg*

Rx ONLY
Recommended Diluent Contains Benzyl Alcohol as a Preservative.

Single Dose Vial Reconstitute with 1.2 mL of Bacteriostatic Water for Injection with benzyl alcohol.

*Each 1 mL (when mixed) contains: Methylprednisolone sodium succinate equiv. to 40 mg methylprednisolone. Lyophilized in container. Protect from light.

Total Care *Pharmaceuticals*

24 Nowhere Street
Anytown, USA 12345-6789

0000-0000-00
Lot
Exp.

Figure 14-11

According to the label and package insert the medication should be reconstituted, with 1.2 mL bacteriostatic water for injection with benzyl alcohol. Once reconstituted, the vial will contain 40 mg/mL.

Methylprednisolone sodium succinate for injection may be administered by intravenous or intramuscular injection or by intravenous infusion, the preferred method for initial emergency use being intravenous injection. To administer by intravenous (or intramuscular) injection, reconstitute the product as follows:

The 40 mg single-dose vial is reconstituted by adding 1.2 mL bacteriostatic water for injection with benzyl alcohol. The 125 mg single-dose vial is reconstituted by adding 2.1 mL bacteriostatic water for injection with benzyl alcohol. The 500 mg single-dose vial is reconstituted by adding 4 mL bacteriostatic water for injection with benzyl alcohol. The 1 gram single-dose vial is reconstituted by adding 7.5 mL bacteriostatic water for injection with benzyl alcohol. The desired dose may be administered intravenously over a period of several minutes.

To prepare solutions for intravenous infusion, first prepare the solution for injection as directed. This solution may then be added to indicated amounts of 5% dextrose in water, isotonic saline solution or 5% dextrose in isotonic saline solution.

Multiple Sclerosis

In treatment of acute exacerbations of multiple sclerosis, daily doses of 200 mg of prednisolone for a week followed by 80 mg every other day for 1 month have been shown to be effective (4 mg of methylprednisolone sodium succinate for injection is equivalent to 5 mg of prednisolone).

STORAGE CONDITIONS

Protect from light.

Store unreconstituted product at 20° to 25°C (68° to 77°F). See USP controlled room temperature.

Store solution at 20° to 25°C (68° to 77°F). See USP controlled room temperature.

Use solution within 48 hours after mixing.

Figure 14-12 Package insert.

According to the package insert, the resulting solution should be used within 48 hours of mixing. If you mix the medication at 9 a.m. on 6/17/14 and store at room temperature, label the vial Exp. 6/19/14 9 a.m., 40 mg/mL. The medication should also be protected from light before and after reconstitution.

Now calculate the amount to administer for Example 3 using a method of your choice:

PROPORTION METHOD

EXAMPLE

Find the amount to administer.

STEP A: GATHER INFORMATION AND CONVERT

Ordered: Methylprednisolone 30 mg IM at 0930

On hand: Refer to the label (Figure 14-11) and package insert (Figure 14-12).

After reconstitution the dosage strength is 40 mg/mL, making the dosage unit Q 1 mL, and the dose on hand H is 40 mg.

The dosage ordered O and the dose on hand H are already expressed in the same units, so the desired dose D is 30 mg.

STEP B: CALCULATE

Follow Procedure Checklist 12-1.

1. Set up the proportion.

$$\frac{H}{Q} = \frac{D}{A}$$

$$\frac{40 \text{ mg}}{1 \text{ mL}} = \frac{30 \text{ mg}}{A}$$

2. Cancel units.

$$\frac{40 \text{ mg}}{1 \text{ mL}} = \frac{30 \text{ mg}}{A}$$

3. Cross-multiply and solve for the unknown.

$$40 \times A = 1 \text{ mL} \times 30$$

$$A = \frac{1 \text{ mL} \times 30}{40}$$

$$A = 0.75 \text{ mL}$$

STEP C: THINK! . . . IS IT REASONABLE?

Since 30 is $\frac{3}{4}$ of 40, and 0.75 is $\frac{3}{4}$ of 1, it is reasonable.

Using a 1 mL tuberculin syringe, we will administer 0.75 mL.

DIMENSIONAL ANALYSIS

Find the amount to administer.

STEP A: GATHER INFORMATION AND CONVERT

Ordered: Methylprednisolone 30 mg IM at 0930

On hand: Refer to the label (Figure 14-11 page 364) and package insert (Figure 14-12 page 365).

After reconstitution the dosage strength is 40 mg/mL, making the dosage unit Q 1 mL, and the dose on hand H is 40 mg.

The dosage ordered O and the dose on hand H are already expressed in the same units, so the desired dose D is 30 mg.

STEP B: CALCULATE
Follow Procedure Checklist 12-2.

1. The unit of measure for the amount to administer will be milliliters.

   A mL $=$

2. No conversion factor is required.

3. The dosage unit is 1 mL. The dose on hand is 40 mg. This is our first factor.

   $A \text{ mL} = \dfrac{1 \text{ mL}}{40 \text{ mg}}$

4. The dosage ordered is 30 mg. Place this over 1 to complete the equation.

   $A \text{ mL} = \dfrac{1 \text{ mL}}{40 \text{ mg}} \times \dfrac{30 \text{ mg}}{1}$

5. Cancel units.

   $A \text{ mL} = \dfrac{1 \text{ mL}}{40 \, \cancel{\text{mg}}} \times \dfrac{30 \, \cancel{\text{mg}}}{1}$

6. Solve the equation.

   $A \text{ mL} = \dfrac{1 \text{ mL}}{40} \times \dfrac{30}{1}$

   $A = 0.75 \text{ mL}$

STEP C: THINK! . . . IS IT REASONABLE?
Since 30 is $\frac{3}{4}$ of 40, and 0.75 is $\frac{3}{4}$ of 1, it is reasonable.

Using a 1 mL tuberculin syringe, we will administer 0.75 mL.

FORMULA METHOD

Find the amount to administer.

STEP A: CONVERT

Ordered: Methylprednisolone 30 mg IM at 0930

On hand: Refer to the label (Figure 14-11 page 364) and package insert (Figure 14-12 page 365).

After reconstitution the dosage strength is 40 mg/mL, making the dosage unit Q 1 mL, and the dose on hand H is 40 mg.

The dosage ordered O and the dose on hand H are already expressed in the same units, so the desired dose D is 30 mg.

STEP B: CALCULATE

Follow Procedure Checklist 12-3.

1. Fill in the formula.

   Desired dose (D) = 30 mg

   Dose on hand (H) = 40 mg

   Quantity (Q) = 1 mL

   $$\frac{D}{H} \times Q = A$$

   $$\frac{30 \text{ mg}}{40 \text{ mg}} \times 1 \text{ mL} = A$$

2. Cancel units.

   $$\frac{30 \text{ m\overline{g}}}{40 \text{ m\overline{g}}} \times 1 \text{ mL} = A$$

3. Solve for the unknown.

   $$\frac{30 \text{ mg}}{40} \times 1 \text{ mL} = A$$

   $$0.75 \text{ mL} = A$$

STEP C: THINK! . . . IS IT REASONABLE?

Since 30 is $\frac{3}{4}$ of 40, and 0.75 is $\frac{3}{4}$ of 1, it is reasonable.

Using a 1 mL tuberculin syringe, we will administer 0.75 mL.

ERROR ALERT!

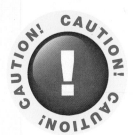

Select the Correct Instructions for the Strength and Route Ordered

The package insert for a 500 mg vial of Maxipime® can be reconstituted for both IM and IV use. Suppose a nurse mistakenly reconstitutes Maxipime® 500 mg IM for 500 mg IV instead. The IV instructions indicate that the nurse should use 5 mL of diluent, producing a solution strength of 100 mg/mL. Calculate the amount to administer.

$$\frac{500 \text{ mg}}{100 \text{ mg}} \times 1 \text{ mL} = A$$

$$\frac{500 \text{ m\overline{g}}}{100 \text{ m\overline{g}}} \times 1 \text{ mL} = A = 5 \times 1 \text{ mL} = 5 \text{ mL}$$

The healthcare professional administers two injections of 2.5 mL each. The patient's discomfort increases, and the number of injection sites available for future injections is reduced. Costs increase because more diluent and syringes than necessary are used. The risk of injection complications is doubled. Correctly reconstituted for IM use, 1.3 mL of diluent will be used to produce a solution with a dosage strength of 280 mg/mL. Calculate the amount to administer.

$$\frac{500 \text{ mg}}{280 \text{ mg}} \times 1 \text{ mL} = A$$

$$\frac{500 \text{ m\overline{g}}}{280 \text{ m\overline{g}}} \times 1 \text{ mL} = A = \frac{50 \text{ mL}}{28} = 1.785 \text{ rounded to } 1.8 \text{ mL}$$

This amount 1.8 mL is the correct IM dose.

Recording Accurate Information

A healthcare professional receives the following order: Somatropin 2 mg IM three times a week.

At 0800 on 10/15/14, the healthcare professional prepares the medication to administer later that day. After reading the label (see Figure 14-13), she draws up all the diluent supplied with the medication (see Figure 14-14) and injects it into the vial. According to the drug label, the remaining medication may be refrigerated for 14 days if protected from light. She labels the vial "Exp: 0800 10/29/14. Refrigerate. 5 mg/mL" and signs it with her initials. The vial will not be exposed to light in the refrigerator. Otherwise, the healthcare professional might wrap it in foil or place it inside a paper bag.

Later that day, the healthcare professional calculates the amount to administer, based on the label,

$$\frac{2 \text{ mg}}{5 \text{ mg}} \times 1 \text{ mL} = A$$

$$\frac{2 \text{ mg}}{5 \text{ mg}} \times 1 \text{ mL} = A = \frac{2}{5} \text{ mL} = 0.4 \text{ mL}$$

She uses a 0.5 mL tuberculin syringe to administer the medication.

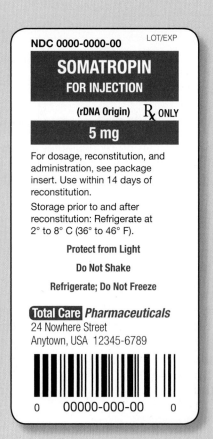

Figure 14-13

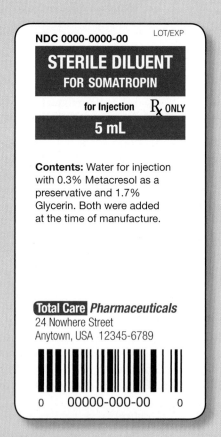

Figure 14-14

Think! . . . Is It Reasonable? What mistake did the healthcare professional make? How could she correct her mistake?

REVIEW AND PRACTICE

14.3 Preparing Parenteral Medication for Administration.

For Exercises 1–4, refer to label A:

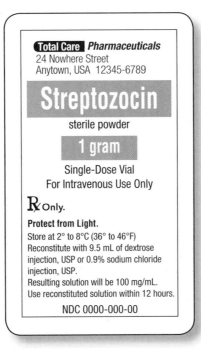

A

1. How much diluent should you add to the 1 gram vial?

2. How would this medication be stored?

3. What can be used to reconstitute the Zanosar?

4. If the dose ordered is 750 mg IV what would be the amount to administer?

For Exercises 5–9, refer to the following order, label B, and package insert C.

Ordered: Synagis® 75 mg IM q8h.

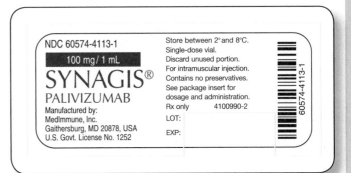

B

Preparation of Lyophilized Product for Administration:

- To reconstitute, remove the tab portion of the vial cap and clean the rubber stopper with 70% ethanol or equivalent.

- Both the 50 mg and 100 mg vials contain an overfill to allow the withdrawal of 50 mg or 100 mg Synagis® respectively when reconstituted following the directions described below.

- SLOWLY add 0.6 mL of sterile water for injection to the 50 mg vial or add 1.0 mL of sterile water for injection to the 100 mg vial. The vial should be tilted slightly and gently rotated for 30 seconds to avoid foaming. DO NOT SHAKE or VIGOROUSLY AGITATE the vial. This is a critical step to avoid prolonged foaming.

- Reconstituted Synagis® should stand undisturbed at room temperature for a minimum of 20 minutes until the solution clarifies.

- Reconstituted Synagis® should be inspected visually for particulate matter or discoloration prior to administration. The reconstituted solution should appear clear or slightly opalescent (a thin layer of micro-bubbles on the surface is normal and will not affect dosage). DO NOT use if there is particulate matter or if the solution is discolored.

- Reconstituted Synagis® does not contain a preservative and should be administered within 6 hours of reconstitution. Administer immediately after withdrawal from vial. Synagis® is supplied in single-use vials. DO NOT re-enter the vial. Discard any unused portion.

C

5. What diluent should you use to reconstitute Synagis®?

6. How much diluent should you add to this vial?

7. How many approximate milligrams are in 1 mL?

8. If Synagis is reconstituted at 1000 on January 3, 2015, what should you write on the label?

9. How much solution should you administer?

For Exercises 10–15, refer to the following order and label D.

Ordered: Gemcitabine 100 mg for IV infusion

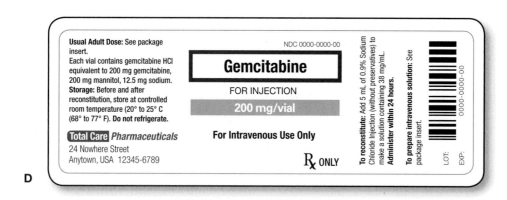

D

10. What diluent should you use to reconstitute this medication?

11. How much diluent should you add to the vial?

12. What solution strength should you write on the label?

13. If the gemcitabine is reconstituted at 2400 on 6/5/2015 and will be stored at room temperature, what expiration date and time should you write on the label?

14. How should the medication be stored?

15. How much solution would be used to administer 100 mg of medication?

For Exercises 16–19, refer to the following order, label E, and package insert F.

Ordered: Penicillin G potassium 1 million units IM q2h

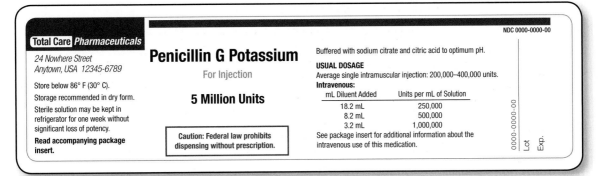

E

Penicillin G Potassium for Injection

R_X ONLY

Reconstitution
Use the following table to determine the amount of solvent to use for various concentrations.

Approx. Desired Concentration (units/mL)	Approx. Volume (mL) 1,000,000 units	Solvent for Vial of 5,000,000 units	Infusion Only 20,000,000 units
50,000	20.0	—	—
100,000	10.0	—	—
250,000	4.0	18.2	75.0
500,000	1.8	8.2	33.0
750,000	—	4.8	11.5
1,000,000	—	3.2	11.5

When the required volume of solvent is greater than the capacity of the vial, dissolve the penicillin by first injecting only a portion of the solvent into the vial. Withdraw the resulting solution and combine it with the rest of the solvent in a larger container.

Buffered penicillin G potassium for injection is highly water-soluble and can be dissolved in small amounts of Water for Injection or Sterile Isotonic Sodium Chloride Solution for Parenteral Use. Store all reconstituted solutions under refrigeration. When refrigerated, penicillin solutions can be stored for up to seven days without significant loss of potency.

Concentrations of 500,000, 1,000,000, and 5,000,000 can be administered IM, by continuous IV drip, or by intrapleural, intra-articular, and other local installations. **THE 20,000,000 UNIT CONCENTRATION MUST BE ADMINISTERED VIA INTRAVENOUS INFUSION ONLY.**

Intramuscular injection: This is the preferred route of administration. Keep total volume of injection small. Solutions containing up to 100,000 units of penicillin per mL cause a minimum of patient discomfort. Greater concentrations are possible, but when large dosages are required, a continuous IV drip should be used.

Continuous Intravenous Infusion: Determine the volume of fluid and rate of administration required in a 24-hour period; then add the appropriate daily dosage of penicillin to this fluid.

Intrapleural or Other Local Infusion: If fluid is aspirated, give infusion in a volume equal to 1/4 or 1/2 the amount of fluid aspirated; otherwise, prepare as for an IM injection.

Intrathecal: The intrathecal use of penicillin in meningitis must be highly individualized and should be used only after consideration of the irritating effects of penicillin given by this route. The preferred route is IV, supplemented by IM injections.

How Supplied
Penicillin G Potassium for Injection is available in vials containing respectively 5,000,000 units x 10's and 20,000,000 units x 1's. Both are buffered with sodium citrate and citric acid to an optimum pH. Store the dry powder below 86° F (30° C).

F

16. To make a solution of 500,000 units/mL, how much diluent should you add to the vial?

17. If the medication in the vial is reconstituted with 4.8 mL of diluent, what solution strength should you write on the label?

18. If the penicillin is reconstituted at 1200 on 11/20/15 and will be stored in the refrigerator, what expiration date and time should you write on the label?

19. When reconstituted with 8.2 mL, how much solution should you administer?

For Exercises 20–24, refer to the following order, label, and package insert.

Ordered: Ceftriaxone 750 mg IM q6h
On hand: See label G.

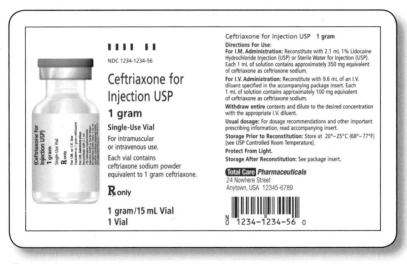

G

20. What diluent will be used to prepare this medication for IM administration?

21. How much diluent should you add to one vial?

22. What is the dosage strength of the solution, once reconstituted?

23. If Ceftriaxone is reconstituted for IM administration at 1600 on October 4, 2015, and will be stored in the refrigerator, what should you write on the label?

24. How much solution should you administer?

COMPATIBILITY AND STABILITY: Ceftriaxone sterile powder should be stored at room temperature—77°F (25°C)—or below and protected from light. After reconstitution, protection from normal light is not necessary. The color of solutions ranges from light yellow to amber, depending on the length of storage, concentration and diluent used.

Ceftriaxone *intramuscular* solutions remain stable (loss of potency less than 10%) for the following time periods:

		Storage	
Diluent	**Concentration mg/ml**	**Room Temp. (25°C)**	**Refrigerated (4°C)**
Sterile Water for Injection	100	2 days	10 days
	250,350	24 hours	3 days
1% Lidocaine Solution (without epinephrine)	100	24 hour	10 days
	250,350	24 hour	3 days

Ceftriaxone *intravenous* solutions, at concentrations of 10, 20 and 40 mg/mL., remain stable (loss of potency less than 10%) for the following time periods stored in glass or PVC containers:

	Storage	
Diluent	**Room Temp. (25°C)**	**Refrigerated (4°C)**
Sterile Water	2 days	10 days
0.9% Sodium Chloride Solution	2 days	10 days
5% Dextrose Solution	2 days	10 days
10% Dextrose Solution	2 days	10 days
5% Dextrose + 0.9% Sodium Chloride Solution*	2 days	Incompatible
5% Dextrose + 0.45% Sodium Chloride Solution	2 days	Incompatible

14.4 Other Parenteral Administration Forms

Calculating dosage for other parenteral administration forms varies slightly depending on the route of administration. For inhalant medications, the medication order includes the solution's strength and the amount of inhalant to administer. For example, the order Mucomyst 20% 3 mL via nebulizer QID is a complete order. In some cases, the order will also include an amount of normal saline to be added to the medication. Suppositories can sometimes be safely divided in half but only according to the manufacturer's directions. However, they are not scored. The order should specify that $\frac{1}{2}$ of a suppository is to be given. For example, if the order reads Tigan 50 mg p.r. TID, ask the physician to clarify whether $\frac{1}{2}$ of a 100 mg suppository is acceptable. The order should then be rewritten: Tigan 100 mg supp. Give $\frac{1}{2}$ supp. For transdermal medication, the dosage rate is usually expressed in milligrams or micrograms per hour. Patches cannot be divided. If a dose is larger than the amount provided by a single patch, you can use multiple patches. When calculations are required, follow the ABCs of dosage calculations and use the proportion method, dimensional analysis, or the formula method.

14.4 Other Parenteral Administration Forms

For Exercises 1-10, find the amount to administer.

1. Ordered: Acetylcysteine 1 g via nebulizer

   On hand: Acetylcysteine 20% solution 10 mL vial

2. Ordered: Albuterol 2.5 mg via nebulizer

   On hand: Albuterol 5 mg/mL

3. Ordered: Atrovent® 250 mcg via nebulizer

   On hand: Atrovent® 0.02% inhalation solution 500 mcg/2.5 mL vial

4. Ordered: Numorphan 10 mg p.r. PRN

   On hand: Numorphan 5 mg suppositories

5. Ordered: RMS morphine supp 15 mg p.r. PRN

   On hand: RMS 5 mg, 10 mg, and 30 mg suppositories

6. Ordered: Phenergan® 12.5 mg pr PRN

   On hand: Phenergan® 25 mg suppositories

7. Ordered: Testoderm 0.8 mg/day top

   On hand: Testoderm 0.4 mg/day patches

8. Ordered: Catapres® 0.5 mg/day top

   On hand: Catapres® TTS-1 (0.1 mg/day), TTS-2 (0.2 mg/day), TTS-3 (0.3 mg/day) transdermal patches

9. Ordered: Alora® 0.15 mg/day

   On hand: Alora® 0.05 mg/day, 0.075 mg/day, and 0.1 mg/day transdermal patches

10. Ordered: Transderm Nitro 0.3 mg/h top

    On hand: Transderm Nitro 0.1 mg/h, 0.2 mg/h, and 0.6 mg/h transdermal patches

14.5 Insulin

Any calculation error may result in patient harm; however some medications that are routinely administered have a higher risk of devastating harm or death, if the dosage is miscalculated. These medications are called **high-alert medications.** Special attention should be used when performing dosage calculation for high-alert medications. One common high-alert medication is insulin.

Insulin is a pancreatic hormone that stimulates glucose metabolism. People who have low or no insulin production may have insulin-dependent diabetes. They often need routine subcutaneous injections of insulin to keep their glucose (blood sugar) from rising to levels that could be life-threatening. These regular injections must be rotated to various sites of the body to prevent scarring of the tissue at a single injection site.

Many types of injectable insulin exist including types produced using genetically engineered bacteria, synthetic forms, and human insulin. Some types of insulin are clear, while other types of insulin are suspensions, causing them to be cloudy.

Timing of Action

Insulins are classified by the timing of their action. Each insulin has an onset, a peak, and a duration time. The **onset** is the time when the insulin begins to lower the glucose level. The **peak** is the time at which the insulin's effect is strongest. Both onset and peak are measured from the time the insulin is administered. The **duration** is the length of time the effect of the insulin lasts. It is measured from the time of onset.

Before you administer insulin, you must know the onset, peak, and duration of action. For example, a dose of regular insulin administered at 0700 will begin to take effect after 30 min, at 0730 (the onset). Its peak will be 2 to 4 hours after it is administered, between 0900 and 1100. Its effect will last until 1530 (the duration), about 8 hours after the onset. Table 14-2 summarizes the action times of many types of insulin, including mixed insulins, which are described later.

TABLE 14-2 Insulin Types and Timing of Action*					
TYPE OF INSULIN	BRAND NAME(S)	GENERIC NAME	ONSET	PEAK	DURATION
Rapid-acting	NovoLog Apidra Humalog	Insulin aspart Insulin glulisine Insulin lispro	15 minutes	30 to 90 minutes	3 to 5 hours
Short-acting	Humulin R Novolin R	Regular (R)	30 to 60 minutes	2 to 4 hours	5 to 8 hours
Intermediate-acting	Humulin N Novolin N	NPH (N)	1 to 3 hours	8 hours	12 to 16 hours
Long-acting	Levemir Lantus	Insulin detmir Insulin glargine	1 hour	Peakless	20 to 26 hours
Pre-mixed NPH (intermediate-acting) and regular (short-acting)	Humulin 70/30 Novolin 70/30	70% NPH and 30% regular	30 to 60 minutes	Varies	10 to 16 hours
	Humulin 50/50	50% NPH and 50% regular	30 to 60 minutes	Varies	10 to 16 hours
Pre-mixed insulin lispro protamine suspension (intermediate-acting) and insulin lispro (rapid-acting)	Humalog Mix 75/25	75% insulin lispro protamine and 25% insulin lispro	10 to 15 minutes	Varies	10 to 16 hours
	Humalog 50/50	50% insulin lispro protamine and 50% insulin lispro	10 to 15 minutes	Varies	10 to 16 hours
Pre-mixed insulin aspart protamine suspension (intermediate-acting) and insulin aspart (rapid-acting)	NovoLog Mix 70/30	70% insulin aspart protamine and 30% insulin aspart	5 to 15 minutes	Varies	10 to 16 hours

*Adapted from the National Diabetes Information Clearinghouse (ndic) http://diabetes.Niddk.Nih.Gov/dm/pubs/medicines_ez/insert_Caspx accessed 11/20/13

Insulin Labels

Like other drug labels, insulin labels identify the manufacturer, the brand name, storage information, and the expiration date (Figures 14-15 and 14-16). The concentration is usually listed twice, as the traditional dosage strength (e.g., 100 units per mL) and as the concentration. In most cases, the concentration is **U-100,** meaning that 100 units of insulin is contained in 1 mL of solution. Occasionally, the concentration is **U-500,** with 500 units per mL. Insulin labels also list the type (e.g., R or Regular) and the origin.

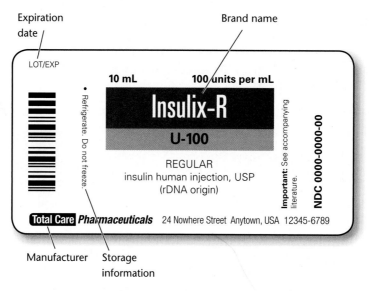

Figure 14-15 Short-acting Insulix-R.

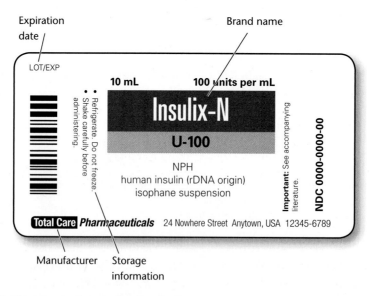

Figure 14-16 Intermediate-acting Insulix-N.

Know Your Insulin Type

The authorized prescriber (AP) ordered "Humulin insulin 20 units subcut, now." The healthcare practitioner, unaware that Humulin insulin is available in both regular and NPH forms, administered Humulin R, regular insulin, at 5 p.m. At 8 p.m. the patient experienced symptoms of hypoglycemia with a blood glucose level of 42. The blood sugar was treated with orange juice and food and rechecked until it was normal (which occurred within 1 hour). The next morning, the fasting blood sugar was elevated, so the AP increased the dose. Again the patient experienced a low blood sugar at bedtime and a high blood sugar in the morning.

1. What error did the AP make?

2. What error did the healthcare practitioner make?

3. How could the healthcare practitioner have prevented this error?

4. Why was the patient's blood sugar low at bedtime?

5. Why was the patient's blood sugar high in the morning?

Insulin Syringes

Insulin is administered with special insulin syringes marked in units. The needlestick safety devices have been removed from the syringes in this chapter so that the visualization of key points will not be obstructed. Review the figures in the chapter "Equipment for Dosage Measurement" for examples of insulin syringes with needlestick safety devices.

LEARNING LINK   Recall from the chapter "Equipment for Dosage Measurement" that insulin syringes should be used only for administration of U-100 insulin.

A standard U-100 insulin syringe holds 100 units or 1 mL of solution (see Figures 14-17 and 14-18). These syringes are calibrated for every 2 units, though some are marked for each unit. Insulin administration is different from the administration of most other injectable medications because the syringe measures units of insulin rather than a volume of solution.

Smaller U-100 insulin syringes, holding up to 50 units (0.5 mL of solution) or 30 units (0.3 mL), are calibrated for each unit (see Figures 14-19 and 14-20). Their larger numbers and expanded calibration scales ensure accuracy with low insulin doses.

RULE 14-7   For more accurate measurements, use a 50 unit capacity insulin syringe for insulin doses of less than 50 units, and a 30 unit capacity insulin syringe for insulin doses less than 30 units if these syringes are available.

Example 1	Ordered: Novolin® N 66 units
	Because this order is for more than 50 units, use a 100 unit insulin syringe. Find the mark for 66 units and fill the syringe to that calibration (see Figure 14-17).
	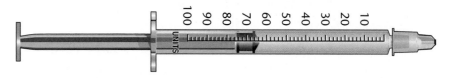
	Figure 14-17 A 100 unit insulin syringe.
Example 2	Ordered: Humulin® R 55 units
	Because this order is for more than 50 units, you will need a U-100 syringe. Your best choice would be a syringe calibrated for each unit (see Figure 14-18). If you use a syringe calibrated for every 2 units, then fill it to the imaginary line between 54 and 56 units.
	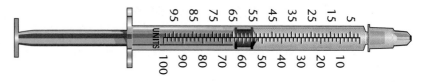
	Figure 14-18 A 100 unit insulin syringe.
Example 3	Ordered: Humulin® R 35 units
	Because this order is for less than 50 units, use a smaller syringe in which each unit is calibrated (see Figure 14-19).
	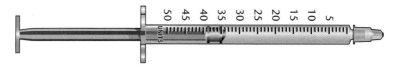
	Figure 14-19 A 50 unit insulin syringe.
Example 4	Ordered: Novolin® R 8 units
	Because this order is for less than 30 units, you may use either a 30 unit or 50 unit insulin syringe in which each unit is calibrated (see Figure 14-20).
	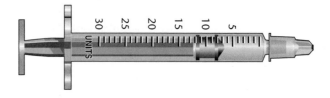
	Figure 14-20 A 30 unit insulin syringe.

U-500 insulin is used for patients who are insulin-resistant and require high dosages of insulin to maintain a normal blood sugar. It is rarely used, and the label includes a warning (Figure 14-21). U-100 insulin is the insulin that is commonly used. Always check how many units are in 1 mL, since accidentally substituting U-500 insulin for U-100 insulin could result in a fatal overdose. When U-500 is ordered or an insulin dose is over 100 units, a tuberculin or standard syringe will be necessary.

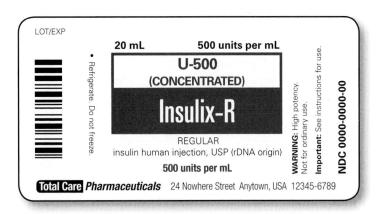

Figure 14-21 U-500 insulin is rarely used. Notice the warning on the label. Check all insulin labels carefully before administering.

RULE 14-8	If the order is for U-500 insulin (which contains 500 units in each milliliter), use a 1-mL tuberculin syringe. Calculate the amount to administer in milliliters.
Example	Ordered: Humulin® R U-500 insulin 80 units

$$\frac{80 \text{ units}}{500 \text{ units}} \times 1 \text{ mL} = A$$

$$\frac{\overset{4}{\cancel{80 \text{ units}}}}{\underset{25}{\cancel{500 \text{ units}}}} \times 1 \text{ mL} = 4 \times \frac{1}{25} \text{ mL} = \frac{4}{25} \text{ mL} = 0.16 \text{ mL}$$

Administer 0.16 mL drawn up in a 0.5 mL tuberculin syringe (Figure 14-22).

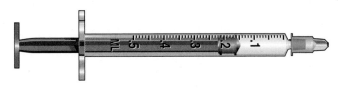

Figure 14-22 0.5 mL tuberculin syringe.

Measuring Insulin Doses

Give the following information to patients:

1. Always wash your hands before handling insulin and syringes.

2. If you are using an intermediate-acting or mixed insulin, roll the vial between your palms to mix the insulin, until all the insulin looks cloudy (Lantus insulin is not a suspension, so it will remain clear and does not need to be rolled).

3. Cleanse the rubber stopper of the vial with an alcohol wipe, using a circular motion. Start at the center of the circle and work outward.

4. Draw up an amount of air equal to your insulin dose in the syringe. Pull back the plunger until the leading ring is aligned with the correct marking on the syringe (Figure 14-23a).

5. Inject the air into the insulin vial; this will make it easier to withdraw the insulin later, without introducing short-acting insulin into the intermediate-acting insulin vial (Figure 14-23b).

6. Keeping the needle inserted through the stopper, turn the vial upside down. Make sure the bevel of the needle is in the insulin. Draw up your ordered dose of insulin (Figure 14-23c).

7. Avoid touching the needle during the procedure.

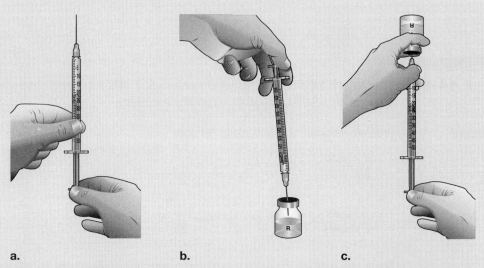

a.   **b.**   **c.**

Figure 14-23 Measuring insulin. **a.** Draw up air. **b.** Inject air into insulin. **c.** Draw up dose of insulin. *Syringe drawings for demonstration purposes only. All syringes should have a safe-needle device.*

Insulin Combinations

In some cases, the physician will prescribe two types of insulin for a patient. For example, the combination of a short-acting insulin and an intermediate-acting insulin provides the patient with the fast onset of the first and the lengthy duration of the second. Two types of insulin may be combined by the drug manufacturer. For example, Novolin® 70/30 is 70 percent intermediate-acting NPH insulin and 30 percent shorter-acting regular insulin (Figure 14-24). Humalog® 50/50 has 50 percent intermediate-acting lispro protamine insulin and 50 percent rapid-acting lispro insulin (Figure 14-25) Humalog® Mix 75/25 has the same types of insulin, but in a different combination (Figure 14-26). In some cases, you will need to prepare the insulin combination yourself.

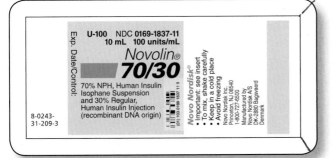

Figure 14-24 This insulin has 70% NPH and 30% R.

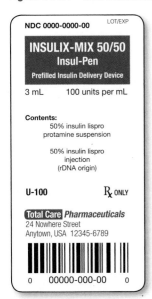

Figure 14-25 This mixed insulin has 50% of two types of insulin.

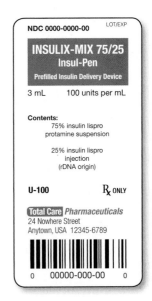

Figure 14-26 Insulin is sometimes self-administered with a pen device. A new needle must be attached for each dose. The manufacturer's directions should be followed carefully to ensure that air is displaced and the entire dose is administered. Patients should not share insulin pens.

RULE 14-9	When you are preparing a combined insulin dose, always draw up the short-acting insulin first. *Remember:* The insulin that will act first is drawn up first. Another way to remember Rule 14-9 is to draw up the clear insulin (short-acting) before the cloudy insulin (intermediate-acting). Keep in mind you must first make sure the types of insulin can be mixed. For example, Lantus is longer acting, clear, and cannot be mixed.
Example	Ordered: Novolin® R 20 units, Humulin® N 15 units subcut now Novolin® R is shorter-acting. Humulin® N is intermediate-acting. The shorter-acting insulin (Novolin® R) will be drawn into the syringe first.

RULE 14-10	To prepare a combined insulin dose (note: not all insulin can be combined): **1.** Calculate the total dose of insulin. Dose of short-acting insulin + dose of intermediate-acting insulin = total dose insulin **2.** Draw up an amount of air equal to the dose of intermediate-acting insulin. Inject it into the intermediate-acting insulin vial but do not draw up the dose. Withdraw the needle from this vial. **3.** Draw up an amount of air equal to the dose of short-acting insulin. Inject it into the short-acting insulin vial.

4. Without withdrawing the needle from the stopper, invert the vial. Draw up the dose of short-acting insulin.

5. Carefully insert the needle through the stopper of the intermediate-acting insulin vial. Invert the vial, without injecting any of the short-acting insulin into the vial.

6. Draw up intermediate-acting insulin until the leading ring reaches the calibration indicating the total dose. The clear insulin is drawn into the syringe first to prevent the cloudy, longer-acting insulin from entering the clear, shorter-acting insulin bottle.

Example

Ordered: Humulin® N 42 units and Humulin® R 10 units subcut daily

First calculate the total dose of insulin:

   10 units of Humulin® R + 42 units Humulin® N = 52 units total

Next draw up 42 units of air and inject it into the vial of Humulin® N. Withdraw the needle from Humulin® N without drawing up the dose. Then draw up 10 units of air and inject it into the vial of Humulin® R. Without withdrawing the needle, invert the vial of Humulin® R and draw up 10 units of insulin (Figure 14-27a). Finally, insert the needle into the vial of Humulin® N and invert the vial. Withdraw 42 units of Humulin® N, until the leading ring of the syringe is at the calibration of 52 units, the total dose (Figure 14-27b).

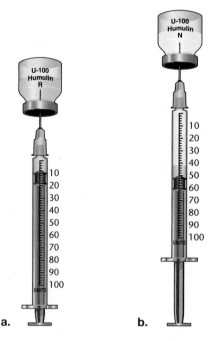

Figure 14-27 a. Draw up the short-acting (clear) insulin first. **b.** Be careful when drawing up the intermediate-acting insulin (cloudy). *Drawings for demonstration purposes only. All syringes should have a safe-needle device.*

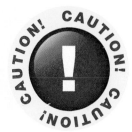

When Two Types of Insulins Are Combined, Measure the Correct Amount of Each

An order reads Novolin® N 37 units and Novolin® R 5 units subcut stat. Suppose you draw up 37 units from the Novolin® R vial and 5 units from the Novolin® N vial. Although the patient receives 42 units of insulin, he receives a much larger dose of regular (shorter-acting) insulin than was ordered—37 units rather than 5 units. The insulin metabolizes the patient's glucose too quickly; he becomes hypoglycemic and loses consciousness; this could lead to brain damage and death. Fortunately, the hypoglycemia is noted in time so glucagon and 50% dextrose are administered, and the patient recovers. This error can be avoided if you carefully check the order against the labels three times.

CRITICAL THINKING ON THE JOB

Timing Is Essential

The authorized prescriber ordered a routine dose of NPH insulin 15 units at 0730 and a prn dose of regular insulin 4 units at 0730, if the patient's blood sugar is greater than 140. The patient's 0730 blood sugar is 141.

Think! . . . Is It Reasonable?

1. What type or types of insulin should be administered?
2. What is the total dose of insulin to be administered?
3. What syringe should be used to administer the insulin?
4. What might happen if you gave the insulin at 0730 and the breakfast tray was delayed until 0930? What could you do to prevent this from happening?

REVIEW AND PRACTICE

14.5 Insulin

For Exercises 1–14, refer to labels A–G. Select the label corresponding to each order. Then mark the desired amount of insulin on the syringe.

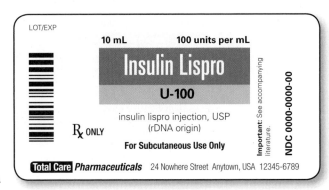

A

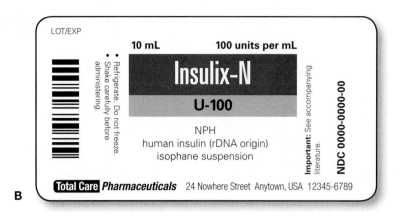

B

LOT/EXP

10 mL   100 units per mL

Insulix-N

U-100

NPH
human insulin (rDNA origin)
isophane suspension

• Refrigerate. Do not freeze.
• Shake carefully before administering.

Important: See accompanying literature.

NDC 0000-0000-00

Total Care *Pharmaceuticals*   24 Nowhere Street Anytown, USA 12345-6789

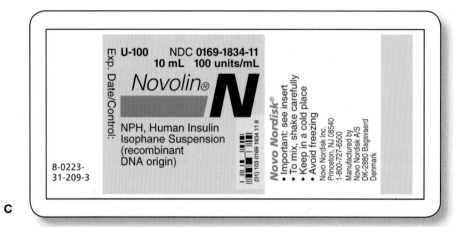

C

Exp. Date/Control:

U-100   NDC **0169-1834-11**
10 mL   100 units/mL

Novolin® **N**

NPH, Human Insulin
Isophane Suspension
(recombinant
DNA origin)

8-0223-
31-209-3

(01) 103 0169 1834 11 8

Novo Nordisk®
• Important: see insert
• To mix, shake carefully
• Keep in a cold place
• Avoid freezing

Novo Nordisk Inc.
Princeton, NJ 08540
1-800-727-6500
Manufactured by
Novo Nordisk A/S
DK-2880 Bagsvaerd
Denmark

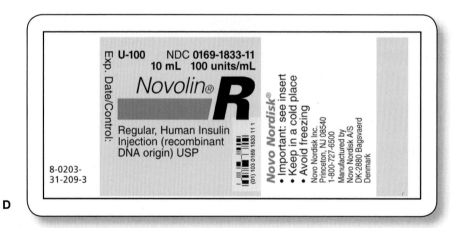

D

Exp. Date/Control:

U-100   NDC **0169-1833-11**
10 mL   100 units/mL

Novolin® **R**

Regular, Human Insulin
Injection (recombinant
DNA origin) USP

8-0203-
31-209-3

(01) 103 0169 1833 11 1

Novo Nordisk®
• Important: see insert
• Keep in a cold place
• Avoid freezing

Novo Nordisk Inc.
Princeton, NJ 08540
1-800-727-6500
Manufactured by
Novo Nordisk A/S
DK-2880 Bagsvaerd
Denmark

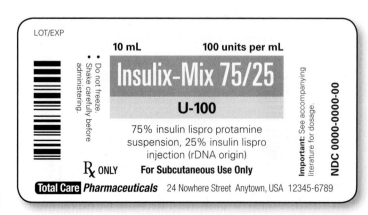

E

LOT/EXP

10 mL   100 units per mL

Insulix-Mix 75/25

U-100

75% insulin lispro protamine
suspension, 25% insulin lispro
injection (rDNA origin)

Rx ONLY   **For Subcutaneous Use Only**

• Do not freeze.
• Shake carefully before administering.

Important: See accompanying literature for dosage.

NDC 0000-0000-00

Total Care *Pharmaceuticals*   24 Nowhere Street Anytown, USA 12345-6789

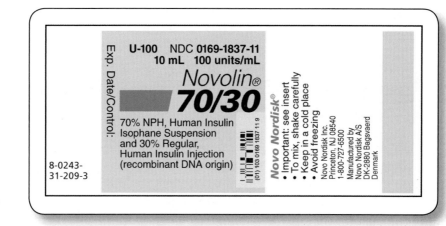

F

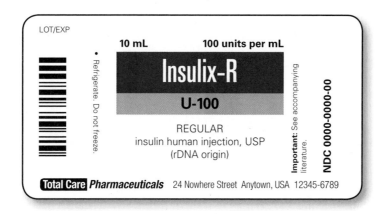

G

1. Ordered: Novolin® R 12 units subcut before breakfast

   Select label: _____

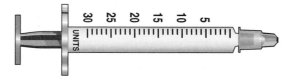

2. Ordered: Insulin lispro injection 5 units subcut 15 min before lunch

   Select label: _____

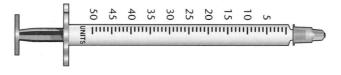

3. Ordered: Novolin® N 35 units subcut daily

   Select label: _____

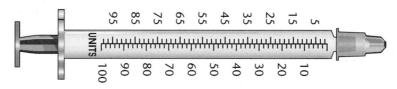

4. Ordered: Insulix-N 72 units subcut daily

Select label: _____

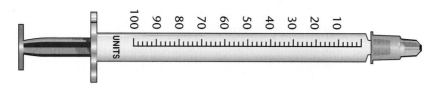

5. Ordered: Insulix-R 42 units subcut before breakfast

Select label: _____

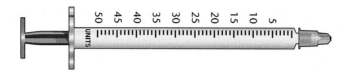

6. Ordered: Insulix-Mix 75/25 17 units subcut before breakfast

Select label: _____

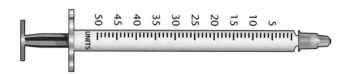

7. Ordered: Novolin® 70/30 53 units subcut before dinner

Select label: _____

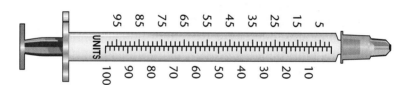

8. Ordered: Novolin® 70/30 R 26 units subcut before breakfast

Select label: _____

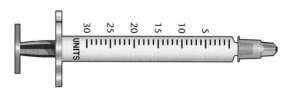

9. Ordered: Insulix-N 44 units subcut before dinner

Select label: _____

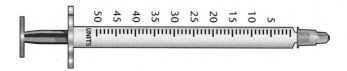

10. Ordered: Insulin lispro injection 15 units subcut before breakfast

Select label: _____

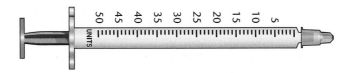

11. Ordered: Novolin® N 64 units subcut daily

Select label: _____

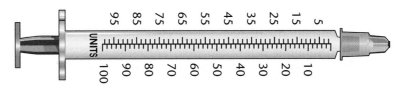

12. Ordered: Insulix-R 36 units subcut before dinner

Select label: _____

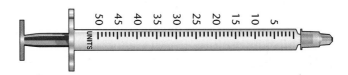

13. Ordered: Insulix-Mix 75/25 7 units subcut stat

Select label: _____

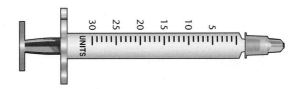

14. Ordered: Novolin® R 14 units subcut before breakfast

Select label: _____

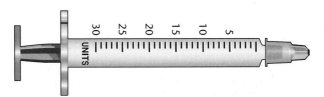

For Exercises 15 and 16, mark and label the syringe, identifying the insulin that will be drawn into the syringe first and second.

15. Novolin® N 65 units and Novolin® R 12 units subcut qam

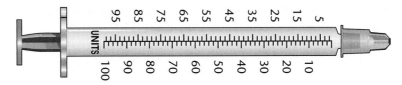

16. Humulin® N 53 units and Humulin® R 4 units subcut qam

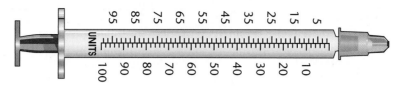

14.6 Heparin

Heparin is another common high-alert medication. This anticoagulant medication decreases the patient's ability to form clots. It is administered in USP units. Patients who receive heparin are at risk of bleeding or hemorrhage. Heparin may be used as an irrigant to keep the blood from clotting in a heparin lock, as discussed in the "Intravenous Calculations" chapter. For this purpose, it is packaged in prefilled syringes, cartridges, or vials of 10 to 100 units (see Figure 14-28). Heparin may also be administered intermittently subcutaneously (subcut) or IV in larger dosages. When multiple injections of heparin are administered subcut, the sites of the injection should be rotated to prevent bruising. Heparin is never administered IM because of the risk of hematoma. Bleeding is a great concern for patients receiving heparin, so the dosage calculations must be accurate.

Even after the identification of heparin as a high-alert medication and the publicity that surrounds heparin dosage errors, heparin dosage errors continue to occur. Some errors have stemmed from mixing up the concentration of the vials; for example, a vial of 10,000 units of heparin/mL was used instead of 10 units/mL. Heparin doses should be written with commas between thousands and hundreds to help prevent this error; for example write 1,000 units, not 1000 units. When administering heparin, it is critically important that you read the information on the drug label and question anything that is unfamiliar. (See Figures 14-29 to 14-34.)

The practitioner chooses which dosage strength of heparin, and volume bottle to use, based on the ordered dose. Heparin dosage strength ranges from 10 USP units/mL to 20,000 USP units/mL, so extreme caution should be used when selecting heparin bottles. For example, if the ordered dose is heparin 5,000 units subcut, the most appropriate concentration and volume would be 5,000 USP units/mL in a 1 mL bottle (see Figure 14-32). This is appropriate because the desired dose is 1 mL, which is easily drawn up, there is no wasted medication, and it is an acceptable volume to administer subcut. It would not be appropriate to use heparin sodium 1,000 USP units/mL in a 1 mL bottle (see Figure 14-29), since it would take 5 bottles to achieve the dose, and the volume of 5 mL is too large to be administered subcut.

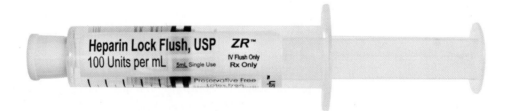

Figure 14-28 Heparin lock flush solution is available in prefilled syringes such as this one. The dosage strength is 100 units/mL and the amount of flush in the syringe is 5 mL.

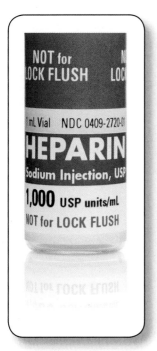

Figure 14-29 Heparin sodium 1,000 USP units/mL in 1 mL bottle.

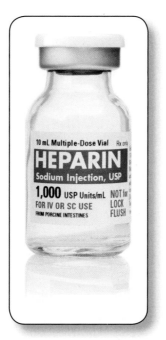

Figure 14-30 Heparin sodium 1,000 USP units/mL in 10 mL bottle.

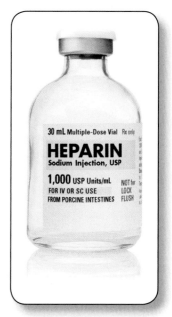

Figure 14-31 Heparin sodium 1,000 USP units/mL in 30 mL bottle.

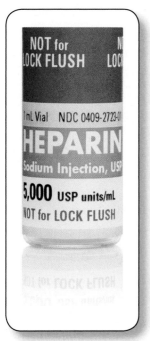

Figure 14-32 Heparin sodium 5,000 USP units/mL in 1 mL bottle.

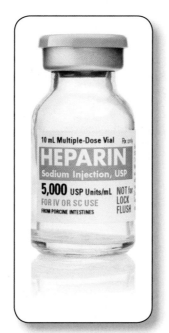

Figure 14-33 Heparin sodium 5,000 USP units/mL in 10 mL bottle.

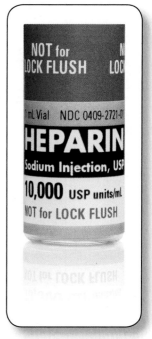

Figure 14-34 Heparin sodium 10,000 USP units/mL in 1 mL bottle.

RULE 14-11	Check the dosage strength on the label to ensure that you are using the correct amount of heparin in your dosage calculation.

Subcutaneous Heparin Dosages

Use the proportion method, dimensional analysis, or the formula method to calculate the volume of heparin to be administered. *Remember to use the ABCs of dosage calculation to ensure your answer is correct.*

PROPORTION METHOD

EXAMPLE

Find the amount (*A*) of subcut heparin to administer.

STEP A: GATHER INFORMATION AND CONVERT

Ordered: heparin 2,500 units subcut

On hand: heparin 5,000 USP units/mL

The desired dose is 2,500 units, the dose on hand (*H*) is 5,000 units, and the dosage unit (*Q*) is 1 mL. Because both the ordered dose and the dose on hand are expressed in units, no conversion is necessary and the dosage ordered (*D*) is 2,500 units.

STEP B: CALCULATE
Follow Procedure Checklist 12-1.

1. Set up the proportion.

$$\frac{H}{Q} = \frac{D}{A}$$

$$\frac{5,000 \text{ units}}{1 \text{ mL}} = \frac{2,500 \text{ units}}{A}$$

2. Cancel units, leaving mL for the answer.

$$\frac{5,000 \text{ units}}{1 \text{ mL}} = \frac{2,500 \text{ units}}{A}$$

3. Cross-multiply and solve for the answer.

$$5,000 \times A = 2,500 \times 1 \text{ mL}$$

$$A = \frac{2,500}{5,000} \times 1 \text{ mL}$$

$$A = \frac{1}{2} \text{ mL}$$

$$A = 0.5 \text{ mL}$$

STEP C: THINK! . . . IS IT REASONABLE?
Since 2,500 units is half as much as 5,000 units and the amount to give is half of 1 mL, the answer is reasonable.

DIMENSIONAL ANALYSIS

EXAMPLE | Find the amount subcut heparin to administer.

STEP A: GATHER INFORMATION AND CONVERT

Ordered: heparin 2,500 units subcut

On hand: heparin 5,000 ISP units/mL

The dose on hand is 5,000 units. The dosage unit is 1 mL. The dosage ordered is 2,500 units. The dose ordered is measured in units and the dosage strength is also measured in units. No conversion factor is needed.

STEP B: CALCULATE
Follow Procedure Checklist 12-2.

1. The unit of measure for the amount to administer will be milliliters.

$$A \text{ mL} =$$

2. No conversion factor is necessary.

3. The dosage unit is 1 mL. The dose on hand is 5,000 units. This is our first factor.

$$A \text{ mL} = \frac{1 \text{ mL}}{5,000 \text{ units}}$$

4. The dosage ordered is 2,500 units. Place this over 1 to finish setting up the equation.

$$A \text{ mL} = \frac{1 \text{ mL}}{5,000 \text{ units}} \times \frac{2,500 \text{ units}}{1}$$

5. Cancel units.

$$A \text{ mL} = \frac{1 \text{ mL}}{5,000 \text{ \st{units}}} \times \frac{2,500 \text{ \st{units}}}{1}$$

6. Solve the equation.

$$A \text{ mL} = \frac{2,500 \text{ mL}}{5,000}$$

$$A = \frac{1}{2} \text{ mL}$$

$$A = 0.5 \text{ mL}$$

STEP C: THINK! . . . IS IT REASONABLE?
Since 2,500 units is half as much as 5,000 units and the amount to give is half of 1 mL, the answer is reasonable.

FORMULA METHOD

EXAMPLE | Find the amount (*A*) of subcut heparin to administer.

STEP A: GATHER INFORMATION AND CONVERT

Ordered (*D*): heparin 2,500 units subcut

On hand (*H/Q*): heparin 5,000 units/mL

The dose on hand is 5,000 units. The dosage unit is 1 mL. The dosage ordered is 2,500 units. The drug is ordered in units, which is the same unit of measure as that of the dose on hand. No conversion is necessary.

STEP B: CALCULATE
Follow Procedure Checklist 12-3

1. Determine the values of D, H, and Q and fill in the formula.

   $D = 2{,}500$ units, $Q = 1$ mL, and $H = 5{,}000$ units.

   $$\frac{2{,}500 \text{ units}}{5{,}000 \text{ units}} \times 1 \text{ mL} = A$$

2. Cancel units.

   $$\frac{2{,}500 \text{ units}}{5{,}000 \text{ units}} \times 1 \text{ mL} = A$$

3. Solve for the unknown.

   $$\frac{1}{2} \times 1 \text{ mL} = A$$

   $$\frac{1}{2} \text{ mL} = A$$

   The amount to administer is 0.5 mL.

STEP C: THINK! . . . IS IT REASONABLE?
Since 2,500 units is half as much as 5,000 units and the amount to give is half of 1 mL, the answer is reasonable.

REVIEW AND PRACTICE

14.6 Heparin

For Exercises 1–3, use Figures 14-29 to 14-34 to determine the appropriate volume bottle and dosage strength for the intended purpose.

1. Heparin 7,500 units subcut

2. Heparin 2,500 units subcut

3. Heparin 10,000 units subcut

For Exercises 4–8, using any one of the described methods, calculate the volume of heparin to be administered.

4. Ordered: Heparin 5,000 units subcut
   On hand: 5,000 USP units/1 mL

5. Ordered: Heparin 7,500 units subcut
   On hand: 10,000 USP units/1 mL

6. Ordered: Heparin 5,000 units subcut
   On hand: Heparin 10,000 USP units/1 mL

7. Ordered: Heparin 8,000 units subcut
   On hand: Heparin 20,000 USP units/1 mL

8. Ordered: Heparin 2,500 units subcut
   On hand: Heparin 5,000 USP units/1 mL

LEARNING OUTCOME	KEY POINTS

14.1 Calculate dosages of parenteral medication in solution and select a syringe based on the dosage calculation. Pages 335–350	▸ Parenteral medication is in solution
	
	▸ Find the dosage strength
	
	▸ Use the ABCs of dosage calculations
	
	   A. Gather information and *convert* to like units of measurement
	
	   B. *Calculate* using the proportion method, dimensional analysis, or formula method (see Chapter 12 for discussion of each method)
	
	   C. *Think!* . . . [about your answer, determine] *Is It Reasonable?*
	
	[following Rules 14-1 to 14-3]
	
	Rule 14-1 Select the proper syringe
	
	▸ If volume to administer is greater than or equal to 1 mL, use a 3 mL syringe
	
	▸ If volume to administer is less than 1 mL, but greater than or equal to 0.5 mL and calculates evenly to the hundredths, use a 1 mL tuberculin syringe or a 3 mL syringe
	
	▸ If the volume to administer is less than 0.5 mL, round to the hundredths and use a 1 mL tuberculin syringe. For amounts less than 0.5 mL, use a 0.5 mL tuberculin syringe, if available.
	
	Rule 14-2 Correctly round the amount of an injection to administer
	
	▸ Round volumes greater than 1 mL to the nearest tenth (3 mL syringe is calibrated in tenths)
	
	▸ Round volumes less than 1 mL to the nearest hundredth (tuberculin syringe is calibrated in hundredths)
	
	Rule 14-3 Do not exceed maximum volume for an injection in a single site.
	
	▸ Intramuscular (IM) injections:
	
	   – Adult, excluding deltoid 3 mL
	
	   – Adult deltoid (arm) 1 mL
	
	   – Child 6–12 years 2 mL
	
	   – Child 0–5 years 1 mL
	
	   – Premature infant 0.5 mL
	
	▸ Subcutaneous (Subcut) injections: 1 mL

LEARNING OUTCOME	KEY POINTS
14.2 Calculate dosages of medications expressed in percent or ratio format. Pages 350–361	*Percent (per 100)* means grams per 100 mL Example: 1% means 1 gram per 100 mL *Ratio* means gram per mL Example 1:2,000 means 1 gram per 2,000 mL Rule 14-4 *Convert* solution strength to standard format of g/mL, mg/mL, or units/mL

14.3 Calculate dosages of reconstituted parenteral medications. Pages 361–373	• Use the appropriate diluent
	• Use the exact volume of diluents recommended by manufacturer, to render the correct dosage strength
	
	Rule 14-5 To reconstitute a powdered medication
	
	   1. Find directions on label or package insert
	   2. Use sterile syringe and aseptic technique
	   3. Inject diluent into the medication vial
	   4. Mix by rolling, inverting, or shaking the vial
	   5. Completely dissolve powdered medication prior to use

14.4 Calculate dosages for other administration forms. Pages 373–374	Inhalant medication orders include the solution strength and the amount of inhalant to administer. Do not divide suppositories unless ordered. Transdermal medications are usually expressed in mcg or mg per hour. Patches are not typically divided. Use the ABCs of dosage calculations to calculate dosages.
14.5 Calculate subcutaneous dosages of the high-alert medication insulin. Pages 374–388	The label identifies insulin type, manufacturer, brand name, storage information, and the expiration date. Insulin labels also contain the concentration written as units/mL (100 units/mL, also called U-100; or 500 units/mL, also called U-500). The standard U-100, 1 mL syringe is calibrated for every 2 units. U-100, 0.5 mL and 0.3 mL syringes are calibrated for every 1 unit; the calibrations and numbers are larger, making them easier for accuracy with smaller doses. Calculate the total dose of insulin (short-acting + intermediate-acting = total dose). Inject correct amount of air into intermediate-acting, then short-acting. Draw up the short-acting insulin first, then the intermediate-acting.
14.6 Calculate subcutaneous dosages of the high-alert medication heparin. Pages 388–392	Heparin is manufactured and labeled in different strengths (10 units/mL; 100 units/mL; 1,000 units/mL; 5,000 units/mL; 10,000 units/mL) and different volumes (1 mL, 10 mL, 30 mL). Harmful and deadly errors have occurred when heparin of the wrong strength has been administered. It is imperative that careful attention be paid to the concentration, and not just the volume of heparin in the bottle. Follow the ABCs of dosage calculation using any of the three methods when preparing subcutaneous dosages of heparin. Pay special attention to the concentration of heparin, so that the total volume of the dose is less than or equal to 1 mL (maximum subcut volume of injection).

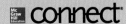
Answer the following questions.

1. What is the correct syringe to select if the amount to be injected is 0.75 mL? (LO 14.1)

2. If the dosage to be administered is 1.75 mL, what syringe would you select and to what amount would the dosage be rounded? (LO 14.1)

3. List the maximum volume for an IM injection for the following patients: an adult, an adult deltoid, a child 6–12 years old. (LO 14.1)

4. If the order for a subcutaneous injection results in an amount of 2.2 mL, what action should be taken before any administration? (LO 14.1)

5. What type of injection is usually less than 0.1 mL? (LO 14.1)

6. List three common diluents used when reconstituting powdered medications. (LO 14.3)

7. Ordered: Acetylcysteine 800 mg via nebulizer q6h

   On hand: Acetylcysteine 10% solution

8. Ordered: Thorazine® 50 mg q6h pr as needed

   On hand: Thorazine® 25 mg and 100-mg suppositories

9. Ordered: Nitro-Dur® 0.3 mg/h top

   On hand: Nitro-Dur® 0.1 mg/h and 0.2 mg/h transdermal patches

Use the identified drug labels to answer the following questions.

10. Refer to Label A. What is the storage information on the label? (LO 14.3)

11. If the order is for 75 mg IM, what amount would be administered? What syringe should be used? (LO 14.1)

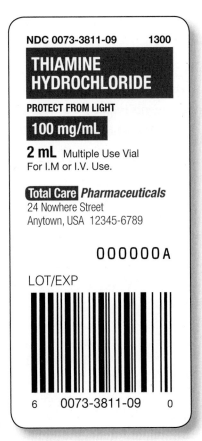

A

12. Refer to Label B. How many units are in each milliliter of this drug? (LO 14.6)

13. If the order is for 800 units subcut, what amount would be administered? (LO 14.6)

14. If the order is for 1,000 units, how many times may this vial be used? (LO 14.6)

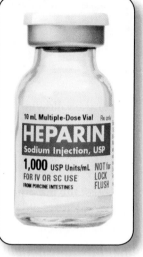

B

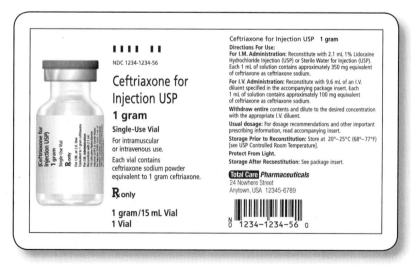

CLINDAMYCIN
INJECTION, USP
600 mg/4mL
(150 mg/mL)
For IM or IV Use   Rx only
DILUTE BEFORE IV USE
4 mL Single Dose Vial
Do not refrigerate.

Total Care *Pharmaceuticals*
24 Nowhere Street
Anytown, USA 12345-6789

LOT/EXP

0   12345-678-90   0

C

15. Refer to Label C. If the order is for 900 mg IM, what amount would be administered? (LO 14.1)

16. What extra preparations would you need to make in order to administer the amount in Question 15? (LO 14.1)

17. Other than IM, what route is acceptable for administration of this drug and what must you do before administration? (LO 14.1)

18. Refer to Label D. What two diluents, and how much of each, are suggested on the label for intramuscular administration? (LO 14.3)

19. Which one of the diluents requires a physician's order? (LO 14.3)

20. If the order is 500 mg IM, what amount would be administered? (LO 14.3)

NDC 1234-1234-56

Ceftriaxone for Injection USP

1 gram

Single-Use Vial

For intramuscular
or intravenous use.

Each vial contains
ceftriaxone sodium powder
equivalent to 1 gram ceftriaxone.

R only

1 gram/15 mL Vial
1 Vial

Ceftriaxone for Injection USP   1 gram
Directions For Use:
For I.M. Administration: Reconstitute with 2.1 mL 1% Lidocaine
Hydrochloride Injection (USP) or Sterile Water for Injection (USP).
Each 1 mL of solution contains approximately 350 mg equivalent
of ceftriaxone as ceftriaxone sodium.
For I.V. Administration: Reconstitute with 9.6 mL of an I.V.
diluent specified in the accompanying package insert. Each
1 mL of solution contains approximately 100 mg equivalent
of ceftriaxone as ceftriaxone sodium.
Withdraw entire contents and dilute to the desired concentration
with the appropriate I.V. diluent.
Usual dosage: For dosage recommendations and other important
prescribing information, read accompanying insert.
Storage Prior to Reconstitution: Store at 20°–25°C (68°–77°F)
[see USP Controlled Room Temperature].
Protect From Light.
Storage After Reconstitution: See package insert.

Total Care *Pharmaceuticals*
24 Nowhere Street
Anytown, USA 12345-6789

N
0   1234-1234-56   0

D

For Exercises 21 and 22, determine the amount to administer and the syringe to use. (LO 14.4)

21. Ordered: Bicillin C-R 1,800,000 units now
    On hand: Bicillin C-R 1,200,000 units/2 mL

22. Ordered: Oxytocin 5 units IM now
    On hand: Oxytocin 10 units/mL

Answer the following questions.

23. Explain what U-100 and U-500 mean when referring to insulin. (LO 14.5)

24. List the steps in preparing a combined insulin dose. (LO 14.5)

25. Calculate the total units of insulin if the order is for 16 units Novolin® R and 30 units of Humulin® N. What type and size of syringe would you select? (LO 14.5)

For Exercises 26–33, refer to labels E to H.

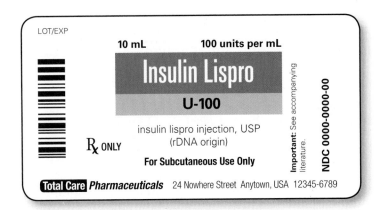

E

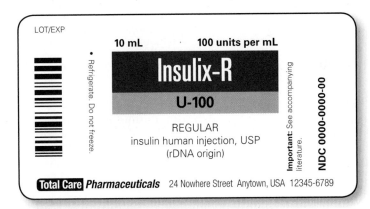

F

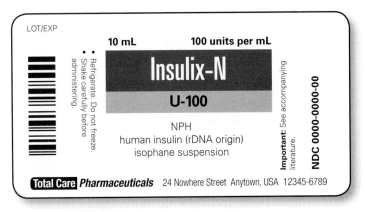

G

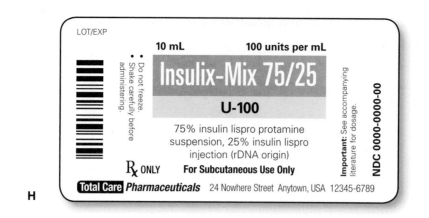

H

26. Administer 20 units of NPH insulin. Use label _____. Demonstrate where the syringe will be filled. (LO 14.5)

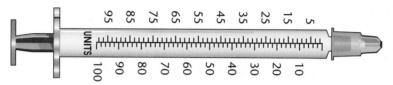

27. Administer 5 units of regular insulin. Use label _____. Demonstrate where the syringe will be filled. (LO 14.5)

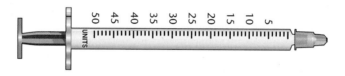

28. Administer 3 units of insulin lispro injection. Use label _____. Demonstrate where the syringe will be filled. (LO14.5)

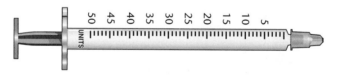

29. Administer 20 units of Insulix-Mix 75/25. Use label _____. In this dose how many units of lispro protamine suspension, and how many units of lispro injection will be administered? Insulin lispro protamine suspension_____, insulin lispro injection _____. (LO 14.5)

30. Administer 10 units short-acting, and 25 units intermediate-acting insulin. Use labels _____. Demonstrate where the syringe will be filled with each of the insulins. (LO 14.5)

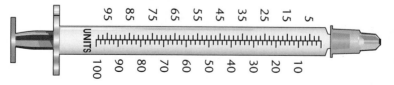

31. Referring to Exercise 30, which insulin will be drawn up first? _____. (LO 14.5)

32. Administer 5 units of rapid-acting insulin and 30 units of intermediate-acting insulin. Use labels _____. Which insulin will be drawn up first? _____ (LO 14.5)

x

33. Refer to Label I. If the order is for 1,500 units heparin subcut, what amount would you administer? (LO 14.6)

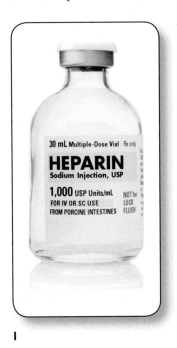

I

CHAPTER 14 REVIEW

CHECK UP

For Exercises 1–10, find the amount to administer, then mark the syringe. (LO 14.1, 14.2)

1. Ordered: INFeD® (iron dextran) 100 mg IM daily
   On hand: INFeD® 50 mg/mL

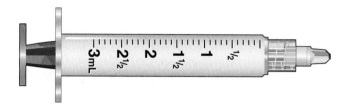

2. Ordered: Haloperidol decanoate 60 mg IM stat
   On hand: Haloperidol decanoate 50 mg/mL

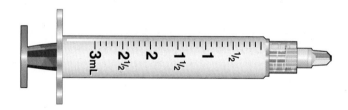

3. Ordered: Loxitane® 30 mg IM bid
   On hand: Loxitane® 50 mg/mL

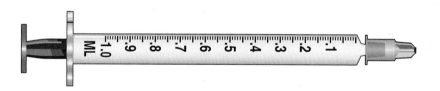

4. Ordered: Epogen® 1,400 units subcut three times per week
   On hand: Epogen® 2,000 units/mL

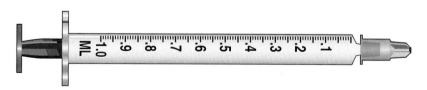

5. Ordered: Lidocaine 300 mg IM stat
   On hand: Lidocaine 20% solution

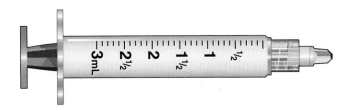

6. Ordered: Magnesium sulfate 250 mg IM daily
   On hand: Magnesium sulfate 10% solution

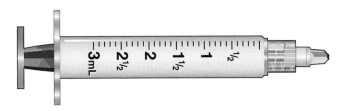

7. Ordered: Levsin® 0.4 mg IM bid
   On hand: Levsin® 0.5 mg/mL

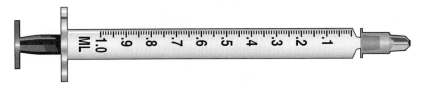

8. Ordered: Robinul® 0.15 mg IM stat
   On hand: Robinul® 0.2 mg/mL

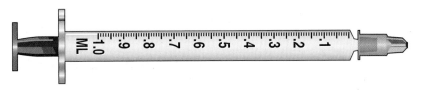

9. Order: Prostigmin 0.75 mg IM q4h
   On hand: Prostigmin 1:1,000 solution

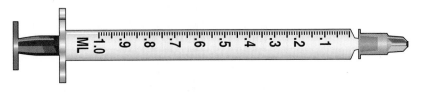

10. Ordered: Epinephrine 0.5 mg subcut stat
   On hand: Epinephrine 1:200 solution

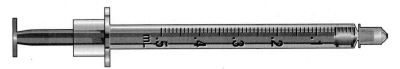

For Exercises 11–21, find the amount to administer, select the proper syringe, and write in the space provided. (LO 14.1, 14.2)

11. Ordered: Adrenalin® 0.2 mg subcut stat
    On hand: Adrenalin® 1:2,000 solution
    Administer: _____ Syringe: _____

12. Ordered: Calciferol 24,000 units IM daily
    On hand: Calciferol 500,000 units/5 mL
    Administer: _____ Syringe: _____

13. Ordered: Heparin sodium 7,500 units subcut q8h
    On hand: Heparin 20,000:1 solution
    Administer: _____ Syringe: _____

14. Ordered: Heparin calcium 7,500 units subcut q8h
    On hand: Heparin calcium 5,000 units/0.2 mL
    Administer: _____ Syringe: _____

15. Ordered: Thiamine 200 mg IM
    On hand: Refer to Label A.
    Administer: _____ Syringe: _____

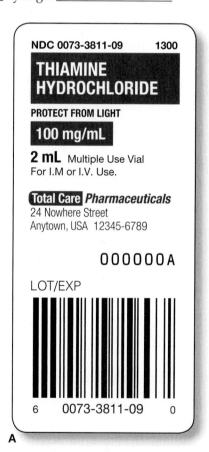

A

16. Ordered: Heparin 400 units subcut daily

On hand: Refer to Label B.

Administer: _____ Syringe: _____

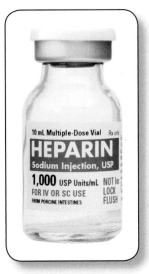

B

17. Ordered: Furosemide 15 mg IM now

On hand: Refer to Label C.

Administer: _____ Syringe: _____

NDC 00000-000-00

FUROSEMIDE

INJECTION

20 mg/2 mL

2 mL   Rx only

Single Dose Vial
Discard unused portion.
Usual Dosage: See insert.

For IM and IV use

Total Care
Pharmaceuticals

24 Nowhere Street
Anytown, USA 12345-6789

LOT/EXP

0 1234-1234-56 0

C

18. Ordered: Oxytocin 20 units IM q 12h prn

On hand: Refer to Label D.

Administer: _____ Syringe: _____

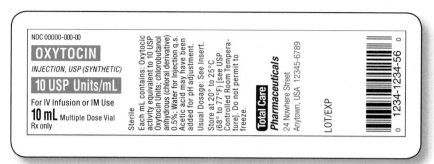

D

19. Ordered: Filgrastim® 2,500 units subcut three times per week

On hand: Refer to Label E.

Administer: _____ Syringe: _____

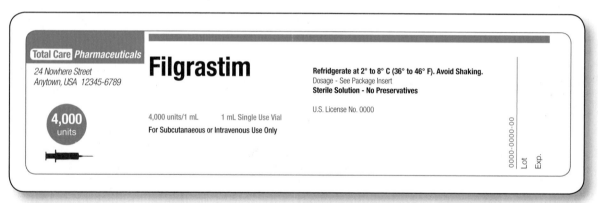

E

20. Ordered: Clindamycin 300 mg IM now

On hand: Refer to Label F.

Administer: _____ Syringe: _____

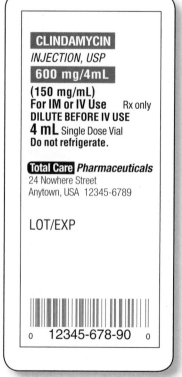

F

21. Ordered: 0.25 mg Sandostatin® subcut daily

On Hand: Refer to Label G.

Administer: _____ Syringe: _____

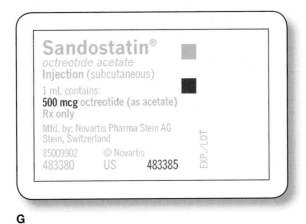

G

22. Explain which vial of medication, Label H or Label I, you would use for the following order. (LO 14.1)

Ordered: Furosemide 40 mg IM

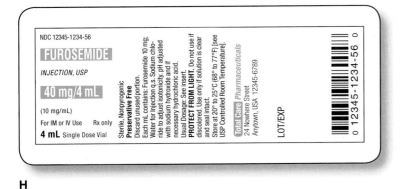

H

I

For Exercises 23–26, refer to Label J and the package insert. (LO 14.3)

23. What diluents may be used to reconstitute Zyprexa® for IM use?

24. How much diluent should be added to the vial?

25. How much would you withdraw for a 5 mg dose?

26. How long will the solution retain its potency at room temperature?

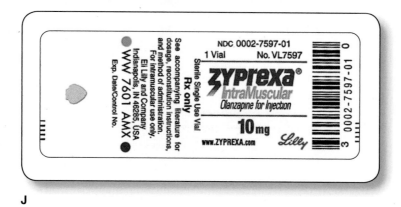

J

ZYPREXA® IntraMuscular (olanzapine for injection) Dosing
ZYPREXA IntraMuscular is approved for the treatment of agitation associated with schizophrenia and bipolar mania.

Dose (mg)	Injection volume (mL)
10.0 mg	Withdraw total contents of vial
7.5 mg	1.5 mL
5.0 mg	1.0 mL
2.5 mg	0.5 mL

10 mg is the recommended dose for agitation associated with bipolar mania and schizophrenia.

Follow the steps below to reconstitute and use ZYPREXA IntraMuscular:

1. Inject 2.1 mL of Sterile Water for Injection into single-packaged vial for up to 10-mg dose.
2. Dissolve contents of vial completely; resulting solution should be clear and yellow.
3. Use solution within 1 hour; discard any unused portion.
4. Refer to table for injection volumes and corresponding doses of ZYPREXA IntraMuscular.
5. Immediately after use, dispose of syringe in approved sharps box.

For Exercises 27–29, find the amount to administer. (LO 14.4)

27. Ordered: Albuterol 1.25 mg via nebulizer q8h
On hand: Albuterol 5 mg/mL

28. Ordered: Dilaudid® 6 mg q4h pr as needed
On hand: Dilaudid® 3 mg suppositories

29. Ordered: Androderm® 5 mg/day top
On hand: Androderm® 2.5 mg/day transdermal patches

For Exercises 30–35, refer to labels K–P. Select the label corresponding to each exercise. Then mark the desired amount of insulin on the syringe. (LO 14.5)

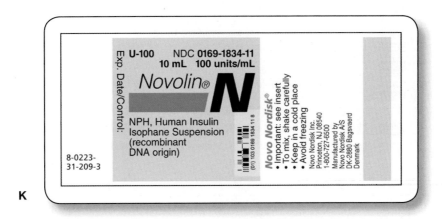

K

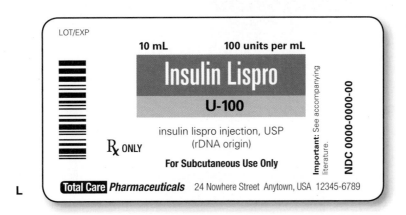

L

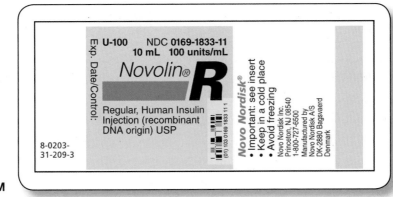

M

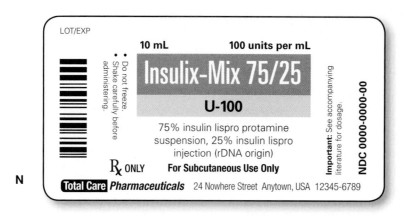

N

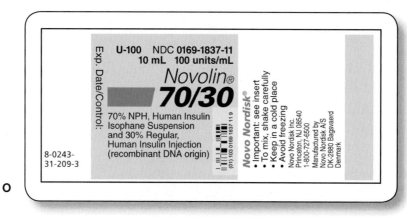

O

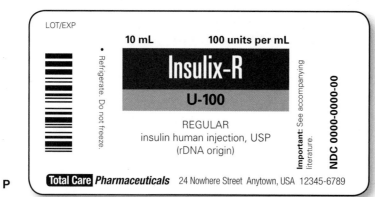

P

30. Ordered: Insulix-R 11 units subcut before breakfast

Select label: _____

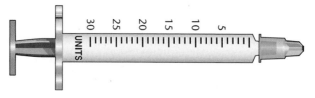

31. Ordered: Insulix-Mix 75/25 48 units subcut before dinner

Select label: _____

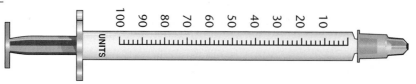

32. Ordered: Novolin® 70/30 57 units subcut before breakfast

Select label: _____

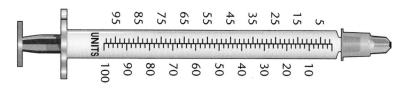

33. Ordered: Insulin lispro injection 24 units subcut daily

Select label: _____

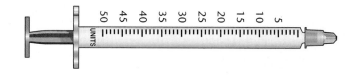

34. Ordered: Novolin® N 65 units subcut before dinner

Select label: _____

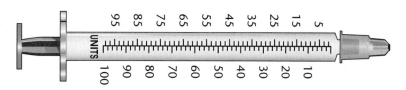

35. Ordered: Novolin® R insulin 21 units subcut before dinner

Select label: _____

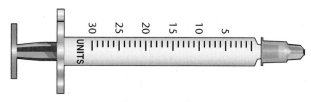

For Exercises 36 and 37, first mark on the syringe the dose of shorter-acting insulin ordered. Then mark where the leading ring will be after you draw up the intermediate-acting insulin into the same syringe. (LO 14.5)

36. Humulin® N 27 units and Humulin® R 8 units subcut qam

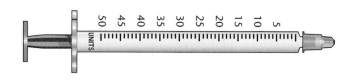

37. Novolin® R 13 units and Novolin® N 57 units subcut qam

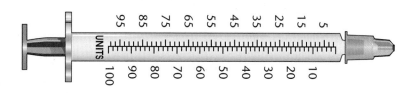

For Exercises 38 and 39, select the correct heparin label. Then calculate the amount of subcutaneous heparin to administer. (LO 14.6)

38. Administer heparin 8,000 units subcut. Label _____ Amount to administer _____

39. Administer heparin 4,000 units subcut. Label _____ Amount to administer _____

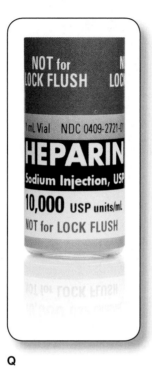

Q

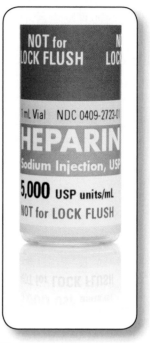

R

CRITICAL THINKING APPLICATIONS

For Questions 1–5 on the next page, refer to the following order, label, and package insert. (LO 14.3)

Ordered: Peginterferon alfa-2b 180 mcg subcut weekly

On hand: Refer to the following label and package insert.

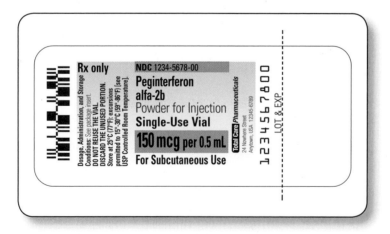

Preparation and Administration
Peginterferon alfa-2B

This package contains a vial of peginterferon alfa-2b 150 mcg/0.5 mL, a 1.25 mL vial of diluent (Sterile Water for Injection, USP), and two safety syringes. The peginterferon alfa-2b is a white to off-white powder or tablet. To reconstitute the medication, use one of the syringes to add exactly 0.7 mL of the supplied diluent to the vial of peginterferon alfa-2b. Invert the vial gently to mix. DO NOT SHAKE. Discard the remaining diluent. The reconstituted solution contains 150 mcg per 0.5 mL. Visually inspect the solution prior to administration. The solution should be clear and colorless. Do not use if it is cloudy or discolored.

After reconstitution, use the remaining syringe to withdraw the appropriate dose and inject subcutaneously. This cartridge contains no preservatives and is for single use only. Dispose of used cartridge in a puncture-resistant sharps container. Do not re-use vial.

Before reconstitution, this medication should be stored at 2°C–8°C (36°F–46°F). The solution should be used immediately after reconstitution. However, it may be stored for up to 24 hours at 2°C–8°C (36°F–46°F). Do not freeze.

Peginterferon alfa-2b package insert

1. How should you prepare this medication?

2. How much diluent is supplied and how much should be used?

3. What should you do with the rest of the diluent?

4. How would this medication most likely be administered?

5. After reconstitution, how should this medication be stored and for how long?

CASE STUDY

For questions 1–3 on the next page, refer to the following labels. (LO 14.2, 14.3)
The physician orders Sandostatin® 75 mcg IM tid.
On hand: See labels A, B, and C.

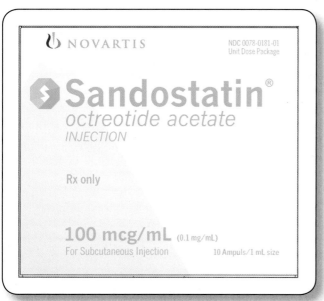

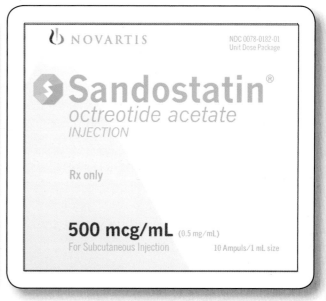

A

B

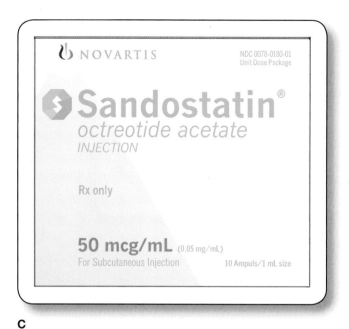

c

Describe what actions you should take before administering the medication. If you were going to administer the medication:

1. Which package would you use and why?

2. What would be the amount to administer?

3. What syringe would you use?

Intravenous Calculations

One must learn by doing the thing, for though you think you know it, you have no certainty until you try.

ARISTOLE

LEARNING OUTCOMES

When you have completed Chapter 15, you will be able to:

15.1 Identify the components and concentrations of IV solutions.

15.2 Distinguish basic types of IV equipment.

15.3 Calculate IV flow rates for electronic devices in mL/h, manually controlled devices in gtt/min, and IV rate adjustments.

15.4 Calculate infusion time and volume.

15.5 Perform calculations for intermittent IV infusions.

KEY TERMS

Central line
Drip chamber
Flow rate
Heparin lock
Hypertonic
Hypotonic
Infiltration
Infusion pumps
Intravenous (IV)
Isotonic
KVO or TKO fluids
Maintenance fluids
Patient-controlled analgesia (PCA)

Peripherally inserted central catheters (PICC)
Phlebitis
Port-A-Cath
Primary line
Rate controllers
Replacement fluids
Saline lock
Secondary line
Syringe pumps
Therapeutic fluids

INTRODUCTION

Intravenous (IV) fluids are solutions, including medications, that are delivered directly into the bloodstream through a vein. Blood, a suspension, is also delivered intravenously. Fluids delivered directly into the bloodstream have a rapid effect, which is necessary during emergencies or other critical care situations when medications are needed. However, the results can be fatal if the wrong medication or dosage is given. Healthcare professionals who administer or monitor IV solutions should know the principles discussed in this chapter.

Many IV drugs are available. Each has its own usage guidelines, based on specifications developed by the manufacturers. The guidelines typically outline recommended dosages, infusion rates, compatibility, and patient monitoring. For example, some medications cannot be combined with others, or must be administered over a specific length of time.

States regulate who may administer IV medications and what training is required. This chapter teaches IV calculations and theory; however, to be proficient, you must obtain the required training and learn by doing.

IV Solutions

IV solutions fall into four functional categories: replacement fluids, maintenance fluids, KVO or TKO fluids, and therapeutic fluids. **Replacement fluids** replace electrolytes and fluids lost or depleted due to hemorrhage, vomiting, or diarrhea. Examples include whole blood, nutrient solutions, or fluids administered to treat dehydration. **Maintenance fluids** help patients maintain normal electrolyte and fluid balance. They include IV fluids such as normal saline given during and after surgery. Some IVs provide access to the vascular system for emergency situations. Fluids prescribed at a very slow rate to maintain open venous access are called **KVO** (keep vein open) **fluids** or **TKO** (to keep open) **fluids**. A commonly used KVO fluid is 0.9% sodium chloride, also called normal saline (NS). **Therapeutic fluids** deliver medication to the patient.

IV Labels

IV solutions are labeled with the name and exact amount of components in the solution. The label in Figure 15-1 is clearly marked as 5% dextrose and lactated Ringer's injection. Table 15-1 summarizes abbreviations often used for IV solutions.

RULE 15-1	In abbreviations for IV solutions, letters identify the component and numbers identify the concentration.
Example 1	An order for 5% dextrose in lactated Ringer's solution might be abbreviated in any of the following ways:
	D5LR D_5LR 5%D/LR D5%LR

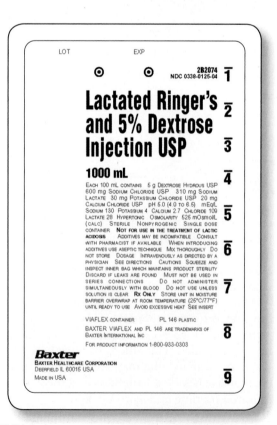

Figure 15-1   1,000 mL D5LR label.

TABLE 15-1 Commonly Used Abbreviations

D10W	10% dextrose in water
D5W	5% dextrose in water
W, H_2O	Water
NS, NSS	Normal saline (0.9% NaCl)
LR	Lactated Ringer's
RL	Ringer's lactate
D5LR, D_5LR, 5%D/LR, D5%LR	5% dextrose in lactated Ringer's solution
$\frac{1}{2}$ NS, $\frac{1}{2}$ NSS	One-half normal saline solution (0.45% NaCl)
$\frac{1}{3}$ NS, $\frac{1}{3}$ NSS	One-third normal saline solution (0.3% NaCl)
$\frac{1}{4}$ NS, $\frac{1}{4}$ NSS	One-fourth normal saline solution (0.225% NaCl)

IV Concentrations

Solutions may have different concentrations of dextrose (glucose) or saline (sodium chloride, or NaCl). For example, 5% dextrose contains 5 g of dextrose per 100 mL (Figure 15-2). Normal saline is 0.9% saline; it contains 900 mg, or 0.9 g, of sodium chloride per 100 mL (Figure 15-3). In turn, 0.45% saline, or $\frac{1}{2}$ NS, has 450 mg of sodium chloride per 100 mL—that is, one-half the amount of normal saline. Other saline concentrations include 0.3% saline (or $\frac{1}{3}$ NS) and 0.225% saline (or $\frac{1}{4}$ NS).

Lactated Ringer's (LR, or Ringer's lactate), also known as Hartmann's solution, contains sodium chloride as well as sodium lactate, potassium chloride, and calcium chloride. LR can also be mixed with 5% dextrose.

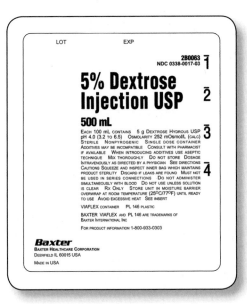

Figure 15-2 500 mL of D5W.

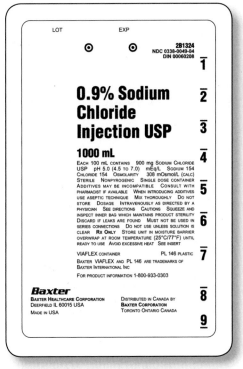

Figure 15-3 1,000 mL of NS.

Example 1	How much dextrose is contained in 500 mL D5W? (Refer to Figure 15-2.) D5W represents 5% dextrose in water; it has 5 g of dextrose per 100 mL of water. Using the proportion method: $$\frac{5 \text{ g}}{100 \text{ mL}} = \frac{x}{500 \text{ mL}}$$ $$100x = 2{,}500 \text{ g}$$ $$x = 25 \text{ g}$$ So 25 g of dextrose is contained in 500 mL D5W.
Example 2	How much sodium chloride is contained in 1,000 mL of NS (see Figure 15-3)? $$\frac{0.9 \text{ g}}{100 \text{ mL}} = \frac{x}{1{,}000 \text{ mL}}$$ $$100x = 900 \text{ g}$$ $$x = 9 \text{ g}$$ So 9 g of sodium chloride is contained in 1,000 mL of NS.
Example 3	How much dextrose and sodium chloride are contained in 1,000 mL of D5 $\frac{1}{2}$ NS (Figure 15-4)? **Dextrose:** $\qquad\qquad$ **Sodium chloride:** $\frac{5 \text{ g}}{100 \text{ mL}} = \frac{x}{1{,}000 \text{ mL}}$ $\qquad$ $\frac{0.45 \text{ g}}{100 \text{ mL}} = \frac{x}{1{,}000 \text{ mL}}$ $100x = 5{,}000 \text{ g}$ $\qquad\qquad$ $100x = 450 \text{ g}$ $x = 50 \text{ g dextrose}$ $\qquad$ $x = 4.5 \text{ g sodium chloride}$ So there are 50 g of dextrose and 4.5 g sodium chloride in 1,000 mL of D5 $\frac{1}{2}$ NS.

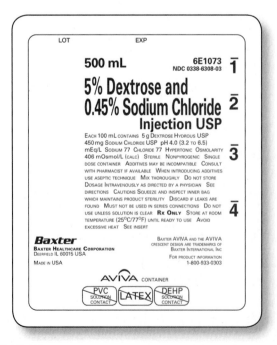

Figure 15-4 D5 1/2 NS.

Calcium, potassium, chloride, phosphorus, and magnesium are electrolytes that can be added to an IV solution to help correct a fluid or chemical imbalance. The concentration of these electrolytes determines the osmolarity of the solution. Solutions with approximately the same osmolarity as the fluid within human body cells are termed **isotonic.** Solutions with a lower osmolarity than intracellular fluid are termed **hypotonic.** Hypotonic solutions are dilute, which results in fluid moving into the cells. Solutions with a higher osmolarity than intracellular fluid are termed **hypertonic.** Hypertonic solutions are concentrated and cause fluid to shift out of the cells. Authorized prescribers use this knowledge to determine which type of IV fluid to administer. If the patient is dehydrated and there is not enough fluid within the body cells, a hypotonic IV fluid is ordered. If the patient has too much fluid in the cells, as in cerebral edema, a hypertonic fluid is ordered. If the patient has a normal fluid balance, but can't take fluids enterally, an isotonic maintenance IV fluid is ordered. Isotonic IV fluid is also used to replace intravascular fluid if the patient is hypovolemic (does not have enough fluid circulating in the blood vessels).

Examples of isotonic solutions are lactated Ringer's, Ringer's lactate, normal saline (0.9% NaCl), and D5W. Although D5W has an osmolarity similar to intracellular fluid while it is in the IV bag, the dextrose quickly moves into the cell after administration, leaving a hypotonic solution in the extracellular fluid. For this reason, D5W is used as a hypotonic solution. Saline solutions with less NaCl than normal saline (less than 0.9% NaCl) are hypotonic. Examples of these are $\frac{1}{2}$ NS (0.45% NaCl), $\frac{1}{3}$ NS (0.3% NS), and $\frac{1}{4}$ NS (0.225% NaCl). Saline solutions with more NaCl than normal saline (greater than 0.9% NaCl) are hypertonic. Examples of these are 3% NaCl and 5% NaCl.

RULE 15-2	Patients with normal electrolyte levels are likely to receive isotonic solutions. Those with high electrolyte levels will receive hypotonic solutions. Those with low electrolyte levels will receive hypertonic solutions.
Example 1	Patient A is a 35-year-old, healthy female who will have an IV infusion during a diagnostic test. She will require an isotonic solution such as NS, or lactated Ringer's.
Example 2	Patient B is an 8-year-old female who has been vomiting and has had diarrhea for 24 hours and is dehydrated. She may require a hypotonic solution such as 0.45% sodium chloride or 0.3% sodium chloride to restore the proper fluid level in her cells and tissues.
Example 3	Patient C is a 50-year-old male with cerebral edema. He may require hypertonic solution such as 3% sodium chloride to help draw fluids from cells and tissues.

Compatibility

Medications, electrolytes, and nutrients are additives that can be combined with IV solutions. Potassium chloride, vitamins B and C, and antibiotics are common additives. While additives are often prepackaged in the solution, you may need to mix the additive and IV solution yourself. The physician's order will tell you how much additive to administer, the amount and type of basic IV solution to use, and the length of time over which the additive/IV mixture should infuse. For example, an order may call for 20 milliequivalents (mEq) of potassium chloride in 1,000 mL of 5% dextrose and normal saline over 8 h, or

1,000 mL D5NS c̄ 20 mEq KCl IV over 8 h

Some incompatible additives may cause the resulting solution to turn cloudy or crystallize, which means it hardens to crystals. If you mix an IV base solution with an additive that is incompatible (Table 15-2), you may place the patient's health at serious risk. Verify compatibility by checking with a compatibility chart, a drug reference book, the pharmacy, the Internet, or a package insert.

TABLE 15-2 Examples of Incompatible IV Combinations

Ampicillin	5% dextrose in water
Cefotaxime sodium	Sodium bicarbonate
Diazepam	Potassium chloride
Dopamine HCl	Sodium bicarbonate
Penicillin	Heparin
Penicillin	Vitamin B complex
Sodium bicarbonate	Lactated Ringer's
Tetracycline HCl	Calcium chloride

RULE 15-3 | Before you combine any medications, electrolytes, or nutrients with an IV solution, be sure the components are compatible.

CRITICAL THINKING ON THE JOB

Checking Compatibility

A patient in respiratory distress with congestive heart failure is started on D5/0.45% NaCl. The next day she is diagnosed with an upper respiratory infection. The physician orders 500 mg ampicillin IVPB q6h.

The healthcare professional begins to administer the ampicillin. She notices that the solution in the tubing has become cloudy.

 Think! . . . Is It Reasonable? Why would the solution in the tubing be cloudy? What should the healthcare professional do?

REVIEW AND PRACTICE

15.1 IV Solutions

For Exercises 1–5, calculate the number of grams of NaCL and/or dextrose in each of the following IV solutions.

1. 1,000 mL $D_{10}W$ _____ g dextrose

2. 500 mL D5 $\frac{1}{2}$ NS _____ g dextrose _____ g NaCl

3. 250 mL D_5NS _____ g dextrose _____ g NaCl

4. 1,000 mL D_5LR _____ g dextrose

5. 500 mL $D_5 \frac{1}{4}$ NS _____ g dextrose _____ g NaCl

15.2 IV Equipment

IV equipment is available in several forms. Most are electronic or have electronic components, while a few are still manual.

The Primary Line

The typical IV setup consists of a bag of IV solution and tubing. IV bags come in different sizes, often containing 500 or 1,000 mL of solution. They should be marked at regular time intervals to help keep track of the amount of solution that is being infused. Your facility will have specific guidelines regarding how IV bags should be marked.

The tubing, which is the **primary line,** usually includes a **drip chamber,** clamp, and injection ports (Figure 15-5). The drip chamber is a transparent enclosure through which the drops of IV fluid can be counted in order to estimate the rate of infusion. The drip chamber attaches to the IV bag. To measure the flow rate, squeeze and release the drip chamber until it is half filled with IV solution. Fluid in the chamber makes it easy to count the drops that fall into it from the bag. Use a roller clamp (Figure 15-6) or a screw clamp to set or adjust the flow rate of the IV solution. A slide clamp shuts off the IV solution flow completely without disturbing the flow rate setting at the roller or screw clamp. Injection ports allow you to inject medications or compatible fluids into the primary line or to attach a second IV line. IV bags may have ports for additives injected directly into the solution.

Tubing is available in two sizes: macrodrip and microdrip. Macrodrip tubing (Figure 15-7) allows larger drops to form before falling into the drip chamber. It is used for infusions of 80 mL/h or more and is always used for operating room infusions. Microdrip tubing allows smaller drops to enter the drip chamber. It is used for flow rates of less than 80 mL/h and is often used for KVO infusions. Microdrip tubing is especially useful for pediatric and critical care IVs, when very small volumes are used and accuracy is extremely important. Accidental increases in volume can be fatal in these situations.

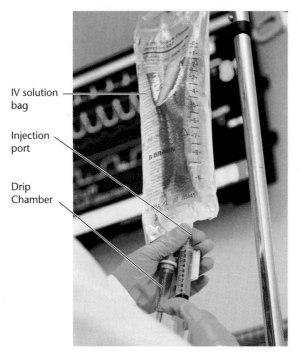

IV solution bag

Injection port

Drip Chamber

Figure 15-5 A bag of IV fluid may have medication added through the injection port before administration.

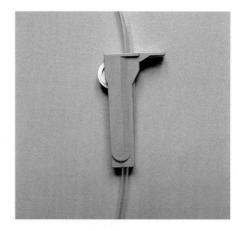

Figure 15-6 Roller clamp.

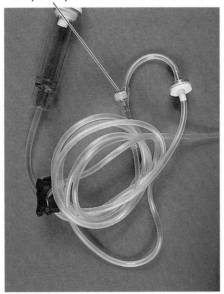

Injection port

Figure 15-7 IV tubing with an injection port.

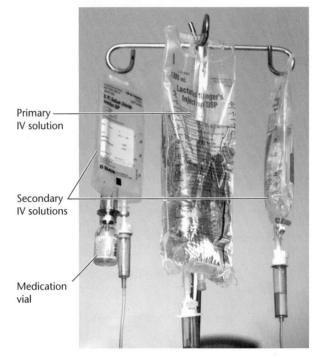

Primary IV solution

Secondary IV solutions

Medication vial

Figure 15-8 Two secondary IV solutions piggybacked to a primary IV solution. The secondary IV solution on the left includes a medication vial attached to the injection port.

Secondary Lines (Piggyback)

A **secondary line,** also known as a piggyback or IVPB, is an IV setup that attaches to a primary line. It can be used to infuse medication or other compatible fluids on an intermittent basis, such as q6h. Although shorter than primary tubing, secondary tubing has the same basic components. IVPB bags are usually smaller, often holding 50, 100, or 150 mL of fluid. (See Figure 15-8.) Some medications require a larger amount of fluid as a diluent, such as 250 mL.

Regulating Intravenous Infusions

IVs may be regulated manually. The bag is hung 36 inches (in.) above the patient's heart to allow gravity to draw the fluid through the tubing and into the vascular system. Whoever administers and monitors the IV adjusts the flow rate, using roller or screw clamps. Manually delivered IV fluids are usually adjusted in drops per minute (gtt/min).

Electronic devices—rate controllers, infusion pumps, syringe pumps, and *patient-controlled analgesia* (PCA) devices—can be used to regulate the flow of IV infusions. These devices often use tubing specific to the equipment. Some types of tubing may be used only with specific pumps.

Rate controllers (Figure 15-9) rely on gravity to infuse the solution, but no clamp is used to adjust the flow rate. Tubing is threaded through the controller, where a pincher maintains a preset flow rate. The controller is attached to a sensor that measures the drops or volume of solution that is delivered. An alarm sounds when the preset flow rate cannot be maintained.

Infusion pumps (Figure 15-10) apply pressure sufficient to deliver a set volume of liquid every minute into the vein. They can introduce liquid into a central vein, where pressure is much higher than in peripheral veins. The desired flow rate is set on an infusion pump, either in milliliters per hour or by dosage. The unit does not rely on gravity, but forces the IV solution through the tubing. A sensor detects when the IV bag is empty or the flow is too rapid and sounds an alarm. An alarm also sounds if the flow rate cannot be maintained or if the bag is empty. A rate that is too slow may indicate too much resistance in the vein, suggesting blockage, a kink in the tubing, or that the IV catheter has come out of the vein. In some cases, the equipment will continue to pump the IV fluid, even though the catheter is out of the vein. Thus, when you use an infusion pump, you must monitor the patient's infusion site regularly for signs of infiltration (such as swelling, coolness, or discomfort).

Syringe pumps allow you to insert a syringe in the pump unit (Figure 15-11). The syringe can deliver medication or fluids that cannot be combined with other medications or solutions. Syringe pumps are useful for pediatric medications as well as for medications that must be administered at a precisely controlled rate. Syringe pumps are often used in cases when a medication must be administered over half an hour or less; however, they can also be used for longer time periods.

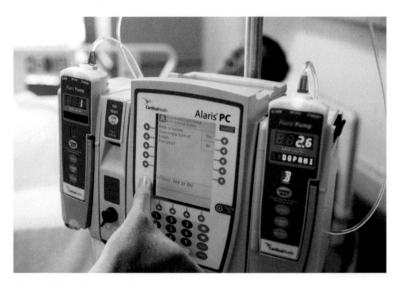

Figure 15-9 Rate controller.

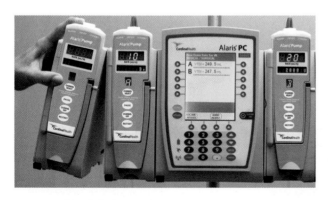

Figure 15-10 Infusion pump.

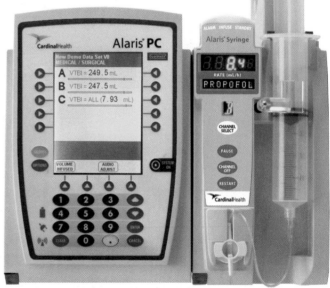

Figure 15-11 Syringe pump.

Copyright © 2016 by McGraw-Hill Education

CHAPTER 15 Intravenous Calculations **421**

Patient-controlled analgesia (PCA) devices are used by patients in pain, including pain from cancer or surgery (Figure 15-12). PCA pumps allow patients to control their own medication within limits preset according to the order of the authorized prescriber. By pressing a button on a hand-held device, a patient administers medication. The PCA device helps monitor the effectiveness of the pain relief prescription, recording the number of times the patient uses the device.

Volume control sets such as Buretrol, Soluset, and Volutrol are used with manual IV setups and electronic rate controllers to improve accuracy, especially for small volumes of medication or fluid (Figure 15-13). They are calibrated in 1 mL increments, with a total volume capacity ranging from 100 to 150 mL. Medication is injected through an injection port into a burette—a chamber that holds a smaller, controlled amount of fluid. An exact amount of IV fluid is added as a diluent to the burette chamber, where it is mixed. The fluid is delivered to the patient in microdrips. Burettes are often used in critical care or pediatric IVs because of their accuracy.

Peripheral and Central IV Therapy

Peripheral IV therapy accesses the circulatory system through a peripheral vein. Sites are usually located in the hand, forearm, foot, and leg. Because peripheral veins can be difficult to locate in small or premature infants, a peripheral IV line may be set up using a vein in the scalp.

Central IV therapy provides direct access to major veins. See Figure 15-14. A **central line** is used when the patient needs large amounts of fluids, a rapid infusion of medication, infusion of highly concentrated solutions, or long-term IV therapy. Central lines can be inserted using a catheter through the chest wall (Figure 15-15) or by threading a catheter through a peripheral vein. In newborn infants, a central line can be inserted into the umbilical vein or artery. These procedures are usually performed by a physician. A **peripherally inserted central catheter (PICC)** is inserted in arm veins and threaded into a central vein, often by specially trained nurses. A **Port-A-Cath** is used to deliver medication to a central vein. It is surgically placed under the skin and accessed through the skin to administer IV medication on an intermittent basis.

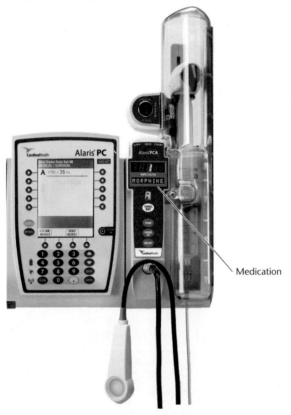

Figure 15-12 Pain medication, such as morphine, is delivered through a PCA pump.

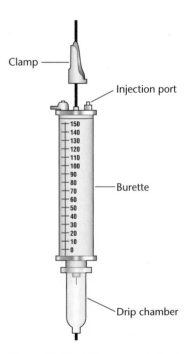

Figure 15-13 Volume control set.

RULE 15-4 | Never flush a sluggish IV with a syringe.

If you flush or irrigate an IV catheter that is clogged, you may be pushing a clot into the circulatory system. This clot, known as an *embolism*, can travel through the bloodstream and block a blood vessel. An obstruction or blockage of any blood vessel in the body is dangerous. An obstruction of a blood vessel in a vital organ such as the heart or lungs can be fatal.

Pain or swelling near an IV site may indicate an infiltration or phlebitis. An **infiltration** occurs when the needle or catheter is dislodged from the vein or penetrates the vein. Fluid is then infused into the surrounding tissue (Figure 15-16). Signs of infiltration include swelling, discomfort, and coolness at the infiltration site, as well as a sizable decrease in flow rate.

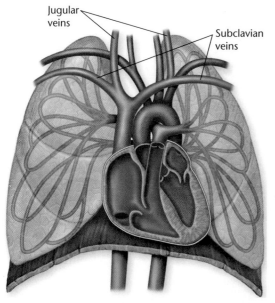

Figure 15-14   A central venous line is usually inserted into the internal jugular or subclavian veins.

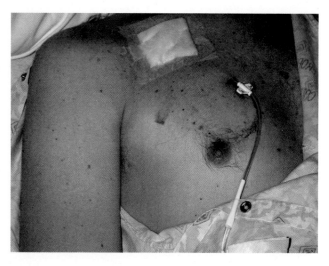

Figure 15-15   Central venous line inserted through the chest wall.

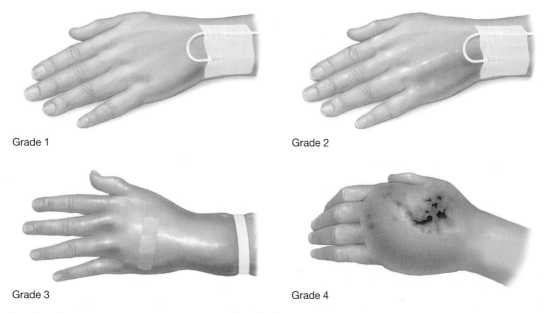

Grade 1

Grade 2

Grade 3

Grade 4

Figure 15-16   The Infusion Nurses Society classifies IV infiltration as pictured here and described in Table 15-3.

Table 15-3 lists the signs associated with varying grades of IV infiltration. **Phlebitis** is an inflammation of the vein. It can develop when the vein is irritated by IV additives, by movement of the needle or catheter, or during long-term IV therapy. In most cases of phlebitis, patients complain of pain at or near the site. Other signs include heat, redness, and swelling of the injection site. In the case of either infiltration or phlebitis, stop the IV infusion and restart it in another limb. In the case of phlebitis, also notify the patient's physician.

TABLE 15-3 Infusion Nurses Society IV INFILTRATION Scale	
GRADE	CLINICAL CRITERIA
0	No symptoms
1	Skin blanched Edema < 1 in. around site Cool to touch With or without pain
2	Skin blanched Edema < 6 in. around site Cool to touch With or without pain
3	Skin blanched and translucent Gross edema > 6 in. around site Cool to touch Mild to moderate pain Possible numbness
4	Skin blanched and translucent Skin tight, leaking Skin discolored, bruised, swollen Gross edema > 6 in. around site Deep pitting tissue edema Circulatory impairment Moderate to severe pain Infiltration of any amount of blood product, irritant, or vesicant

REVIEW AND PRACTICE

15.2 IV Equipment

For Exercises 1–8, identify the IV equipment that you would use in each instance.

1. Add a dose of medication to an existing line.

2. Adjust the flow rate of an IV solution.

3. Stop the IV flow without disturbing the flow rate.

4. Introduce IV fluid into a central vein.

5. Set up tubing to infuse D5W at the rate of 40 mL/h.

6. Allow patient to self-administer medication for pain.

7. Administer a small amount of fluid over 15 minutes.

8. Administer an exact amount of IV fluid added as a diluent that is mixed and delivered in microdrips to a pediatric patient.

Provide a brief response to each of the following questions.

9. When would central IV therapy be used?

10. What are some problems that can occur with an IV?

11. How might you recognize infiltration?

12. What are three possible causes of phlebitis?

13. How high should the IV bag be hung?

14. What four electronic devices can be used to regulate the flow of IV infusions?

15. When is an injection port used?

15.3 Calculating Flow Rates

An order for IV fluids indicates the amount of an IV fluid to be administered and the length of time over which it is to be given. Before you can administer the IV, you must calculate a **flow rate** for the intravenous solution from these two values. For most electronic devices that regulate the flow of IV solutions, the flow rate will be expressed in milliliters per hour (mL/h).

RULE 15-5

To calculate flow rates in milliliters per hour, identify the following:

- V (volume) is expressed in milliliters.

- T (time) must be expressed in hours. (Convert the units when necessary by using the proportion method or dimensional analysis.)

- F (flow rate) will be rounded to the nearest whole number.

Use the formula $F = \frac{V}{T}$ to determine the flow rate in milliliters per hour.

FORMULA METHOD

EXAMPLE 1   Find the flow rate.

Ordered: 500 mg ampicillin in 100 mL NS to infuse over 30 minutes

STEP A: GATHER INFORMATION AND CONVERT
In this case the volume is expressed in milliliters, and $V = 100$ mL.

Since time is expressed in minutes, you must first convert 30 minutes (min) to hours to find T. In this example, the proportion method is used.

$$\frac{1\ h}{60\ min} = \frac{x}{30\ min}$$

$$\frac{1\ h}{60\ \cancel{min}} = \frac{x}{30\ \cancel{min}}$$

$$60 \times x = 1\ h \times 30$$

$$x = \frac{1\ h \times 30}{60}$$

$$x = 0.5\ h$$

We now have the information needed in the proper units.

$$V = 100 \text{ mL} \quad \text{and} \quad T = 0.5 \text{ h}$$

STEP B: CALCULATE

Using the formula $F = \frac{V}{T}$, we find that

$$F = \frac{100 \text{ mL}}{0.5 \text{ h}}$$

$$F = \frac{200 \text{ mL}}{\text{h}}$$

STEP C: THINK! . . . IS IT REASONABLE?

If 100 mL infuses in $\frac{1}{2}$ hour then 200 mL would infuse in 1 hour.

| EXAMPLE 2 | Find the flow rate. |

Ordered: 500 mL D5 1/2 NS over 3 h

STEP A: GATHER INFORMATION AND CONVERT

In this case the units are already expressed in milliliters and hours; $V = 500$ mL and $T = 3$ h.

No conversion is needed.

STEP B: CALCULATE

Using the formula $F = \frac{V}{T}$, we have

$$F = \frac{500 \text{ mL}}{3 \text{ h}}$$

$$F = 166.7 \text{ mL/h}$$

$$F = 167 \text{ mL/h} \quad \text{rounded to nearest whole number}$$

STEP C: THINK! . . . IS IT REASONABLE?

If 500 mL is divided by 3 hours it equals 166.7, rounded to 167 mL/h.

For a manually regulated IV, the flow rate needs to be calculated as the number of drops per minute (gtt/min). Before this can be calculated, you must first know how many drops are in a milliliter. IV tubing packages are labeled with a drop factor, which tells you how many drops of IV solution are equal to 1 mL when using that tubing (Figures 15-17 and 15-18). Macrodrip tubing has larger drops and usually one of three typical drop factors: 10 gtt/mL, 15 gtt/mL, or 20 gtt/mL. Microdrip tubing has a drop factor of 60 gtt/mL. See Figure 15-19. After you have determined the desired flow rate in gtt/mL, you can adjust the roller or screw clamp so that the drops fall at the desired rate.

Most electronic devices are set at a flow rate of milliliters per hour. However, if you need to check an electronic device manually, then convert milliliters per hour to drops per minute so that you can compare the actual rate (the drops delivered to a patient in 1 minute) with the ordered flow rate in mL/h.

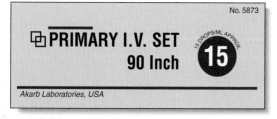

Figure 15-17　15 gtt/mL calibrated macrodrip tubing.

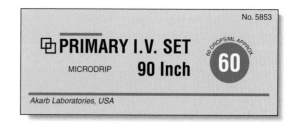

Figure 15-18　60 gtt/mL calibrated microdrip tubing.

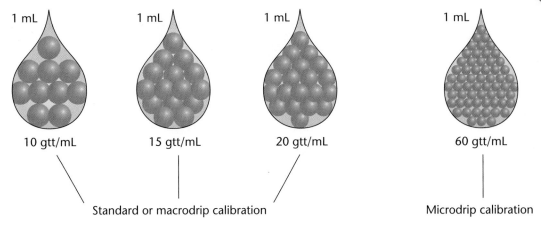

1 mL   1 mL   1 mL   1 mL

10 gtt/mL   15 gtt/mL   20 gtt/mL   60 gtt/mL

Standard or macrodrip calibration   Microdrip calibration

Figure 15-19 Macrodrip and microdrip calibration.

RULE 15-6	To convert the flow rate in milliliters per hour (F) to drops per minute (f), use the formula:

$$f = \frac{F \times C}{60}$$

where F = flow rate, mL/h
C = calibration factor of tubing, gtt/mL
60 = number of minutes in 1 h

Round your answer to the nearest whole number.

FORMULA METHOD

EXAMPLE 1

Find the flow rate in drops per minute that is equal to 75 mL/h when you are using 20 gtt/mL macrodrip tubing.

STEP A: GATHER INFORMATION AND CONVERT

$F = 75$ mL/h

$C = 20$ gtt/mL

No conversion is necessary.

STEP B: CALCULATE

Substituting into the formula gives:

$$f = \frac{F \times C}{60 \text{ min/h}}$$

$$f = \frac{75 \text{ mL/h} \times 20 \text{ gtt/mL}}{60 \text{ min/h}}$$

Cancel units.

$$f = \frac{75 \text{ mL/h} \times 20 \text{ gtt/mL}}{60 \text{ min/h}}$$

Solve the equation.

$$f = 25 \text{ gtt/min}$$

STEP C: THINK! . . . IS IT REASONABLE?

If the flow rate is 75 mL/h and you need to determine the rate in minutes, you can divide by 60 min/h, which equals 1.25 mL/min. Then you multiply by the drop factor of 20 gtt/mL, which equals 25 gtt/min. The answer 25 gtt/min is reasonable.

EXAMPLE 2

Find the flow rate in drops per minute that is equal to 35 mL/h when you are using 60 gtt/mL microdrip tubing.

STEP A: GATHER INFORMATION AND CONVERT

$$F = 35 \text{ mL/h}$$

$$C = 60 \text{ gtt/mL}$$

No conversion is necessary.

STEP B: CALCULATE

Substituting into the formula gives:

$$f = \frac{F \times C}{60}$$

$$f = \frac{35 \text{ mL/h} \times 60 \text{ gtt/mL}}{60 \text{ min/h}}$$

Cancel the units.

$$f = \frac{35 \text{ mL/h} \times 60 \text{ gtt/mL}}{60 \text{ min/h}}$$

$$f = 35 \text{ gtt/min}$$

STEP C: THINK! . . . IS IT REASONABLE?

The value of the flow rate is the same in drops per minute or milliliters per hour when 60 gtt/mL microdrip tubing is used. In other words, for microdrop tubing, $F = f$. In this case, the value calculated for f equals the value for F, so the answer is reasonable.

Adjusting Flow Rates

Counting drops and timing are not always precise. What you calibrated as 25 drops per minute may actually be 25.4 drops per minute. Therefore, adjustments to flow rates sometimes need to be made. You should check at least once every hour that the IV is infusing to see if it is behind or ahead of schedule. The policy at the facility where you are employed will dictate whether you may adjust the IV flow rate and how much you can adjust it or whether you should notify the physician instead. Always check this policy before you adjust a flow rate. If an adjustment is to be made, always double-check your calculations, especially when a large adjustment is indicated.

RULE 15-7

To adjust the flow rate:

- Check the guidelines at your facility to determine whether you are allowed to adjust the flow rate.

- To recalculate the infusion rate in gtt/min (f), use the volume remaining in the IV and the time remaining in the order in minutes. Use the following formula:

$$f = C \times \frac{V}{T}$$

where C = calibration factor of tubing, in gtt/mL
V = the volume remaining in the IV, in mL
T = time remaining from original order (original infusion time—time elapsed), in minutes

- To recalculate the infusion rate in mL/h (F), use the volume remaining in the IV and the time in hours remaining for the order. Use the following formula.

$$F = \frac{V}{T}$$

FORMULA METHOD

EXAMPLE 1 Calculate the adjustment in gtt/min.

Original order: 1,500 mL NS over 12 h

The IV was infused at an ordered rate of 42 gtt/min using 20 gtt/mL macrodrip tubing. After 3 h, 1,200 mL remains in the bag.

STEP A: GATHER INFORMATION AND CONVERT

$V = 1{,}200$ mL (volume remaining)

$T = 12$ h original $- 3$ h elapsed $= 9$ h remaining

$C = 20$ gtt/mL

Notice that, unlike the formula to convert mL/h to gtt/min, this formula requires the time in minutes. Before we can use the formula, we must first convert 9 h to minutes. Using the proportion method with ratios, we find:

$$\frac{60 \text{ min}}{1 \text{ h}} = \frac{T}{9 \text{ h}}$$

$$\frac{60 \text{ min}}{1 \cancel{h}} = \frac{T}{9 \cancel{h}}$$

$$T \times 1 = 60 \text{ min} \times 9$$

$$T = 540 \text{ min}$$

Now we have all of the information needed for the formula: $C = 20$ gtt/mL, $V = 1{,}200$ mL, and $T = 540$ min.

STEP B: CALCULATE

Insert the appropriate numbers into the formula.

$$f = C \times \frac{V}{T}$$

$$f = 20 \text{ gtt/mL} \times \frac{1{,}200 \text{ mL}}{540 \text{ min}}$$

Cancel units.

$$f = 20 \text{ gtt/}\cancel{mL} \times \frac{1{,}200 \cancel{mL}}{540 \text{ min}}$$

Solve for the unknown.

$$f = 20 \text{ gtt} \times \frac{1{,}200}{540 \text{ min}}$$

$$f = 44.4 \text{ gtt/min}$$

Round to the nearest whole number.

$$f = 44 \text{ gtt/min} = \text{adjusted flow rate}$$

Note: You can also determine the IV rate adjustment in mL/h by dividing the remaining hours into the remaining volume.

STEP C: THINK!. . .IS IT REASONABLE?
The policy states that the flow rate cannot be adjusted by more than 10 gtt/min. Since the original flow rate is 42 gtt/min and the new flow rate is 44 gtt/min, the change in the gtt/min is reasonable.

EXAMPLE 2

Calculate the adjustment in gtt/min.

Original order: 1,500 mL NS over 12 h

Using 15 gtt/mL macrodrip tubing, the IV should have infused at 31 gtt/min. After 4 h, 1,100 mL remains in the bag.

STEP A: GATHER INFORMATION AND CONVERT

V = 1,100 mL (volume remaining)

T = 12 h − 4 h = 8 h remaining

C = 15 gtt/mL

Before we can use the formula $f = C \times \dfrac{V}{T}$, we must convert 8 h to minutes. Using the proportion method with fractions, we have:

$$\frac{1 \cancel{h}}{60 \text{ min}} = \frac{8 \cancel{h}}{x}$$

$$1 \times x \text{ min} = 60 \times 8$$

$$x \text{ min} = 480$$

Now we have all of the information needed for the formula: C = 15 gtt/mL, V = 1,100 mL, and T = 480 min.

STEP B: CALCULATE

Insert the appropriate numbers into the formula.

$$f = 15 \text{ gtt/mL} \times \frac{1{,}100 \text{ mL}}{480 \text{ min}}$$

Cancel units.

$$f = 15 \text{ gtt/}\cancel{\text{mL}} \times \frac{1{,}100 \ \cancel{\text{mL}}}{480 \text{ min}}$$

Solve for the unknown.

$$f = 15 \text{ gtt} \times \frac{1{,}100}{480 \text{ min}}$$

$$f = 34.4 \text{ gtt/min}$$

Round to the nearest whole number.

$$f = 34 \text{ gtt/min} = \text{adjusted flow rate}$$

STEP C: THINK!. . .IS IT REASONABLE?

The policy states that the flow rate cannot be adjusted by more than 10 gtt/min. The original flow rate is 42 gtt/min. The adjusted flow rate is 33 gtt/min. In this case, the answer is reasonable.

EXAMPLE 3

Calculate the adjustment in mL/h.

Original order: 1,500 mL NS over 12 h

After 4 h, 1,100 mL remains in the bag.

STEP A: GATHER INFORMATION AND CONVERT

V = 1,100 mL (volume remaining)

T = 12 h − 4 h = 8 h remaining

We have all the information needed for the formula. No conversion is necessary.

V = 1,100 mL T = 8 h

STEP B: CALCULATE

Insert the appropriate numbers into the formula.

$$F = \frac{V}{T}$$

$$F = \frac{1{,}100 \text{ mL}}{8 \text{ h}}$$

Solve for the unknown.

$F = 137.5$ mL/h

Round to the nearest whole number.

$F = 138$ mL/h

STEP C: THINK!. . .IS IT REASONABLE?
The policy states the flow rate cannot be adjusted more than 20 mL/h. Calculate the original flow rate of 1,500 mL/12 h, which equals 125 mL/h. The new flow rate is 138 mL/h. Since 138 mL/h is only 13 mL/h greater than the original rate, the adjustment can be made.

CRITICAL THINKING ON THE JOB

Adjusting the Flow Rate

Earlier in the day, Pat set up an IV based on the following physician's order: 750 mL D5NS to infuse over 8 h. Pat calculated that the patient should receive 94 mL of fluid per hour, with a flow rate of 16 gtt/min using 10 gtt/mL tubing.

After 4 h (one-half the time ordered for the infusion), Pat observed that 450 mL remained in the IV bag. Only one-half of the fluid, or 375 mL, should have remained in the bag. The patient had received 75 mL less fluid than expected. Pat decided to reset the flow rate for the next hour so that the patient would receive the original 94 mL/h plus the 75 mL that should have already been administered, for a total of 169 mL. After the next hour, Pat planned to reset the IV to the original flow rate of 16 gtt/min. Pat calculated the new flow rate as

$$\frac{10 \text{ gtt}}{1 \text{ mL}} \times \frac{169 \text{ mL}}{1 \text{ h}} \times \frac{1 \text{ h}}{60 \text{ min}} =$$

$$\frac{28.17 \text{ gtt}}{1 \text{ min}} = 28 \text{ gtt/min}$$

Thus, Pat adjusted the flow rate to 28 gtt/min.

Think! . . . Is It Reasonable? What mistake did Pat make? What should Pat have done to avoid the mistake?

REVIEW AND PRACTICE

15.3 Calculating Flow Rates

For Exercises 1–4, find the flow rate in milliliters per hour.

1. Ordered: 1,000 mL LR over 6 h

2. Ordered: 300 mL NS over 2 h

3. Ordered: 3,000 mL 1/2 NS q24h

4. Ordered: 40 mEq KCl in 100 mL NS over 45 min

For Exercises 5–10, calculate the flow rate for IVs using electronic devices.

5. Ordered: 1,500 mL RL over 12 h, using an infusion pump

6. Ordered: 1,000 mL NS over 12 h, using an infusion pump

7. Ordered: 750 mL NS over 8 h, using an electronic controller set in milliliters per hour

8. Ordered: 20 mEq KCl in 50 mL NS over 30 min, using an electronic rate controller set in milliliters per hour

9. Ordered: 1,800 mL 1/2 NS per day by infusion pump

10. Ordered: 250 mL D5W over 3 h by infusion pump

For Exercises 11–16, calculate the flow rate for manually regulated IVs.

11. Ordered: 1,000 mL NS over 24 h, tubing is 20 gtt/mL

12. Ordered: 400 mL RL over 8 h, tubing is 10 gtt/mL

13. Ordered: 1,500 mL 0.45% S over 12 h, tubing is 15 gtt/mL

14. Ordered: 250 mL D5W over 3 h, tubing is 10 gtt/mL

15. Ordered: 40 mEq KCl in 100 mL NS over 40 min, tubing is 20 gtt/mL

16. Ordered: 500 mL NS over 8 h, tubing is 15 gtt/mL

For Exercises 17–20, look at the drop factor (gtt/mL) on labels A–D to calculate flow rates.

17. Ordered: 3,000 mL NS over 24 h, refer to Label A.

18. Ordered: 50 mL penicillin IV over 1 h, refer to Label B.

19. Ordered: 750 mL 5%D NS over 5 h, refer to Label C.

20. Ordered: 100 mL gentamicin over 30 min, refer to Label D.

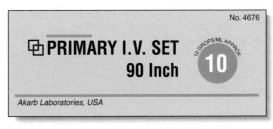

A

For Exercises 21 and 22, calculate the flow rate in drops per minute.

21. Ordered: 1,000 mL D5W over 9 h, using an electronic controller set in drops per minute, tubing calibration is 15 gtt/mL

22. Ordered: 750 mL RL over 8 h by electronic rate controller set in drops per minute, tubing calibration is 15 gtt/mL

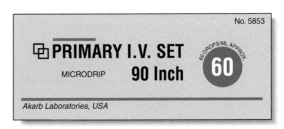

B

For Exercises 23–25, calculate the ordered flow rate in gtt/min and mL/h. Then determine if an adjustment is necessary and calculate the adjusted flow rate in gtt/min and mL/h.

23. Ordered: 375 mL RL over 3 h (10 gtt/mL tubing). After 1 h, 175 mL has infused.

24. Ordered: 1,000 mL NS over 8 h (20 gtt/mL tubing). With 5 h remaining, 550 mL of NS remains in the IV bag.

25. Ordered: 500 mL D5W over 4 h (15 gtt/mL tubing). After 2 h, 200 mL has infused

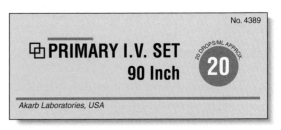

C

For Exercises 26–30, you must manually check the IV infusion rate. Calculate the rate in drops per minute.

26. Rate controller set at 200 mL/h, tubing 10 gtt/mL

27. Infusion pump set at 125 mL/h, tubing 15 gtt/mL

28. Electronic pump set at 150 mL/h, tubing 15 gtt/mL

29. Pediatric infusion set at 75 mL/h, tubing 60 gtt/mL

30. Rate controller set at 100 mL/h, tubing 10 gtt/mL

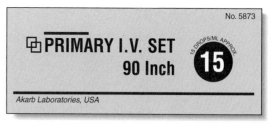

D

15.4 Infusion Time and Volume

An order may call for a certain amount of fluid to infuse at a specific rate, without specifying the duration. In this case you will need to calculate the duration or amount of time the IV will take to infuse, so that you can monitor the IV properly. In other cases, you may know the duration and the flow rate, and you will need to calculate the fluid volume.

Calculating Infusion Time

In the previous section, you calculated the rate of infusion when given the volume and time. Sometimes the infusion rate and volume are given in the order, and you will need to calculate the duration or amount of time the infusion will take to be administered.

RULE 15-8	To calculate infusion time in hours *T*, identify:

- *V* (volume) expressed in milliliters.

- *F* (flow rate) expressed in milliliters per hour.

- Fractional hours expressed in minutes by multiplying by 60.

Use the formula $T = \frac{V}{F}$ to find *T*, the infusion time in hours.

FORMULA METHOD

EXAMPLE 1	**Find the total time to infuse.**

Ordered: 1,000 mL NS to infuse at a rate of 75 mL/h

STEP A: GATHER INFORMATION AND CONVERT
The volume $V = 1,000$ mL. The flow rate *F* is : $F = 75$ mL/h. No conversions are necessary to use the formula.

STEP B: CALCULATE
Substitute the values into the formula $T = \frac{V}{F}$.

$$T = \frac{1,000 \text{ mL}}{75 \text{ mL/h}}$$

Cancel the units.

$$T = \frac{1,000 \text{ mL}}{75 \text{ mL/h}}$$

$$T = 13.33 \text{ h} = \text{total time to infuse 1,000 mL}$$

Note that 0.33 h does not represent 33 minutes. Because there are 60 min in 1 h, you must multiply the fractional hour by 60 to convert it to minutes.

$$0.33 \text{ h} \times 60 \text{ min/h} = 20 \text{ min}$$

The total time to infuse the solution is 13 h 20 min.

STEP C: THINK!. . .IS IT REASONABLE?

Check your math to determine whether the answer is reasonable: multiply your answer, 13.33 h, by the flow rate, 75 mL/h. The answer should equal the volume to be infused. In this case, 13.33 h × 75 mL/h = 999.8 mL, which rounds to 1,000 mL, so the answer is reasonable.

EXAMPLE 2   Find the total time to infuse.

Ordered: 750 mL LR to infuse at a rate of 125 mL/h started at 11 p.m.

STEP A: GATHER INFORMATION AND CONVERT
The volume $V = 750$ mL. The flow rate F is expressed in milliliters per hour, $F = 125$ mL/h. No conversion is necessary.

STEP B: CALCULATE
Substitute the values into the formula $T = \frac{V}{F}$.

$$T = \frac{750 \text{ mL}}{125 \text{ mL/h}}$$

$T = 6$ h = total time to infuse 750 mL

STEP C: THINK!. . .IS IT REASONABLE?
Multiply your answer by the flow rate to see if your answer is reasonable. The answer should equal the volume to be infused. In this case, 6 h × 125 mL/h = 750 mL, so the answer is reasonable.

In some cases, you will need to determine the time an infusion will be completed.

RULE 15-9   To calculate the time when an infusion will be completed, you must first know the time the infusion started in military time and the total time, in hours and minutes, required to infuse the solution ordered. Since each day is only 24 hours long, when the sum is greater than 2400 (midnight), you must start a new day by subtracting 2400. This will determine the time of completion, which will be the next calendar day.

Example 1   Determine when the following infusion will be completed.

Ordered: 1,000 mL NS to infuse at a rate of 75 mL/h

You start the infusion at 7 a.m. on 6/06/14. First determine the start time in military or international time: 7 a.m. = 0700.

 LEARNING LINK   Recall from the "Temperature and Time" chapter the rule about how to use the 24-hour clock.

Next, calculate the infusion time using the formula: $T = \frac{V}{F}$

$$T = \frac{1,000 \text{ mL}}{75 \text{ mL/h}}$$

$T = 13.33$ h or 13 h 20 min

Now, add the total amount of time (in hours and minutes) writing the hours followed by minutes. Since the infusion time is 13 h 20 min, add 1320.

	0700 time started in military or international time
	+1320 total amount of time in hours and minutes
	2020

The infusion will be completed at 2020, which is 8:20 p.m.

| **Example 2** | Determine when the infusion will be completed.

Ordered: 750 mL LR to infuse at a rate of 125 mL/h, started at 11 p.m. on 8/04/15

First, determine the start time using international or military notation: 11 p.m. = 2300.

Next, calculate the infusion time, $T = \frac{V}{F}$:

$$T = \frac{750 \text{ mL}}{125 \text{ mL/h}}$$

$$T = 6 \text{ h}$$

Add the total amount of time to infuse, which was determined as 6 h, 00 minutes; therefore add 600 to the starting time.

    2300   time started in military or international time
+ 600   total amount of time of infusion in hours and minutes
    2900   sum is greater than 2400
−2400   subtract 2400
     500

The infusion will be complete at 0500, or 5:00 a.m., on 8/05/15. |

Calculating Infusion Volume

When infusion rate and infusion time are given in the order, the volume infused over a given period of time can be calculated so that you can monitor the IV properly.

| **RULE 15-10** | To calculate infusion volume:
Use the formula $V = T \times F$ or dimensional analysis to find the infusion volume V in milliliters, where:

- T (time) must be expressed in hours.
- F (flow rate) must be expressed in milliliters per hour. |

FORMULA METHOD

EXAMPLE 1	Find the total volume infused in 5 h if the infusion rate is 35 mL/h.
	STEP A: GATHER INFORMATION AND CONVERT
The total infusion time $T = 5$ h. The flow rate F is expressed in milliliters per hour: $F = 35$ mL/h. No conversion is necessary.

STEP B: CALCULATE
$$T = 5 \text{ h}$$
$$F = 35 \text{ mL/h}$$ |

Substitute the values into the formula $V = T \times F$.

$$V = 5\text{ h} \times 35\text{ mL/h}$$

$$V = 175\text{ mL} = \text{volume that will infuse over 5 h}$$

STEP C: THINK!. . .IS IT REASONABLE?
Divide your answer by the total time specified in the order to see if your answer is reasonable. The answer should equal the specified flow rate. In this case, 175 mL divided by 5 hours equals 35 mL/h, so the answer is reasonable.

| **EXAMPLE 2** | Find the total volume infused in 12 h if the infusion rate is 200 mL/h. |

STEP A: GATHER INFORMATION AND CONVERT
The total infusion time $T = 12$ h. The flow rate F is expressed in milliliters per hour: $F = 200$ mL/h. No conversion is necessary.

STEP B: CALCULATE
Substitute the values into the formula.

$$V = 12\text{ h} \times 200\text{ mL/h}$$

$$V = 2{,}400\text{ mL} = \text{volume that will infuse over 12 h}$$

STEP C: THINK!. . .IS IT REASONABLE?
Divide your answer by the total time specified in the order to see if your answer is reasonable. The answer should equal the specified flow rate. In this case, 2,400 mL divided by 12 hours equals 200 mL/h, so the answer is reasonable.

DIMENSIONAL ANALYSIS

| **EXAMPLE 1** | Find the total volume infused in 5 h if the infusion rate is 35 mL/h. |

STEP A: GATHER INFORMATION AND CONVERT
The total infusion time $T = 5$ h. The flow rate F is expressed in milliliters per hour: $F = 35$ mL/h. No conversion factor is necessary.

STEP B: CALCULATE
1. Determine the unit of measure for the answer V, and place it as the unknown on the left side of the equation.

   $$V\text{ mL} =$$

2. The first factor is the length of time of the infusion over 1.
   $$V\text{ mL} = \frac{5\text{ h}}{1}$$

3. Multiply the first factor by the flow rate to finish setting up the equation.
   $$V\text{ mL} = \frac{5\text{ h}}{1} \times \frac{35\text{ mL}}{1\text{ h}}$$

4. Cancel units on the right side of the equation. The remaining unit of measure on the right side of the equation should match the unit of measure on the left side of the equation.
   $$V\text{ mL} = \frac{5\,\cancel{\text{h}}}{1} \times \frac{35\text{ mL}}{\cancel{\text{h}}}$$

5. Solve the equation.

   $$V\text{ mL} = 175\text{ mL to be infused in 5 h}$$

STEP C: THINK!. . .IS IT REASONABLE?
Divide 175 mL by 5 hours. The answer equals the specified flow rate of 35 mL/h, so the answer is reasonable.

| EXAMPLE 2 | Find the total volume infused in 12 h if the infusion rate is 200 mL/h. |

STEP A: GATHER INFORMATION AND CONVERT

The total infusion time $T = 12$ h. The flow rate F is expressed in milliliters per hour: $F = 200$ mL/h. No conversion is necessary.

STEP B: CALCULATE

1. Determine the unit of measure for the answer (V), and place it as the unknown on the left side of the equation.

$$V \text{ mL} =$$

2. The first factor is the length of time of the infusion over 1.

$$V \text{ mL} = \frac{12 \text{ h}}{1}$$

3. Multiply the first factor by the flow rate.

$$V \text{ mL} = \frac{12 \text{ h}}{1} \times \frac{200 \text{ mL}}{\text{h}}$$

4. Cancel units on the right side of the equation. The remaining unit of measure on the right side of the equation should match the unit of measure on the left side of the equation.

$$V \text{ mL} = \frac{12 \cancel{\text{h}}}{1} \times \frac{200 \text{ mL}}{\cancel{\text{h}}}$$

5. Solve the equation.

$$V \text{ mL} = 2{,}400 \text{ mL to be infused in 12 h}$$

STEP C: THINK!. . .IS IT REASONABLE?

Divide 2,400 mL by 12 hours. The answer equals the specified flow rate of 200 mL/h, so the answer is reasonable.

REVIEW AND PRACTICE

15.4 Infusion Time and Volume

For Exercises 1–5, find the total time to infuse.

1. Ordered: 1,000 mL NS at 83 mL/h using an infusion pump

2. Ordered: 500 mL LR at 125 mL/h using microdrip tubing

3. Ordered: 750 mL 1/2 NS at 31 mL/h

4. Ordered: 1,000 mL NS at 200 mL/h

5. Ordered 250 mL D5W at 100 mL/h using an infusion pump

For Exercises 6–10, find when the infusion will be completed.

6. Ordered: 1,500 mL D5W with 30 mEq KCl/L at a rate of 75 mL/h. You start the infusion at noon.

7. Ordered: 2,000 mL NS via infusion pump at 100 mL/h. You start the infusion at 3:30 p.m.

8. Ordered: 750 mL RL at 50 mL/h. You start the IV at 1000.

9. Ordered: 250 mL via a microdrip set at 40 mL/h. You start the infusion at 9:45 p.m.

10. Ordered: 500 mL $\frac{1}{2}$ NS at 75 mL/h. The infusion started at 1615.

For Exercises 11–14, find the total volume to administer.

11. 75 mL/h 1/2 NS for 2 h 30 min using a rate controller

12. D5RL set at 100 mL/h for 8 h

13. D5W at 125 mL/h for 12 h using an infusion pump

14. An antibiotic solution infused over 2 h at 75 mL/h

15.5 Intermittent IV Infusions

IV medications are sometimes delivered on an intermittent basis. Intermittent medications can be delivered through an IV secondary line or a saline or heparin lock. Intermittent IV infusions are usually delivered through an IV secondary line when the patient is receiving continuous IV therapy. Intermittent IV infusions or IV push medications can also be delivered through a saline or heparin lock when the patient does not require continuous or replacement fluids.

Secondary Lines (Piggyback)

As stated in Section 15.2, a secondary line is used to infuse medications through an intravenous piggyback (IVPB) system. IVPB medications are typically infused via mini-bags of 50, 100, 150, 200, or 250 mL of fluid. (See Figure 15-20.)

Intermittent Peripheral Infusion Devices

You can administer medication to a patient on a regular, though not continuous, schedule by using an *intermittent peripheral infusion device*. These devices are more commonly known as **heparin locks** or **saline locks.** To create a lock, attach an infusion port to an already inserted IV catheter. This port allows you to inject medication directly into the vein by using a syringe or to infuse medication intermittently. (See Figure 15-21.) Physicians' orders will list IV push or bolus for medication that is injected into an IV line or through a saline or heparin lock.

Fluids do not flow continuously through the IV needle or catheter when a lock is used. To prevent blockage of the line, the device must be flushed 2 or 3 times a day or after administering medication. A saline lock is flushed or irrigated with saline. A heparin lock is flushed or irrigated with saline mixed with heparin, an anticoagulant that retards clot formation. The policy of the facility and the device will dictate the amount and concentration of solution to use. Saline or saline and heparin fills the infusion port and IV catheter, preventing blood from entering and becoming trapped. If blood were trapped, a clot would form, blocking the catheter.

Preparing and Calculating Intermittent Infusions

Frequently, intermittent medications are already reconstituted and prepared for administration by piggyback or through a heparin or saline lock. The flow rate for prepared medications is calculated in the same manner as regular IV infusions. The amount of fluid may be less and the amount of time to infuse may be less than an hour, so to calculate the flow rate you will need to change the number of minutes into hours (see Example 1 for Rule 15-5).

In some cases, you will be required to reconstitute and prepare a medication for IV infusion or calculate the amount to administer for an IV push medication.

When intermittent IV infusions are given through a saline or heparin lock, the lock should be irrigated or flushed before and after administration. If you meet resistance when flushing a saline or heparin lock, stop the procedure immediately so that you do not force a clot into the bloodstream.

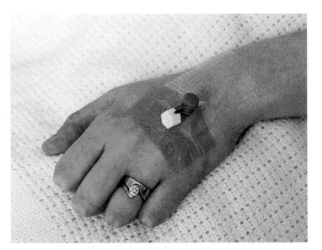

5%
Dextrose
Injection USP

LOT
EXP
2B0087
NDC 0338-0017-48

100mL SINGLE DOSE CONTAINER EACH 100 mL CONTAINS 5 g DEXTROSE HYDROUS USP pH 4.0 (3.2 TO 6.5) OSMOLARITY 252 mOsmol/L (CALC) STERILE NONPYROGENIC READ PACKAGE INSERT FOR FULL INFORMATION ADDITIVES MAY BE INCOMPATIBLE DOSAGE INTRAVENOUSLY AS DIRECTED BY A PHYSICIAN CAUTIONS MUST NOT BE USED IN SERIES CONNECTIONS DO NOT ADMINISTER SIMULTANEOUSLY WITH BLOOD DO NOT USE UNLESS SOLUTION IS CLEAR **Rx ONLY** VIAFLEX CONTAINER PL 146 PLASTIC BAXTER VIAFLEX AND PL 146 ARE TRADEMARKS OF BAXTER INTERNATIONAL INC

Baxter
BAXTER HEALTHCARE CORPORATION
DEERFIELD IL 60015 USA
MADE IN USA

Figure 15-20 A 100 mL bag of IV fluid with a label like this one may be used to mix and administer intermittent IV infusions.

Figure 15-21 Intermittent peripheral infusion device—also called saline lock or heparin lock.

RULE 15-11	When you prepare medication for an intermittent IV infusion:
	• Reconstitute the medication, using the label and package insert.
	• Calculate the amount to administer and the flow rate.
Example	Ordered: Eloxatin® 75 mg in 250 mL D5W IV piggyback over 90 min
	On hand: Eloxatin® (oxaliplatin injection) 5 mg/mL injection 100 mg single-use vial
	According to the package insert, Eloxatin® should be reconstituted with 20 mL of water for injection or 5% dextrose for injection. The dosage strength of the medication will be 100 mg/20 mL. First, calculate the amount of medication to administer using the proportion method, dimensional analysis, or the formula method.

PROPORTION METHOD

EXAMPLE	Calculate the amount to administer.
	STEP A: GATHER INFORMATION AND CONVERT
	Refer to the information in the example for Rule 15-11. Since the dosage ordered is 75 mg, you will calculate the amount to administer using the following information:
	D (desired dose) = 75 mg
	H (dose on hand) = 100 mg
	Q (dosage unit) = 20 mL
	Because the dosage ordered and the desired dose are both in milligrams, no unit conversion is necessary.

STEP B: CALCULATE
Follow Procedure Checklist 12-1.

1. Set up the proportion using fractions.

$$\frac{H}{Q} = \frac{D}{A}$$

$$\frac{100 \text{ mg}}{20 \text{ mL}} = \frac{75 \text{ mg}}{A}$$

2. Cancel units.

$$\frac{100 \text{ m\cancel{g}}}{20 \text{ mL}} = \frac{75 \text{ m\cancel{g}}}{A}$$

3. Cross-multiply and solve for the unknown.

$$100 \times A = 20 \text{ mL} \times 75$$

$$A = 20 \text{ mL} \times \frac{75}{100}$$

$$A = 15 \text{ mL}$$

STEP C: THINK . . . IS IT REASONABLE?
Since the ordered dose is $\frac{3}{4}$ of the supply dose, the ordered volume, 15 mL, is reasonable as it is $\frac{3}{4}$ of the supply volume (dosage unit).

DIMENSIONAL ANALYSIS

EXAMPLE

Calculate the amount to administer.

STEP A: GATHER INFORMATION AND CONVERT

Refer to the information in the example for Rule 15-11 on page 439. Since the dosage ordered is 75 mg, you will calculate the amount to administer using the following information:

D (desired dose) = 75 mg

H (dose on hand) = 100 mg

Q (dosage unit) = 20 mL

Because the dosage ordered and the desired dose are both in milligrams, no conversion factor is necessary.

STEP B: CALCULATE
Follow Procedure Checklist 12-2.

1. The unit of measure for the amount to administer will be milliliters.

A mL =

2. Since the unit of measurement for the dosage ordered is the same as that for the dose on hand, no conversion factor is necessary.

3. The dosage unit is 20 mL. The dose on hand is 100 mg. This is the first factor.

$$A \text{ mL} = \frac{20 \text{ mL}}{100 \text{ mg}}$$

4. The dosage ordered is 75 mg.

$$A \text{ mL} = \frac{20 \text{ mL}}{100 \text{ mg}} \times \frac{75 \text{ mg}}{1}$$

5. Cancel units.

$$A \text{ mL} = \frac{20 \text{ mL}}{100 \text{ m\cancel{g}}} \times \frac{75 \text{ m\cancel{g}}}{1}$$

6. Solve the equation.

$$A \text{ mL} = \frac{20 \text{ mL}}{100} \times \frac{75}{1}$$
$$A = 15 \text{ mL}$$

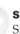

STEP C: THINK . . . IS IT REASONABLE?

Since the ordered dose is $\frac{3}{4}$ of the supply dose, the ordered volume, 15 mL, is reasonable as it is $\frac{3}{4}$ of the supply volume (dosage unit).

FORMULA METHOD

EXAMPLE

Calculate the amount to administer.

STEP A: GATHER INFORMATION AND CONVERT

Refer to the information in the example for Rule 15-11 on page 439. Since the dosage ordered is 75 mg, you will calculate the amount to administer using the following information:

D (desired dose) = 75 mg

H (dose on hand) = 100 mg

Q (dosage unit) = 20 mL

Because the dosage ordered and the desired dose are both in milligrams, no conversion factor is necessary.

STEP B: CALCULATE

Follow Procedure Checklist 12-3.

1. Fill in the formula.

$$\frac{D}{H} \times Q = A$$

$$\frac{75 \text{ mg}}{100 \text{ mg}} \times 20 \text{ mL} = A$$

2. Cancel units.

$$\frac{75 \text{ mg}}{100 \text{ mg}} \times 20 \text{ mL} = A$$

3. Solve for the unknown.

$$\frac{75}{100} \times 20 \text{ mL} = A$$

$$15 \text{ mL} = A$$

STEP C: THINK . . . IS IT REASONABLE?

Since the ordered dose is $\frac{3}{4}$ of the supply dose, the ordered volume, 15 mL, is reasonable as it is $\frac{3}{4}$ of the supply volume (dosage unit).

Once you have determined the amount of medication to administer, you will need to calculate the flow rate.

From the package insert (Figure 15-22), you determine that the reconstituted solution must be further diluted with an infusion solution of 250 to 500 mL of 5% dextrose injection, USP. The order reads to use 250 mL of D5W; so using a sterile needle and proper aseptic technique, you withdraw 15 mL of the diluted medication and inject it into the 250 mL bag of D5W. Now you have a solution of 75 mg of Eloxatin® in 250 D5W, which you must deliver over 90 min.

Add 15 mL medication plus 250 mL of D5W for a total volume of 265 mL. Calculate the flow rate in milliliters per hour, using Rule 15-5.

Note: Check your facility policy. In some cases, 15 mL of IV solution is withdrawn from the IV bag before adding the 15 mL of medication. This will allow the calculation to be based on the original volume of IV fluid, 250 mL.

ELOXATIN™ Prescribing Information
(oxaliplatin for injection)

Preparation of Infusion Solution
  RECONSTITUTION OR FINAL DILUTION MUST NEVER BE PERFORMED WITH A SODIUM CHLORIDE SOLUTION OR OTHER CHLORIDE-CONTAINING SOLUTIONS.

  The lyophilized powder is reconstituted by adding 10 mL (for the 50 mg vial) or 20 mL (for the 100 mg vial) of Water for Injection, USP or 5% Dextrose Injection, USP. Do not administer the reconstituted solution without further dilution. The reconstituted solution must be further diluted in an infusion solution of 250–500 mL of 5% Dextrose Injection, USP.

  After reconstitution in the original vial, the solution may be stored up to 24 hours under refrigeration (2–8°C [36–46°F]). After final dilution with 250–500 mL of 5% Dextrose Injection, USP, the shelf life is 6 hours at room temperature (20–25°C [68–77°F]) or up to 24 hours under refrigeration (2–8°C [36–46°F]). ELOXATIN is not light sensitive.

Figure 15-22

FORMULA METHOD

EXAMPLE

Calculate the flow rate in mL/h.

STEP A: GATHER INFORMATION AND CONVERT

Ordered: Eloxatin® 75 mg in 250 mL D5W IV piggyback over 90 min

Since time is expressed in minutes, you must first convert 90 min to hours to find *T*. (In this example, we will use the proportion method to convert.)

$$\frac{1\,h}{60\,min} = \frac{x}{90\,min}$$

$$\frac{1\,h}{60\,\cancel{min}} = \frac{x}{90\,\cancel{min}}$$

$$60 \times x = 1\,h \times 90$$

$$x = \frac{1\,h \times 90}{60}$$

$$x = 1.5\,h$$

For this example, we will use the volume $V = 265$.

We now have the information needed in the proper units.

$$V = 265\,mL \quad \text{and} \quad T = 1.5\,h$$

STEP B: CALCULATE THE FLOW RATE IN MILLILITERS PER HOUR

Using the formula $F = \frac{V}{T}$, we find that

$$F = \frac{265\,mL}{1.5\,h}$$

$$F = 177\,mL/h$$

You would set the infusion pump to 177 mL/h.

STEP B: CALCULATE THE FLOW RATE IN DROPS PER MINUTE

If an infusion pump is not used, you will need to calculate the drops per minute. For this example we will use standard tubing that is 15 gtt/mL. Always check the drop factor on the tubing packaging.

To determine the flow rate f in drops per minute, use the formula $f = F \times \frac{C}{60}$.

Where: f = flow rate in gtt/min

F = flow rate in mL/h

C = drop factor of the tubing

60 = # minutes in 1 hour

Fill in the formula.

$$f = \frac{177 \text{ mL/h} \times 15 \text{ gtt/min}}{60 \text{ min}}$$

$$f = \frac{177 \text{ mL/h} \times 15 \text{ gtt/mL}}{60 \text{ min}}$$

$$f = 2{,}655 \text{ gtt}/60 \text{ min}$$

$$f = 44.25 \text{ rounded the nearest whole number is 44 gtt/min}$$

STEP C: THINK!. . .IS IT REASONABLE?

Since 177 times 1.5 equals 265, the rate of 177 mL/h is reasonable.

Since there are 60 minutes in 1 hour and the tubing drop factor is 1/4 of the number of minutes in an hour, the rate in gtt/min should be about 1/4 of the rate in mL/h. In this case, 177 divided by 4 equals 44.25, so the answer of 44 gtt/min is reasonable.

PATIENT EDUCATION

Instruct patients who are sent home with a saline or heparin lock to care for the device and administer their medications. Teach them about infiltration and phlebitis, and to contact their physician immediately should signs of either problem arise.

1. Avoid getting the injection site wet when bathing or washing hands.

2. Collect all necessary supplies before irrigating the lock or administering medication.

3. Irrigate the device at least twice a day to prevent clotting around the needle or catheter. Develop a schedule.

4. Clean the injection port with an antiseptic swab before injecting the irrigant or prescribed medication.

5. Before administering medication, flush a heparin lock with 1 to 10 mL NS to clear any residual heparin.

6. Attach the syringe to the lock, and pull the plunger back. Watch for blood in the chamber to confirm access to the vein. This step must be followed for every injection with the device.

7. After injecting the saline, withdraw the syringe. Inject the medication according to the physician's instructions.

8. After withdrawing the syringe, flush any residual medication from the device.

9. If heparin is used as an irrigant, inject it according to the physician's instructions. Then withdraw the syringe.

10. After completing the injections, swab the port with an antiseptic wipe.

Select the Correct Strength of Heparin for an Intermittent IV Flush

A heparin flush is a diluted solution of heparin administered to maintain patency of an intravenous line. The concentration of a heparin flush is 10 units/mL or 100 units/mL See Figure 15-23 Label C. Heparin to be administered for therapeutic purposes is available in 1,000 units/mL (see Figure 15-23, Label A), 5,000 units/mL, and 10,000 units/mL. If the medication technician administered 1 mL of the 10,000:1 solution instead of the 100:1 solution, the patient would receive 100 times the dose ordered! Serious, sometimes fatal, errors have occurred as a result of administering the wrong concentration of heparin.

REVIEW AND PRACTICE

15.5 Intermittent IV Infusions

For Exercises 1–4, refer to Labels A through C in Figure 15-23.

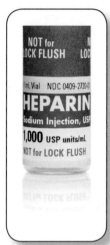

A

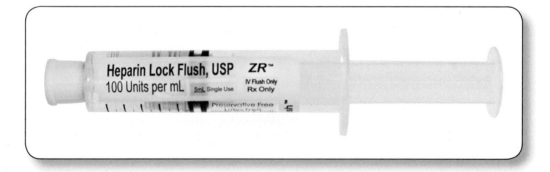

C

Figure 15-23   Heparin injection solution, saline lock flush, and heparin lock flush.

1. Which would be used to flush a saline lock?

2. Which would be used to flush a heparin lock?

3. Standing order reads 3 mL saline lock flush q8h. Calculate the amount to administer.

4. Standing order reads heparin 5,000 units IV q12h. Calculate the amount to administer.

For Exercises 5–10, determine the amount to administer and calculate the flow rate in milliliters per hour and drops per minute. For these exercises, if the volume of medication is 15 mL or more, then add the volume of medication to the total volume of the infusion before calculating the infusion rate.

Ordered: Gemzar® 150 mg in 500 mL NS over 2 h

On hand: Refer to IV tubing packaging D, label E, and package insert F (Figure 15-24).

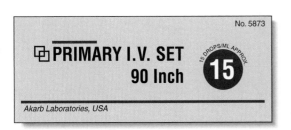

D

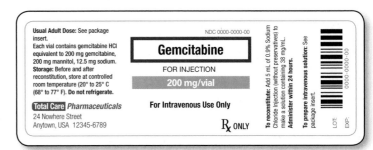

E

Gemcitabine

Instructions for Use and Handling

The recommended diluent for reconstitution of gemcitabine is 0.9% Sodium Chloride Injection without preservatives. The maximum concentration after reconstitution is 40 mg/mL, because reconstitution at concentrations above 40 mg/mL may result in incomplete dissolution.

Reconstitution

To reconstitute gemcitabine, add 5 mL of 0.9% Sodium Chloride Injection, without preservatives, to the 200 mg vial, or add 25 mL of 0.9% Sodium Chloride Injection, without preservatives, to the 1 g vial. Each of these dilutions produces a gemcitabine concentration of 38 mg/mL. The total volume after reconstitution is 5.26 mL or 26.3 mL, respectively. Complete withdrawal of vial content will provide 200 mg or 1 g of gemcitabine, respectively. The appropriate amount of medication may be administered as prepared or further diluted to concentrations as low as 0.1 mg/mL using 0.9% Sodium Chloride Injection.

After reconstitution, gemcitabine is a clear, colorless to light straw-colored solution with a pH of 2.7 to 3.3. Inspect visually for particulates and discoloration prior to administration. Do not administer if particulates or discoloration are present.

Stability

When prepared as directed, gemcitabine is stable for 24 hours at controlled room temperature [see USP]. Discard unused portion. To avoid crystalization, do not refrigerate.

F

Figure 15-24 IV tubing packaging, Gemcitabine HCl label, and package insert information.

5. Amount to administer: _____

6. Flow rate in milliliters per hour: _____

7. Flow rate in drops per minute: _____

Ordered: Doxycycline 75 mg IVPB in 100 mL of D5W over 1 hour

On hand: Refer to label G, package insert H, and IV tubing packaging I (Figure 15-25).

8. Amount to administer: _____

9. Flow rate in milliliters per hour: _____

10. Flow rate in drops per minute: _____

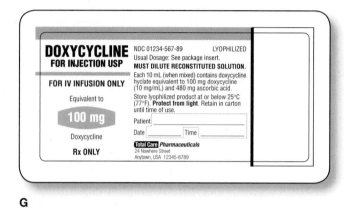

G

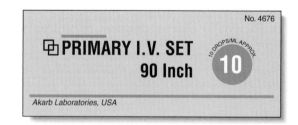

Doxycycline Reconstitution

Preparation of Solution: To prepare a solution containing 10 mg/mL, the contents of the vial should be reconstituted with 10 mL of Sterile Water for Injection USP, or any of the six intravenous infusion solutions listed below. Each 100 mg of doxycycline (i.e., withdraw entire solution from the 100 mg vial) is further diluted with 100 to 1,000 mL of the intravenous solutions listed below:

   1. 0.9% Sodium Chloride Injection USP

   2. 5% Dextrose Injection USP

   3. Ringer's Injection USP

   4. Invert Sugar, 10% in Water

   5. Lactated Ringer's Injection USP

   6. Dextrose 5% in Lactated Ringer's

This will result in desired concentrations of 0.1 to 1 mg/mL. Concentrations lower than 0.1 mg/mL or higher than 1 mg/mL are not recommended.

H   I

Figure 15-25 Doxycycline label, package insert information, and IV tubing package.

LEARNING OUTCOME	KEY POINTS
15.1 Identify the components and concentrations of IV solutions. Pages 414–418	D = Dextrose; W = Water D5W = Dextrose 5% in Water Percent = grams/100 mL, therefore 1,000 mL D5W contains 50 g Dextrose calculated: $$\frac{1\text{ g}}{100\text{ mL}} = \frac{x}{1,000\text{ mL}}$$ NS = Normal saline (0.9% NaCl, i.e., 0.9 g/100 mL) $\frac{1}{2}$NS = 0.45% NS (0.45 g/100 mL) $\frac{1}{4}$NS = 0.225% NS (0.225 g/100 mL) LR or RL = Lactated Ringers or Ringer's lactate IV solutions are ordered for: Replacement fluids—replace fluids and electrolytes lost due to hemorrhage, illness, surgery Maintenance fluids—maintain normal fluid and electrolyte balance KVO fluids—fluids delivered at a very slow rate to keep vein open Therapeutic fluids—deliver medication
15.2 Distinguish basic types of IV equipment. Pages 419–425	Primary line—larger IV bag (e.g., 500 mL or 1,000 mL) connected to long tubing with a drip chamber (to count drops), roller clamp (to adjust the flow rate), and injection ports (to inject medications, fluids, or attach a secondary line) Secondary line—smaller IV Bag (e.g., 250 mL) or mini-bag (e.g., 50 mL, 100 mL) connected to shorter tubing with similar tubing components as primary line; aka IVPB or intravenous piggyback because it is hung higher than the primary line in order to infuse or piggyback an intermittent infusion into the primary line Rate controller—sensor applied to the drip chamber to measure drops or volume that is delivered Infusion pump—device that delivers a set volume per minute or per hour; equipped with alarm to indicate tubing blockage or empty bag Syringe pump—infusion device to which a syringe is attached for delivery of intravenous medications PCA device (patient-controlled analgesia)—pump in which the patient presses a button to deliver pain medication within preset limits per order of authorized prescriber

LEARNING OUTCOME	KEY POINTS
	Volume control set—a burette chamber (calibrated in 1 mL increments) with an injection port to which up to 150 mL fluid and medications can be added
	Peripheral line—IV access through a peripheral vein
	Central line—IV access through a large vessel, such as the jugular vein or femoral vein
	PICC line—peripherally inserted (central catheter) line threaded into a central vein
	Port-A-Cath—device implanted under the skin connected to a central vein used for long-term intermittent medication administration
15.3 Calculate IV flow rates. Pages 425–433	mL/h (F) Calculate 250 mL over 2 hours in mL/h: **Formula method:** Flow rate $(F) = \dfrac{\text{Volume (mL)}}{\text{Time (hours)}}$; $\dfrac{250 \text{ mL}}{2 \text{ h}} = 125 \text{ mL/h}$ Calculate 100 mL over 45 minutes in mL/h: **Formula method:** convert 45 min to 0.75 h using the proportion method $(\dfrac{60 \text{ min}}{1 \text{ h}} = \dfrac{45 \text{ min}}{x})$, then apply the formula $F = \dfrac{V}{T}$. $F = \dfrac{100 \text{ mL}}{0.75 \text{ h}} = 133.33 \text{ or } 133 \text{ mL/h}$ gtt/min (f): Calculate 125 mL/h using a drop factor (calibration) of 15 gtt/mL **Formula method:** $f \text{ (gtt/min)} = \dfrac{F \text{ (mL/h)} \times C}{60 \text{ min/h}}$; $f = \dfrac{(125 \text{ mL/h} \times 15 \text{ gtt/mL})}{60 \text{ min/h}}$; cancel units: $f = \dfrac{125}{4} = 31.25 \text{ or } 31 \text{ gtt/min}$ IV Rate Adjustment $= \dfrac{\text{Volume left}}{\text{Time left}}$

LEARNING OUTCOME	KEY POINTS
15.4 Calculate infusion time and volume. Pages 433–438	Time: ▸ **Formula Method:** Time $= \dfrac{\text{Volume (mL)}}{F \text{ (mL/h)}}$; convert fractional hours to minutes by multiplying by 60 Calculate time to infuse 500 mL at 60 mL/h: $T = \dfrac{500 \text{ mL}}{60 \text{ mL/h}} = 8.33$ h or 8 h, 20 min (0.33 h $\times$ 60 min/h = 20 min) Volume: ▸ **Formula Method:** $V = T \times F$ Calculate the volume infused in 2 hours 30 minutes for IV running at 150 mL/h $V = 2.5$ h $\times$ 150 mL/h $= 375$ mL ▸ **Dimensional Analysis:** V mL $= \dfrac{2.5 \cancel{h}}{1} \times \dfrac{150 \text{ mL}}{\cancel{h}} = 375$ mL/h
15.5 Perform calculations for intermittent IV infusions. Pages 438–446	Saline lock—a port through which a medication can be injected directly into the vein or to which an intermittent infusion can be attached; flushed intermittently with saline to maintain patency Heparin lock—similar to a saline lock except it is flushed intermittently with low-dose heparin to maintain patency Calculations: 1. Use formula method, proportion method, or dimensional analysis (from "Parenteral Dosages" chapter) to determine amount to administer after medication is reconstituted 2. Use formula method or dimensional analysis to calculate flow rate: a. First convert minutes to hours, if necessary, then apply formula: • To calculate mL/h: $F = V/T$ • To calculate gtt/min: $f = \dfrac{F \times C}{60 \text{ min/h}}$

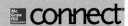
Answer the following questions.

1. List the four functional categories of IV solutions. (LO 15.1)

2. In the IV label abbreviation D5W, which component identifies the concentration level? (LO 15.1)

3. Define the terms *isotonic, hypertonic,* and *hypotonic.* (LO 15.1)

4. Before combining any medication with an IV solution, what must be verified? (LO 15.1)

5. List the four parts of a primary IV line. (LO 15.2)

6. List four types of electronic infusion devices. (LO 15.2)

7. Under what circumstances would a patient most likely need central line IV therapy? (LO 15.2)

8. What is the drop factor for microdrip tubing? (LO 15.2)

9. How is the flow rate measured when an infusion pump is used? (LO 15.2)

10. Name and explain two types of intermittent IV infusion methods. (LO 15.2)

11. If the order is 1,000 mL to infuse over 12 hours (10 gtt/mL tubing), calculate the manual flow rate. (LO 15.3)

12. If the order is 50 mL to infuse over 90 minutes (microdrip tubing), calculate the manual flow rate. (LO 15.3)

13. If the order is 500 mL to infuse at 150 mL/hour (10 gtt/mL tubing), how long will it take to infuse? (LO 15.3)

14. If an IV is infusing at 20 gtt/minute with a drop factor (calibration) of 20 gtt/mL and the volume of the IV bag is 500 mL, how many hours will it take to infuse? (LO 15.4)

15. An IV of 500 mL is begun at 11 a.m. and the flow rate is 15 gtt/minute (10 gtt/mL tubing). At what time will the infusion be complete? (LO 15.4)

16. If the order is 250 mL over 3 hours, what mL/hour setting will you use on an infusion pump? (LO 15.4)

17. If the order is 150 mL over 30 minutes, how many mL/hour will you set on the infusion pump? (LO 15.4)

18. What is the total volume to be infused for an IV infusing at 80 mL/hour for 6 hours? (LO 15.4)

19. At the end of 4 hours, what is the total volume infused for an IV infusing at 20 drops per minute (10 gtt/mL tubing)? (LO 15.4)

20. If the order is 500 mL over 4 hours (10 gtt/mL tubing), after 1 hour there should be how much remaining in the bag? (LO 15.4)

CHECK UP

For Exercises 1–7, match the term to its description. Write the answer in the space provided. (LO 15.1, 15.2)

_____ **1.** Roller clamp   **a.** type of solution that causes fluid to move out of the cell

_____ **2.** KVO fluids   **b.** type of fluid given to a patient who is dehydrated

_____ **3.** Hypertonic   **c.** the patient is in charge of delivering his or her own pain medications

_____ **4.** Phlebitis   **d.** provide access to the vascular system for emergency situations

_____ **5.** PCA   **e.** redness, swelling, and pain at an IV site

_____ **6.** Infusion pump   **f.** applies pressure to administer an IV fluid

_____ **7.** Hypotonic   **g.** used to control the rate of an IV infusion

For Exercises 8–13, calculate the flow rate for orders to be administered by an infusion pump. (LO 15.3)

8. 3,000 mL D5W IV q24h

9. 500 mL LR IV q8h

10. 1,200 mL 1/2 NS IV q12h

11. 250 mL NS IV q4h

12. 1 g claforan in 100 mL D5W IV over 90 min

13. 500 mg ampicillin in 50 mL D5W IV over 30 min

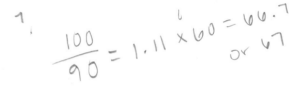

For Exercises 14–19, find the flow rate for the orders, rounded to the nearest drop/min. (LO 15.3)

14. 2,200 mL IV RL q24h (15 gtt/mL tubing)

15. 300 mL IV NS q8h (10 gtt/mL tubing)

16. 1,000 mL IV D5W q6h (15 gtt/mL tubing)

17. 1,800 mL IV D5/$\frac{1}{2}$ NS q12h (20 gtt/mL tubing)

18. 1,500 mL IV $\frac{1}{3}$ NS q8h (10 gtt/mL tubing)

19. 300 mL D5LR IV q6h (microdrip tubing)

For Exercises 20–22, calculate the ordered flow rate in gtt/min and mL/h. Then determine if an adjustment is necessary and calculate the adjusted flow rate. Determine if the rate can be adjusted safely. For this exercise, flow rate adjustment can be no more than 10 gtt/min or 50 mL/h. (LO 15.3)

20. Ordered: 1,000 mL RL over 8 h (15 gtt/mL tubing)

After 2 h, 125 mL has infused.

Ordered rate _____ mL/h _____ gtt/min

Adjusted rate _____ mL/h _____ gtt/min

Is it safe to adjust? _____ yes _____ no

21. Ordered: 2,500 mL NS over 24 h (10 gtt/mL tubing)

    After 3 h, 200 mL has infused.

    Ordered rate _____ mL/h _____ gtt/min

    Adjusted rate _____ mL/h _____ gtt/min

    Is it safe to adjust? _____ yes _____ no

22. Ordered 500 mL $\frac{1}{2}$ NS over 8 h (60 gtt/mL tubing)

    After 2 h, 450 mL is remaining in the IV bag.

    Ordered rate _____ mL/h _____ gtt/min

    Adjusted rate _____ mL/h _____ gtt/min

    Is it safe to adjust? _____ yes _____ no

For Exercises 23–26, find the total time to infuse. (LO 15.4)

23. Ordered: 1,000 mL D5/0.45% NS at 125 mL/h via infusion pump

24. Ordered: 800 mL $\frac{1}{4}$ NS at 50 mL/h via rate controller

25. Ordered: 600 mL LR IV at 25 mL/h

26. Ordered: 1,200 mL D5/NS IV at 70 mL/h

For Exercises 27–30, find when the infusion will be completed. (LO 15.4)

27. 800 mL via infusion pump at 90 mL/h, starting at 0820

28. 1,000 mL at 125 mL/h, starting at 1 p.m.

29. 500 mL at 175 mL/h, starting at 2230

30. 750 mL at 35 mL/h, starting at 4 p.m.

For Exercises 31–34, find the total volume to administer. (LO 15.4)

31. $\frac{1}{4}$ NS at 125 mL/h over 5 h 30 min via infusion pump

32. RL at 25 mL/h over 12 h

33. NS at 125 mL/h over 7 h 30 min

34. D5W at 80 mL/h over 8 h 20 min

CRITICAL THINKING APPLICATIONS

The physician has ordered an adult patient with *Pneumocystis carinii* pneumonia to have clindamycin 500 mg IV q8h.

On hand: See clindamycin label A and package insert B. (LO 15.5)

  1. Calculate the amount to administer.

  2. How would you prepare the medication?

  3. Is this the correct dose for treatment of pneumonia? Why or why not?

  4. What fluid should not be used as a diluent for neonates?

  5. The medication cannot be administered immediately because the patient is having a diagnostic test. What should you do?

  6. Calculate the flow rate of the infusion.

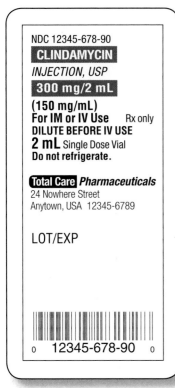

A

CLINDAMYCIN PHOSPHATE INJECTION USP

Usual adult and adolescent dose

Antibacterial
Intramuscular or intravenous, 300 to 600 mg (base) every six to eight hours; or 900 mg every eight hours.

[Babesiosis (treatment)][1]
Intravenous, 300 to 600 mg clindamycin (base) four times a day with concurrent oral administration of 650 mg of quinine, three or four times a day for seven to ten days.

[Pneumonia, *Pneumocystis carinii* (treatment)]
Intravenous, 2,400 to 2,700 mg (base) per day in divided doses in combination with 15 to 30 mg of primaquine daily.

[Toxoplasmosis, central nervous system (CNS) (treatment)]
Intravenous, 1,200 to 4,800 mg (base) per day in divided doses in combination with 50 to 100 mg of pyrimethamine daily.

Usual adult prescribing limits
Up to 2.7 grams (base) daily.

Note: Doses up to 4.8 grams daily have been used. However, some medical experts recommend a maximum dose of 2.7 grams daily.

Preparation of dosage form:
To prepare initial dilution for intravenous use, each dose must be diluted as follows (it must not be administered undiluted as a bolus):

Dose (mg)	Diluent (mL)	Duration of administration (min)
300	50	10
600	100	20
900	100	30

Caution: Products containing benzyl alcohol are not recommended for use in neonates. A fatal toxic syndrome consisting of metabolic acidosis, CNS depression, respiratory problems, renal failure, hypotension, and possibly seizures and intracranial hemorrhages has been associated with this use.

Stability:
Clindamycin phosphate retains its potency for 24 hours at room temperature in intravenous infusions containing sodium chloride, dextrose, potassium, vitamin B complex, cephalothin, kanamycin, gentamicin, penicillin, or carbenicillin.

Incompatibilities:
Clindamycin phosphate is physically incompatible with ampicillin, phenytoin sodium, barbiturates, aminophylline, calcium gluconate, and magnesium sulfate.

B

CASE STUDY

A patient has a PCA pump with morphine sulfate 50 mg in 500 mL D5W. Hospital policy requires you to document the dose of morphine administered during your shift. When you came on duty, the pump showed that 227 mL had infused. At the end of your shift the pump shows that 272 mL has infused. How much morphine did the patient receive during your shift? (LO 15.3)

connect

Now that you have completed the materials in the chapter text, go to CONNECT and complete any chapter activities you have not yet done.

For Questions 1–2, refer to labels A–E.

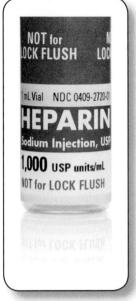

Label A Heparin Sodium 1,000 USP units/mL, 1 mL bottle

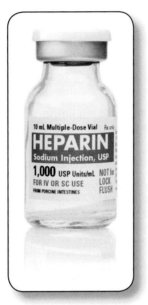

Label B Heparin Sodium 1,000 USP units/mL, 10 mL bottle

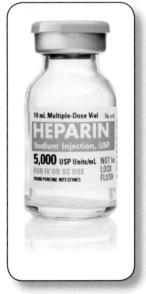

Label C Heparin Sodium 5,000 USP units/mL, 10 mL bottle

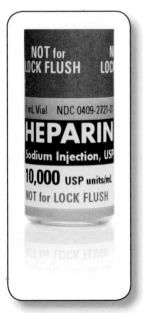

Label D Heparin Sodium 10,000 USP units/mL, 1 mL bottle

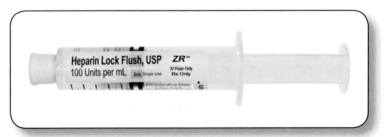

Label E Heparin Lock Flush 100 units/ mL, USP

For questions 1 and 2, refer to the following:

Ordered: Heparin 8,000 units subcut

1. Which concentration of heparin should you choose? Label _____

2. How much heparin will you administer? _____ mL

3. What is the dose of insulin in the following syringe?

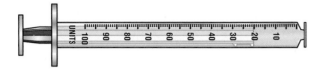

For Questions 4–6 refer to labels through F to I.

Order: Insulin lispro injection 7 units subcut and Insulix-N 30 units subcut

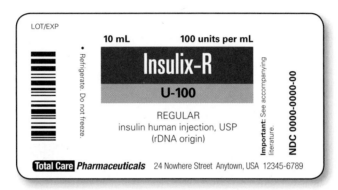

Label F   Insulix-R

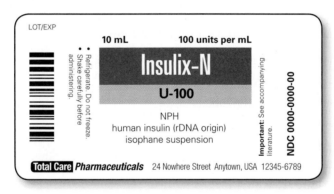

Label G   Insulix-N

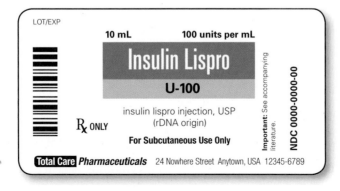

Label H   Insulin lispro injection

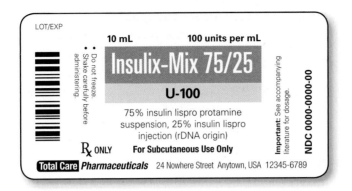

Label I Insulix-Mix 75/25

4. Which insulin would you draw up first?   Label _____

5. Which insulin would you inject air into first? Label _____

6. Mark on the syringe how many units of each insulin you administer.

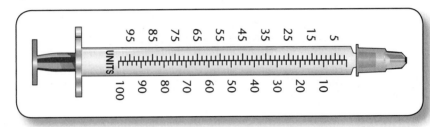

7. What would be the best syringe to administer 1.5 mL of fluid IM?

8. What would be the best syringe to administer 8 mL of fluid IV?

9. What would be the best syringe to administer 50 units of U-100 insulin?

10. What would be the best syringe to administer 0.1 mL of fluid ID?

Calculate one dose of the following medication orders.

11. Ordered: levothyroxine 75 mcg PO daily
    On hand: levothyroxine 0.15 mg scored tablets
    Administer: _____ tablet(s)

12. Ordered: cefadroxil 1 g PO q6h
    On hand: cefadroxil 500 mg tablets
    Administer: _____ tablet(s)

13. Ordered: cefprozil 1 g PO daily
    On hand: cefprozil 250 mg/5 mL
    Administer: _____ tsp

14. Ordered: potassium chloride 60 mEq PO daily
    On hand: potassium chloride 20 mEq/15 mL
    Administer: _____ oz

15. Ordered: azithromycin 0.5 g PO daily
    On hand: azithromycin 200 mg/5 mL
    Administer: _____ mL

16. Determine the concentration of dextrose and/or sodium chloride in each of the following intravenous solutions:

    a. D5NS   b. D10W   c. D5 $\frac{1}{2}$ NS   d. D5 $\frac{1}{4}$ NS

17. Match the IV equipment to the most appropriate description:
    a. Primary line _____   i. The calibration is 60 gtt/mL.
    b. Central line _____   ii. This device is surgically implanted under the skin.
    c. Secondary line _____   iii. This tubing has injection ports for additional lines.
    d. Port-a-Cath _____   iv. This device can be peripherally inserted and provides direct access to major veins.
    e. Microdrip tubing _____   v. Intravenous piggyback (IVPB) medications are given through this device.

18. Calculate the following IV flow rates:
    a. Ordered: 3000 mL D5NS over 24 h using an infusion pump
       Rate: _____ mL/h
    b. Ordered: 50 mL D5W over 45 min using an infusion pump
       Rate: _____ mL/h
    c. Ordered: 1000 mL NS over 10 h; tubing is 15 gtt/mL
       Rate: _____ gtt/min
    d. Ordered: 80 mg tobramycin in 100 mL D5W over 20 min
       Rate: _____ mL/h
    e. Ordered: 1,000 mL D5 ½ NS to run at 85 mL/h; tubing is 10 gtt/mL
       Rate: _____ gtt/min

19. Calculate the IV infusion time or volume as indicated:
    a. Ordered: 1000 mL NS at 125 mL/h started at 1500
       At what time will the IV finish? _____
    b. Ordered: D5W at 50 mL/h started at 0730 and finished at 1230
       What volume infused? _____
    c. Ordered: 1000 mL D5 $\frac{1}{2}$ NS at 100 mL/h started at 2145
       At what time will the IV finish? _____
    d. Ordered: $\frac{1}{2}$ NS at 80 mL/h infused for 3 h 45 min
       What volume infused? _____

20. Determine the IV flow rate for the following intermittent infusion orders:
    a. Ordered: ampicillin 125 mg in 50 mL D5W to be administered over 20 min
       Rate: _____ mL/h
    b. Ordered: cefazolin 1 g in 100 mL NS to be administered over 40 min
       Rate: _____ mL/h
    c. Ordered: gentamicin 35 mg in 25 mL D5W to be administered over 15 min; tubing is 60 gtt/mL
       Rate: _____ gtt/min
    d. Ordered: oxacillin sodium 500 mg in 50 mL NS to be administered over 10 min
       Rate: _____ mL/h

UNIT 5

Performing Advanced Dosage Calculations

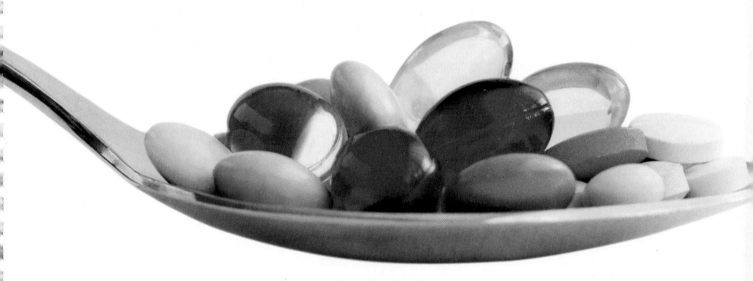

CHAPTER 16

Calculations for Special Populations

Perfection consists not in doing extraordinary things, but in doing ordinary things extraordinarily well.

ANGELIQUE ARNAULD

LEARNING OUTCOMES

When you have completed Chapter 16, you will be able to:

16.1 Identify factors that impact drug dosing in special populations.

16.2 Calculate safe dosages based on body weight.

16.3 Calculate dosages based on body surface area (BSA).

KEY TERMS

Absorption

Body surface area

Distribution

Elimination

Geriatric

Metabolism

Nomogram

Pediatric

Pharmacokinetics

Polypharmacy

INTRODUCTION

There are two special populations that require extra consideration when you are calculating medication dosages. These are pediatric (children) and geriatric (mature adult) patients. Generally speaking, **pediatric** patients are under the age of 18, and **geriatric** patients are 65 and over. See Figures 16-1 and 16-2. The risk of harm to these populations is far greater because of how they break down and absorb medications. You must clarify all confusing drug orders, calculate with absolute accuracy, verifying that the dose is safe, and seek assistance from your supervisor if you have concerns. No matter how rushed you may feel, you may not take shortcuts with medication calculations for patients from special populations; rather, you must calculate their dosages extraordinarily well!

16.1 Factors that Impact Dosing and Medication Administration

For most drugs, there is a normal recommended dose standardized for an average adult weighing approximately 150 pounds. This standardized dose of a medication is based on a number of assumptions about the patient's body and age. It is assumed that the body systems are fully developed and functioning at a certain level. While these assumptions hold true for most patients, there are many situations in which the dose needs to be adjusted. If the liver or kidneys are not functioning normally, for example, the dose of many drugs needs to be decreased. If the digestive system is not functioning normally, the dose of oral medications may need to be adjusted. These changes in dosage are necessary because the drug is affecting each patient's body differently.

Pharmacokinetics—How Drugs Are Used by the Body

Pharmacokinetics is the study of what happens to a drug after it is administered to a patient. There are four processes that affect a drug after it is administered: *absorption, distribution, metabolism* (biotransformation), and *elimination*. Pharmacokinetics is the study of these four processes, which you can remember using the acronym ADME. Understanding the processes allows adjustments to be made for patients whose body systems are not fully developed or are not functioning at a certain level.

Absorption is the process that moves a drug from the site where it is given into the bloodstream. Intravenous medications bypass the absorption process because they are administered directly into the bloodstream. Oral medications are absorbed through the digestive system, while topical medications are absorbed through the skin.

Distribution is the process that moves a drug from the bloodstream into other body tissues and fluids. The blood and each of these other areas are called *compartments*. Some compartments include blood, fat, cerebrospinal fluid, and the target site. The *target site* is the site where the drug produces its desired effect. The compartments that a drug will go to are different for different drugs, and depend on the chemical nature of the drug.

Metabolism, or biotransformation of a medication, is the process that chemically changes a drug either before or after it performs its intended task. These changes occur primarily in the liver.

Elimination is the process in which the drug leaves the body. Most drugs are eliminated through the urine, although they can also be eliminated in the air that we exhale, sweat, feces, breast milk, or any other body secretion.

The dose of a drug may need to be adjusted if one of the four pharmacokinetic processes is not functioning within certain limits. Certain conditions affect these four processes, thus affecting the dose. Some examples are found in Table 16-1. A dose adjustment is made based upon the nature and severity of the patient's condition. Thus, the dose ordered might be lower or higher than normal in some circumstances, yet still be the proper dose for the patient. These dosing considerations for various conditions are normally included in the package insert and are considered when the order for the medication is written. As an entry-level healthcare professional, you will not be making the dosage adjustments; however, understanding these processes will make you *aware* of the many factors that need to be taken into consideration when determining the appropriate dose for an individual.

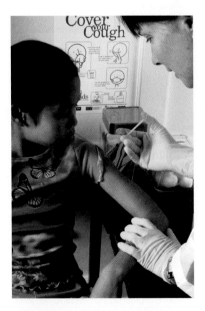

Figure 16-1 Pediatric patients, less than 18 years, require extra attention to detail when performing calculations.

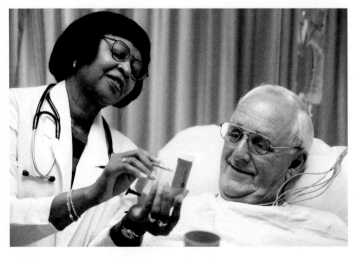

Figure 16-2 Dosage calculations for geriatric patients, those 65 years and older, require extraordinary accuracy.

TABLE 16-1 Conditions That May Impact Dosing

CONDITION	PROCESS AFFECTED	EFFECT ON DOSING
Stomach or intestinal disorders	Absorption	Dose of oral medications may need to be changed.
Liver disorders	Metabolism (biotransformation)	The dose of some drugs needs to be decreased.
Obesity	Distribution	Dose of drugs distributed to fat may need to be increased.
Kidney disease	Elimination	Dose of drugs eliminated in urine may need to be changed.

The function of many body systems changes over the life of a person. In newborns, some systems are not yet fully developed. This is especially true for premature infants. In geriatric patients, those 65 and over, the function of some body systems begins to deteriorate. Skin and veins become more fragile. The functions of the digestive and urinary systems may be affected. Table 16-2 describes examples of age-related factors that can affect dosing.

There are other things to consider when working with special populations. Pediatric and geriatric patients may have a parent or caretaker who will administer or assist them with medications. These individuals will need education. You may be called upon to teach the patients or the caregivers about the medications they will be taking. Table 16-3 provides a list of what each patient or caregiver should know about medications. Geriatric patients may require extra consideration based upon their level of awareness and understanding.

TABLE 16-2 Age-Related Factors That May Impact Dosing

AGE GROUP	CONDITION	PROCESS AFFECTED	EFFECT ON DOSING
Pediatric	pH of stomach is lower	Absorption	Dose of oral medications may need to be changed.
	Thinner skin	Absorption	Dose of topical medications may need to be decreased.
	Liver still developing	Metabolism	Dose of some drugs needs to be decreased.
	Less circulation to muscles	Absorption	Dose of IM medications may need to be increased.
Geriatric	Thinner skin	Absorption	Dose of topical medications may need to be decreased.
	Decreased liver function	Metabolism	Dose of some drugs needs to be decreased.
	Decreased kidney function	Elimination	Dose of drugs eliminated in the urine may need to be decreased.
	Poor circulation	Absorption and distribution	Dose of some drugs needs to be adjusted.
	Decreased HCl in stomach (pH is slightly higher)	Absorption	Dose of oral acidic drugs needs to be adjusted.

TABLE 16-3 What Patients and Caregivers Should Know about Medications

Name of the medication
Purpose of taking the medication
How to store the medication
How long the patient will need to take the medication
How and when to take the medication
How to know if the medication is effective
Required follow-up (lab tests, doctor appointments)
Possible side effects and what to do about them
Interactions with other drugs and foods
Symptoms to report to the doctor
What to do if a dose is missed
Keeping a list of all medications
When the medication expires

Pediatric Patients

Physiological differences between children and adults make children more susceptible to the effects and adverse reactions of medications. Not only the difference in body size and composition but also the immaturity of organ systems contribute to increased risks associated with pediatric medication administration. As seen in Table 16-2, because children have an increased metabolism and a higher percentage of water per kilogram of body weight, the pharmacokinetic processes—absorption, distribution, metabolism (biotransformation), and excretion—are different in children than they are in adults. Appropriate drug dosages in children are typically calculated based on body weight or body surface area (BSA). Rules for calculating drug dosages based on body weight and body surface area will be explored later in this chapter.

Geriatric Patients

When you work with geriatric patients, show them respect. Encourage them, if they are able, to participate in planning their schedule. Listen to their concerns. Recommend that they use the same pharmacy to fill all prescriptions. Encourage them to have one doctor as their primary physician to monitor and approve all medications. Remind them to keep a list of all their medications including vitamins, herbals, and alternative medications. They should take the list or their medication bottles when they see their primary physician and all their specialists.

In some cases, geriatric patients may have decreased manual dexterity that can interfere with their ability to inject medications, administer eye drops, or even open bottles. Patients may need to specifically ask their pharmacist for bottle caps that are not childproof. Patients with difficulty swallowing will need information about which medications may be crushed and mixed with applesauce or pudding. In addition, they need information about which medications may *not* be broken or crushed.

Many patients cannot read small print. Medications may need labels that can easily be read and will clearly describe the purpose of each medication. Do not assume that patients can distinguish between colors of tablets; white and yellow may be confused, as may blue and green, or orange and pink. Make a chart for the patient with the medications, time, and description to prevent errors.

Family members or others who care for special population patients at home must understand and follow directions when they administer drugs. Talk to parents or caretakers about the following:

1. Explain how much medication to administer at one time, how often during the day, and for how many days. Give parents or caretakers this information in writing. Have them repeat this information, especially if their English or literacy skills are limited.

2. Discuss expected side effects. Provide a telephone number or resource for them to call in case of unexpected or serious side effects. Explain how to reach a Poison Control Center.

3. No one should ever be given someone else's medication. Patients may react differently to medications than expected.

4. Over-the-counter, herbal, and alternative remedies should never be given to a child under age 2 without first speaking to a healthcare provider.

5. Parents or caregivers must check dosage information on over-the-counter medications. The amount to administer changes with age and weight. Some medications may *not* be administered to children below a certain age (often 2) without first checking with a physician.

6. Demonstrate how to measure doses accurately. Calibrated equipment should be used. Droppers are not interchangeable between medications.

7. The full course of prescription medications such as antibiotics must be administered, even if the patient appears to be well or resists taking the medication.

8. Never refer to medication as candy or physically force a patient to take a medication. In some cases, you may mix the medication with a liquid or food, but check with the pharmacist before doing so. The patient's healthcare practitioner should be notified when medications are not taken on a consistent basis.

9. Replace childproof caps properly and keep medications out of reach of children or patients with mental confusion.

Geriatric patients often have some form of hearing loss. They may even try to hide their hearing loss from you. Have patients repeat to you the information that you give them. They may also have short-term memory loss. Determine if they need written directions and explanations. Help them work with memory tools, such as medication calendars that tell them which medications to take each day. Pharmacies often sell weekly dispensers that have a container for each day of the week; patients or family members can prepare in advance the medications for the week (see Figure 16-3).

Instruct patients who regularly take prescription medications not to take over-the-counter or herbal medications without first checking with their physician. They should not take more of any medication than is indicated by the label. They should avoid any medications that have expired (show them how to read the expiration date). They should never borrow medications, especially prescription ones, from anyone else.

Liver and kidney functions are often reduced in geriatric patients. Decreased liver function results in slower metabolism of certain drugs, delaying or prolonging the desired effect of the medication. It can also lead to a higher level of drug in the blood system, producing more intense results.

Decreased kidney function, along with decreased cardiac output, slows the excretion of medications from the body. The effects of slower excretion (resulting from decreased kidney function) and reduced metabolism (resulting from decreased liver function) may combine,

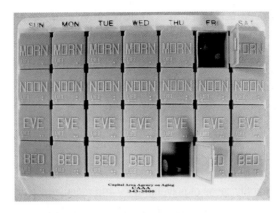

Figure 16-3 A medication container like this one would be very useful for a patient taking multiple daily medications.

causing medication to accumulate in the body. This may cause increased side effects or even toxicity. Many chronic diseases common in the elderly can damage the kidneys. These diseases include hypertension, diabetes, and congestive heart failure. Also, some commonly used drugs, such as Lasix® and aminoglycoside antibiotics, can further impair kidney function. In addition, long-term use of over-the-counter anti-inflammatory medications such as ibuprofen and naproxen can cause impaired kidney function. Geriatric patients who have these diseases or are taking these medications must be monitored especially closely for their kidney functions.

CREATININE CLEARANCE Many package inserts discuss safe dosage levels based on creatinine clearance. Creatinine is a by-product of muscle metabolism and is found in the blood. The kidneys filter creatinine from the blood, and the rate at which creatinine is excreted through the urine is called creatinine clearance (CL_{CR}). A person's creatinine clearance is considered an indicator of the rate at which the kidneys filter the blood.

Creatinine clearance often decreases with age as a normal part of the aging process. For example, normal values usually drop by 6 mL/min for every 10 years past the age of 20. If a patient has decreased kidney function, however, the creatinine clearance will decrease beyond the normal effect of aging. At the same time, the amount of creatinine in the blood (serum creatinine level) may increase.

The creatinine clearance level is calculated using information that comes from an analysis of blood and urine samples. You may not know this information for every patient. The authorized prescriber will usually factor in a patient's creatinine clearance when preparing a drug order. If you have any questions about administering a medication when creatinine clearance is a factor, speak with your supervisor or authorized prescriber.

POLYPHARMACY The practice of taking many medications at one time is called **polypharmacy**. Many geriatric patients take several medications. They may take more than a dozen prescription medications, as well as numerous over-the-counter medications or natural supplements. They often have more than one physician and one or more specialists who treat very specific diseases and ailments. Because of this, some medications may be prescribed without consideration of their interaction with other medications the patient is already taking.

Because of financial pressures, elderly patients may attempt to limit physician costs by using older medications instead of visiting the physician. They may use medications that were initially prescribed years earlier and are past their expiration date. They may borrow medications. They may also order medications by mail or through the Internet, without having direct contact with the pharmacist.

Each additional medication a patient takes increases the likelihood of a drug interaction. These interactions can interfere with the effectiveness of one or more medications. They can also cause serious or even fatal side effects.

Elderly patients often take more than one medication to treat the same problem. Sometimes they have neglected to inform a new physician about medications prescribed by other physicians. Sometimes multiple medications are needed to bring a problem under control. The patient may then continue to take all the medications, even though only one or two are still needed. This overuse is especially common with patients being treated for high blood pressure, constipation, or behavioral problems that occur with dementia. Healthcare providers should periodically review with their elderly patients the list of medications the patients are taking. They should look especially for medications that are no longer needed as well as for multiple medications being used to treat the same condition.

RULE 16-1	To identify cases of polypharmacy and reduce the risk of drug interactions, ask elderly patients about:

- All medications they take that are prescribed by all of their physicians and specialists.
- Any over-the-counter medications they take, including vitamins, laxatives, and allergy medications.
- Any social drugs that they use, including alcohol, tobacco, and marijuana.
- Medications that they borrow from family and friends.
- Herbal and home remedies that they use, including natural supplements such as ginseng, gingko biloba, and St. John's wort.
- Bringing all the medications they take to be checked. This includes prescriptions, over-the-counter drugs, vitamins, minerals, and herbals.

ADDITIONAL CONSIDERATIONS   Adverse drug reactions can be caused by a variety of factors. These include advanced age, small body size, multiple illnesses (including chronic problems), multiple medications, living alone (patients with failing memories or mental capacities), and malnutrition. All of these factors must be taken into consideration by the authorized prescriber. In addition, certain medications should not be taken by patients with specific diseases. Table 16-4 provides a list of some of these medications.

TABLE 16-4 Drugs to Be Avoided in Specific Diseases

These drugs are likely to cause significant adverse effects in elderly patients with the diseases noted.

SEVERE RISK	DRUGS	LESS SEVERE RISK	DRUGS
Benign prostatic hypertrophy	Antihistamines, anti-Parkinson's drugs, GI antispasmodics, antidepressants	Benign prostatic hypertrophy	Narcotics
Cardiac dysrhythmia	Tricyclic antidepressants	Constipation	Antihistamines, anti-Parkinson's drugs, GI antispasmodics, antidepressants
Clotting disorders	Antiplatelet drugs, ASA (aspirin)	Diabetes mellitus	Steroids, beta blockers
COPD	Hypnotics, sedatives, beta blockers	GI diseases	Aspirin, potassium supplements
GI diseases	NSAIDs, ASA (aspirin)	Insomnia	Decongestants, bronchodilators, some antidepressants
Seizures	Metoclopramide (Reglan)	Seizures	Antipsychotics

16.1 Factors that Impact Dosing and Medication Administration

For Exercises 1–10, match the terms with the definition.

1. Process that moves a drug into the bloodstream

2. Chemical changing of a drug in the body

3. Process in which a drug is removed from the body

4. Movement of a drug from the bloodstream to body tissues and fluids

5. The study of what happens to a drug after it is administered

6. The rate at which the kidneys filter the blood

7. When a patient takes multiple medications

8. Patients under the age of 18

9. Alteration of the effects or pharmacokinetics of a drug due to another drug

10. Patients over the age of 65

a. metabolism

b. pharmacokinetics

c. distribution

d. elimination

e. absorption

f. geriatric

g. drug interaction

h. polypharmacy

i. creatinine clearance

j. pediatric

For Exercises 11–15, identify the special population with a G (geriatric), P (pediatric), or B (both) that may be impacted by age-related factors.

11. Decreased liver function _____

12. Poor circulation _____

13. Lower stomach pH _____

14. Less circulation to muscles _____

15. Thinner skin _____

16.2 Dosages Based on Body Weight

Many medication orders, especially pediatric and geriatric orders, are based on body weight. This is especially common for small children. An order based on body weight may state an amount of medication per weight of the patient per unit of time. For example, the order may read 8 mg/kg/day PO q6h. This order says that, over the course of the day, the patient is to be administered 8 mg of medication for every kilogram that he or she weighs. It also says that the total daily dosage is to be divided into 4 doses given at 6-hour intervals. You will calculate the amount to administer from the information on the drug order, the patient's weight, and the dose on hand.

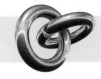

LEARNING LINK   Recall from the chapter "Other Systems of Measurement," in the table of approximate equivalent measures, that 1 kg = 2.2 lb.

Calculating Dosage Based on Body Weight

1. Convert the patient's weight to kilograms. Round body weight according to facility policy. If your institution does not have a policy for rounding, round to the nearest tenth.

2. Calculate the total ordered dose:

   Total ordered dose = ordered dose × patient weight (kg)

Remember that the ordered dose will be the amount of drug per unit body weight, so the first element in the equation will be a fraction. Examples:

$$D = \frac{mg}{kg} \times kg \qquad or \qquad D = \frac{mcg}{kg} \times kg$$

3. Check the label, package insert, or product literature to determine whether the ordered dose is safe. If it is unsafe, consult the authorized prescriber.

4. Use Steps A, B, and C from Rule 12-2 to calculate the amount to administer using the proportion method, dimensional analysis, or the formula method.

PROPORTION METHOD

EXAMPLE 1

Calculate the amount to administer to a 3-year-old who weighs 34 lb.

Ordered: Hyoscyamine sulfate 5 mcg/kg subcut 1 h preanesthesia

On hand: Hyoscyamine sulfate 0.5 mg/mL

1. Convert the patient's weight to kilograms.

$$\frac{1\ kg}{2.2\ lb} = \frac{x}{34\ lb} \qquad or \qquad 1\ kg : 2.2\ lb = x : 34\ lb$$

$$2.2 \times x = 34 \times 1\ kg$$

$$x = \frac{34\ kg}{2.2}$$

$$x = 15.5\ kg = \text{patient's weight in kilograms}$$

2. Calculate the ordered dose.

$$\frac{5\ mcg}{kg} \times 15.5\ kg = 77.5\ mcg \text{ rounded to } 78\ mcg$$

3. Confirm that the ordered dose is safe.

   Checking a reputable drug reference, you find that 5 mcg/kg is the recommended dosage for pediatric patients over 2 years of age.

4. Calculate the amount to administer.

STEP A: GATHER INFORMATION AND CONVERT

Gather the information necessary to calculate the amount to administer: $H = 0.5$ mg and $Q = 1$ mL. Convert ordered dose 78 mcg to mg, the same unit of measurement as dose on hand, using the proportion method:

$$\frac{1\ mg}{1,000\ mcg} = \frac{x}{78\ mcg}$$

$$1,000 \times x = 78 \times 1\ mg$$

$$x = \frac{78\ mg}{1,000}$$

$$x = 0.078\ mg$$

STEP B: CALCULATE

Follow Procedure Checklist 12-1.

$$\frac{H}{Q} = \frac{D}{A} \qquad \text{or} \qquad H:Q = D:A$$

$$\frac{0.5 \text{ mg}}{1 \text{ mL}} = \frac{0.078 \text{ mg}}{A}$$

$$\frac{0.5 \text{ mg}}{1 \text{ mL}} = \frac{0.078 \text{ mg}}{A}$$

$$0.5 \times A = 0.078 \times 1 \text{ mL}$$

$$0.5A = 0.078 \text{ mL}$$

$$A = 0.16 \text{ mL}$$

STEP C: THINK! . . . IS IT REASONABLE?

Since the ordered dose, 0.078 mg, is a lot less than the dose on hand, 0.5 mg, the amount administered should be a lot less than the volume on hand, 1 mL, so 0.16 mL is a reasonable answer.

DIMENSIONAL ANALYSIS

EXAMPLE 1

Calculate the amount to administer to a 3-year-old who weighs 34 lb.

Ordered: Hyoscyamine sulfate 5 mcg/kg subcut 1 h preanesthesia

On hand: Hyoscyamine sulfate 0.5 mg/mL

1. Convert the patient's weight to kilograms.

$$x = \frac{1 \text{ kg}}{2.2 \text{ lb}} \times 34 \text{ lb}$$

$$x = 15.5 \text{ kg}$$

2. Calculate the ordered dose.

$$\frac{5 \text{ mcg}}{\text{kg}} \times 15.5 \text{ kg} = 77.5 \text{ mcg rounded to 78 mcg}$$

3. Confirm that the ordered dose is safe.
   Checking a reputable drug reference, you find that 5 mcg/kg is the recommended dose for pediatric patients over 2 years of age.

4. Calculate the amount to administer.

STEP A: GATHER INFORMATION AND CONVERT

Gather the information necessary to calculate the amount to administer: $H = 0.5$ mg and $Q = 1$ mL. Since the ordered dose is not in the same unit of measurement as the dose on hand, you will need to determine the conversion factor. The unit of measure for the dosage ordered is mcg. The unit of measure for the dose on hand is mg. Use the conversion factor 1 mg = 1,000 mcg. Since we will be converting the dosage ordered to mg, place mg in the numerator.

STEP B: CALCULATE

Follow Procedure Checklist 12-2. Set up the conversion factor as the first factor in the equation:

$$A \text{ mL} = \frac{1 \text{ mg}}{1,000 \text{ mcg}}$$

The dosage unit is 1 mL; the dose on hand is 0.5 mg. This is the second factor.

$$A \text{ mL} = \frac{1 \text{ mg}}{1,000 \text{ mcg}} \times \frac{1 \text{ mL}}{0.5 \text{ mg}}$$

The ordered dose is 78 mcg. Place this over 1 to complete the equation.

$$A \text{ mL} = \frac{1 \text{ mg}}{1,000 \text{ mcg}} \times \frac{1 \text{ mL}}{0.5 \text{ mg}} \times \frac{78 \text{ mcg}}{1}$$

$$A = \frac{78 \text{ mL}}{1,000} \times 0.5$$

$$A = 0.156 \text{ mL}$$

Since the volume of the injection is less than 1 mL, we round to the nearest hundredth (two decimal places).

$$A = 0.16 \text{ mL}$$

STEP C: THINK! . . . IS IT REASONABLE?
Since the ordered dose, 0.078 mg is a lot less than the dose on hand, 0.5 mg, the amount administered should be a lot less than the volume on hand, 1 mL, so 0.16 mL is a reasonable answer.

FORMULA METHOD

EXAMPLE 1

Calculate the amount to administer to a 3-year-old who weighs 34 lb.

Ordered: Hyoscyamine sulfate 5 mcg/kg subcut 1 h preanesthesia
On hand: Hyoscyamine sulfate 0.5 mg/mL

1. Convert the patient's weight to kilograms.

$$x \text{ kg} = \frac{1 \text{ kg}}{2.2 \text{ lb}} \times 34 \text{ lb}$$

$$x = 15.5 \text{ kg}$$

2. Calculate the ordered dose.

$$\frac{5 \text{ mcg}}{\text{kg}} \times 15.5 \text{ kg} = 77.5 \text{ mcg rounded to } 78 \text{ mcg}$$

3. Confirm that the ordered dose is safe. Checking a reputable drug reference, you find that 5 mcg/kg is the recommended dose for pediatric patients over 2 years of age.

4. Calculate the amount to administer.

STEP A: GATHER INFORMATION AND CONVERT
Because the unit of measure for the dose on hand is milligrams, the desired dose must also be expressed in milligrams. Convert the desired dose to mg:

$$\frac{1 \text{ mg}}{1,000 \text{ mcg}} = \frac{x}{78 \text{ mcg}}$$

$$1,000 \times x = 78 \times 1 \text{ mg}$$

$$x = \frac{78 \text{ mg}}{1,000}$$

$$x = 0.078 \text{ mg}$$

We now have all the information necessary to calculate the amount to administer:

$$D = 0.078 \text{ mg}$$

$$H = 0.5 \text{ mg}$$

$$Q = 1 \text{ mL}$$

STEP B: CALCULATE
Calculate the amount to administer, using Procedure Checklist 12-3.

$$\frac{D}{H} \times Q = A$$

1. Fill in the formula.
$$\frac{0.178 \text{ mg}}{0.5 \text{ mg}} \times 1 \text{ mL} = A$$

2. Cancel units.
$$\frac{0.178 \text{ m\cancel{g}}}{0.5 \text{ m\cancel{g}}} \times 1 \text{ mL} = A$$

3. Solve for the unknown.
$$\frac{0.178}{0.5} \times 1 \text{ mL} = A$$

$A = 0.156$ mL rounded to 0.16, since the volume of the injection is less than 1 mL.

STEP C: THINK! . . . IS IT REASONABLE?

Since the ordered dose, 0.078 mg is a lot less than the dose on hand, 0.5 mg, the amount administered should be a lot less than the volume on hand, 1 mL, so 0.16 mL is a reasonable answer.

The total volume of a pediatric injection is limited based on the size and the age of the child. (See the table in the "Parenteral Dosages" chapter.) The length and gauge of the needle used will also vary with the age and size of the patient as well as the location of the injection. Smaller muscles need smaller needles. The depth of an injection may also vary for geriatric patients due to their reduced muscle size. You must be aware of all these factors when administering injections to special populations. Additional details regarding these injection techniques are outside the scope of this book. Please review injection techniques before you administer any injection.

Ensuring Safe Dosages

Drug orders may be written in several ways. If you measure or administer the medication, you have the responsibility to check whether the dose is the standard recommended dose. The recommended dose is sometimes written as a range, with a minimum and a maximum recommended dose. In this case, you will need to determine whether the ordered dose is within the recommended range.

PROCEDURE CHECKLIST 16-2

Calculations to Ensure Safe Dosages

When you are working with special populations, always check the package insert, drug label, or product literature to ensure the safety of the dose to be administered.

When the recommended dose is written as a range, follow these steps to ensure that the dosage is safe.

1. Perform any necessary conversions:

   a. If the patient's weight is stated in pounds, convert the weight to kilograms.

   b. If the ordered dose is divided into more than one administration per day, convert the ordered dose to the total ordered dose per day by multiplying the number of doses per day by the amount per dose.

2. Check the drug label, package insert, or product literature for the recommended dosage range.

3. Calculate the minimum and maximum recommended dosage for the patient using the patient's weight and Checklist 16-1.

4. Check the ordered dose to see if it falls within the range you calculated in steps 3 and 4. If it does, proceed to calculate the amount to administer. If it does not, contact the authorized prescriber.

Example 1

Determine whether the following order is safe. If safe, calculate the amount to administer.

Patient: Child who weighs 14.5 kg

Ordered: Erythromycin 125 mg PO q4h

On hand: Refer to the label in Figure 16-4.

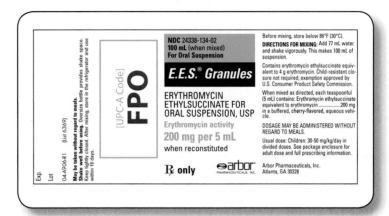

Figure 16-4

1. Since the patient's weight is already in kg, no conversion is needed. However, since the ordered dose is divided into 6 doses per day (q4h), we must calculate the total dose per day:

$$\text{Dosage ordered} = \frac{125 \text{ mg}}{\cancel{\text{dose}}} \times \frac{6 \cancel{\text{ doses}}}{\text{day}} = 750 \text{ mg/day}$$

2. Check the label to find the recommended dosage range. In this case, the range is 30–50 mg/kg/day.

3. Calculate the recommended dose range for this patient mg/kg/day × kg

$$\text{Minimum recommended dosage} = \frac{30 \text{ mg}}{\cancel{\text{kg}}} \times 14.5 \cancel{\text{ kg}} = 435 \text{ mg/day}$$

$$\text{Maximum recommended dosage} = \frac{50 \text{ mg}}{\cancel{\text{kg}}} \times 14.5 \cancel{\text{ kg}} = 725 \text{ mg/day}$$

4. In this case, the ordered dose of 750 mg/day is not within the recommended dosage range of 435–725 mg/day. You should contact the authorized prescriber.

Example 2

Determine whether the following order is safe. If it is safe, calculate the amount to administer.

Patient: 1-year-old child who weighs 27 lb

Ordered: Amoxicillin oral suspension 120 mg po q8h

On hand: Refer to the label in Figure 16-5.

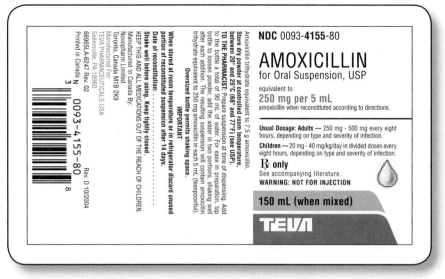

This label is for US only, and cannot be altered or translated.

Figure 16-5

1. Convert lb to kg:

$$27 \text{ lb} \times \frac{1 \text{ kg}}{2.2 \text{ lb}} = 12.3 \text{ kg}$$

Next, since the ordered dose is divided into 3 doses per day (q8h), we must calculate the total ordered dosage per day:

$$\text{Dosage ordered} = \frac{120 \text{ mg}}{\text{dose}} \times \frac{3 \text{ doses}}{\text{day}} = 360 \text{ mg/day}$$

2. Check the label to find the recommended dosage range. In this case, the range is 20–40 mg/kg/day.

3. Calculate the recommended dose range: mg/kg/day × kg

$$\text{Minimum recommended dosage} = \frac{20 \text{ mg}}{\text{kg}} \times 12.3 \text{ kg} = 246 \text{ mg/day}$$

$$\text{Maximum recommended dosage} = \frac{40 \text{ mg}}{\text{kg}} \times 12.3 \text{ kg} = 492 \text{ mg/day}$$

4. The dosage ordered, 360 mg/day, falls within the recommended range of 246 mg/day to 492 mg/day. We can now proceed to calculate the amount to administer in each dose.

$$D = 120 \text{ mg} \qquad H = 250 \text{ mg} \qquad Q = 5 \text{ mL}$$

PROPORTION METHOD

EXAMPLE 2

Calculate the amount to administer.

Patient: 1-year-old child who weighs 27 lb

Ordered: Amoxicillin oral suspension drops 120 mg po q8h

On hand: Refer to the label in Figure 16-5.

STEP A: GATHER INFORMATION AND CONVERT
In this case, the desired dose and the dose on hand are both stated in milligrams, so no conversion is necessary; $D = 120$ mg, $H = 250$ mg, and $Q = 5$ mL.

STEP B: CALCULATE
Follow Procedure Checklist 12-1.

1. Set up the proportion.

$$\frac{H}{Q} = \frac{D}{A}$$

$$\frac{250 \text{ mg}}{5 \text{ mL}} = \frac{120 \text{ mg}}{A}$$

2. Cancel units.

$$\frac{250 \text{ m\cancel{g}}}{5 \text{ mL}} = \frac{120 \text{ m\cancel{g}}}{A}$$

3. Cross-multiply and solve for the unknown.

$$250 \times A = 5 \text{ mL} \times 120$$

$$A = 5 \text{ mL} \times \frac{120}{250}$$

$$A = 2.4 \text{ mL}$$

STEP C: THINK! . . . IS IT REASONABLE?
Since the ordered dose 120 mg is less than the dose on hand, 250 mg, then the ordered volume should be less than the supply volume, 5 mL, so an answer of 2.4 mL is a reasonable answer.

DIMENSIONAL ANALYSIS

EXAMPLE 2

Calculate the amount to administer.

Patient: 1-year-old child who weighs 27 lb

Ordered: Amoxicillin oral suspension drops 120 mg po q8h

On hand: Refer to the label in Figure 16-5.

STEP A: GATHER INFORMATION AND CONVERT
In this case, the desired dose and the dose on hand are both stated in milligrams, so no conversion factor is necessary; $D = 120$ mg, $H = 250$ mg, and $Q = 5$ mL.

STEP B: CALCULATE
Follow Procedure Checklist 12-2.

1. The unit of measure will be milliliters.

   A mL =

2. No conversion factor is needed.

3. The dosage unit is 5 mL; the dose on hand is 250 mg.

$$A \text{ mL} = \frac{5 \text{ mL}}{250 \text{ mg}}$$

4. The desired dose is 120 mg. Place this over 1 to finish setting up the equation.

$$A \text{ mL} = \frac{5 \text{ mL}}{250 \text{ mg}} \times \frac{120 \text{ mg}}{1}$$

$$A = 5 \text{ mL} \times \frac{120}{250}$$

$$A = 2.4 \text{ mL}$$

STEP C: THINK! . . . IS IT REASONABLE?
Since the ordered dose 120 mg is less than the dose on hand, 250 mg, then the ordered volume should be less than the supply volume, 5 mL, so an answer of 2.4 mL is a reasonable answer.

FORMULA METHOD

| EXAMPLE 2 | **Calculate the amount to administer.** |

Patient: 1-year-old child who weighs 27 lb

Ordered: Amoxicillin oral suspension drops 120 mg po q8h

On hand: Refer to the label in Figure 16-5.

STEP A: GATHER INFORMATION AND CONVERT
In this case, the desired dose and the dose on hand are both stated in milligrams, so no conversion is necessary; $D = 120$ mg, $H = 250$ mg, and $Q = 5$ mL.

STEP B: CALCULATE
Follow Procedure Checklist 12-3.

1. Fill in the formula.

$$\frac{120 \text{ mg}}{250 \text{ mg}} \times 5 \text{ mL} = A$$

2. Cancel units.

$$\frac{120 \text{ mg}}{250 \text{ mg}} \times 5 \text{ mL} = A$$

3. Solve for the unknown.

$$\frac{120}{250} \times 5 \text{ mL} = A$$

$$A = 2.4 \text{ mL}$$

STEP C: THINK! . . . IS IT REASONABLE?
Since the ordered dose 120 mg is less than the dose on hand, 250 mg, then the ordered volume should be less than the supply volume, 5 mL, so an answer of 2.4 mL is a reasonable answer.

Example 3

Determine whether the following order is safe. If it is safe, calculate the amount to administer.
Patient: 6-year-old child who weighs 49 lb
Ordered: Midazolam 0.025 mg/kg IV now
On hand: Midazolam HCL 2 mg/2 mL. According to the label pediatric patients 6 to 12 years should have an initial dose of up to 0.4 mg/kg increased up to 10 mg to reach the desired effect.

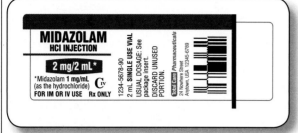

Figure 16-6a

1. Pediatric Patients Less Than 6 Months of Age:
   Limited information is available in non-intubated pediatric patients less than 6 months of age. It is uncertain when the patient transfers from neonatal physiology to pediatric physiology, therefore the dosing recommendations are unclear. Pediatric patients less than 6 months of age are particularly vulnerable to airway obstruction and hypoventilation, therefore titration with small increments to clinical effect and careful monitoring are essential.

2. Pediatric Patients 6 Months to 5 Years of Age:
   Initial dose 0.05 to 0.1 mg/kg; total dose up to 0.6 mg/kg may be necessary to reach the desired endpoint but usually does not exceed 6 mg. Prolonged sedation and risk of hypoventilation may be associated with the higher doses.

3. Pediatric Patients 6 to 12 Years of Age: Initial dose 0.025 to 0.05 mg/kg; total dose up to 0.4 mg/kg may be needed to reach the desired endpoint but usually does not exceed 10 mg. Prolonged sedation and risk of hypoventilation may be associated with the higher doses.

4. Pediatric Patients 12 to 16 Years of Age: Should be dosed as adults. Prolonged sedation may be associated with higher doses; some patients in this age range will require higher than recommended adult doses but the total dose usually does not exceed 10 mg.

Figure 16-6b

1. Convert the patient's weight to kilograms.

$$x \text{ kg} = \frac{1 \text{ kg}}{2.2 \text{ lb}} \times 49 \text{ lb}$$

$$x = 22.3 \text{ kg}$$

Only one dose is ordered, so the total ordered dose per day is 0.025 mg/kg. The ordered dose for this patient is:

$$\frac{0.025 \text{ mg}}{1 \text{ kg}} \times 22.3 \text{ kg} = 0.5575 \text{ mg}$$

2. Check the label and package insert in Figure 16-6 to determine the recommended dosage range. Notice in this case that several pediatric ranges are specified, depending on the age of the child. The patient is 6 years old, so follow the pediatric range for patients 6 to 12 years of age. The range for an initial dose is 0.025–0.05 mg/kg, with a total dose of up to 0.4 mg/kg, not to exceed 10 mg.

3. Calculate the recommended dosage range for this patient:

$$\text{Minimum recommended dosage} = \frac{0.025 \text{ mg}}{1 \text{ kg}} \times 22.3 \text{ kg} = 0.5575 \text{ mg/day}$$

$$\text{Maximum recommended dosage} = \frac{0.05 \text{ mg}}{1 \text{ kg}} \times 22.3 \text{ kg} = 1.115 \text{ mg/day}$$

4. In this case, the ordered dose of 0.5575 mg is at the low end of the recommended range of 0.5575–1.115 mg/day, so the ordered dose is safe. We can proceed to calculate the amount to administer.

PROPORTION METHOD

| EXAMPLE 3 | Find the amount to administer. |

Patient: 6-year-old child who weighs 49 lb

Ordered: Midazolam 0.025 mg/kg IV now

On hand: Refer to the label in Figure 16-6a

STEP A: GATHER INFORMATION AND CONVERT

As calculated previously, the ordered dose of midazolam for this patient is 0.5575 mg. The dose on hand is also in milligrams: $H = 2$ mg, so no conversion is necessary and the desired dose $D = 0.5575$ mg. The dosage unit is 2 mL.

STEP B: CALCULATE

Follow Procedure Checklist 12-1.

1. Set up the proportion.

$$\frac{H}{Q} = \frac{D}{A}$$

$$\frac{2 \text{ mg}}{2 \text{ mL}} = \frac{0.5575 \text{ mg}}{A}$$

2. Cancel units.

$$\frac{2 \text{ m\cancel{g}}}{2 \text{ mL}} = \frac{0.5575 \text{ m\cancel{g}}}{A}$$

3. Cross-multiply and solve for the unknown.

$$2 \times A = 2 \text{ mL} \times 0.5575$$

$$A = 2 \text{ mL} \times \frac{0.5575}{2}$$

$$A = 0.5575 \text{ mL or } 0.56 \text{ mL rounded to the nearest hundredth.}$$

STEP C: THINK! . . . IS IT REASONABLE?

Since the ordered dose, 0.5575 mg, is about one-fourth of the dose on hand, 2 mg, the amount administered should be approximately one-fourth of the dosage unit, 2 mL. Since 0.56 mL is approximately one-fourth of 2 mL, the answer is reasonable.

DIMENSIONAL ANALYSIS

| EXAMPLE 3 | Find the amount to administer. |

Patient: 6-year-old child who weighs 49 lb

Ordered: Midazolam 0.025 mg/kg IV now

On hand: Refer to the label in Figure 16-6a

STEP A: GATHER INFORMATION AND CONVERT

As calculated previously, the ordered dose of midazolam for this patient is 0.5575 mg. The dose on hand is also in milligrams: $H = 2$ mg, so no conversion is necessary. The desired dose is 0.5575 mg. The dosage unit is 2 mL.

STEP B: CALCULATE

Follow Procedure Checklist 12-2.

1. The amount to administer A will be in milliliters.

$$A \text{ mL} =$$

2. No conversion factor is needed.

3. The first factor has the dosage unit Q in the numerator and the dose on hand H in the denominator:

$$A \text{ mL} = \frac{2 \text{ mL}}{2 \text{ mg}}$$

4. The second factor is the desired dose over 1. Finish setting up the equation:

$$A \text{ mL} = \frac{2 \text{ mL}}{2 \text{ mg}} \times \frac{0.5575 \text{ mg}}{1}$$

$A = 0.5575$ mL or 0.56 mL rounded to the nearest hundredth.

STEP C: THINK! . . . IS IT REASONABLE?

Since the ordered dose, 0.5575 mg, is about one-fourth of the dose on hand, 2 mg, the amount administered should be approximately one-fourth of the dosage unit, 2 mL. Since 0.56 mL is approximately one-fourth of 2 mL, the answer is reasonable.

FORMULA METHOD

EXAMPLE 3   Find the amount to administer.

Patient: 6-year-old child who weighs 49 lb

Ordered: Midazolam 0.025 mg/kg IV now

On hand: Refer to the label in Figure 16-6a

STEP A: GATHER INFORMATION AND CONVERT

As calculated previously, the ordered dose of midazolam for this patient is 0.5575 mg. The dose on hand is also in milligrams: $H = 2$ mg, so no conversion is necessary. The desired dose $D = 0.5575$ mg. The dosage unit (Q) is 2 mL.

STEP B: CALCULATE

Follow Procedure Checklist 12-3.

1. Fill in the formula.

$$\frac{D}{H} \times Q = A$$

$$\frac{0.5575 \text{ mg}}{2 \text{ mg}} \times 2 \text{ mL} = A$$

2. Cancel units.

$$\frac{0.5575 \text{ mg}}{2 \text{ mg}} \times 2 \text{ mL} = A$$

3. Solve for the unknown.

$$\frac{0.5575}{2} \times 2 \text{ mL} = A$$

$A = 0.5575$ mL or 0.56 mL rounded to the nearest hundredth.

STEP C: THINK! . . . IS IT REASONABLE?

Since the ordered dose, 0.5575 mg, is about one-fourth of the dose on hand, 2 mg, the amount administered should be approximately one-fourth of the dosage unit, 2 mL. Since 0.56 mL is approximately one-fourth of 2 mL, the answer is reasonable.

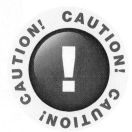

ERROR ALERT!

Converting Ounces Carefully

When infants are weighed in pounds and ounces, you will need to convert the weight to kilograms to perform safe dose calculations. Before converting pounds to kilograms, convert ounces to pounds. Remember 16 oz = 1 lb. An ounce is *not* one-tenth of a pound. A baby whose weight is 8 lb 6 oz does not weigh 8.6 lb. Convert 6 oz to pounds, using the conversion factor of $\frac{1 \text{ lb}}{16 \text{ oz}}$.

Here, $6 \text{ oz} \times \frac{1 \text{ lb}}{16 \text{ oz}} = 0.375 \text{ lb}$. Thus, 8 lb 6 oz = 8.375 lb.

CRITICAL THINKING ON THE JOB

Consider the Safe Dose

While transcribing orders for Mrs. Bekins, who is 83 years old and weighs 118 lb, Karen notes that one of Mrs. Bekins' diagnoses is chronic renal failure. Mrs. Bekins has been given the following drug order: Tazidime 1 g IV q8h for pneumonia. Karen knows that safe doses of antibiotics are often lower for patients with kidney disease than usual pre-scribed doses. From the package insert, she knows the recommended maintenance dose for Tazidime should be adjusted based on CL_{CR}. According to a table in the insert, for creatinine clearance levels of 31 to 50 mL/min, the recommended dosage is 1 g q12h; for levels of 16 to 30 mL/min, the dosage is 1 g q24h; for levels 6 to 15 mL/min, the dosage is 500 mg q24h; and for levels < 5 mL/min, the dosage is 500 mg q48h. Karen is able to determine that the patient's creatinine clearance level is 9.5 mL/min. This value is between 6 and 15 mL/min. Therefore, the safe dose of Tazidime for the patient is 500 mg q24h. This amount is considerably less than the one indicated by the drug order.

Think! . . . Is It Reasonable? What should Karen do? By using critical thinking skills, what patient problem was avoided?

REVIEW AND PRACTICE

16.2 Dosages Based on Body Weight

For Exercises 1–10, convert the following weights to kilograms. Round to the nearest tenth.

1. 66 lb   **2.** 77 lb   **3.** 54 lb   **4.** 37 lb

5. 152 lb   **6.** 202 lb   **7.** 16 lb 4 oz   **8.** 11 lb 10 oz

9. 9 lb 14 oz   **10.** 14 lb 5 oz

For Exercises 11–22, determine if the order is safe. If it is, then determine the amount to administer.

11. The patient is a 3-day-old newborn who weighs 6 lb 5 oz.

    Ordered: Nebcin® 5 mg IM q12h

    On hand: Nebcin® multidose vial, 20 mg/2 mL. According to the package insert, a premature or full-term neonate up to 1 week of age may be administered up to 4 mg/kg/day in 2 equal doses every 12 h.

12. The patient is a 4-year-old child who weighs 32 lb.

    Ordered: Proventil® 1 tsp syrup po tid

    On hand: Proventil® Syrup, 2 mg/5 mL. According to the package insert, for children 2 to 6 years of age, dosing should be initiated at 0.1 mg/kg of body weight 3 times a day.

13. The patient is a 3-year old child who weighs 32 lb and has a severe infection.

    Ordered: Amoxicillin 750 mg PO q8h

    On hand: Refer to label A. According to the package label, the dosing regimen for children is 20 to 40 mg/kg/day q8h.

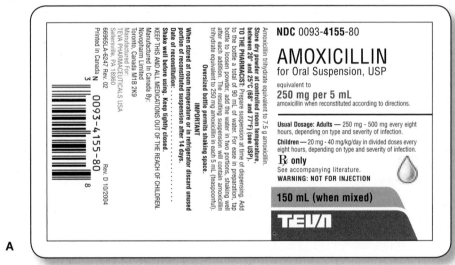

A

This label is for US only, and cannot be altered or translated.

14. The patient is a 5-month-old child who weighs 14 lb.

    Ordered: Kaletra oral solution 40 mg/10 mg PO BID

    On hand: Refer to label B and package insert information C.

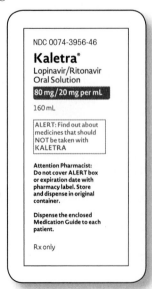

B

14 Days to 6 Months:

In pediatric patients 14 days to 6 months of age, the recommended dosage of lopinavir/ritonavir using KALETRA oral solution is 16/4 mg/kg or 300/75 mg/m^2 twice daily. Prescribers should calculate the appropriate dose based on body weight or body surface area.

Because no data exists for dosage when administered with efavirenz, nevirapine, or nelfinavir, it is recommended that KALETRA not be administered in combination with these drugs in patients < 6 months of age.

C

15. The patient is an 8-year-old child who weighs 55 lb and is being treated for streptococcal pharnygitis.
Ordered: Cephalexin Susp. 200 mg PO q6h

On hand: See label D and package insert information E below.

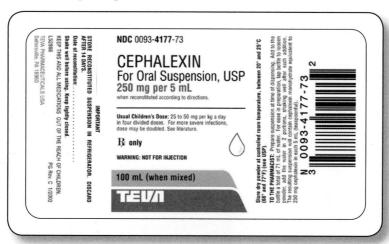

D

This label is for US only, and cannot be altered or translated.

Pediatric Patients The usual recommended daily dosage for pediatric patients is 25 to 50 mg/kg in divided doses. For streptococcal pharyngitis in patients over 1 year of age and for skin and skin structure infections, the total daily dose may be divided and administered every 12 hours.

E

16. The patient is a 44 lb child who is $5\frac{1}{2}$ years old.
Ordered: Tolectin 100 mg po qid

On hand: Tolectin 200 mg scored tablets. The package insert indicates that for children 2 years and older, the usual dose ranges from 15 to 30 mg/kg/day.

17. The patient is a 44 lb child who is $5\frac{1}{2}$ years old.
Ordered: Midazolam 1.5 mg IV

On hand: Refer to label F. The package insert indicates that for children the usual dose ranges from 0.05–0.4 mg/kg.

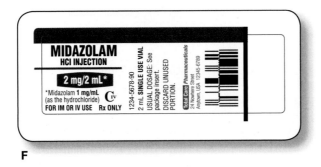

F

18. The patient is a 33 lb child who is 2 years old.

    Ordered: Midazolam 1 mg IV.

    On hand: Refer to label F. The package insert indicates that for children the usual dose ranges from 0.05–0.4 mg/kg.

19. The patient is a 4-month-old child who weighs 12 lb.

    Ordered: Erythromycin suspension 65 mg po q12h

    On hand: Erythromycin oral suspension 100 mg/2.5 mL. According to the package insert, the following are usual dosages for children over 3 months of age: For mild to moderate ear, nose, throat infections, either 25 mg/kg/day in divided doses every 12 h, or 20 mg/kg/day in divided doses every 8 h.

20. The patient is a 1-year-old child who weighs 18 lb.

    Ordered: Erythromycin suspension 160 mg po q8h.

    On hand: Refer to label G.

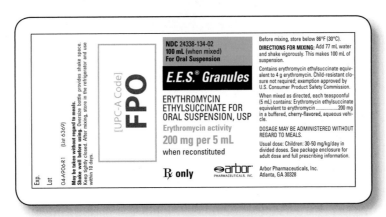

G

21. The patient weighs 47 lb.
    Ordered: Cipro 500 mg PO BID

    On hand: Cipro 250 mg tablets. According to the package insert, the medication can be given 10 to 20 mg/kg every 12 hours.

22. The patient weighs 27 kg.

    Ordered: Somatropin 0.5 mg subcut daily for 1 week

    On hand: 22.5 mg vial with the dosage strength of 1 mg/mL. The recommended weekly dose is 0.18 mg/kg to 0.3 mg/kg body weight. The dose should be divided into equal daily doses given 6 or 7 times per week subcutaneously.

16.3 Dosages Based on Body Surface Area (BSA)

Some medications are prescribed based on a patient's body weight. Other medication orders factor in both weight and height to determine a patient's **body surface area (BSA)**. Many pediatric medications use a patient's BSA to determine the daily dosage. BSA is also important for burn victims and for patients undergoing chemotherapy, radiation treatments, and open-heart surgery. BSA calculations are used to provide more accurate dosage calculations specific to the patient's size and the severity of the illness.

Calculating a Patient's BSA

A patient's BSA is stated in square meters (m^2). You can calculate the BSA by using one of the two formulas listed in Procedure Checklist 16-3. Your calculator should have a program or button that will help you find a square root ($\sqrt{}$). You can also use a special chart called a *nomogram*. **Nomograms** provide an estimate of BSA and are easier to use. Nomograms are available for children and adults. See Figures 16-7 and 16-8.

PROCEDURE CHECKLIST 16-3	Calculating the Body Surface Area Using a Formula To determine a patient's BSA (body surface area):
	1. If you know the height in centimeters and weight in kilograms, calculate $$BSA = \sqrt{\frac{\text{height (cm)} \times \text{weight (kg)}}{3,600}} \text{ m}^2$$ **2.** If you know the height in inches and weight in pounds, calculate $$BSA = \sqrt{\frac{\text{height (in)} \times \text{weight (lb)}}{3,131}} \text{ m}^2$$ *Note: When using a formula to calculate BSA, if the result is less than 1, round to the nearest hundredth. When the result is greater than 1, round to the nearest tenth.*
Example 1	Find the body surface area for a child who is 85 cm tall and weighs 13.9 kg. Use the first of the formulas from Procedure Checklist 16-3. $$BSA = \sqrt{\frac{85 \times 13.9}{3,600}} \text{ m}^2 = \sqrt{\frac{1,181.5}{3,600}} \text{ m}^2 = 0.572 \text{ m}^2 = 0.57 \text{ m}^2$$
Example 2	Find the body surface area for a baby who is 24 in. tall and weighs 12 lb 4 oz. Use the second of the formulas from Procedure Checklist 16-3. First, convert the pounds and ounces to pounds. Recall that there are 16 oz in 1 lb. So $\frac{4}{16} = 0.25$ oz rounded to 0.3 12 lb 4 oz = 12.3 lb $$BSA = \sqrt{\frac{24 \times 12.3}{3,131}} \text{ m}^2 = \sqrt{\frac{295.2}{3,131}} \text{ m}^2 = 0.307 \text{ m}^2 = 0.31 \text{ m}^2$$
Example 3	Find the body surface area for an adult who is 5 ft 6 in. tall and weighs 168 lb. First, convert the height to inches. Since 1 ft equals 12 in., multiply the number of feet by 12 and then add the inches. $5 \times 12 = 60$ $60 + 6 = 66$ in. $$BSA = \sqrt{\frac{66 \times 168}{3,131}} \text{ m}^2 = \sqrt{\frac{11,088}{3,131}} \text{ m}^2 = 1.88 \text{ m}^2 = 1.9 \text{ m}^2$$

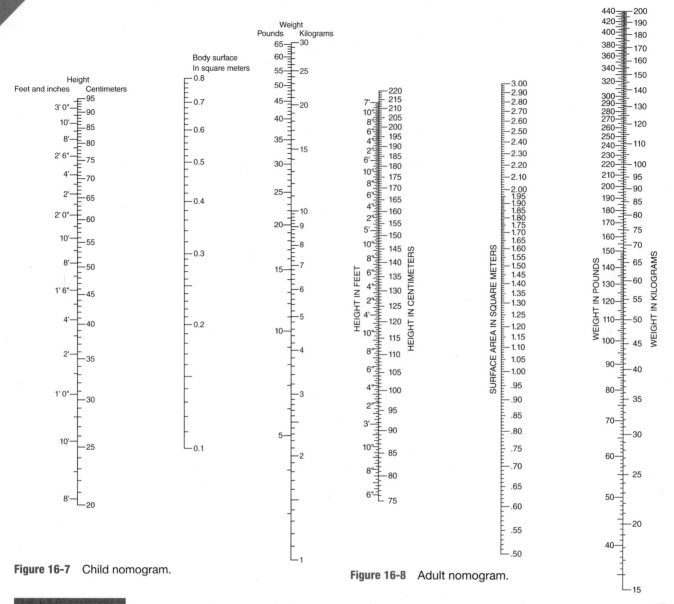

Figure 16-7 Child nomogram.

Figure 16-8 Adult nomogram.

RULE 16-2	Finding the Body Surface Area Using a Nomogram
	Using a straightedge (such as a ruler or piece of paper), align the straightedge so that it intersects at the patient's height and weight. Doing so will create an intersection in the BSA scale. *Note: Read the calibrations carefully, because the spaces and lines vary based upon where the BSA scale is intersected.*
Example 1	Find the body surface area for a child who is 95 cm tall and weighs 13.9 kg, using the child nomogram (Figure 16-9). BSA = 0.60 m^2
Example 2	Find the body surface area for a baby who is 24 in. tall and weighs 12 lb 3 oz, using the child nomogram (Figure 16-10). BSA = 0.29 m^2
Example 3	Find the body surface area for an adult who is 5 ft 6 in. tall and weighs 168 lb, using the adult nomogram (Figure 16-11). BSA = 1.9 m^2

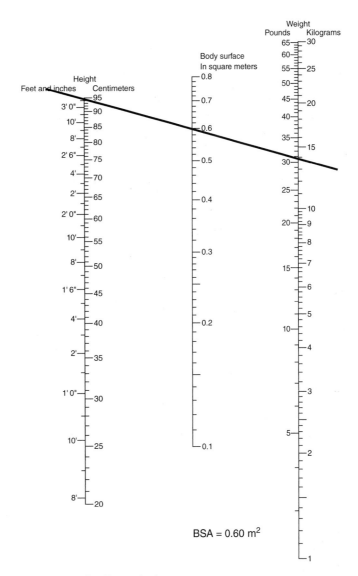

Weight
Pounds   Kilograms

Body surface
In square meters

Height
Feet and inches   Centimeters

BSA = 0.60 m²

Figure 16-9 Child nomogram for Example 1.

PROCEDURE CHECKLIST 16-4	Calculating Dosage Based on BSA
	1. Convert the height and weight into BSA (m²).
	2. Calculate the desired dose: $D =$ dose based on BSA $\times$ BSA mg/m² $\times$ m² (or mcg/m² $\times$ m² or units/m² $\times$ m² . . . .)
	3. Confirm whether the desired dose is safe. If it is unsafe, consult the physician who wrote the order.
	4. If the dose is safe, calculate the amount to administer, using the proportion method, dimensional analysis, or the formula method.
Example 1	Ordered: CeeNU® (first dose) 140 mg now for a patient whose height is 38 in. and weight is 47 lb. On hand: CeeNU® 10 mg, 40 mg, and 100 mg capsules. According to the package insert, the first recommended dose of CeeNU® is a single oral dose providing 130 mg/m². Determine if the dosage ordered is safe, and if safe, calculate the amount to administer.

1. Convert the height and weight into BSA (m^2).

   Because the recommended dose is per square meter (m^2), you need to find the patient's BSA. You know the patient's height and weight in inches and pounds. Use the second formula in Procedure Checklist 16-3 or a nomogram.

   $$BSA = \sqrt{\frac{height\ (in.) \times weight\ (lb)}{3{,}131}}\ m^2$$

   $$BSA = \sqrt{\frac{38 \times 47}{3{,}131}}\ m^2 = \sqrt{\frac{1{,}786}{3{,}131}}\ m^2 = 0.76\ m^2$$

2. Calculate the desired dose.

   $$\frac{130\ mg}{m^2} \times 0.76\ m^2 = 98.8\ mg$$

3. The dose ordered, 140 mg, is above the first recommended dose of 98.8 mg. Consult the authorized prescriber who wrote the order.

4. No calculation is necessary at this time.

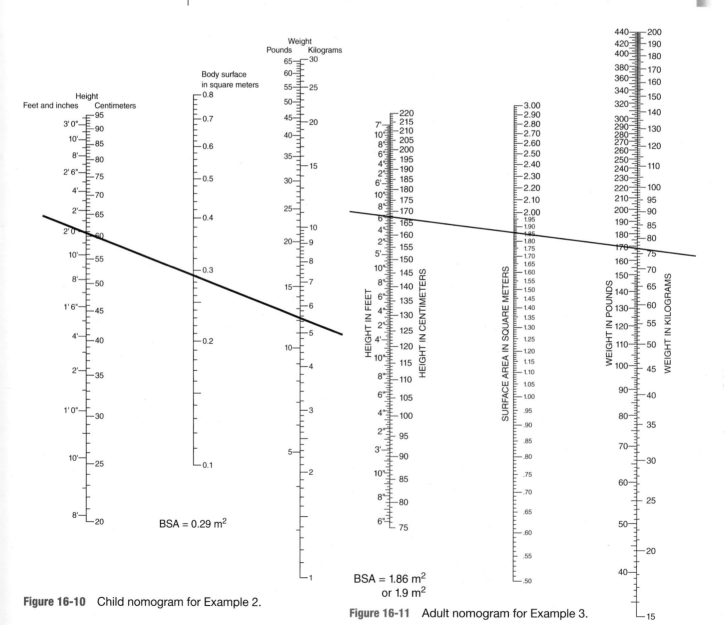

Figure 16-10   Child nomogram for Example 2.

BSA = 0.29 m²

BSA = 1.86 m²
or 1.9 m²

Figure 16-11   Adult nomogram for Example 3.

Example 2

Ordered: CeeNU® (first dose) 150 mg now for a patient who is 99 cm tall and weighs 50 kg.
On hand: CeeNU® 10 mg, 40 mg, and 100 mg capsules. According to the package insert, the first recommended dose of CeeNU® is a single oral dose providing 130 mg/m². Determine if the dosage ordered is safe, and if safe, calculate the amount to administer.

1. Convert the height and weight into BSA m².

   Use the first formula in Procedure Checklist 16-3.

   $$BSA = \sqrt{\frac{99 \times 50}{3,600}}\ m^2 = \sqrt{\frac{4,950}{3,600}}\ m^2 = 1.2\ m^2$$

2. Calculate the desired dose.

   $$\frac{130\ mg}{m^2} \times 1.2\ m^2 = 156\ mg$$

3. The dose ordered is safe since the ordered dose of 150 mg is less than the calculated recommended dose of 156 mg.

4. Calculate the amount to administer. Thinking critically and realizing the capsules cannot be divided, you administer 1 capsule of each strength, 100 mg + 40 mg + 10 mg.

REVIEW AND PRACTICE

16.3 Dosages Based on Body Surface Area (BSA)

For Exercises 1–8, use the appropriate formula to calculate the BSA for patients with the following heights and weights.

1. 88 cm and 13.2 kg
2. 58 cm and 21 kg
3. 38 cm and 6 kg
4. 48 cm and 10 kg
5. 52 in. and 64 lb
6. 43 in. and 35 lb
7. 22 in. and 18 lb
8. 26 in. and 21 lb

For Exercises 9–12, calculate the recommended dosage in the appropriate unit.

9. The child's BSA is 0.82 m². The recommended dosage is 175 mcg/m².

10. The child's BSA is 0.65 m². The recommended dosage is 0.4 mg/m².

11. The child's height is 62 cm and weight is 5 kg. The recommended dosage is 50 mcg/m².

12. The child's height is 41 in. and weight is 63 lb. The recommended dosage is 0.2 mg/m².

For Exercises 13–16, calculate the amount to administer.

13. The patient is 42 in. tall and weighs 71 lb.
    Ordered: Chemotherapy medication 6 mg/m²/day IV q12h
    On hand: Chemotherapy medication 200 mcg/mL for IV use.

14. The patient is 86 cm tall and weighs 12 kg.
    Ordered: Antibiotic 25 mg/m²/day IM q6h
    On hand: Antibiotic 2 mg/mL for IM use.

15. The patient is 34 cm tall and weighs 5 kg.
Ordered: Cerubidine® 25 mg/m² IV weekly
On hand: Cerubidine® for injection. When reconstituted, each milliliter contains 5 mg of drug. The recommended pediatric dosage is 25 mg/m² IV the first day every week.

16. The patient, who is over 1 year old, is 42 in. tall and weighs 45 lb.
Ordered: Oncaspar® 2,500 units/m² IM every 14 days
On hand: Oncaspar® 5 mL/vial, 750 units/mL. The recommended pediatric dosage is 2,500 units/m² for children whose BSA is greater than or equal to 0.6 m² and 82.5 units/kg for children whose BSA is less than 0.6 m².

For Exercises 17–18, determine if the order is safe. If so, calculate the amount to administer.

17. The patient is 125 cm tall and weighs 45 kg.
Ordered: Gemcitabine 800 mg IV weekly.
On hand: Refer to Label A. The usual dose is 1,000 mg/m² over 30 min IV.

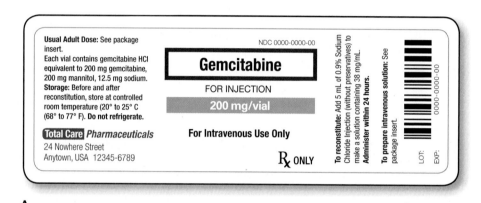

A

18. The patient is 63 in. tall and weighs 125 lb.
Ordered: Cisplatin 125 mg IV every four weeks
On hand: Refer to Label B. The usual dose is 75–100 mg/m².

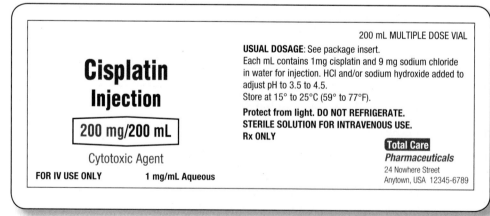

B

CHAPTER 16 SUMMARY

LEARNING OUTCOME	KEY POINTS

16.1 Identify factors that impact drug dosing in special populations. Pages 460–467	1. Pharmacokinetics—the study of how drugs are used by the body.
	
	  a. Absorption—movement of drug into the bloodstream
	
	  b. Distribution—movement of drug from bloodstream into body fluids/tissues
	
	  c. Biotransformation—chemical changing of a drug in the body (liver)
	
	  d. Elimination—excretion of a drug via exhalation or body secretions (urine, sweat, feces, breast milk)
	
	2. Age-related variables
	
	  a. Pediatric (age <18)—increased metabolism, more stomach acid causes lower pH, thinner skin, immature liver, decreased circulation to muscles
	
	  b. Geriatric—(age 65 and older)
	
	    i. Creatinine clearance (CL_{CR})—an indicator of the rate at which kidneys excrete waste; CL_{CR} decreases with age
	
	    ii. Polypharmacy—the practice of taking multiple medications at the same time; polypharmacy may lead to drug interactions.

16.2 Calculate safe dosages based on body weight. Pages 467–482	To calculate a safe dosage based on body weight: 1. Convert weight to kg 2. Calculate the desired dose: mg/kg × kg (or mcg/kg × kg or units/kg × kg ...) 3. Confirm the desired dose is safe. 4. If the dose is safe, calculate the amount to administer using the proportion method, dimensional analysis, or the formula method.

16.3 Calculate dosages based on body surface area (BSA). Pages 483–488	Body surface area incorporates both the height and weight of the patient and can be determined in one of two ways:
	
	1. Using a formula:
	
	  a. BSA in $m^2 = \sqrt{\dfrac{(\text{ht (cm)} \times \text{wt (kg)})}{3{,}600}}$
	
	  b. BSA in $m^2 = \sqrt{\dfrac{(\text{ht (in)} \times \text{wt (lb)})}{3{,}131}}$
	
	2. Using a nomogram by aligning the height and weight with a straightedge and locating the BSA in the center

LEARNING OUTCOME	KEY POINTS
	Safe dose calculations using BSA are used for medications that require very precise amounts.
	To calculate safe doses based on BSA, follow these steps:
	1. Convert the height and weight into BSA (m²).
	2. Calculate the desired dose by multiplying the patient's BSA by the dosage per BSA.
	3. Determine whether the desired dose is safe. If it is unsafe, consult the authorized prescriber.
	4. If the dose is safe, calculate the amount to administer using the proportion method, dimensional analysis, or the formula method.

HOMEWORK ASSIGNMENT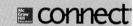

Answer the following questions.

1. List and explain the four processes in the body that affect a drug after it is administered. (LO 16.1)

2. Name two special populations of patients who require extra consideration when calculating medication dosages. (LO 16.1)

3. List four age-related factors that may affect the dosage of a medication for a pediatric patient. (LO 16.1)

4. List four age-related factors that may affect the dosage of a medication for a geriatric patient. (LO 16.1)

5. Explain the impact of creatinine clearance on drug dosages. (LO 16.1)

6. Explain the term "recommended dosage range." (LO 16.2)

7. Body surface area (BSA) uses what two body measurements to provide a more accurate dosage? (LO 16.3)

8. Define the term *polypharmacy* and explain how it would increase the risk of drug interactions in a geriatric patient. (LO 16.1)

For Exercises 9–15, use the identified drug labels and package insert information to answer the following questions. (LO 16.2)

9. What is the safe initial dosage range of valproic acid for a 4-year-old child weighing 41.8 lb? See label A and package insert information.

10. If 850 mg of valproic acid is ordered, what amount would you administer to the child described in the previous question? See label A and package insert information.

Valproic acid package insert information:

> PO (children) initial dose of 15–45 mg/kg/day
>
> If dose is >250 mg/day, it must be administered in divided doses.

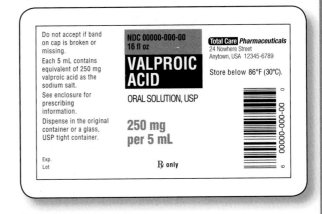

Label A

11. Calculate the correct dosage of granisetron HCl and amount to administer for a 7-year-old child weighing 61.6 lb. See label B and package insert information.

Granisetron HCl package insert information:

> IV (adults & children 2–16 yr.) 10 mcg/kg within 30 min. prior to chemotherapy

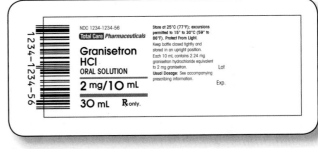

Label B

12. Calculate the safe IM dosage range of clindamycin for a 3-week-old infant weighing 6 lb 12 oz. See label C and package insert information.

13. Calculate the safe IM dosage range of clindamycin for a 3-year-old weighing 33 lb. See label C and package insert information.

Clindamycin package insert information:

> IM, IV (infants <1 month)
> 3.75–5 mg/kg every 6 hours
> IM, IV (children >1 month)
> 5–13.3 mg/kg every 8 hours

14. Calculate the safe dosage range of Gammagard Liquid for a 66-year-old woman weighing 110 lb. See label D and package insert information. (LO 16.2)

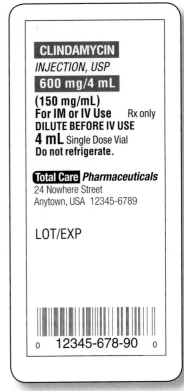

Label C

15. If the order for Gammagard is 15 g, what amount would you administer? See label D and package insert information. (LO 16.2)

Gammagard Liquid package insert information:

Monthly doses of approximately 300–600 mg/kg infused at 3 to 4 week intervals are commonly used.

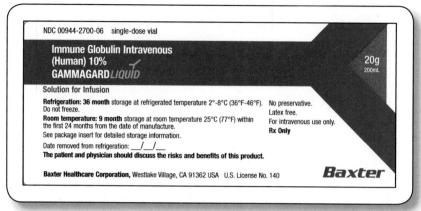

Label D

16. Using the blank nomogram, label E, and the package insert information, calculate the correct dosage of Camptosar® for a 5 ft 8 in. tall, 70-year-old man weighing 170 lb. (LO 16.3)

NOMOGRAM

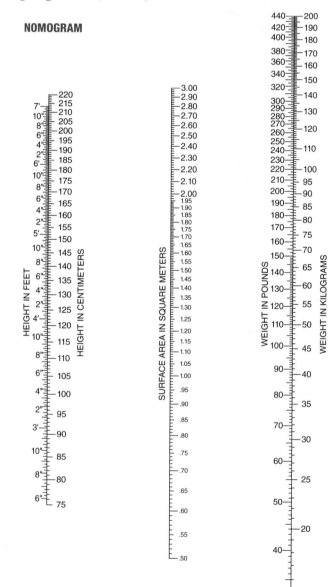

Camptosar® package insert information

The usual dose of CAMPTOSAR® is 180 mg/m² as a 90-minute infusion

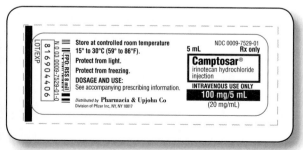

Label E

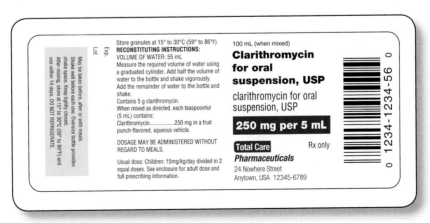

CHAPTER 16 REVIEW

CHECK UP

In Exercises 1–6, convert the following weights to kilograms. Round to the nearest tenth. (LO 16.2)

1. 49 lb

2. 61 lb

3. 6 lb 9 oz

4. 12 lb 13 oz

5. 145 1/4 lb

6. 54 lb 10 oz

In Exercises 7–12, calculate the BSA for patients with the following heights and weights. (LO 16.3)

7. 105 cm and 19 kg

8. 74 cm and 12.1 kg

9. 41 in. and 33 lb

10. 30 in. and 23 lb

11. 66 in. and 165 lb

12. 92 cm and 16.5 kg

In Exercises 13–20, determine if the order is safe. If it is, then determine the amount to administer.

13. The child weighs 30 lb. (LO 16.2)

Ordered: Depakene® syrup 100 mg po q12h

On hand: Depakene® syrup 250 mg/5 mL. According to the package insert, the initial daily dose for pediatric patients is 15 mg/kg/day.

14. The patient is a 4-year-old child who weighs 16 kg. (LO 16.2)

Ordered: Ventolin syrup 1.6 mg po tid

On hand: Ventolin syrup 2 mg/5 mL. According to the package insert, for children from 2 to 6 years of age, dosing should be initiated at 0.1 mg/kg of body weight 3 times a day. This starting dosage should not exceed 2 mg 3 times a day.

15. The patient is 72 cm tall and weighs 16 kg. (LO 16.3)

Ordered: Oncaspar® 1,300 units IM every 14 days

On hand: Oncaspar® 5 mL/vial, 750 units/mL. The recommended pediatric dosage is 2,500 units/m² for children whose BSA is greater than or equal to 0.6 m² and 82.5 units/kg for children whose BSA is less than 0.6 m².

16. The child weighs 31 kg. (LO 16.2)

Ordered: Clarithromycin susp 225 mg po q12h × 10

On hand: Refer to label A. According to the package insert, the usual recommended daily dosage for children is 15 mg/kg/day for 10 days.

A

17. The child weighs 66 lb. (LO 16.2)

Ordered: Oxcarbazepine 150 mg po BID

On hand: Refer to label B. According to the package insert, treatment should be initiated at a daily dose of 8–10 mg/kg generally not to exceed 600 mg/day, given in a BID regimen. The target maintenance dose of Trileptal® should be achieved over 2 weeks and is dependent upon patient weight, according to the following chart:

20–29 kg	900 mg/day
29.1–39 kg	1,200 mg/day
39 kg	1,800 mg/day

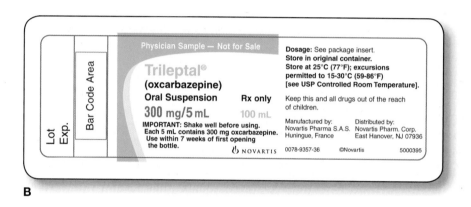

B

18. The patient is a 58 lb child with severe infection. (LO 16.2)

Ordered: Erythromycin 650 mg PO tid.

On hand: Refer to label C. According to the package insert, in mild to moderate infections the usual dosage of erythromycin ethylsuccinate for children is 30 to 50 mg/kg/day in equally divided doses every 6 hours. For more severe infections this dosage may be doubled. If twice-a-day dosage is desired, one-half of the total daily dose may be given every 12 hours. Doses may also be given three times daily by administering one-third of the total daily dose every 8 hours.

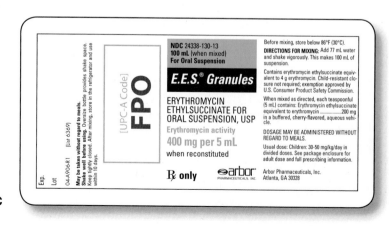

C

19. The patient is a 25 kg child receiving myelosuppressive chemotherapy. (LO 16.2)

Ordered: Filgrastim 125 mcg IVPB over 30 min

On hand: Refer to label D. According to the package insert, for patients receiving myelosuppressive chemotherapy, the recommended daily starting dose is 5 mcg/kg/day, administered as a single daily injection by subcut bolus injection, by short IV infusion (15 to 30 min), or by continuous subcut or continuous IV infusion.

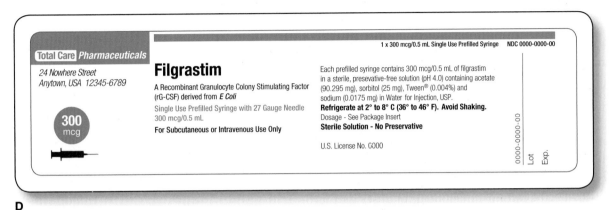

D

20. A 22 lb. 18-month-old child is being treated for hypothyroidism. (LO 7.2)

Ordered: Levothyroxine 50 mcg PO daily

On hand: 25, 50, 75, 88, and 100 mcg tablets. According to the package insert Synthroid (levothyroxine sodium) may be administered to infants and children who cannot swallow intact tablets by crushing the tablet and suspending the freshly crushed tablet in a small amount (5–10 mL or 1–2 tsp) of water. The dosing guidelines indicate that children 1 to 5 years should have 5 to 6 mcg/kg/day.

CRITICAL THINKING APPLICATIONS

A 45-year-old female patient who is 152 lb and 5 ft 6 in. is receiving her Day 1 treatment for ovarian cancer.

Ordered: DAY 1

Cisplatin 150 mg IV

Cyclophosphamide 1080 mg IV

On hand: Cisplatin multiple dose vials 200 mg/200 mL, 100 mg/100 mL, and 50 mg/50 mL and cyclophosphamide 500 mg, 1 g, and 2 g for injection.

According to the package insert the usual cisplatin dose for the treatment of metastatic ovarian tumors in combination with cyclophosphamide is 75 to 100 mg/m2 IV per cycle once every four weeks (DAY 1).

The dose of cyclophosphamide when used in combination with Cisplatin (cisplatin injection) is 600 mg/m2 IV once every four weeks (DAY 1).

For direct IV injection you must gently swirl the vial to dissolve the drug completely. Reconstitute with 0.9% sodium chloride. Sterile water should not be used for reconstitution. Use the following table to determine the volume and dosage strength.

Strength	Volume of 0.9% Sodium Chloride	Cyclophosphamide Concentration
500 mg	25 mL	20 mg per mL
1 g	50 mL	
2 g	100 mL	

1. Are the doses for each drug (cisplatin and cyclophosphamide) ordered within the recommended dose range for this patient?

2. What is the amount to administer of each medication?

CASE STUDY

You are working in a pediatric ICU where your patient is a 3-year-old boy who has a staphylococcal skin infection in the area surrounding his incision. His attending physician has prescribed the following treatment. You know from his chart that he weighs 40 lb. (LO 16.2)

Ordered: Ceftriaxone 600 mg IV over 30 min bid

On hand: Refer to label E. According to the package insert, for pediatric patients with skin infections, the recommended total daily dose is 50 to 75 mg/kg/day given once a day (or in equally divided doses twice a day). The total daily dose should not exceed 2 g. The ceftriaxone is reconstituted to a dosage strength of 40 mg/mL.

1. What is the recommended range of doses for this patient?

2. Is this order a safe dose for your patient? If it is not a safe dose, what steps should you take?

3. Calculate the flow rate for the infusion pump used to deliver this order.

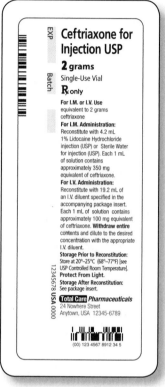

Ceftriaxone for Injection USP

2 grams
Single-Use Vial
R only

For I.M. or I.V. Use
equivalent to 2 grams
ceftriaxone
For I.M. Administration:
Reconstitute with 4.2 mL
1% Lidocaine Hydrochloride
injection (USP) or Sterile Water
for injection (USP). Each 1 mL
of solution contains
approximately 350 mg
equivalent of ceftriaxone.
For I.V. Administration:
Reconstitute with 19.2 mL of
an I.V. diluent specified in the
accompanying package insert.
Each 1 mL of solution contains
approximately 100 mg equivalent
of ceftriaxone. **Withdraw entire**
contents and dilute to the desired
concentration with the appropriate
I.V. diluent.
Storage Prior to Reconstitution:
Store at 20°–25°C (68°–77°F) [see
USP Controlled Room Temperature].
Protect From Light.
Storage After Reconstitution:
See package insert.
Total Care *Pharmaceuticals*
24 Nowhere Street
Anytown, USA 12345-6789

(00) 123 4567 8912 34 5

E

Critical IV Calculations

Great works are performed not by strength but by perseverance.

SAMUEL JOHNSON

LEARNING OUTCOMES

Upon completion of Chapter 17, you will be able to:

17.1 Calculate daily maintenance fluid needs.

17.2 Determine safe doses based on weight and renal function.

17.3 Calculate the hourly flow rate for IV infusions ordered in dosage per time.

17.4 Calculate safe IV heparin dosages.

17.5 Calculate IV flow rates for medications ordered based on body weight over a specified period of time.

17.6 Calculate IV flow rates for titrated medications.

KEY TERMS

Antiarrhythmic (antidysrhythmic) medications

Daily maintenance fluid needs (DMFN)

Dry weight

Hemodynamics

Heparin protocol

Ideal body weight (IBW)

Loading dose

Titrate

Vasoactive medications

INTRODUCTION

Critical dosage calculations surround patients who require close monitoring, have a chronic illness, or are critically ill. For example, children and critically or chronically ill patients are both at risk for an overload of fluid from an IV. Patients with less lean body mass or poor kidney function may need to have their dose of medication adjusted. Controlling vital functions of critically ill patients is difficult and requires constant intervention. Often **vasoactive medications** (medications that cause the blood vessels to dilate or constrict) are administered IV to keep the patient's blood pressure within the normal range. These medications may have a side effect on the patient's heart rate. While these medications are administered, the healthcare professional continuously monitors the patient's blood pressure, heart rhythm, and rate—to **titrate** (adjust) the dosage of medication in response to the patient's vital signs.

In addition to vasoactive medications, **antiarrhythmic (antidysrhythmic) medications** may be given to regulate the patient's heart rate and/or rhythm; and analgesics to relieve pain, sedatives to relieve anxiety, and paralytics to decrease oxygen consumption may also be infused. These medications may be administered at a constant rate, or the rate may be titrated to patient response. Other IV medications, such as antibiotics or electrolyte replacements, must be administered no faster than a specified rate to prevent serious or life-threatening side effects.

For example, a too-rapid infusion of potassium will result in death, and too much heparin can result in severe bleeding. These two high-alert medications and many others require special attention when performing dosage calculations. In these cases, a separate healthcare professional should calculate the dosage independently to verify the dosage before administering the medication or changing the rate of IV administration. These medications are administered by an electronic infusion pump. See Figure 17-1. Critical dosage calculations require a high level of expertise and extra attention to detail to ensure the safety of the patient.

17.1 Daily Maintenance Fluid Needs (DMFN)

Children's bodies contain a higher percentage of water than adults' bodies. Children, as well as critically ill patients, are at greater risk for fluid overload, dehydration, or electrolyte imbalances. Therefore, you must monitor not only the amount of medication but also the amount of fluid the patient receives. Fluids may be calculated based on body weight, body surface area (BSA), metabolism, or age.

Daily maintenance fluid needs (DMFN) represent the fluid a patient needs over 24 h. It combines maintenance fluids (both orally and parenterally), medications, diluent for medications, and fluids used to flush the injection port. The amount of maintenance fluid required varies according to weight, with the smallest children requiring 100 mL/kg/day. DMFN does not include fluids needed to replace those lost to vomiting, diarrhea, or fever. These are called *replacement fluids* and are based on each patient's condition.

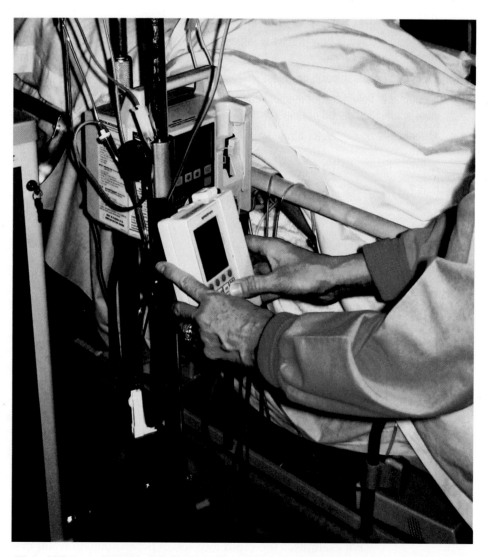

Figure 17-1   Using an electronic infusion pump, a critical care nurse may need to titrate (adjust the dose of a medication) in response to the patient's vital signs.

RULE 17-1	To calculate daily maintenance fluid needs (DMFN) based on weight, use one of the following formulas.

- If the patient weighs up to 10 kg:

$$\frac{100 \text{ mL}}{1 \text{ kg}} \times \text{kg} = \text{DMFN mL}$$

- If the patient weighs 10 to 20 kg:

$$1{,}000 \text{ mL} + \left[\frac{50 \text{ mL}}{1 \text{ kg}} \times (\text{kg} - 10)\right] = \text{DMFN mL}$$

- If the patient weighs over 20 kg:

$$1{,}500 \text{ mL} + \left[\frac{20 \text{ mL}}{1 \text{ kg}} \times (\text{kg} - 20)\right] = \text{DMFN mL}$$

Example 1

Find the DMFN for a patient who weighs

a. 7 kg

The child weighs less than 10 kg.

$$\frac{100 \text{ mL}}{1 \text{ kg}} \times 7 \text{ kg} = 700 \text{ mL}$$

b. 16 kg

The child weighs between 10 and 20 kg.

$$1{,}000 \text{ mL} + \left[\frac{50 \text{ mL}}{1 \text{ kg}} \times (16 \text{ kg} - 10)\right]$$

$$1{,}000 \text{ mL} + \left[\frac{50 \text{ mL}}{1} \times 6\right]$$

$$1{,}000 \text{ mL} + 300 \text{ mL} = 1{,}300 \text{ mL}$$

c. 24 kg

The child weighs over 20 kg.

$$1{,}500 \text{ mL} + \left[\frac{20 \text{ mL}}{1 \text{ kg}} \times (24 \text{ kg} - 20)\right]$$

$$1{,}500 \text{ mL} + \left[\frac{20 \text{ mL}}{1} \times 4\right]$$

$$1{,}500 \text{ mL} + 80 \text{ mL} = 1{,}580 \text{ mL}$$

d. 108 lb

First convert the weight to kg. Recall that 1 lb = 2.2 kg.

$$108 \text{ lb} \times \frac{1 \text{ kg}}{2.2 \text{ lb}} = 49 \text{ kg}$$

The patient weighs over 20 kg.

$$1{,}500 \text{ mL} + \left[\frac{20 \text{ mL}}{1 \text{ kg}} \times (49 \text{ kg} - 20)\right]$$

$$1{,}500 + [20 \text{ mL} \times 29]$$

$$1{,}500 + 580 \text{ mL} = 2{,}080 \text{ mL}$$

RULE 17-2	For pediatric and critically ill patients, you must consider the amount of solution in the IV tubing when you determine infusion times and volumes.
	Five feet of standard IV tubing contains about 10 mL of solution. If this tubing is used along with a volume control chamber, a child will not begin receiving medication until the 10 mL of solution already in the tubing has infused. Low-volume (small-diameter) tubing contains only 0.3 mL of solution per 5 ft and effectively eliminates this problem. Additionally, most medical facilities use electronic flow regulators or infusion pumps to ensure accuracy of medications delivered.

PROCEDURE CHECKLIST 17-1	To determine IV flow rates using the DMFN amount.
	1. Calculate the DMFN using the appropriate formula.
	2. Determine the IV portion of the DMFN by subtracting the daily fluid taken by mouth.
	(Although not always necessary, this step is essential for patients with restricted fluid intake.)
	3. Add the fluid from the IV tubing if a volume control chamber is used.
	4. Calculate the IV flow rate in mL/h or gtt/min using the appropriate formula.

Example 1	What is the flow rate using microdrip tubing for DMFN for a child who weighs 14 kg? The child is NPO and has had nothing by mouth. The IV has a volume control chamber with low-volume, microdrip tubing.

1. Find the DMFN. The patient weighs between 10 and 20 kg.

$$1{,}000 \text{ mL} + \left[\frac{50 \text{ mL}}{1 \text{ kg}} \times (14 \text{ kg} - 10) \right]$$

$$1{,}000 \text{ mL} + \left[\frac{50 \text{ mL}}{1} \times 4 \right]$$

$$1{,}000 \text{ mL} + 200 \text{ mL} = 1{,}200 \text{ mL}$$

2. The child has had nothing by mouth, so the IV DMFN is 1,200 mL.

3. Since low-volume tubing is being used, fluid does not need to be added.

4. Calculate the IV flow rate for 1,200 mL/day.

STEP A: GATHER INFORMATION AND CONVERT

$V = 1{,}200$

$T = 24$ hours

No conversion is needed.

STEP B: CALCULATE

Calculate the IV flow rate in mL/h by substituting into the formula $F = \frac{V}{T}$.

$$F = \frac{1{,}200 \text{ mL}}{24 \text{ h}}$$

$$F = 50 \text{ mL/h}$$

LEARNING LINK   Recall from the "Intravenous Calculations" chapter that microdrip tubing has a drop factor of 60 gtt/mL.

Calculate the IV flow rate in gtt/min by substituting into the formula $f = F \times \dfrac{C}{60}$.

$$f = \frac{50 \text{ mL/h} \times 60 \text{ gtt/mL}}{60 \text{ min/h}}$$

$$f = \frac{50 \text{ m\cancel{L}/\cancel{h}} \times 60 \text{ gtt/m\cancel{L}}}{60 \text{ min/\cancel{h}}}$$

$$f = 50 \text{ gtt/min}$$

STEP C: THINK!. . .IS IT REASONABLE?
The DMFN was calculated using the proper formula. No additions or subtractions were necessary. The flow rate f should equal F because microdrip tubing is being used. So the answer is reasonable if all calculations were performed accurately.

Example 2

Find the DMFN for a patient who weighs 154 lb. The patient is on a fluid restriction and has taken 1,000 mL by mouth. What would be the IV flow rate (F) in mL/h?

1. First convert 154 lb to kilograms.

$$154 \text{ \cancel{lb}} \times \frac{1 \text{ kg}}{2.2 \text{ \cancel{lb}}} = 70 \text{ kg}$$

The patient weighs over 20 kg.

$$1,500 + \left[\frac{20 \text{ mL}}{1 \text{ \cancel{kg}}} \times (70 \text{ \cancel{kg}} - 20)\right] = \text{DMFN mL}$$

$$2,500 \text{ mL} = \text{DMFN}$$

2. Subtract the 1,000 mL of fluid taken by mouth.

$$2,500 - 1,000 = 1,500 \text{ mL IV fluids needed in 24 h}$$

3. A volume control chamber is not being used, so no fluid needs to be added.

4. Calculate the IV flow rate in mL/h.

STEP A: GATHER INFORMATION AND CONVERT

$$V = 1,500$$

$$T = 24 \text{ hours}$$

No conversion is needed.

STEP B: CALCULATE

Use the formula $F = \dfrac{V}{T}$

$$F = 1,500 \text{ mL/24 h}$$

$$F = 62.5, \text{ rounded to } 63 \text{ mL/h}$$

STEP C: THINK!. . .IS IT REASONABLE?
The weight was converted to kg. The DMFN was calculated using the proper formula. The oral fluids were subtracted. The flow rate was calculated using the correct formula. If all calculations were done accurately, the answer is reasonable.

REVIEW AND PRACTICE

17.1 Daily Maintenance Fluid Needs (DMFN)

For Exercises 1–5, calculate the daily maintenance fluid needs, based on the following weights.

1. 8 kg	**2.** 33 kg	**3.** 37 lb	**4.** 58 lb	**5.** 121 lb

In Exercises 6–10, find the microdrip tubing flow rate for DMFN for patients, based on the following weights.

6. 21 kg	**7.** 15 kg	**8.** 17 lb	**9.** 41 lb	**10.** 165 lb

For Exercises 11 and 12, determine the recommended IV flow rate.

11. A patient who weighs 180 lb has an oral intake of 1,000 mL. What should be the flow rate of his IV per hour to maintain his fluids?

12. A patient weighs 31 kg and has an oral intake of 200 mL. What would be the flow rate of his IV per hour to maintain fluids?

17.2 Dosages Based on Ideal Weight

A geriatric patient's body generally has a decreased proportion of lean body mass and water, along with an increased proportion of body fat. These proportions alter the distribution of drugs. Some water-soluble drugs, such as aminoglycosides (antibiotics) and digitalis preparations (cardiac medications), are strongly bound to lean tissues. Because the elderly have less lean tissue, more of these water-soluble drugs remain in the circulating blood. Higher levels can lead to toxicity. Thus, serum drug levels (the level of drug dissolved in the blood) must be monitored.

Fat-soluble drugs are distributed to body fat. Because the elderly have a larger proportion of body fat, these drugs are distributed to more tissues. The drugs do not remain in the body fat, but are slowly released back into circulation. Thus, fat-soluble drugs have a longer duration of action, resulting in residual effects such as drowsiness.

For medications strongly bound to lean tissues (water-soluble), the dose for an overweight patient should be based on the ideal body weight. For patients whose weight is below ideal, the actual weight should be used. For medications strongly bound to body fat (fat-soluble), the dose is based on the actual weight. Note that **ideal body weight (IBW)** is unique for each individual and is based upon many things, such as weight, height, gender, body type, body frame, and age. Use a medically accepted IBW calculator to determine the IBW when needed.

PROCEDURE CHECKLIST 17-2

Determining Safe Dosage Based on Ideal Weight

1. Check the package insert or product literature.

2. Determine if the dose is safe based on renal function and ideal or actual body weight.

3. Determine the dose based on ideal weight.

4. If the dose is safe, calculate the amount to administer.

| **Example** | A 78-year-old male, 5 ft 4 in. tall and weighing 180 lb, is given the following order. He has normal renal function and is being treated for a serious, but not life-threatening, infection. |

Ordered: Garamycin® 70 mg IM q8h

On hand: Garamycin® Injectable, 40 mg/mL

1. According to the package insert, for patients with normal renal function, the usual dosage for serious infections is 1 mg/kg q8h.

2. The dosage for obese patients should be based on lean body mass. Using an IBW calculator, you find that for a 5 ft 4 in. patient, the ideal weight range is 122 to 157 lb.

3. Determine the dose based on the patient's ideal weight.

Convert the weight to kg and multiply by the usual dose.

$$122 \text{ lb}/2.2 \text{ kg/lb} = 55.45 \text{ rounded to } 55 \text{ kg} \times 1 \text{ mg/kg} = 55 \text{ mg}$$

$$157 \text{ lb}/2.2 \text{ kg/lb} = 71.36 \text{ rounded to } 71 \text{ kg} \times 1 \text{ mg/kg} = 71 \text{ mg}$$

The dosage ordered, 70 mg, falls within the safe range.

4. The dose is safe, so calculate the amount to administer. Using the formula method. $\frac{D}{H} \times Q = A$

$$\frac{70 \text{ mg}}{40 \text{ mg}} \times 1 \text{ mL} = 1.75 \text{ mL; round to } 1.8 \text{ mL}$$

LEARNING LINK Recall the importance of creatinine clearance (CL_{CR}) from the chapter "Calculations for Special Populations".

ERROR ALERT!

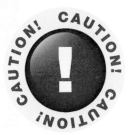

Calculations for Overweight Patients

For Medications That Are Strongly Bound to Lean Body Tissue, Calculate an Overweight Patient's Dose on Ideal Body Weight, Not Actual Weight.

Suppose a 75-year-old female, 5 ft 1 in. tall, 190 lb with a CL_{CR} of 30 mL/min is prescribed an initial daily dose of 0.25 mg of Lanoxin® injection. According to the package insert, the level of Lanoxin® is based on the patient's creatinine clearance and ideal body weight, not actual body weight. The patient's safe dose is 125 mcg/day (0.125 mg/day), one-half the amount prescribed. By getting too much medication, the patient could suffer digoxin toxicity. The physician who initially ordered the Lanoxin® made the first error. Still, the healthcare professional who administers the Lanoxin® should check the safety of the amount and verify the order with the authorized prescriber before administration.

Selecting the Safest Medication

You are preparing medication for two patients. Patient A has healthcare-acquired pneumonia and a creatinine clearance of 37 mL/min. He has been ordered Zosyn® 4.5 grams q6h IV. Patient B has pelvic inflammatory disease and a normal creatinine clearance. She has been ordered Zosyn® 3.375 grams IV q6h. You have the following Zosyn® medication vials and package insert information.

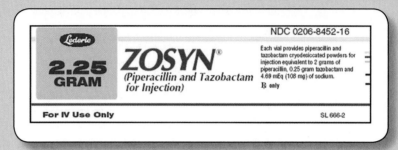

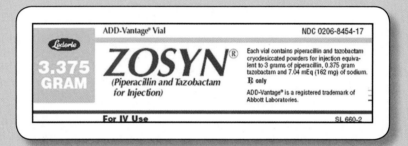

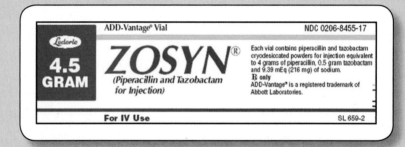

Directions for Reconstitution and Dilution for Use Intravenous Administration

For conventional vials, reconstitute Zosyn® per gram of piperacillin with 5 mL of a compatible reconstitution diluent from the list provided below.

2.25 g, 3.375 g, and 4.5 g Zosyn® should be reconstituted with 10 mL, 15 mL, and 20 mL, respectively. Swirl until dissolved.

Pharmacy vials should be used immediately after reconstitution. Discard any unused portion after 24 hours if stored at room temperature [20°C to 25°C (68°F to 77°F)], or after 48 hours if stored at refrigerated temperature [2°C to 8°C (36°F to 46°F)].

Compatible Reconstitution Diluents

0.9% sodium chloride for injection
Sterile water for injection

Dextrose %
Bacteriostatic saline/parabens
Bacteriostatic water/parabens
Bacteriostatic saline/benzyl alcohol
Bacteriostatic water/benzyl alcohol
Reconstituted Zosyn® solution should be further diluted (recommended volume per dose of 50 mL to 150 mL) in a compatible intravenous diluent solution listed below. Administer by infusion over a period of at least 30 minutes. During the infusion it is desirable to discontinue the primary infusion solution.

Recommended Dosing of Zosyn in Patients with Normal Renal Function and Renal Insufficiency (As total grams piperacillin/tazobactam)

Renal Function (Creatinine Clearance, mL/min)	All Indications (except healthcare-acquired pneumonia)	Healthcare-acquired Pneumonia
> 40 mL/min	3.375 q 6 h	4.5 q 6 h
20-40 mL/min*	2.25 q 6 h	3.375 q 6 h
< 20 mL/min*	2.25 q 8 h	2.25 q 6 h
Hemodialysis**	2.25 q 12 h	2.25 q 8 h
CAPD	2.25 q 12 h	2.25 q 8 h

*Creatinine clearance for patients not receiving hemodialysis

** 0.75 g should be administered following each hemodialysis session on hemodialysis days

1. Are the dosages for Patient A and Patient B safe?

2. If safe, what medication will you use and how will you prepare the medication?

3. If not safe, what action should you take?

4. According to the package insert, you further dilute each medication with 150 mL of sterile water for injection. To infuse the medication over 30 minutes, what would the IV flow rate be in mL per hour for administration of the medication to Patient B?

REVIEW AND PRACTICE

17.2 Dosages Based on Ideal Weight

For Exercises 1–4, determine if the dosage ordered is safe.

1. The patient: 92-year-old female, 5 ft 6 in. tall, 130 lb, and CL_{CR} of 61 mL/min. Patient is in ideal weight range and has normal renal function.

   Ordered: Amikacin 375 mg IM q12h

   According to the package insert, patients with normal renal function may be administered up to 7.5 mg/kg q12h or 5 mg/kg q8h.

2. The patient: 76-year-old female, 5 ft 2 in. tall, 126 lb, and CL_{CR} of 50 mL/min. Patient is in ideal weight range.

Ordered: Tazidime 1 g IV q12h

According to the package insert, for creatinine clearance levels of 31 to 50 mL/min, the recommended dosage is 1 g q12h; for levels of 16 to 30 mL/min, the dosage is 1 g q24h; for levels of 6 to 15 mL/min, the dosage is 500 mg q24h; and for levels less than 5 mL/min, the dosage is 500 mg q48h.

3. The patient: 68-year-old male, 5 ft 7 in. tall, 188 lb, CL_{CR} of 60 mL/min, and impaired renal function. Ideal weight should be 172 lb.

Ordered: Vancocin® HCl 150 mg IV q6h

According to the package insert, the daily dosage for patients with normal renal function is 2 g divided into doses q6h or q12h. The daily dosage for patients with impaired renal function is 1,545 mg/24 h for creatinine clearance of 100 mL/min; 1,390 mg/24 h for 90 mL/min; 1,235 mg/24 h for 80 mL/min; 1,080 mg/24 h for 70 mL/min; 925 mg/24 h for 60 mL/min; 770 mg/24 h for 50 mL/min; 620 mg/24 h for 40 mL/min; 425 mg/24 h for 30 mL/min; 310 mg/24 h for 20 mL/min; and 155 mg/24 h for 10 mL/min.

4. The patient: 79-year-old female, 5 ft tall, 110 lb, CL_{CR} of 90 mL/min, and normal renal function. Patient is within ideal weight range.

Ordered: Vancocin® HCl 0.5 g IV q6h

See Exercise 3 above for information about the recommended daily dosage.

For Exercises 5 and 6, determine if the dosage ordered is safe. If the dosage is safe, find the amount to administer.

5. The patient: 75-year-old female, 5 ft 3 in. tall, 198 lb, CL_{CR} of 30 mL/min, diagnosed with hypertension and renal impairment. Ideal weight should be 152 lb.

Ordered: Vasotec® 5 mg po daily

On hand: Vasotec® 5-mg scored tablets

According to the package insert, the usual dose for patients with normal renal function (over 80 mL/min creatinine clearance) is 5 mg/day; for mild impairment (over 30 and up to 80 mL/min), 5 mg/day; for moderate to severe impairment (30 or less mL/min), 2.5 mg/day.

6. The patient: 81-year-old male, 5 ft tall, 138 lb, CL_{CR} of 63 mL/min, and renal impairment. Patient is within ideal weight range.

Ordered: Ticarcillin 2 g IV q4h

On hand: Ticar 1 g vial, 200 mg/mL when reconstituted

According to the package insert, the usual dose, after the initial loading dose, for patients with infections complicated by renal insufficiency, is 3 g q4h with creatinine clearance over 60 mL/min; 2 g q4h for 30 to 60 mL/min; 2 g q8h for 10 to 30 mL/min; 2 g q12h for less than 10 mL/min; other amounts for patients with complications.

▌17.3▐ Hourly Flow Rates for Dosage per Time Infusions

Dosage per Hour

When you know the amount of medication in an amount of solution and the amount of medication to be delivered in a specific amount of time, you can determine the hourly flow rate of the medication.

RULE 17-3	Calculate the rate to administer a solution with medication using an electronic device in mL/h where: D = rate of desired dose (mcg/h, mg/h, g/h, units/h) Q = dosage unit (mL) H = dose on hand (total number of mcg, mg, g, units) A = amount to administer (mL/h) Use the proportion method, dimensional analysis, or formula method to find the hourly flow rate.

PROPORTION METHOD

Copyright © 2016 by McGraw-Hill Education

EXAMPLE 1

Find the hourly rate at which to administer IV morphine sulfate.

Ordered: morphine sulfate 4 mg/h
On hand: morphine sulfate 10 mg/100 mL D5W

STEP A: GATHER INFORMATION AND CONVERT

The rate of the desired dose D is 4 mg/1h. The dosage unit Q is 100 mL. The dose on hand H is 10 mg. A is the amount (volume) to administer/h.

The desired dose and dose on hand are both in mg, so no conversion factor is necessary.

STEP B: CALCULATE

Follow Procedure Checklist 12-1.

1. Set up the proportion.

$$\frac{H}{Q} = \frac{D}{A}$$

$$\frac{10 \text{ mg}}{100 \text{ mL}} = \frac{4 \text{ mg/h}}{A}$$

2. Cancel the units, leaving mL/h

$$\frac{10 \text{ m\cancel{g}}}{100 \text{ mL}} = \frac{4 \text{ m\cancel{g}/h}}{A}$$

3. Cross-multiply and solve for the unknown.

$$10 \times A = 100 \text{ mL} \times 4/h$$

$$A = \frac{400 \text{ mL/h}}{10}$$

$$A = 40 \text{ mL/h}$$

STEP C: THINK! . . . IS IT REASONABLE?

Since the dosage strength is 1 mg to 10 mL, and 4 × 10 is 40, it is reasonable that a 4 mg/h dose would equal 40 mL/h.

EXAMPLE 2

Find the hourly rate at which to administer IV heparin.

Ordered: 1,000 units/h IV heparin using an infusion pump
On hand: 25,000 units heparin in 500 mL of D5W

STEP A: GATHER INFORMATION AND CONVERT

The rate of the dosage ordered D is 1,000 units/h. The dose on hand H is 25,000 units, and the dosage unit Q is 500 mL.

The dosage ordered and the dose on hand have the same units; no conversion is necessary.

STEP B: CALCULATE

Follow Procedure Checklist 12-1.

1. Set up the proportion.

$$\frac{25,000 \text{ units}}{500 \text{ mL}} = \frac{1,000 \text{ units/h}}{A}$$

2. Cancel units, leaving mL/h for the answer.

$$\frac{25,000 \text{ \cancel{units}}}{500 \text{ mL}} = \frac{1,000 \text{ \cancel{units}/h}}{A}$$

3. Cross-multiply and solve for the answer.

$$25,000 \times A = 500 \text{ mL} \times 1,000/\text{h}$$

$$25,000 \times A = 500,000 \text{ mL}/\text{h}$$

$$A = \frac{500,000 \text{ mL}/\text{h}}{25,000}$$

$$A = 20 \text{ mL}/\text{h}$$

STEP C: THINK! . . . IS IT REASONABLE?

Since the dosage strength of a 25,000 units/500 mL solution is 50 units/1 mL, and 50×20 is 1,000, it is reasonable.

DIMENSIONAL ANALYSIS

EXAMPLE 1 | Find the hourly rate at which to administer IV morphine sulfate.

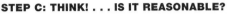

Ordered: morphine sulfate 4 mg/h
On hand: morphine sulfate 10 mg/100 mL D5W

STEP A: GATHER INFORMATION AND CONVERT

The rate of the desired dose D is 4 mg/h. The dosage unit Q is 100 mL. The dose on hand H is 10 mg. Follow Procedure Checklist 12-2.

The desired dose and dose on hand are both in mg, so no conversion factor is needed.

STEP B: CALCULATE

1. The unit of measure will be in milliliters per hour

A mL/h

2. No conversion factor is needed.

3. The dosage unit is 100 mL; the dose on hand is 10 mg. This is the first factor.

$$A \text{ mL}/\text{h} = \frac{100 \text{ mL}}{10 \text{ mg}}$$

4. The desired dose is 4 mg/h. This is the second factor. Complete the equation.

$$A \text{ mL}/\text{h} = \frac{100 \text{ mL}}{10 \text{ mg}} \times \frac{4 \text{ mg}}{\text{h}}$$

5. Cancel units.

$$A \text{ mL}/\text{h} = \frac{100 \text{ mL}}{10 \text{ mg}} \times \frac{4 \text{ mg}}{\text{h}}$$

Since the remaining units are mL/h and the unit of measure for the amount to administer is mL/h, the equation is set up correctly.

6. Solve the equation.

$$A \text{ mL}/\text{h} = \frac{100 \text{ mL} \times 4}{10 \text{ h}}$$

$$A \text{ mL}/\text{h} = \frac{400 \text{ mL}}{10 \text{ h}}$$

$$A = 40 \text{ mL}/\text{h}$$

STEP C: THINK! . . . IS IT REASONABLE

Since the dosage strength is 1 mg to 10 mL, and 4 × 10 is 40, it is reasonable that a 4 mg/h dose would equal 40 mL/h.

EXAMPLE 2

Find the hourly rate at which to administer IV heparin.

Ordered: 1,000 units/h IV heparin using an infusion pump

On hand: 25,000 units heparin in 500 mL of D5W

STEP A: GATHER INFORMATION AND CONVERT

The rate of the desired dose D is 1,000 units/h. The dosage unit Q is 500 mL. The dose on hand H is 25,000 units.

Follow Procedure Checklist 12-2.

No conversion factor is necessary because the desired dose and dose on hand are both in units.

STEP B: CALCULATE

1. The unit of measure will be milliliters per hour.

   A mL/h =

2. No conversion factor is needed.

3. The dosage unit is 500 mL; the dose on hand is 25,000 units. This is your first factor.

   $$A \text{ mL/h} = \frac{500 \text{ mL}}{25,000 \text{ units}}$$

4. The desired dose is 1,000 units/h. This is the second factor. Complete the equation.

   $$A \text{ mL/h} = \frac{500 \text{ mL}}{25,000 \text{ units}} \times \frac{1,000 \text{ units}}{1 \text{ h}}$$

5. Cancel units. The remaining units on the right side of the equation should be milliliters per hour. The equation is set up correctly.

   $$A \text{ mL/h} = \frac{500 \text{ mL}}{25,000 \text{ units}} \times \frac{1,000 \text{ units}}{1 \text{ h}}$$

6. Solve the equation.

   $$A \text{ mL/h} = 500 \text{ mL} /25 \times 1\text{h}$$

   $$A = 20 \text{ mL/h}$$

STEP C: THINK! . . . IS IT REASONABLE?

Since the dosage strength of a 25,000 unit/500 mL solution is 50 units/1 mL, and 50 × 20 is 1,000, it is reasonable.

FORMULA METHOD

EXAMPLE 1

Find the hourly rate at which to administer IV morphine sulfate.

Ordered: morphine sulfate 4 mg/h
On hand: morphine sulfate 10 mg/100 mL D5W

STEP A: GATHER INFORMATION AND CONVERT

The rate of the desired dose D is 4 mg/h. The dosage unit Q is 100 mL. The dose on hand H is 10 mg. The desired dose and dose on hand are both in mg, so no conversion is necessary.

STEP B: CALCULATE

Follow Procedure Checklist 12-3.

1. Fill in the formula:

$$\frac{D}{H} \times Q = A$$

$$\frac{4 \text{ mg/h}}{10 \text{ mg}} \times 100 \text{ mL} = A$$

2. Cancel units.

$$\frac{4 \cancel{\text{mg}}/h}{10 \cancel{\text{mg}}} \times 100 \text{ mL} = A$$

3. Solve for the unknown.

$$\frac{400 \text{ mL/h}}{10} = A$$

$$\frac{40 \text{ mL}}{h} = A$$

STEP C: THINK! . . . IS IT REASONABLE?

Since the dosage strength is 1 mg to 10 mL, and 4×10 is 40, it is reasonable that a 4 mg/h dose would equal 40 mL/h.

EXAMPLE 2

Find the hourly rate at which to administer IV heparin.

Ordered: 1,000 units/h IV heparin using an infusion pump
On hand: 25,000 units heparin in 500 mL of D5W

STEP A: GATHER INFORMATION AND CONVERT

The rate of the desired dose D is 1,000 units/h. The dosage unit Q is 500 mL. The dose on hand is 25,000 units. The desired dose and dose on hand are both in mg, so no conversion is necessary.

STEP B: CALCULATE

Follow Procedure Checklist 12-3.

1. Fill in the formula:

$$\frac{D}{H} \times Q = A$$

$$\frac{1,000 \text{ units/h}}{25,000 \text{ units}} \times 500 \text{ mL} = A$$

2. Cancel units

$$\frac{1,000 \cancel{\text{units}}/h}{25,000 \cancel{\text{units}}} \times 500 \text{ mL} = A$$

3. Solve the equation.

$$\frac{1,000 \text{ h}}{25,000} \times 500 \text{ mL} = A$$

$$20 \text{ mL/h} = A$$

STEP C: THINK!. . .IS IT REASONABLE?

Since the dosage strength of 25,000 units/500 mL solution equals 50 units/1 mL, and 50×20 is 1,000, it is reasonable.

Dosage per Minute

Potent medications may be ordered in amounts per minute. Amounts per minute need to be converted to milliliters per hour in order to program the infusion pump.

RULE 17-4

To calculate an hourly flow rate from a per-minute order:

1. Convert mg/min to mg/hr. Multiply mg/min $\times$ 60 min/h. For dimensional analysis, use 60 min/1 h as the first conversion factor.

2. Use the proportion method or dimensional analysis to calculate the flow rate in mL/h.

PROPORTION METHOD

EXAMPLE

Find the hourly flow rate.

Ordered: 5,000 mg Esmolol in 500 mL of D5W at 8 mg/min via infusion pump

STEP A: GATHER INFORMATION AND CONVERT

Dosage unit Q is 500 mL. Dose on hand H is 5,000 mg. The dosage ordered is 8 mg/min. We must convert mg/min to mg/h to obtain the desired dose D.

Convert mg/min to mg/h

There are 60 minutes in an hour so

$$\text{mg/min} \times 60 \text{ min/h} = \text{mg/h}$$

$$8 \text{ mg/\cancel{min}} \times 60 \text{ \cancel{min}/h} = 480 \text{ mg/h}$$

The rate of the desired dose D is now 480 mg/h.

STEP B: CALCULATE

Follow Procedure Checklist 12-1.

1. Fill in the proportion.

$$\frac{H}{Q} = \frac{D}{A}$$

$$\frac{5,000 \text{ mg}}{500 \text{ mL}} = \frac{480 \text{ mg/h}}{A}$$

2. Cancel the units leaving mL/h

$$\frac{5,000 \text{ \cancel{mg}}}{500 \text{ mL}} = \frac{480 \text{ \cancel{mg}/h}}{A}$$

3. Cross-multiply and solve for the unknown.

$$5,000 \times A = 500 \text{ mL} \times 480/h$$

$$A = \frac{500 \text{ mL} \times 480/h}{5,000}$$

$$A = 48 \text{ mL/h}$$

STEP C: THINK! . . . IS IT REASONABLE?

Since the concentration of 5,000 mg/500 mL equals 10 mg/mL, and 480 mg/10 = 48, the answer is reasonable.

DIMENSIONAL ANALYSIS

EXAMPLE	**Find the hourly flow rate.**

Ordered: 5,000 mg Esmolol in 500 mL of D5W at 8 mg/min via infusion pump

STEP A: GATHER INFORMATION AND CONVERT
The rate of the desired dose D is 8 mg/min. The dosage unit Q is 500 mL. The dose on hand H is 5,000 mg. The desired dose D in mg/min should be converted to mg/h, so the conversion factor 60 min/1 h is required.

STEP B: CALCULATE
Follow Procedure Checklist 12-2.

1. The unit of measure will be milliliters per hour.

   A mL/h =

2. The conversion factor is 60 min/1 h. This is your first factor.

   $A \text{ mL/h} = \dfrac{60 \text{ min}}{1 \text{ h}}$

3. The dosage unit is 500 mL; the dose on hand is 5,000 mg. This is the second factor.

   $A \text{ mL/h} = \dfrac{60 \text{ min}}{1 \text{ h}} \times \dfrac{500 \text{ mL}}{5,000 \text{ mg}}$

4. The desire dose is 8 mg/min. This is the third factor. Complete the equation.

   $A \text{ mL/h} = \dfrac{60 \text{ min}}{1 \text{ h}} \times \dfrac{500 \text{ mL}}{5,000 \text{ mg}} \times \dfrac{8 \text{ mg}}{1 \text{ min}}$

5. Cancel units. The remaining units on the right side of the equation should be milliliters per hour.

   $A \text{ mL/h} = \dfrac{60 \text{ \cancel{min}}}{1 \text{ h}} \times \dfrac{500 \text{ mL}}{5,000 \text{ \cancel{mg}}} \times \dfrac{8 \text{ \cancel{mg}}}{1 \text{ \cancel{min}}}$

6. Solve the equation.

   $A \text{ mL/h} = \dfrac{60}{1 \text{ h}} \times \dfrac{500 \text{ mL}}{5,000} \times \dfrac{8}{1}$

   $A = 48 \text{ mL/h}$

STEP C: THINK! . . . IS IT REASONABLE?
Since the concentration of 5,000 mg/500 mL equals 10 mg/mL, and 480 mg/10 = 48, the answer is reasonable.

REVIEW AND PRACTICE

17.3 Hourly Flow Rates for Dosage per Time Infusions

For Exercises 1–15, find the flow rate in mL/h via infusion pump.

1. Ordered: Heparin 1,000 units/h

   On hand: 20,000 units in 1,500 mL of 5% DW

2. Ordered: Heparin 1,000 units/h

   On hand: 20,000 units in 500 mL of D5W

3. Ordered: Heparin 850 units/h

   On hand: 40,000 units in 1,500 mL of 5% DW

4. Ordered: Heparin 1,500 units/h

   On hand: 30,000 units 500 mL of 5% D 0.45% NS

5. Ordered: Heparin 750 units/h

   On hand: 30,000 units in 1,000 mL of 5% DW

6. Ordered: xylocaine 2 mg/min IV

   On hand: xylocaine 1 g/500 mL D5W

7. Ordered: nitroglycerin 10 mcg/min IV

   On hand: nitroglycerin 50 mg/250 mL NS

8. Ordered: vasopressin 0.04 units/min IV

   On hand: vasopressin 60 units/50 mL NS

9. Ordered: diltiazem 5 mg/h IV

   On hand: diltiazem 125 mg/125 mL D5W

10. Ordered: epinephrine 2 mcg/min IV

    On hand: epinephrine 1 mg/500 mL NS

11. Ordered: nitroglycerin 10 mcg/min IV

    On hand: nitroglycerin 25 mg in 250 mL D5W

12. Ordered: procainamide 3 mg/min IV

    On hand: procainamide hydrochloride 1 g/250 mL D5W

13. Ordered: morphine 4 mg/h IV

    On hand: morphine 50 mg/100 mL NS

14. Ordered: midazolam 0.5 mg/h

    On hand: midazolam 25 mg/50 mL NS

15. Ordered: nicardipine 7.5 mg/h

    On hand: nicardipine 25 mg/250 mL D5W

17.4 Safe Heparin Dosages

Heparin, as you should know, is a high-alert medication. As such, it requires special attention to ensure that it is administered safely. To prevent dosage and administration errors, many hospitals use a **heparin protocol**. A heparin protocol is a preprinted order set that guides the administration of IV heparin based on the patient's weight and serum activated partial thromboplastin time (aPTT), a blood clotting value measured in seconds. Look at the sample weight-based heparin protocol in Table 17-1. Tables like this one are used for high-intensity conditions, such as deep vein thrombosis (DVT) or pulmonary embolism (PE). The **loading dose**, which is the initial bolus dose given to achieve a therapeutic blood level of heparin, is based on the patient's weight. A maximum dose is provided, so that the patient will not receive a toxic dose of heparin. If the calculated dose of heparin, based on the patient's weight, exceeds the maximum bolus dosage, then only the maximum bolus dosage will be administered, followed by the heparin infusion. Notice too, that the infusion rate and all subsequent changes are based on the patient's weight in kg. Adjustments to the IV will be discussed in Section 17.6.

TABLE 17-1 Heparin Protocol for DVT, PE, and High-Intensity Indications
GOAL: aPTT 70–100

Use heparin sodium 1,000 USP units/mL for bolus dose. Use premixed heparin sodium 25,000 USP units in 5% dextrose in water 500 mL (50 units/mL) for infusion. Obtain baseline CBC and aPTT prior to administering heparin. Obtain aPTT 6 hours after each rate change. If the aPTT is at goal, repeat the aPTT until two consecutive aPTT are at goal, draw aPTT daily while receiving heparin, and aPTT remains between 70 and 100.
Initial bolus dose: 80 units/kg (maximum 8,000 units)
Initial rate: 18 units/kg/h (maximum 1,800 units/h = 36 mL/h)

aPTT RESULT	IV BOLUS DOSE	# MINUTES TO HOLD INFUSION	AMOUNT TO CHANGE CURRENT INFUSION RATE
Less than 54 Notify AP	80 units/kg (max. 8,000 units)	Do not hold	Increase by 4 units/kg/h
54–59	40 units/kg (max. 4,000 units)	Do not hold	Increase by 2 units/kg/h
60–69	40 units/kg (max. 4,000 units)	Do not hold	Increase by 1 unit/kg/h
70–100 goal	**No bolus dose**	**Do not hold**	**Do not change current infusion rate**
101–115	No bolus dose	Do not hold	Decrease by 1 unit/kg/h
116–135	No bolus dose	30	Decrease by 2 units/kg/h
136–150	No bolus dose	60	Decrease by 3 units/kg/h and repeat aPTT 6 hours after infusion resumed
151–200 Notify AP	No bolus dose	90	Decrease by 4 units/kg/h and repeat aPTT 6 hours after infusion resumed

Adapted for calculation purposes only, from (2008) ACCP guidelines; **not to be used in clinical practice.**

Weight-Based Bolus Dose Calculations

When a heparin protocol is started, an initial IV bolus dose of heparin is usually calculated for each patient based upon the patient's weight. This dose is typically administered directly into the IV, also known as *IV push.*

PROPORTION METHOD

EXAMPLE

The patient weighs 154 lb. Using the heparin protocol in Table 17-1, calculate the loading dose.

STEP A: GATHER INFORMATION AND CONVERT

According the Table 17-1, the loading dose (initial bolus dose) should be 80 units/kg. First convert the patient's weight in pounds to kilograms.

$$\frac{1\,\text{kg}}{2.2\,\text{lb}} = \frac{x}{154\,\text{lb}}$$

Cross multiply and solve the equation.

$$1\,\text{kg} \times 154 = 2.2 \times x$$

$$\frac{154\,\text{kg}}{2.2} = x$$

$$70\,\text{kg} = x$$

STEP B: CALCULATE

Calculate the bolus dose.

$$\frac{80 \text{ units}}{1 \text{ kg}} = \frac{x}{70 \text{ kg}}$$

Cancel kg and multiply

$$\frac{80 \text{ units}}{1 \text{ kg}} \times 70 \text{ kg} = x$$

$$5{,}600 \text{ units} = A$$

STEP C: THINK! . . . IS IT REASONABLE?

5,600 units is less than the maximum dose of 8,000 units, so it is reasonable.

Once you know the bolus dose, you will need to calculate the amount of heparin to administer in mL. The bolus dose is the desired dose *D* for this calculation.

PROPORTION METHOD

EXAMPLE

Following the heparin protocol in Table 17-1, calculate the amount to administer in mL for a bolus dose of 5,600 units, using a supply dose of 1,000 units/mL.

STEP A: GATHER INFORMATION AND CONVERT

$D = 5{,}600$ mL (the bolus dose for a patient weighing 70 kg using Table 17-1 heparin protocol)
The dose on hand *H* is 1,000 units. The dosage unit *Q* is 1 mL.
No conversion necessary

STEP B: CALCULATE

Follow Procedure Checklist 12-1.

1. Set up the proportion.

$$\frac{H}{Q} = \frac{D}{A}$$

$$\frac{1{,}000 \text{ units}}{1 \text{ mL}} = \frac{5{,}600 \text{ units}}{A}$$

2. Cancel units.

$$\frac{1{,}000 \text{ units}}{1 \text{ mL}} = \frac{5{,}600 \text{ units}}{A}$$

3. Cross-multiply and solve.

$$1{,}000 \times A = 1 \text{ mL} \times 5{,}600$$

$$1{,}000 \, (A) = 5{,}600 \text{ mL}$$

$$A = \frac{5{,}600 \text{ mL}}{1{,}000}$$

$$A = 5.6 \text{ mL}$$

STEP C: THINK! . . . IS IT REASONABLE?

Since you want to give 5,600 units, and 5,600 units is 5.6 times larger than 1,000 units, giving 5.6 mL is reasonable. Administer an IV bolus of 5.6 mL heparin sodium 1,000 USP units/mL from a 10 mL bottle.

DIMENSIONAL ANALYSIS

EXAMPLE

Following the heparin protocol in Table 17-1, calculate the amount to administer in mL for a bolus dose of 5,600 units, using a supply dose of 1,000 units/mL.

Find the amount to administer.

STEP A: GATHER INFORMATION AND CONVERT

$D = 5,600$ mL (the bolus dose for a patient weighing 70 kg using Table 17-1 heparin protocol)
The dose on hand H is 1,000 units. The dosage unit Q is 1 mL.
The ordered dose and the supply dose are both measured in units. No conversion factor is necessary.

STEP B: CALCULATE

Follow Procedure Checklist 12-2.

1. The unit of measure for the amount to administer will be in milliliters.

   A mL $=$

2. No conversion factor necessary.

3. The dosage unit is 1 mL. The dose on hand is 1,000 units. This is the first factor.

   A mL $= \dfrac{1 \text{ mL}}{1,000 \text{ units}}$

4. The dosage ordered is 5,600 units. Complete the equation.

   A mL $= \dfrac{1 \text{ mL}}{1,000 \text{ units}} \times \dfrac{5,600 \text{ units}}{1}$

5. Cancel units.

   A mL $= \dfrac{1 \text{ mL}}{1,000 \text{ units}} \times \dfrac{5,600 \text{ units}}{1}$

6. Solve the equation.

   $A = \dfrac{5,600 \text{ mL}}{1,000}$

   $A = 5.6$ mL

STEP C: THINK! . . . IS IT REASONABLE?

Since you want to give 5,600 units, and 5,600 units 5.6 times larger than 1,000 units, giving 5.6 mL is reasonable. Administer an IV bolus of 5.6 mL heparin sodium 1,000 USP units/mL from a 10 mL bottle.

FORMULA METHOD

EXAMPLE

Following the heparin protocol in Table 17-1, calculate the amount to administer in mL for a bolus dose of 5,600 units, using a supply dose of 1,000 units/mL.

STEP A: GATHER INFORMATION AND CONVERT

$D = 5,600$ mL (the bolus dose for a patient weighing 70 kg using Table 17-1 heparin protocol)
The dose on hand H is 1,000 units. The dosage unit Q is 1 mL.
The ordered dose and the dose on hand are both measured in units; no conversion is necessary.

STEP B: CALCULATE

Follow Procedure Checklist 12-3

1. Fill in the formula.

   $\dfrac{5,600 \text{ units}}{1,000 \text{ units}} \times 1 \text{ mL} = A$

2. Cancel units.

$$\frac{5{,}600 \ \cancel{\text{units}}}{1{,}000 \ \cancel{\text{units}}} \times 1 \ \text{mL} = A$$

3. Solve for the unknown.

$$5.6 \ \text{mL} = A$$

STEP C: THINK! . . . IS IT REASONABLE?

Since you want to give 5,600 units, and 5,600 units is 5.6 times larger than 1,000 units, giving 5.6 mL is reasonable. Administer an IV bolus of 5.6 mL heparin sodium 1,000 USP units/mL from a 10 mL bottle.

Determining the Hourly Dose

With heparin and other critical medications that require close monitoring, you may need to determine the hourly dose of medication a patient is receiving. This is done to ensure that the maximum and/or safe dose is not exceeded. In these cases, you already know the rate of the amount to administer. You will use the proportion method or dimensional analysis to determine D (desired hourly dose).

PROPORTION METHOD

EXAMPLE

What is the hourly dose?

Ordered: 30,000 units of IV heparin in 500 mL of D5W to infuse at 25 mL/h

STEP A: GATHER INFORMATION AND CONVERT

$H = 30{,}000$ units (dose on hand or total amount to administer)

$Q = 500$ mL (dosage unit for total amount)

$A = 25$ mL/h (amount to administer or flow rate of infusion)

Since the dosage unit is mL and the amount to administer is in mL, no conversion is necessary.

STEP B: CALCULATE
Follow Procedure Checklist 12-1.

1. Set up the proportion. Recall that:

$$\frac{H}{Q} = \frac{D}{A} \quad \text{or} \quad \frac{\text{dose on hand}}{\text{dosage unit}} = \frac{\text{desired dose}}{\text{amount to administer}}$$

Thinking critically, we realize we know the amount to administer A or flow rate of the infusion and we need to determine the hourly dose D or desired dose.

$$\frac{30{,}000 \ \text{units}}{500 \ \text{mL}} = \frac{D}{25 \ \text{mL/h}}$$

2. Cancel units.

$$\frac{30{,}000 \ \text{units}}{500 \ \cancel{\text{mL}}} = \frac{D}{25 \ \cancel{\text{mL}}/\text{h}}$$

3. Cross-multiply and solve for the unknown.

$$500 \times D = 30{,}000 \ \text{units} \times 25/\text{h}$$

$$D = \frac{30{,}000 \ \text{units}}{500} \times 25/\text{h}$$

$$D = \frac{30{,}0\cancel{00} \ \text{units}}{5\cancel{00}} \times 25/\text{h}$$

$$D = 1{,}500 \ \text{units/h}$$

STEP C: THINK! . . . IS IT REASONABLE?

Since a dosage strength of 30,000 unit/500 mL provides 60 units/1 mL, and $60 \times 25 = 1{,}500$, it is reasonable.

DIMENSIONAL ANALYSIS

EXAMPLE	**What is the hourly dose?**

Ordered: 30,000 units of IV heparin in 500 mL of D5W to infuse at 25 mL/h

STEP A: GATHER INFORMATION AND CONVERT

H = 30,000 units (dose on hand or total amount to administer)

Q = 500 mL (dosage unit for total amount)

A = 25 mL/h (amount to administer or flow rate of infusion)

The dosage unit and the amount to administer are both mL, so no conversion factor is necessary.

STEP B: CALCULATE
Follow Procedure Checklist 12-2.

1. Thinking critically, you determine that the hourly dose for the unknown D will be in units per hour. Place this on the left side of the equation.

   D units/h =

2. No conversion is needed.

3. The dose on hand is 30,000 units. The dosage unit is 500 mL. This is your first factor.

   $$D \text{ units/h} = \frac{30,000 \text{ units}}{500 \text{ mL}}$$

4. The flow rate of the infusion is 25 mL/h. Use this as your second factor. Finish the equation.

   $$D \text{ units/h} = \frac{30,000 \text{ units}}{500 \text{ mL}} \times \frac{25 \text{ mL}}{1 \text{ h}}$$

5. Cancel units. The remaining units on the right side of the equation must match those on the left side of the equation.

   $$D \text{ units/h} = \frac{30,000 \text{ units}}{500 \text{ m\cancel{L}}} \times \frac{25 \text{ m\cancel{L}}}{1 \text{ h}}$$

6. Solve the equation.

   $$D \text{ units/h} = \frac{30,000 \text{ units}}{500} \times \frac{25}{1 \text{ h}}$$

   D = 1,500 units/h

STEP C: THINK! . . . IS IT REASONABLE?
Since a dosage strength of 30,000 unit/500 mL provides 60 units/1 mL, and 60 × 25 = 1,500, it is reasonable.

REVIEW AND PRACTICE

17.4 Safe Heparin Dosages

For Exercises 1–6, calculate the requested bolus doses and amount to administer using the heparin protocol in Table 17-1 for a patient who weighs 50 kg.

1. Initial bolus (loading) dose _____

2. Amount to administer _____

3. Bolus dose for an aPTT of 57 _____

4. Amount to administer for an aPTT of 57 _____

5. Bolus dose for an aPTT of 70 _____

6. Amount to administer for an aPTT of 70 _____

For Exercises 7–8, calculate the requested bolus doses and amount to administer using the heparin protocol in Table 17-1 for a patient who weighs 264 lb.

7. What is the initial loading dose? _____

8. What is the amount to administer? _____

9. The physician wants to give a bolus dose of 80 units/kg using the heparin shown in Label A. The patient weighs 189 lb. How many units will the patient receive?

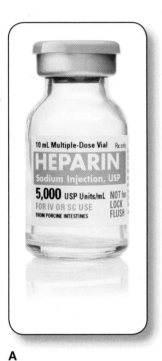

A

10. What is the amount to administer for the patient in question 9?

For Exercises 11–15, find the hourly dosage for the heparin orders.

11. An IV with 60,000 units in 1,500 mL of 5% DW infusing at 25 mL/h

12. An IV setup delivering 45 mL/h from 25,000 units in 2,500 mL of D5NS

13. 40,000 units in 1,800 mL of 5% DW delivered at 25 mL/h

14. 30,000 units in 1,500 mL of 5% D 0.45% NS delivered at 20 mL/h

15. 50,000 units in 500 mL NS infusing at 25 mL/h

17.5 IV Flow Rates Based on Body Weight per Time

Many infusions administered to the critically ill patient are ordered by an amount based upon the patient's weight for a certain length of time. This is written as amount/patient's weight/time. For example, heparin is calculated in units/kg/h.

PROCEDURE CHECKLIST 17-3

To find the flow rate based on weight per time:

1. Convert pounds to kilograms, if needed.

2. Convert the unit of measure of the dose on hand to the same unit of measure as the dose ordered, if needed.

3. Calculate the desired dose:

   ordered dose × weight in kg = desired dose

   unit of measurement/kg/h × kg = unit of measurement/h = D

4. Convert unit of measurement of the desired dose, if needed.

5. Calculate the flow rate in mL/h.

PROPORTION METHOD

EXAMPLE

Find the hourly rate at which to administer dopamine to a 220 lb patient.

Ordered: dopamine 5 mcg/kg/min
On hand: dopamine 400 mg/250 mL NS

STEP A: GATHER INFORMATION AND CONVERT

1. Convert the weight to kilograms.

$$\frac{1 \text{ kg}}{2.2 \text{ lb}} = \frac{x}{220 \text{ lb}}$$

$$\frac{220 \text{ lb} \times 1 \text{ kg}}{2.2 \text{ lb}} = x$$

$$100 \text{ kg} = x$$

The patient weighs 100 kg.

2. The dose on hand is in mg. The dosage ordered is in mcg. So, you need to convert milligrams to micrograms.

$$\frac{1,000 \text{ mcg}}{1 \text{ mg}} = \frac{x}{400 \text{ mg}}$$

$$\frac{400 \text{ mg} \times 1,000 \text{ mcg}}{1 \text{ mg}} = x$$

$$400,000 \text{ mcg} = x$$

Therefore 400 mg in 250 mL = $\dfrac{400,000 \text{ mcg}}{250 \text{ mL}}$

STEP B: CALCULATE

3. Calculate the desired dose of dopamine.

$$5 \text{ mcg/kg/min} \times 100 \text{ kg} = \frac{500 \text{ mcg}}{\text{min}}$$

4. Convert the unit of measure of the desired dose. The desired dose is in mcg/min and you need to calculate mcg/h. Convert mcg/min to mcg/h using Rule 17-4. Recall that you multiply by 60 min/h to convert units per minute to units per hour.

$$\frac{500 \text{ mcg}}{\text{min}} \times \frac{60 \text{ min}}{\text{h}} = \frac{30,000 \text{ mcg}}{\text{h}}$$

The desired dose D is 30,000 mcg/h

5. Calculate the flow rate in mL/h using Procedure Checklist 12-1.

$$\frac{400,000 \text{ mcg}}{250 \text{ mL}} = \frac{30,000 \text{ mcg/h}}{A}$$

$$400,000 \text{ mcg} \times A = 30,000 \text{ mcg/h} \times 250 \text{ mL}$$

$$400,000 \, A = 7,500,000 \text{ mL/h}$$

$$A = 18.75 \text{ mL/h (round to the nearest tenth)}$$

The flow rate is 18.8 mL/h.

STEP C: THINK ! . . . IS IT REASONABLE?
Since the ordered dose, 400,000 mcg, is more than 10 times the desired dose, 30,000 mcg/h, and the quantity 250 mL is more than 10 times 18.8 mL, the flow rate is reasonable.

DIMENSIONAL ANALYSIS

EXAMPLE

Find the hourly rate at which to administer dopamine to a 220 lb patient.

Ordered: dopamine 5 mcg/kg/min
On hand: dopamine 400 mg/250 mL NS

STEP A: GATHER INFORMATION AND CONVERT

1. Convert the weight to kilograms.

$$1 \text{ kg/2.2 lb} = x/220 \text{ lb}$$

$$220 \times 1 \text{ kg/2.2} = x$$

$$100 \text{ kg} = x$$

The patient weighs 100 kg.

2. The desired dose is in micrograms and the dose on hand is in milligrams, so a conversion factor, 1 mg/1,000 mcg, is necessary.

STEP B: CALCULATE

3. Calculate the desired dose of dopamine.

$$5 \text{ mcg/kg/min} \times 100 \text{ kg} = 500 \text{ mcg/min}$$

The desired dose D is 500 mcg/min.

4. Convert the unit of measure of the desired dose. The desired dose is in mcg/min and you need to calculate mcg/h. Convert as indicated in Rule 17-4 using 60 min/1 h as a conversion factor.

5. Follow Procedure Checklist 12-2.

Add each of the needed factors to the equation.

- 1 mg/1,000 mcg converts the desired dose to the dose on hand.
- 60 min/1 h converts the desired dose from mcg/min to mcg/h.
- 250 mL/400 mg is the dosage unit over the dose on hand.
- 500 mcg/1 min is the dosage ordered over 1.

$$A \text{ mL/h} =$$

$$A \text{ mL/h} = \frac{1 \text{ mg}}{1,000 \text{ mcg}} \times \frac{60 \text{ min}}{1 \text{ h}} \times \frac{250 \text{ mL}}{400 \text{ mg}} \times \frac{500 \text{ mcg}}{1 \text{ min}}$$

$$A \text{ mL/h} = \frac{1 \text{ mg}}{1,000 \text{ mcg}} \times \frac{60 \text{ min}}{1 \text{ h}} \times \frac{250 \text{ mL}}{400 \text{ mg}} \times \frac{500 \text{ mcg}}{1 \text{ min}}$$

The units remaining on the right side of the questions match the unknown unit of measure, so the equation is set up correctly.

$$A \text{ mL/h} = 18.75$$

Round to the nearest tenth.
The flow rate is 18.8 mL/h.

STEP C: THINK! . . . IS IT REASONABLE?
Since the ordered dose, 400,000 mcg, is more than 10 times the desired dose, 30,000 mcg/h, and the quantity 250 mL is more than 10 times 18.8 mL per hour, the flow rate is reasonable.

RULE 17-5	Sometimes it is necessary to convert the rate from mL/h to mL/min to verify a safe dosage. Since there are 60 minutes in 1 hour, to calculate the rate in mL/minute, you divide the rate in mL/h by 60 min/h or multiply the rate in mL/h by the conversion factor 1 h/60 min.
Example	If the rate = 18.8 mL/h, the rate in mL/min is calculated: 18.8 mL/h̶ ÷ 60 min/h̶ = 0.31 mL/min OR 18.8 mL/h̶ × 1h̶/60 min = 0.31 mL/min

RULE 17-6	If you know the total amount of medication in the total volume of solution (dose on hand), as well as the volume of solution that the patient has received, then you can use a proportion to calculate the amount of medication the patient has received (the dose). $$\frac{\text{Total amount of medication}}{\text{Total volume of solution}} = \frac{\text{amount of medication received}}{\text{volume of solution received}}$$
Example 1	A pregnant patient has been given increasing rates of Pitocin® to induce labor. Since her arrival at the hospital, she has received 50 mL of a solution of Pitocin® that contains 20 units in 1,000 mL LR. How much Pitocin® has she received? The total amount of medication is 20 units, the total volume of solution is 1,000 mL, and the volume of solution received is 50 mL. $$\frac{20 \text{ units}}{1{,}000 \text{ mL}} = \frac{x \text{ units}}{50 \text{ mL}}$$ 20 units × 50 = 1,000 × x 1,000 units = 1,000 × x 1 unit = x The patient has received 1 unit of Pitocin®.
Example 2	Your patient is receiving dopamine titrated to maintain his blood pressure. His infusion started with dopamine 800 mg/D5W 250 mL at a rate of 5 mL/h. Over the last 3 hours you have titrated the dopamine up to 12 mL/h to maintain the blood pressure. He has received 112 mL of the solution. How much dopamine has the patient received? The total amount of medication is 800 mg. The total volume of solution is 250 mL. The volume of solution received is 112 mL. $$\frac{800 \text{ mg}}{250 \text{ mL}} = \frac{x}{112 \text{ mL}}$$ 800 mg × 112 = 250 × x $$\frac{800 \text{ mg} \times 112}{250} = x$$ 358.4 mg = x The patient has received 358.4 mg of dopamine.

17.5 IV Flow Rates Based on Body Weight per Time

For Exercises 1–4 refer to the following order for a 185 lb patient.

Ordered: vecuronium 1 mcg/kg/min IV
On hand: vecuronium 10 mg/100 mL NS

1. What is the patient's weight in kg?

2. What is the desired dose?

3. What is the flow rate in mL/h?

4. What is the rate in mL/min?

For Exercises 5–8 refer to the following order for a 140 lb patient.

Ordered: nitroprusside 0.5 mcg/kg/min IV
On hand: nitroprusside 50 mg/250 mL D5W

5. What is the patient's weight in kg?

6. What is the desired dose?

7. What is the flow rate in mL/min?

8. What is the rate in mL/hr?

For Exercises 9–12 refer to the following order for a 113 lb patient.

Ordered: nesiritide 0.02 mcg/kg/min IV
On hand: nesiritide 1.5 mg/250 mL D5W

9. What is the patient's weight in kg?

10. What is the desired dose?

11. What is the flow rate in mL/min?

12. What is the rate in mL/h?

For Exercises 13–16 refer to the following order for a 150 lb patient.

Ordered: dobutamine 1 mcg/kg/min IV
On hand: dobutamine HCl 250 mg/500 mL D5W

13. What is the patient's weight in kg?

14. What is the desired dose?

15. What is the flow rate in mL/min?

16. What is the rate in mL/hr?

For Exercises 17–18, find the amount of medication that has already been administered to the patient.

17. Ordered: Lidocaine® 2 g in 1,000 mL of D5W.

    The patient has received 400 mL.

18. Ordered: Remicade® 300 mg in 250 mL of NaCl.

    The patient has received 150 mL.

17.6 IV Flow Rate Adjustments and Titrated Medications

IV flow rates of heparin and other medications may need to be adjusted. The goal is to administer the least amount of medication to achieve the desired effect. The amount of medication needed to achieve the desired effect varies. For example, looking at Table 17-1 on page 514, you will see that heparin is given to achieve an aPTT test result between 70 and 100. After you have given the bolus dose and calculated the flow rate, the patient's blood is monitored and adjustments to the IV flow rate are made based upon the results of this blood test.

RULE 17-7

To calculate a weight-based intravenous rate adjustment.

1. Determine the rate change needed, using the current infusion rate, protocol result, and the patient's weight.

2. Subtract the rate adjustment from the current IV rate.

3. Find the flow rate based upon weight per time, using Procedure Checklist 17-3.

PROPORTION METHOD

EXAMPLE

Find the hourly flow rate adjustment using the heparin protocol in Table 17-1 on page 514.

Current infusion rate is 25.2 mL/h and the aPTT protocol result was 120 seconds. The patient weighs 70 kg.

1. Reviewing the protocol, you find that for an aPTT test result of 116–135, the rate should be decreased by 2 units/kg/h.

2. Subtract the rate adjustment from the initial or current IV rate of 18 units/kg/h:

$$18 \text{ units/kg/h} - 2 \text{ units/kg/h} = 16 \text{ units/kg/h}$$

3. Find the flow rate for 16 units/kg/h. Follow the steps in Procedure Checklist 17-3.

STEP A: GATHER INFORMATION AND CONVERT

1. The patient is 70 kg.

2. The dose on hand is found in the heparin protocol in Table 17-1. It is 50 units/mL. No conversion is necessary because both the dose on hand and the dose ordered are in units.

STEP B: CALCULATE

3. Calculate the desired dose by multiplying the weight in kg by the ordered dose.

$$16 \text{ units/kg/h} \times 70 \text{ kg} = 1,120 \text{ units/h}$$

4. Calculate the flow rate using Procedure Checklist 12-1.

$$50 \text{ units}/1 \text{ mL} = 1,120 \text{ units/h}/A$$

$$50 \cancel{\text{ units}}/1 \text{ mL} = 1,120 \cancel{\text{ units}}/h/A$$

$$50 A = 1,120 \text{ mL/h}$$

$$A = 22.4 \text{ mL/h}$$

STEP C: THINK!. . .IS IT REASONABLE?

If you divide the original rate of 18 by the new rate of 16, you get 1.125. If you divide the original flow rate of 25.2 by the new flow rate of 22.4, you get 1.125. So the answer is reasonable.

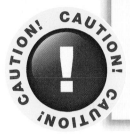

ERROR ALERT!

Dry Weight for Weight-Based Calculations

Be aware that a patient's weight may fluctuate frequently due to changes in volume status. Base calculations on the patient's "**dry weight**" (weight when properly hydrated) when titrating IV rates. Sometimes this can be determined by noting the patient's weight when discharged from the last hospital stay.

Titrated Medications

Many critical care IV medication dosages are also titrated (changed) based on the effect on the patient's **hemodynamics** (forces of blood flow), and/or heart rhythm. This requires constant observation of the patient's response, and frequent titration (altering of) the rate.

When the dosage of a medication is to be titrated, the AP orders the drug, dosage range (the maximum dose and the minimum dose), the starting dose (which is often the minimum dose), and the desired effect. There also may be limitations that would stop an increased dose, even though the desired effect has not been achieved. For example, an order might read:

> Dopamine 400 mg in 500 mL NS, to infuse at 5–20 mcg/kg/min IV to keep systolic blood pressure greater than 90 mm Hg. Keep HR less than 100. Start at 5 mcg/kg/min and titrate to effect.

For this order, the vital signs should be monitored and if the patient's systolic blood pressure goes below 90 mm Hg and the heart rate exceeds 100 bpm, the dose would be left at the current rate and not be increased, even though the desired effect of keeping the systolic blood pressure greater than 90 mm Hg has not been achieved.

RULE 17-8	For safe titration:
	1. Calculate the starting flow rate using Procedure Checklist 17-3.
	2. Calculate the minimum allowable flow rate using Procedure Checklist 17-3.
	3. Calculate the maximum allowable flow rate using Procedure Checklist 17-3.
	4. Begin infusion at the starting flow rate.
	5. Titrate (adjust) dosage, based on patient response.
	6. Do not exceed maximum rate (call AP for new order if the patient does not have the desired response at the maximum rate).
	7. If the patient's response exceeds the prescribed parameters at the minimum dose, discontinue the infusion and notify the AP.
Example	Perform safe titration for the following order. Ordered: Dopamine 400 mg in 500 mL NS (1,600 mcg/mL), to infuse at 5–20 mcg/kg/min IV to keep systolic blood pressure greater than 90. Keep heart rate less than 100. Start at 5 mcg/kg/min and titrate according to blood pressure (BP) and heart rate (HR). You are using an infusion pump and the patient weighs 80 kg. Calculate the flow rates for steps 1, 2, and 3 following Procedure Checklist 17-3 using the proportion method or dimensional analysis.

Rule 17-8 Safe Titration Step 1. Calculate the starting flow rate following Procedure Checklist 17-3. In this example, we will calculate using the proportion method.

PROPORTION METHOD

EXAMPLE

Ordered: Dopamine 400 mg in 500 mL NS to infuse at 5–20 mcg/kg/min IV to keep systolic blood pressure greater than 90. Keep heart rate less than 100. Start at 5 mcg/kg/min and titrate according to blood pressure and heart rate. You are using an infusion pump and the patient weighs 80 kg.

STEP A: GATHER INFORMATION AND CONVERT

According to the order the starting flow rate is 5 mcg/kg/min.

1. The patient weighs 80 kg.

2. Convert milligrams to micrograms because the dose on hand is in mg and dose ordered is in mcg.

$$\frac{1{,}000 \text{ mcg}}{1 \text{ mg}} = \frac{x \text{ mcg}}{400 \text{ mg}}$$

$$1{,}000 \text{ mcg} \times 400 \text{ mg} = 1 \text{ mg} \times x$$

$$400{,}000 \text{ mcg} = x$$

Therefore the 400 mg in 500 mL equals 400,000 mcg/500 mL, which can be reduced to 800 mcg/1 mL. This is the dose on hand (H) over the dosage unit (Q)

STEP B: CALCULATE

3. Calculate the starting rate (desired dose) of dopamine.

$$5 \text{ mcg/kg/min} \times 80 \text{ kg} = D$$

$$400 \text{ mcg/min} = D$$

The desired dose $D = 400$ mcg/min.

4. Since the desired dose is in mcg/min and you need to determine mcg/h, convert mcg/min to mcg/h:

$$\frac{400 \text{ mcg}}{\text{min}} \times \frac{60 \text{ min}}{\text{h}} = 24{,}000 \text{ mcg/h}$$

The desired dose D is 24,000 mcg/h.

5. Calculate the flow rate using Procedure Checklist 12-1.

$$\frac{H}{Q} = \frac{D}{A}$$

$$\frac{800 \text{ mcg}}{1 \text{ mL}} = \frac{24{,}000 \text{ mcg/h}}{A}$$

$$\frac{800 \text{ mcg}}{1 \text{ mL}} = \frac{24{,}000 \text{ mcg/h}}{A}$$

$$800 \times A = 24{,}000 \text{ mL/h}$$

$$A = 30 \text{ mL/h}$$

The starting flow rate is 30 mL/h.

STEP C: THINK! . . . IS IT REASONABLE?

Since the ordered dose, 400,000 mcg, is more than 10 times the desired dose, 24,000 mcg/h, and the quantity 500 mL is more than 10 times 30 mL per hour, the flow rate is reasonable.

Rule 17-8 Safe Titration Step 2. Calculate the minimum allowable flow rate. Reviewing the order, you note that the starting rate of 5 mcg/kg/min is the same as the minimum rate of 5 mcg/kg/min. So the minimum flow rate will be 30 mL/h.

Rule 17-8 Safe Titration Step 3. Calculate the maximum allowable flow rate using Procedure Checklist 17-3. In this example we will calculate using dimensional analysis.

DIMENSIONAL ANALYSIS

EXAMPLE

Ordered: Dopamine 400 mg in 500 mL NS to infuse at 5–20 mcg/kg/min IV to keep systolic blood pressure greater than 90. Keep heart rate less than 100. Start at 5 mcg/kg/min and titrate according to blood pressure and heart rate. You are using an infusion pump and the patient weighs 80 kg.

STEP A: GATHER INFORMATION AND CONVERT

According to the order, the maximum allowable flow rate is 20 mcg/kg/min.

1. The weight of 80 kg does not need to be converted.
2. The desired dose is in mcg and the dose on hand is in mg, so a conversion factor of $\frac{1\,mg}{100\,mcg}$ is necessary.

STEP B: CALCULATE

3. Determine the maximum desired dose.

   $20\ \text{mcg}/\text{kg}/\text{min} \times 80\ \text{kg} = D$

   $20\ \text{mcg}/\text{min} \times 80 = D$

   $1{,}600\ \text{mcg}/\text{min} = D$ (desired dose)

4. Since the desired dose is in mcg/min and you need to calculate mcg/h, you will need to use a conversion factor of $\frac{60\,min}{1\,h}$.

5. Calculate the flow rate using each of the factors you have identified:

   - $\frac{1\,mg}{1{,}000\,mcg}$ converts the desired dose to the same unit of measure as the dose on hand.

   - $\frac{60\,min}{1\,h}$ converts the desired dose from mcg/min to mcg/h since your flow rate needs to be in mL/h for the infusion pump.

   - $\frac{500\,mL}{400\,mg}$ is the dosage unit over the dose on hand.

   - $\frac{1{,}600\,mcg}{min}$ is the desired dose over 1.

   $$A\ \text{mL/h} = \frac{1\,mg}{1{,}000\,mcg} \times \frac{60\,min}{1\,h} \times \frac{500\,mL}{400\,mg} \times \frac{1{,}600\,mcg}{min}$$

   $$A\ \text{mL/h} = \frac{1\,\cancel{mg}}{1{,}000\,\cancel{mcg}} \times \frac{60\,\cancel{min}}{1\,h} \times \frac{500\,mL}{400\,\cancel{mg}} \times \frac{1{,}600\,\cancel{mcg}}{\cancel{min}}$$

   $$A\ \text{mL/h} = \frac{1}{1{,}000} \times \frac{60}{1\,h} \times \frac{500\,mL}{400} \times 1{,}600$$

   The units remaining on the right side of the equation match the unknown unit of measure, so the equation is set up correctly.

   $A\ \text{mL/h} = 120\ \text{mL/h}$

STEP C: THINK! . . . IS IT REASONABLE?

Since the maximum dose is four times the size of the minimum dose and 120 is four times larger than 30, the answer is reasonable.

Rule 17-8 Safe Titration Step 4. The starting flow rate is 30 mL/h and in this case is the same as the minimum flow rate, so you start the IV at at 30 mL/h.

Rule 17-8 Safe Titration Step 5. For this order, the systolic blood pressure must not go below 90 and the heart rate should not go above 100. The blood pressure and pulse should be monitored at frequent intervals.

Rule 17-8 Safe Titration Step 6. Based on the patient's blood pressure and heart rate, the rate of dopamine may be titrated up to 75 mL/h and be within the prescribed guidelines.

Rule 17-8 Safe Titration Step 7. If the systolic blood pressure goes below 80 or the HR goes above 100, the infusion should be stopped and the AP notified.

When working with critically ill patients, some nurses create a titration table to make dose changes quickly and easily. Each of the flow rate calculations is performed and recorded based on the order and the patient. Table 17-2 shows a titration table for the following example.

Ordered: Dopamine 400 mg in 250 mL NS, to infuse at 5-20 mcg/kg/min IV to keep systolic blood pressure greater than 90 mm Hg. Keep HR less than 100. Start at 10 mcg/kg/min and titrate to effect. The patient weighs 220 lb (100 kg) and an IV infusion pump is being used.

TABLE 17-2 Titration Table with Dopamine Dosages for a Patient Who Weighs 100 kg

DOPAMINE DOSAGE (mcg/100 kg)	IV RATE (mL/h) 1,600 mcg/1 mL
5 mcg/kg/min	18.8 mL/h
10 mcg/kg/min	37.5 mL/h
15 mcg/kg/min	56.3 mL/h
20 mcg/kg/min	75 mL/h

REVIEW AND PRACTICE

17.6 IV Flow Rate Adjustments and Titrated Medications

For Exercises 1–7, use the heparin protocol in Table 17-1 for a patient who weighs 166 lb. Round patient weights and IV flow rates to the nearest tenth.

1. Calculate the loading dose, including the amount (volume) to administer.

2. Calculate the initial flow rate.

3. An aPTT test was done after 6 hours and the result was 55. What is the bolus dose and amount to administer now?

4. What is the new flow rate?

5. Another aPTT test was done and the result was 69. What is the bolus dose and amount to administer now?

6. What is the new flow rate?

7. The next aPTT test showed a result of 127. What is the new flow rate?

For Exercises 8–10, refer to the following order.

Ordered: Dopamine 400 mg in 500 mL NS (1,600 mcg/mL), to infuse at 5–20 mcg/kg/min IV to keep systolic blood pressure greater than 90. Keep heart rate less than 100. Start at 5 mcg/kg/min and titrate according to blood pressure and heart rate. The patient weighs 220 lb and you are using an infusion pump. Use Table 17-2 to determine the following:

8. Starting mL/h flow rate

9. Minimum mL/h flow rate

10. Maximum mL/h flow rate

For Exercises 11–13 refer to the following order and calculate the requested rates.

Ordered: xylocaine 1 g in 250 mL D5W; start IV infusion at 2 mg/min and titrate to absence of ventricular dysrhythmia; dosage range 1 mg/min–4 mg/min.

11. Calculate the minimum dose rate in mL/h.

12. Calculate the maximum dose rate in mL/h.

13. Calculate the starting dose rate in mL/h.

For Exercises 14–15, the following order applies:

Ordered: dopamine: Begin infusion of 2 mcg/kg/min for bradycardia and systolic BP less than 90. Increase infusion up to 10 mcg/kg/min as needed.

You have a premixed bag of dopamine with 200 mg in 500 ml of D5W. The patient weighs 165 lb.

14. At what flow rate in milliliters per hour should you start the IV?

15. The BP remains low, and you increase the flow rate to 35 mL/h. What is the dosage that the patient is receiving at this time?

For Exercises 16–20 calculate the IV flow rate in mL/h based on the following order:

Ordered: nicardipine 25 mg/250 mL normal saline IV; start at 5 mg/h and infuse for 30 minutes. Titrate to systolic BP greater than or equal to 90 by increasing rate 3 mg/h every 5 to 15 minutes during the infusion. Maximum infusion rate 15 mg/h.

Maintenance rate: After 30 minutes, while systolic BP is greater than or equal to 90 mm Hg, decrease rate to 3 mg/h; may increase rate by 2.5 mg every 5 to 15 minutes until systolic BP is greater than or equal to 90. Maximum infusion rate 15 mg/h.

16. Calculate the minimum flow rate.

17. Calculate the maximum flow rate.

18. Calculate the starting flow rate.

19. The nicardipine has been infusing at 80 mL/h for 15 minutes. The patient's systolic BP is 74. Should the infusion be titrated? If so, what is the new rate?

20. The patient's systolic BP is 94, and the nicardipine infusion has been infusing for 30 minutes. How many mL/h should be infused now?

LEARNING OUTCOMES	KEY POINTS
17.1 Calculate daily maintenance fluid needs. Pages 498–502	Calculation of DMFN is based on weight in kilograms: ▸ Up to 10 kg: 100 mL/kg ▸ 10–20 kg: 1,000 mL + [50 mL/kg × (kg − 10)] ▸ Over 20 kg: 1,500 mL + [20 mL/kg × (kg − 20)] Determine the IV DMFN by subtracting any fluids taken by mouth Add fluid from the IV tubing if a volume control chamber is used
17.2 Determine safe doses based on weight and renal function. Pages 502–506	For water-soluble medications that are strongly bound to lean tissues, safe dosage should be based on ideal body weight, unless the patient's weight is below ideal body weight. In that case, the actual body weight should be used. For fat-soluble medications, which are strongly bound to body fat, the dose should be based on the patient's actual weight.
17.3 Calculate the hourly flow rate for IV infusions ordered in dosage per time. Pages 506–513	▸ Refer to Rule 17-3. D = rate of desired dose (mcg/h, mg/h, units/h) Q = dosage units (mL) H = dose on hand (total number of mcg, mg, units) A = amount to administer (mL/h) Follow Procedure Checklist 12-1 or 12-2 to calculate the flow rate. Refer to Rule 17-4. To calculate an hourly flow rate from a per minute order: Multiply per minute order by 60 min/h. For dimensional analysis, use the conversion factor 60 min/1 h.

17.4 Calculate safe IV heparin dosages. Pages 513–519	To calculate weight-based heparin bolus doses:
	1. Convert the patient's weight to kg:
	  1 kg/2.2 lb = x/patient's weight in lb
	2. Calculate the desired dose:
	  Ordered dose/1 kg = deisred dose/patient's weight
	3. Calculate the amount to administer in mL using one of the three methods.
	
	Calculate the hourly dose of medication a patient is receiving to ensure that the maximun and/or safe dose is not exceeded. To do this, you know the amount to administer and you use dimensional analysis or the proportion method to determine the desired hourly dose.

LEARNING OUTCOMES	KEY POINTS
17.5 Calculate IV flow rates for medications ordered based on body weight over a specified period of time. Pages 519–523	Refer to Procedure Checklist 17-3. 1. Convert pounds to kilograms, if needed 2. Convert the unit of measure of the dose on hand to the same unit of measure as the dose ordered, if needed 3. Calculate the desired dose: ordered dose × weight in kg = desired dose unit of measurement/kg/h × kg = unit of measurement/h = D 4. Convert unit or measurement of the desired dose, if needed 5. Calculate the flow rate in mL/h
17.6 Calculate IV flow rates for titrated medications. Pages 524–529	▶ Refer to Rule 17-8. For safe titration: 1. Calculate the starting rate 2. Calculate the maximum allowable rate 3. Calculate the minimum allowable rate 4. Begin infusion at the starting rate 5. Titrate (adjust) dosage based on patient response 6. Do not exceed maximum rate (call AP for new order if the patient does not have the desired response at the maximum rate) 7. If the patient's response exceeds the prescribed parameters at the minimum dose, discontinue the infusion and notify the AP

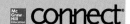
Answer the following questions.

1. Explain the difference between daily maintenance fluids and replacement fluids. (LO 17.1)

2. A patient weighs 13 kg and is not taking any fluids by mouth. What would be the DMFN and the IV flow rate using microdrip tubing? (LO 17.1)

3. What type of medication is strongly bound to lean tissue? (LO 17.2)

4. When would the dose of a medication be calculated on ideal body weight rather than actual weight? (LO 17.2)

5. Explain why a medication dosage may be altered based on the result of a patient's creatine clearance test. (LO 17.2)

For Exercises 6–8, find the flow rates for an infusion pump. (LO 17.3)

6. Ordered: Vasopressin 60 units/50 mL NS infusing at 0.3 units/min

7. Ordered: 250 mg dobutamine HCl in 50 mL LR infusing at 1.5 mg/min

8. Ordered: 2,000 mg lidocaine in 500 mL NS infusing at 2 mg/min

For Exercises 9–10, find the appropriate flow rate for using an infusion pump. (LO 17.5)

9. Nitroglycerin 50 mg/250 mL D5W infusing at 27 mcg/min.

10. Levophed® 8 mg/250 mL D5W infusing at 10 mcg/min

11. Find the amount of medication that has already been administered to the patient. (LO 17.5)

    Ordered: Dobutrex® 250 mg in 1,000 mL of D5W.

    The patient has received 120 mL.

12. Based on the following, what dosage is the patient receiving at this time? (LO 17.6)

    Ordered: dopamine: begin infusion of 2 mcg/kg/min for bradycardia and systolic BP < 90 mmHg. Increase infusion up to 10 mcg/kg/min as needed.

    You have a premixed bag of dopamine with 200 mg in 500 mL of D5W. The patient weighs 195 lb. The blood pressure remains low and you increase the rate to 65 mL/h.

For Exercises 13–14, calculate the flow rate in mL/h.

13. Ordered: procainamide 2 mg/min IV. On hand: procainamide 2 g/500 mL D5W. (LO 17.3)

14. Ordered: nesritide 1.8 mcg/kg/h. On hand: nesritide 1.5 mg/250 mL D5W; the patient weighs 70 kg. (LO 17.5)

15. Calculate the flow rate in mL/h for the following titrated dose:

    Dobutamine 250 mg/500 mL D5W, 2.5 mcg/kg/min–20 mcg/kg/min IV to keep cardiac index greater than 1.8. Start at 2.5 mcg/kg/min.

    The dobutamine is currently infusing at 2.5 mcg/kg/min in a 50 kg patient. The new cardiac index is 1.4 and the infusion needs to be titrated to 4 mcg/kg/min. What is the new hourly rate? (LO 17.6)

16. Find the flow rate for using an infusion pump.

Ordered: heparin 1,500 units/h

On hand: heparin 50,000 units in 1,000 mL D5W (LO 17.4)

For Exercises 17–18, find the hourly dosage for the heparin orders.

17. Heparin 20,000 units in 1,000 mL D5W infusing at 30 mL/h (LO 17.4)

18. Heparin 30,000 units in 1,000 mL NS infusing at 10 mL/h (LO 17.4)

19. Refer to Label A. If the bolus dose was heparin 40 units/kg and the patient weighed 80 kg, how many units would you administer and how many mL would you administer? (LO 17.4)

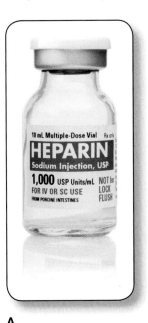

A

20. Per weight-based heparin protocol, the 90 kg patient has heparin 25,000 units in 500 mL D5W (50 units/mL) infusing at 24 units/kg/h. The aPTT is 130 and the protocol is to decrease the rate by 2 units/kg/h. What is the new infusion rate in mL/h? (LO 17.6)

CHECK UP

For Exercises 1–3, find the flow rates for an infusion pump. (LO 17.3)

1. Ordered: 3,000 mg lidocaine in 750 mL D5W to infuse at 3 mg/min

2. Ordered: 500 mg dobutamine HCl in 100 mL of D5W to infuse at 2.4 mg/min

3. Ordered: epinephrine 1 mg/500 mL to infuse at 3 mcg/min

For Exercises 4–6, find the appropriate flow rate for an infusion pump. Round all answers to the nearest tenth. (LO 17.5)

4. Ordered: Neosynephrine® 0.5 mcg/kg/min. On hand: Neosynephrine® 40 mg/250 mL 0.9% NaCl. The patient weighs 214 lb.

5. Ordered: Inocor® 8 mcg/kg/min. On hand: Inocor® 300 mg/120 mL 0.9% NaCl. The patient weighs 152 lb.

6. Primacor® 0.375 mcg/kg/min. On hand: Primacor® 20 mg/100 mL D5W. The patient weighs 165 lb.

7. Find the amount of medication that has already been administered to the patient. (LO 17.5)

    Ordered: procainamide 1 g/250 mL D5W

    The patient has received 105 mL.

For Exercises 8–9, the following order applies (LO 17.6):

Ordered: dopamine: begin infusion of 2 mcg/kg/min for bradycardia and systolic BP < 90 mm Hg. Increase infusion up to 10 mcg/kg/min as needed.

You have a premixed bag of dopamine with 200 mg in 500 mL of D5W. The patient weighs 185 lb. Round all answers to the nearest tenth.

8. At the end of your shift the patient has received 425 mL of the premixed bag of 200 mg in 500 mL of D5W. What is the total amount of dopamine the patient has received on your shift?

9. What is the maximum flow rate at which the IV should run?

For Exercises 10–15, calculate the flow rate in mL/h (LO 17.3, 17.5)

10. Ordered: nitroglycerin 15 mcg/min IV. On hand: nitroglycerin 25 mg in 500 mL D5W

11. Ordered: xylocaine 3 mg/min IV. On hand: xylocaine 2 g/500 mL D5W

12. Ordered: epinephrine 4 mcg/min. On hand: epinephrine 1 mg in 500 mL of NS

13. Ordered: nesritide 0.6 mcg/kg/h (the patient weighs 80 kg). On hand: nesritide 1.5 mg/250 mL D5W

14. Ordered: dobutamine 4 mcg/kg/min (the patient weighs 95 kg). On hand: dobutamine 1,000 mg/250 mL D5W

15. Ordered: amiodarone 0.5 mg/min. On hand: amiodarone 450 mg/250 mL D5W

For Exercises 16–20, calculate the hourly flow rate in mL/h; refer to the following order to titrate the dosage: (LO 17.6)

While receiving mechanical ventilation: to achieve Richmond Agitation Sedation Scale (RASS) Level 0, administer lorazepam loading dose 1 mg IVP. Begin lorazepam 50 mg/250 mL D5W IV to infuse at 0.5 mg–2 mg/h. Titrate q 1–2 h, as needed, in 0.5 mg/h increments, to achieve RASS level 0. Rebolus with lorazepam 1 mg IVP prior to making each rate increase.

16. Calculate the minimum flow rate.

17. Calculate the maximum flow rate.

18. The patient's RASS is 2, so the patient needs increased sedation. The current infusion rate is 5 mL/h. What is the new rate? _____ Should the patient receive a bolus dose?

19. Two hours have passed since the rate change in question 18, and the patient's RASS is 1, so the patient needs increased sedation. Should the patient receive more lorazepam? If so, how much?

20. Two hours have passed since the rate change in question 19, and the patient's RASS is −1, so the patient needs less sedation. What is the new rate? Should the patient receive a bolus dose prior to this rate adjustment?

In Exercises 21–23, calculate the daily maintenance fluid needs, based on the following weights. Then find the flow rate in milliliters per hour (F) for the DMFN. (LO 17.1)

21. 24 kg

22. 39 lb

23. 110 lb (The patient has taken 800 mL fluid orally.)

For Exercises 24–28, determine if the dosage ordered is safe. If the order is safe, then find the amount to administer. Assume that the patients have impaired renal functions. (LO 17.2)

24. The patient: 85-year-old male, 6 ft 1 in. tall, 210 lb, CL_{CR} of 64 mL/min. Ideal weight should be 195 lb.

    Ordered: Cartrol 2.5 mg PO q24h

    On hand: Cartrol 2.5 mg/tablet

    According to the package insert, the usual dosage interval for 2.5 mg is as follows: for patients with creatinine clearance above 60 mL/min, 24 h; for 20 to 60 mL/min, 48 h; and for less than 20 mL/min, 72 h.

25. The patient: 68-year-old female, 5 ft 5 in. tall, 166 lb, CL_{CR} of 60 mL/min. Ideal weight should be 162 lb.

    Ordered: Capastat 600 mg IM qd

    On hand: Capastat sulfate, diluted to 300 mg/mL

    According to the package insert, the estimated daily dosage required to maintain a steady level of drug is 1.29 mg/kg for creatinine clearance of 0 mL/min; 2.43 mg/kg for 10 mL/min; 3.58 mg/kg for 20 mL/min; 4.72 mg/kg for 30 mL/min; 5.87 mg/kg for 40 mL/min; 7.01 mg/kg for 50 mL/min; and 8.16 mg/kg for 60 mL/min.

26. The patient: 82-year-old female, 4 ft 10 in. tall, 102 lb, CL_{CR} of 26 mL/min. Patient is within ideal weight range.

    Ordered: Acyclovir sodium (Zovirax®) 450 mg IV q12h infused over 1 h

    On hand: Zovirax® for injection, 50 mg/mL when reconstituted

    According to the package insert, the recommended dose for patients with normal renal function is 10 mg/kg q8h. The dose is adjusted as follows for patients with impaired renal function: for creatinine clearance over 50 mL/min, 100 percent of the recommended dose every 8 h; from 25 to 50 mL/min, 100 percent of the recommended dose every 12 h; from 10 to 25 mL/min, 100 percent of the recommended dose every 24 h; for 0 to 10 mL/min, 50 percent of the recommended dose every 24 h.

27. The patient: 73-year-old male, 5 ft 8 in. tall, 154 lb, CL_{CR} of 49 mL/min, diagnosed with a complicated urinary tract infection. Patient is within ideal weight range.

    Ordered: Fortaz® 1 g IV q12h

    On hand: Fortaz® for injection, reconstituted at 10 mg/mL

    According to the package insert, the usual recommended dosage for patients with complicated urinary tract infections is 500 mg to 1 g given q8–12h. For patients with renal insufficiency, the following maintenance dosages are recommended (however, if the usual dosage is less, administer the lower amount): for creatinine clearance of 31 to 50 mL/min, 1 g q12h; for 16 to 30 mL/min, 1 g q24h; for 6 to 15 mL/min, 500 mg q24h; for less than 5 mL/min, 500 mg q48h.

28. The patient: 79-year-old male, 5 ft 9 in. tall, 149 lb, CL_{CR} of 55 mL/min. The patient does not have a life-threatening infection. Patient is within ideal weight range.

    Ordered: Mandol 2 g IV q6h

    On hand: Mandol reconstituted to 1 g/10 mL

    According to the package insert, for patients with renal impairment and less severe infections, the following maintenance dosages are recommended: for creatinine clearance of over 80 mL/min, 1 to 2 g q6h; for 50 to 80 mL/min, 0.75 to 1.5 g q6h; for 25 to 50 mL/min, 0.75 to 1.5 g q8h; for 10 to 25 mL/min, 0.5 to 1 g q8h; for 2 to 10 mL/min, 0.5 to 0.75 g q12h; for less than 2 mL/min, 0.25 to 0.5 g q12h.

29. The patient: 92-year-old female, 5 ft 1 in. tall, 112 lb, CL_{CR} of 32 mL/min. Patient is within ideal weight range.
    Ordered: Timentin® 2 g IV q4h

    On hand: Timentin® reconstituted to 20 mg/mL

    According to the package insert, for patients with renal impairment, the following maintenance dosages are recommended: for creatinine clearance over 60 mL/min, 3.1 g q4h; for 30 to 60 mL/min, 2 g q4h; for 10 to 30 mL/min, 2 g q8h; for less than 10 mL/min, 2 g q12h. For patients with more advanced impairments, lower dosages are recommended.

For Exercises 30–32, refer to the weight-based heparin protocol in Table 17-1; the 60 kg patient currently has heparin 25,000 units in 500 mL D5W (50 units/mL) infusing at 18 units/kg/h. The aPTT is 65 seconds, and the protocol is to bolus with heparin 40 units/kg (max. 4,000 units) and to increase the infusion by 1 unit/kg/h. (LO 17.4)

30. How many units is the bolus dose?

31. Using heparin 1,000 units/mL, how many mL of heparin would be administered?

32. What is the new infusion rate in mL/h?

For Exercises 33–34, find the hourly dosage for the heparin orders. (LO 17.4)

33. 40,000 units in 1,000 mL NS infusing at 40 mL/h

34. 50,000 units in 500 mL D5W infusing at 10 mL/h

For Exercises 35–36, use the following information to calculate the answer in units and mL: The patient weighs 165 lb, the concentration of heparin for bolus dose is 1,000 units/mL, and the concentration of the heparin infusion is 25,000 units/500 mL (50 units/mL). (LO 17.3, 17.4)

35. Administer a bolus dose of heparin 80 units/kg (max. 8,000 units).

36. Administer a heparin infusion at 18 units/kg/h (max. 1,800 units/h).

CRITICAL THINKING APPLICATIONS

A patient with malignant hypertension is being treated in the critical care unit. The physician writes the following order: nitroprusside 50 mg in 250 mL D5W to start at 1 mcg/kg/min, and titrate to maintain the systolic BP under 180. (When you measure a patient's blood pressure, the first number represents the systolic blood pressure.) The patient weighs 176 lb. According to the product insert, the maximum safe dose of nitroprusside is 8 mcg/kg/min (for no longer than 10 minutes) and the average dose is 3 mcg/kg/min. Nitroprusside's effect on BP can be seen in 1–2 minutes. (LO 17.6)

1. At what flow rate should you initially set the infusion?

2. What is the maximum safe flow rate for the infusion?

3. At 1600, the patient's BP is 220/110. The nitroprusside infusion is running at 165 mL/h. What should you do?

4. At 1610, the patient's BP is 198/96. The nitroprusside infusion is running at 192 mL/h. What should you do?

CASE STUDY

A patient has a PCA pump with fentanyl 1,500 mcg in 30 mL in D5W. Hospital policy requires you to document the dose of fentanyl administered every 4 hours. When you came on duty, the pump showed that 13 mL had infused. After 4 hours, the pump shows that 21 mL has infused. How much fentanyl did the patient receive during your shift? (LO 17.5)

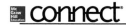

Now that you have completed the materials in the chapter text, go to CONNECT and complete any chapter activities you have not yet done.

For Questions 1–4, refer to the heparin protocol in the table below. The patient's aPTT is 50, weight is 70 kg, and currently heparin is infusing at 1,200 units/h.

You have the following concentrations of heparin available:

Heparin sodium injection, 1,000 USP units/mL, 1 mL vial

Heparin sodium injection, 1,000 USP units/mL, 10 mL vial

Heparin sodium injection, 5,000 USP units/mL, 10 mL vial

Heparin sodium injection, 10,000 USP units/mL, 1 mL vial

1. Which of these should be used for the bolus?

2. What is the bolus dose of heparin? _____ units

3. What is the current rate? _____ mL/h rounded the nearest whole number.

4. What is the new rate? _____ mL/h rounded the nearest whole number.

HEPARIN PROTOCOL for DVT, PE, and High-Intensity Indications
GOAL: APTT 70–100

Use heparin sodium 1,000 USP units/mL for bolus dose.
Use premixed heparin sodium 25,000 USP units in 5% dextrose in water 500 mL (50 units/ mL) for infusion.
Obtain baseline CBC and aPTT prior to administering heparin. Obtain aPTT 6 hours after each rate change.
If the aPTT is at goal, repeat the aPTT until two consecutive aPTT are at goal, draw aPTT daily while receiving heparin, and aPTT remains between 70 and 100.
Initial bolus dose: 80 units/kg (maximum 8,000 units)
Initial rate: 18 units/kg/h (maximum 1,800 units/h = 36 mL/h)

aPTT result	IV bolus dose	Number of minutes to hold infusion	Amount to change current infusion rate
Less than 54 Notify AP	80 units/kg (max. 8,000 units)	Do not hold	Increase by 4 units/kg/h
54–59	40 units/kg (max. 4,000 units)	Do not hold	Increase by 2 units/kg/h
60–69	40 units/kg (max. 4,000 units)	Do not hold	Increase by 1 unit/kg/h
70–100 goal	**No bolus dose**	**Do not hold**	**Do not change current infusion rate**
101–115	No bolus dose	Do not hold	Decrease by 1 unit/kg/h
116–135	No bolus dose	30	Decrease by 2 units/kg/h
136–150	No bolus dose	60	Decrease by 3 units/kg/h and repeat aPTT 6 hours after infusion resumed
151–200 Notify AP	No bolus dose	90	Decrease by 4 units/kg/h and repeat aPTT 6 hours after infusion resumed

Adapted for calculation purposes only, from (2008) ACCP guidelines; not to be used in clinical practice.

5. Using the heparin protocol in the table, how many units of heparin will a patient who weighs 120 kg receive in the initial bolus? _____ units

6. Identify the pharmacokinetic process described below:
   a. The process by which a medication leaves the body
   b. The process that moves a medication from the site where it is given into the bloodstream
   c. The process that chemically changes the medication in the body
   d. The process that moves a medication into other body tissues and fluids

7. Ordered: tobramycin 3 mg/kg/day given in three divided doses to a 15 kg child
   Administer: _____ mg/day or _____ mg/dose

8. Ordered: cephalexin 150 mg PO q6h for a child who weighs 44 lb
   Recommended dose range: 25–50 mg/kg/day in four divided doses
   What is the minimum and maximum safe dosages? What is the daily ordered dose, and is it safe? _____

9. Ordered: enalapril 2.5 mg PO daily for a 76-year-old patient, 5 ft 3 in. tall, 195 lb, with a CL_{CR} of 55 mL/min, who is diagnosed with hypertension and renal impairment and whose ideal weight is 152 lb.
   On hand: enalapril 5 mg (scored) tablets
   According to the package insert, the usual dose for patients with normal renal function (over 80 mL/min creatinine clearance) is 5 mg/day; for mild impairment (30 to 80 mL/min)—2.5 mg/day; for moderate to severe impairment (< 30 mL/min)—2.5 mg/day
   Is the dose ordered safe? _____ If the dose is safe, administer _____ tablet(s)

10. What is the safe dose of interferon for a child with a BSA of 0.28 m^2 if the recommended dose is 2 million units/m^2? _____ units

11. Calculate the daily maintenance fluid needs (DMFN) for a child who weighs 24 kg. _____ mL

12. An 11 lb, 8 oz infant is taking 3 oz formula every 4 hours. What is the child's DMFN? Is he meeting his DMFN? _____

13. Ordered: Ticarcillin 2 g IV q4h for an 82-year-old male, 5 ft 8 in. tall, 161 lb, with a CL_{CR} of 28 mL/min. Patient is in ideal weight range.
   On hand: Ticarcillin 1 g vial, 200 mg/mL when reconstituted
   According to the package insert, the usual dose, after the initial loading dose, for patients with infections complicated by renal insufficiency is as follows: creatinine clearance over 60 mL/min: 3 g q4h; 30 to 60 mL/min: 2 g q4h; 10 to 30 mL/min: 2 g q8h; and less than 10 mL/min: 2 g q12h.
   Is the ordered dose safe? If the dose is safe, what is the amount to administer?

14. Ordered: Heparin 600 units/h
    On hand: Heparin 20,000 units in 500 mL of D5W
    What is the hourly flow rate?

15. Ordered: lidocaine 3 mg/min IV
    On hand: lidocaine 0.5 g in 250 mL D5W
    What is the hourly flow rate?

16. Ordered: nitroglycerin 30 mcg/min IV
    On hand: 50 mg nitroglycerin in 250 mL D5W
    What is the hourly flow rate?

17. Ordered: dobutamine 3 mcg/kg/min IV; the patient weighs 187 lb
    On hand: dobutamine HCl 200 mg in 500 mL NS
    What is the hourly flow rate?

18. Ordered: nitroprusside 25 mg in 500 mL D5W. The patient has received 325 mL. How much medication has the patient received?

For Exercises 19–20, refer to the following order:
   Ordered: Levophed 4 mg in 1,000 mL D5W; start IV infusion at 8 mcg/min and infuse for 30 minutes. Titrate to systolic BP greater than or equal to 90 mm Hg by increasing the rate by 1 mcg/min every 15 minutes. Maximum infusion rate is 12 mcg/min.

19. What is the starting flow rate in mL/h?

20. What is the maximum flow rate in mL/h?

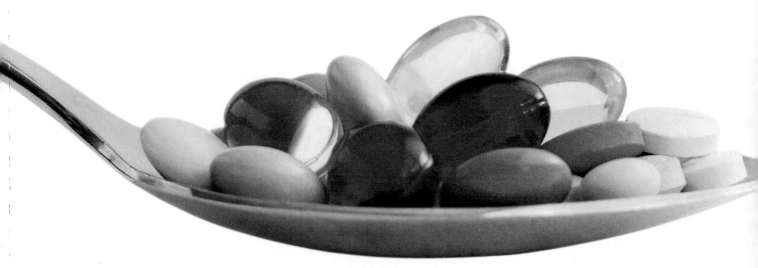

UNIT 6

Performing, Dispensing, and Compounding Calculations

Amount to Dispense and Days' Supply

CHAPTER

> *Math is like going to the gym for your brain. It sharpens your mind.*

DANICA MCKELLAR

LEARNING OUTCOMES

When you have completed Chapter 18, you will be able to:

18.1 Calculate the amount of a medication to dispense.

18.2 Calculate the days' supply of a medication.

KEY TERM

days' supply

INTRODUCTION
In earlier chapters you learned how to interpret medication orders and calculate the amount to administer. These skills allow you to determine the dose to be given and how often it will be given. In this chapter, you will use similar skills to calculate how much medication will be needed to last a given number of days, and how many days a given amount of medication will last the patient.

18.1 Calculating the Amount to Dispense

While medication orders often state the amount of medication that is to be dispensed, some orders are written for a certain number of days rather than for a specific quantity of medication. In these cases, it is necessary to calculate the amount to dispense before you can fill the order. For example, a physician may write an order for an antibiotic that is to be taken for 10 days. You will also need to calculate the amount to dispense when filling an order for a patient with prescription insurance. Insurance companies usually limit the amount of medication the patient can receive at one time to a certain number of days.

In these situations, the amount to dispense must be determined by the pharmacist or technician. In order to perform the calculations, you will need three pieces of information:

- The amount to administer for a single dose
- The number of doses per day
- The days' supply needed

PROCEDURE CHECKLIST 18-1	Calculating the Amount of Medication to Dispense
	1. Multiply the amount to administer for each dose by the number of doses given in 1 day to find the amount of medication that the patient needs each day.
	2. Multiply the amount of medication needed each day by the number of days the medication is to be taken to find out the amount of medication to be dispensed.
Example 1	Ordered: Erythromycin 300 mg q6h for 10 days

On hand: See Figure 18-1.

Calculate the amount of erythromycin needed to fill the order.

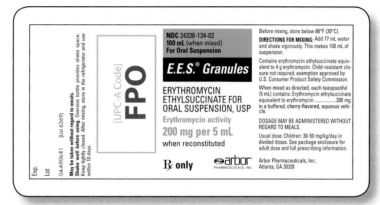

Figure 18-1

1. Multiply the amount to administer by the number of doses per day.

7.5 mL × 4 doses/day = 30 mL/day

2. Multiply the amount needed for 1 day by the number of days needed.

30 mL/day × 10 days = 300 mL

The amount to dispense is 300 mL.

Example 2	Ordered: Welchol 1,875 mg bid for 60 days

On hand: Welchol 625 mg tabs

Calculate the number of Welchol tablets to dispense. Note that in this case you must first determine the number of 625 mg tablets to administer for each dose.

1,825 mg/625 mg = 3 tabs per dose

1. Multiply the amount to administer by the number of doses per day.

3 tablets × 2 doses/day = 6 tablets/day

2. Multiply the amount needed for 1 day by the number of days needed.

6 tablets/day × 60 days = 360 tablets

The amount to dispense is 360 tablets.

In the examples above, the medication can be dispensed in the exact quantity needed. This is not always the case, however. Some medications come in packages that cannot be divided. Insulin, for example, comes in a vial, and is dispensed as whole vials. The same is true for any injectable medication. Many common antibiotics come in bottles that contain a powder to be reconstituted. Once it has been reconstituted, the entire bottle is dispensed to the patient. When a medication is packaged in this way, you will need to calculate the number of containers that need to be dispensed.

<table>
<tr>
<td>

PROCEDURE CHECKLIST 18-2

</td>
<td>

Calculating the Amount of Medication to Dispense for Prepackaged Products

1. Multiply the amount to administer for each dose by the number of doses given in 1 day to find the amount of medication the patient needs each day.

2. Multiply the amount of medication needed each day by the number of days of medication needed to find the amount of medication needed to last the days ordered.

3. Divide the amount of medication needed (answer from step 2) by the amount of medication in one package of the product.

4. Round your answer *up* to the nearest whole number. This is the number of packages to be dispensed.

</td>
</tr>
<tr>
<td>

Example 1

</td>
<td>

Ordered: Amoxicillin 250 mg tid for 10 days

On hand: 100 mL bottles of amoxicillin. See Figure 18-2.

Calculate the number of bottles of amoxicillin needed to fill the order. Partial bottles are not dispensed.

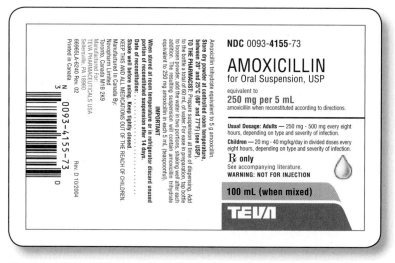

This label is for US only, and cannot be altered or translated.

Figure 18-2

1. Multiply the amount to administer by the number of doses per day.

5 mL × 3 doses/day = 15 mL/day

2. Multiply the amount needed for 1 day by the number of days needed.

15 mL/day × 10 days = 150 mL

3. Divide the amount of medication needed by the amount of medication in one bottle.

150 mL ÷ 100 mL/bottle = 1.5 bottles

4. Round your answer up to the nearest whole number.

1.5 bottles → 2 bottles

The amount to dispense is 2 bottles.

</td>
</tr>
</table>

Example 2

Ordered: 35 units insulin lispro injection subcut tid for 90 days

On hand: 1,000 unit vials of insulin lispro U-100

Calculate the number of vials of insulin needed to fill the order. Partial vials are not dispensed.

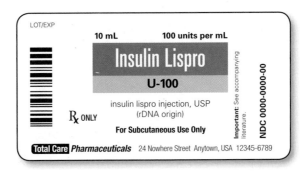

1. Multiply the amount to administer by the number of doses per day.

   35 units × 3 doses/day = 105 units/day

2. Multiply the amount needed for 1 day by the number of days needed.

   105 units/day × 90 days = 9,450 units

3. Divide the amount of medication needed by the amount of medication in one bottle.

   9,450 units ÷ 1,000 units/vial = 9.45 vials

4. Round your answer up to the nearest whole number.

   9.45 vials → 10 vials

   The amount to dispense is 10 vials.

CRITICAL THINKING ON THE JOB

Dispense the Correct Medication and Amount

A prescription reads: Cephalexin oral suspension 175 mg q6h for 7 days.
The pharmacy technician preparing the medication has the following two bottles of medication on hand.

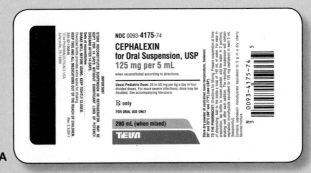

A

This label is for US only, and cannot be altered or translated.

(Continued)

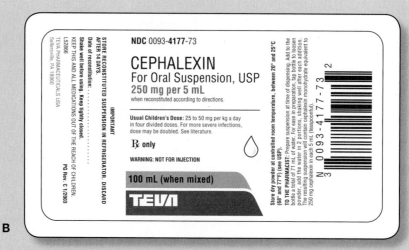

This label is for US only, and cannot be altered or translated.

The pharmacy technician must determine the amount to dispense but is unsure which bottle to use. He decides to use Label A because the order is for seven days and he sees that it reconstitutes to the larger volume of 200 mL. Performing his calculations, he determines that each dose will be 7 mL and the patient will need 4 doses per day for a total of 28 mL. The patient must take 28 mL for 7 days, so he needs to dispense 198 mL of medication. He reconstitutes the medication in Label A and dispenses the entire bottle.

 Think! . . . Is It Reasonable? Did the pharmacy technician dispense the correct medication and amount?

REVIEW AND PRACTICE

18.1 Calculating the Amount to Dispense

Calculate the amount to dispense for each of the following orders. When more than one dosage strength is available, choose the most appropriate.

1. Ordered: Cephalexin 500 mg po 3 times a day for 7 days

   On hand: Cephalexin 500 mg capsules

2. Ordered: Baclofen 5 mg po tid for 4 days

   On hand: Baclofen 10 mg and 20 mg scored tablets

3. Ordered: Furosemide 80 mg po daily for 90 days

   On hand: Furosemide 40 mg/5 mL oral solution

4. Ordered: Fosamax® 10 mg po daily for 30 days

   On hand: Fosamax® 5 mg tablets

5. Ordered: Celexa® 15 mg po BID for 30 days

On hand: Celexa oral solution 10 mg/5 mL

6. Ordered: See Prescription A

On hand: Synthroid 50 mcg, 88 mcg, 100 mcg, and 150 mcg tablets

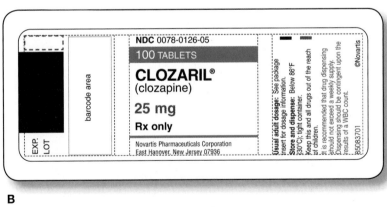

Mark DeSantis
123 Baker Drive
Owosso, MI 48867
989-555-1234

Prescribed Date _1/23/2014_

Name _Jeannies Kucharek_   DOB _8/10/1939_

Address _____

Rx: _Synthroid 0.1 mg_

QUANTITY: _#30_

SIG: _tab i po tid_

Refills: _0_

_____MD1234567_____   _Mark Desantis, MD_
Prescriber ID #   Signature

A

7. Ordered: Clozaril 50 mg po q6h for 7 days

On hand: See Label B

B

NDC 0078-0126-05

100 TABLETS

CLOZARIL®
(clozapine)

25 mg

Rx only

Novartis Pharmaceuticals Corporation
East Hanover, New Jersey 07936

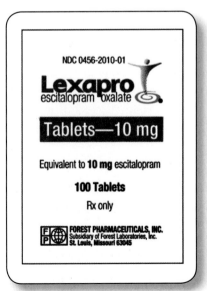

NDC 0456-2010-01

Lexapro
escitalopram oxalate

Tablets—10 mg

Equivalent to **10 mg** escitalopram

100 Tablets

Rx only

FOREST PHARMACEUTICALS, INC.
Subsidiary of Forest Laboratories, Inc.
St. Louis, Missouri 63045

8. Ordered: Lexapro 20 mg po daily for 30 days

On hand: See Label C

C

9. Ordered: Vistaril oral suspension 25 mg tid for 21 days

   On hand: See Label D

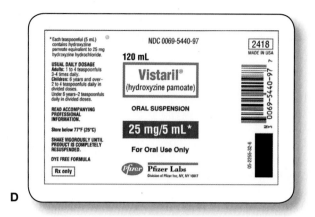

D

10. Ordered: Prandin 0.5 mg by mouth three times daily before meals for 30 days

    On hand: See Labels E and F

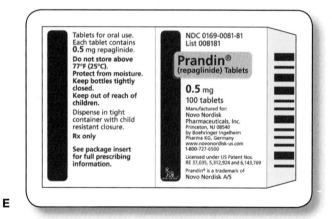

E

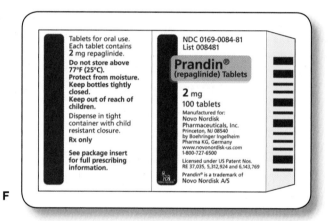

F

11. Ordered: Zemplar 2 mcg po every other day for 90 days

    On hand: See Label G

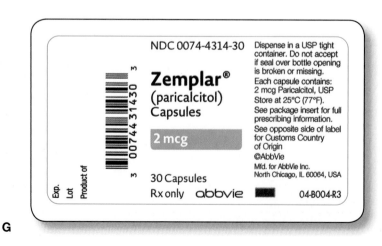

G

12. Ordered: Norvir 300 mg po bid with meals for 30 days

On hand: See Label H

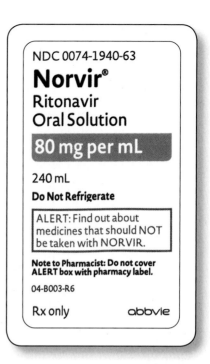

NDC 0074-1940-63

Norvir®
Ritonavir
Oral Solution

80 mg per mL

240 mL

Do Not Refrigerate

ALERT: Find out about
medicines that should NOT
be taken with NORVIR.

**Note to Pharmacist: Do not cover
ALERT box with pharmacy label.**

04-B003-R6

Rx only   abbvie

H

Calculate the number of containers to dispense. Assume that partial containers are not dispensed.

13. Ordered: Advair® Diskus 250/50, 1 puff bid for 90 days

On hand: Advair® Diskus 250/50, each Diskus provides 60 puffs

14. Ordered: Insulin lispro 22 units subcut 4 times daily, with meals and at bedtime, for 60 days

On hand: 1,000 unit vials of insulin lispro

15. Ordered: Amoxicillin suspension 500 mg po tid for 14 days

On hand: Amoxicillin suspension 250 mg per 5 mL; each bottle contains 150 mL when reconstituted

16. Ordered: Vantin® 100 mg po q12h for 7 days

On hand: See Label I

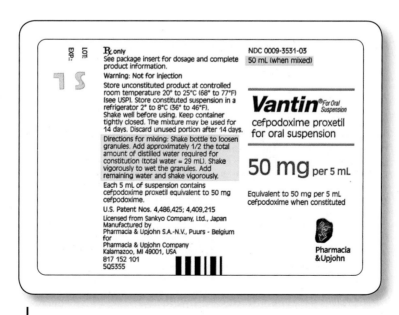

Rx only
See package insert for dosage and complete
product information.

Warning: Not for injection

Store unconstituted product at controlled
room temperature 20° to 25°C (68° to 77°F)
[see USP]. Store constituted suspension in a
refrigerator 2° to 8°C (36° to 46°F).
Shake well before using. Keep container
tightly closed. The mixture may be used for
14 days. Discard unused portion after 14 days.
Directions for mixing: Shake bottle to loosen
granules. Add approximately 1/2 the total
amount of distilled water required for
constitution (total water = 29 mL). Shake
vigorously to wet the granules. Add
remaining water and shake vigorously.
Each 5 mL of suspension contains
cefpodoxime proxetil equivalent to 50 mg
cefpodoxime.
U.S. Patent Nos. 4,486,425; 4,409,215
Licensed from Sankyo Company, Ltd., Japan
Manufactured by
Pharmacia & Upjohn S.A.-N.V., Puurs - Belgium
for
Pharmacia & Upjohn Company
Kalamazoo, MI 49001, USA
817 152 101
5Q5355

NDC 0009-3531-03
50 mL (when mixed)

Vantin® For Oral Suspension
cefpodoxime proxetil
for oral suspension

50 mg per 5 mL

Equivalent to 50 mg per 5 mL
cefpodoxime when constituted

Pharmacia
&Upjohn

I

17. Ordered: Cefprozil 250 mg po q12h for 10 days

On hand: See Label J

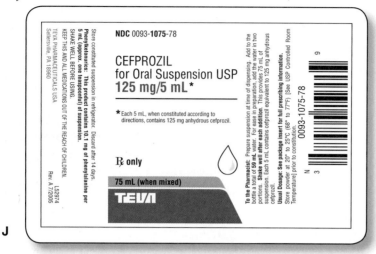

J

This label is for US only, and cannot be altered or translated.

18. Ordered: Amoxicillin 500 mg po q8h for 10 days

On hand: See Label K

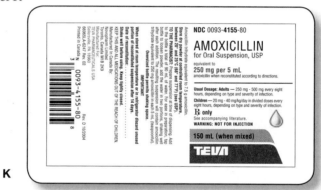

K

This label is for US only, and cannot be altered or translated.

19. Ordered: Insulin lispro injection 18 units qid subcut before each meal and at bedtime, for 90 days

On hand: See Label L

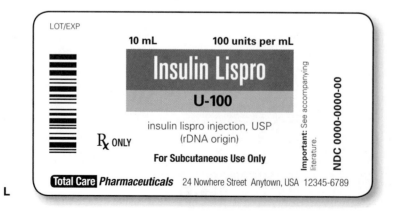

L

20. Ordered: Cephalexin 500 mg po q6h for 14 days

On hand: See Label M

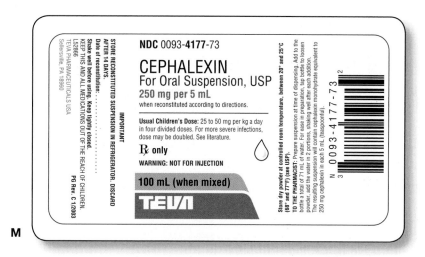

M

This label is for US only, and cannot be altered or translated.

18.2 Calculating the Days' Supply

Another calculation that sometimes needs to be performed before filling an order is the **days' supply**—number of days that the order should last. This is most commonly needed when you are refilling a prescription that is to be billed to an insurance company. If the patient originally received a 30 day supply of medication, for example, the insurance company will not pay for a refill until the 30 days are nearly completed. The insurance company may have a policy that an order cannot be refilled until the patient is down to 5 days of medication or less. In these situations, you will need to determine how many days have elapsed since the prescription was originally filled and how many days the previous order should last. In order to perform the calculations, you will need three pieces of information:

- The amount to administer for a single dose
- The number of doses per day
- The amount of medication that was originally dispensed

PROCEDURE CHECKLIST 18-3

Calculating the Days' Supply of Medication Dispensed

1. Multiply the amount to administer for each dose by the number of doses given in 1 day to find the amount of medication the patient needs each day.

2. Divide the amount of medication dispensed by the amount needed each day.

3. Round the answer from step 2 *down* to the nearest whole number to find the number of full days that the order will last the patient.

Example 1

Ordered: 500 mL acetaminophen 160 mg/5 mL infant/children's suspension; take 7.5 mL every 6 hours PRN.

On hand: See Figure 18-3.

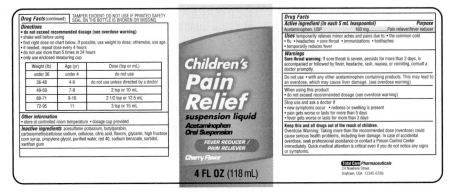

Figure 18-3

Calculate how many days the order will last the patient.

1. Multiply the amount to administer by the number of doses per day.

7.5 mL × 4 doses/day = 30 mL/day

2. Divide the amount of medication dispensed by the amount needed each day.

500 mL ÷ 30 mL/day = 16.67 days

3. Round down to the nearest whole number to determine the number of full days that the order will last.

16.67 days → 16 full days

The order will last the patient 16 full days.

Example 2

Ordered: eight 1,000 unit vials of insulin lispro; inject 35 units subcutaneously 4 times a day, with meals and at bedtime.
Calculate how many days the order will last the patient.

1. Multiply the amount to administer by the number of doses per day.

35 units × 4 doses/day = 140 units/day

2. Divide the amount of medication dispensed by the amount needed each day.

8,000 units ÷ 140 units/day = 57.14 days

3. Round down to the nearest whole number to determine the number of full days that the order will last.

57.14 days → 57 full days

The order will last the patient 57 full days.

18.2 Calculating the Days' Supply

Calculate the days' supply for each of the following medication orders.

1. Ordered: Diltiazem 30 mg tablets #120; take 1 tab po bid

2. Ordered: 240 mL Augmentin® 250 mg/5 mL suspension; take 5 mL po q8h

3. Ordered: 210 mL Acyclovir 200 mg/5 mL; take 400 mg po tid

4. Ordered: Erythromycin Base Filmtab® 250 mg #50; take 1 tab po q6h

5. Ordered: Ranitidine 150 mg tablets #28; 1 tab po q6h

6. Ordered: 200 mL Benadryl®; take $1\frac{1}{2}$ tsp po every 6 hours

7. Ordered: Fluconazole 40 mg/mL, disp 60 mL; take 80 mg po daily

8. Directions: Inject 1.2 mL Depo-Testosterone deep IM once a day; quantity dispensed: one 15 mL vial

9. Ordered: Allopurinol 300 mg tablets #60; take 1 tab po bid

10. Ordered: Gemfibrozil 600 mg tabs #40, 1 tab po q12h

11. Ordered: Phenazopyridine 100 mg tablets #6, 1 tab po tid after meals

12. Ordered: Tylenol 120 mg/5 mL, disp 150 mL; 60 mg po q4h prn

13. Ordered: four 800 unit vials Novolin® R (insulin); inject 18 units subcut 4 times a day

14. Ordered: Metoclopramide 10 mg tablets #56; 1 tab po qid 30 min before meals and at bedtime

15. Ordered: See prescription A

Alan Capsella, MD
Westtown Medical Clinic
989-555-1234

Prescribed Date _April 10, 2014_

Name _Mark Ward_   DOB _8/12/10_

Address _____

Rx: _Amoxil – oral susp_

QUANTITY: _100 mL_

SIG: _i tsp po q8h_

Refills: _0_

_MD398475_   _Alan Capsella MD_
Prescriber ID #   Signature

A

16. Ordered: Artane 2 mg/5 mL, disp
    8 fl oz; 3 mg po daily

17. Ordered: Dilaudid® 8 mg scored
    tablets #16; 4 mg po q6h

18. Ordered: Duricef® 1 g scored tabs
    #30; take 500 mg po bid

19. Ordered: Biaxin® liquid 125 mg/5 mL,
    disp 25 mL; 62.5 mg po q12h

20. Ordered: See prescription B

B

Mark DeSantis
123 Baker Drive
Owosso, MI 48867
989-555-1234

Prescribed Date _1/23/2014_

Name _Jeannies Kucharek_   DOB _8/10/1939_

Address _____

Rx: Synthroid 0.1 mg

QUANTITY: #30

SIG: tab i po tid

Refills: 0

_____MD1234567_____   _Mark Desantis, MD_
Prescriber ID #   Signature

CHAPTER 18 SUMMARY

LEARNING OUTCOME	KEY POINTS
18.1 Calculate the amount of a medication to dispense. Pages 540–549	To calculate the amount to dispense, you need to know the amount to administer for a single dose, the number of doses per day, and the days' supply needed.
	Some medications are packaged in containers that cannot be divided. Examples include inhalers, injectables, and reconstituted antibiotics. For these products, it is necessary to calculate the number of containers (vials, bottles, or inhalers) that need to be dispensed.
	When calculating the number of containers to be dispensed, round up to ensure the patient has enough medication to last the number of days needed.
18.2 Calculate the days' supply of a medication. Pages 549–552	To calculate the number of days a medication order will last the patient, you need to know the amount to administer for a single dose, the number of doses per day, and the amount of medication that was dispensed.
	When calculating the number of days an order will last, round your answer down to find the number of full days that the order will last the patient.

Calculate the amount to dispense for each of the following orders. When more than one dosage strength is available, choose the most appropriate.

1. Ordered: Azithromycin 1 g po daily for 5 days

   On hand: Azithromycin 500 mg tablets

2. Ordered: Zyrtec 2.5 mg po daily for 60 days

   On hand: Zyrtec syrup 1 mg/mL

3. Ordered: Baclofen 5 mg po daily for 60 days

   On hand: Baclofen 10 mg scored tablets

4. Ordered: Furosemide oral solution 75 mg daily for 60 days

   On hand: Furosemide oral solution 40 mg per 4 mL

5. Ordered: Robaxin®-750, 2 tablets po q6h for 10 days

   On hand: Robaxin®-750 tablets

6. Ordered: Amitriptyline 75 mg po at bedtime for 15 days

   On hand: Amitriptyline 25 mg, 50 mg, and 75 mg tablets

7. Ordered: Xanax 1 mg po tid for 8 days

   On hand: See Label A

   Note: Tablets are scored in fourths.

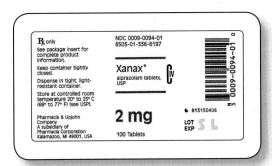

A

8. Ordered: Diazepam 7 mg po bid for 5 days

   On hand: See Labels B, C, and D

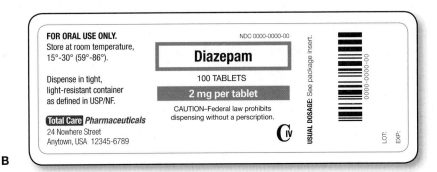

B

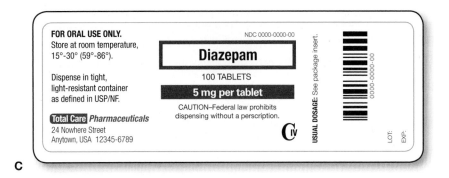

C

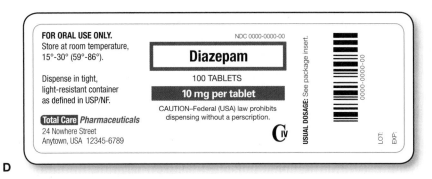

D

9. Ordered: Trileptal 600 mg po bid for 30 days

On hand: See Label E

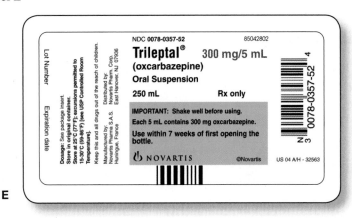

E

10. Ordered: Zoloft 50 mg po daily for 21 days

On hand: See Labels F and G

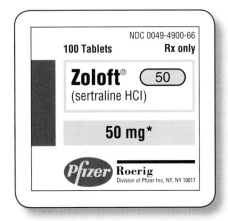

F

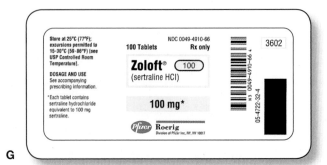

G

Calculate the number of containers to dispense. Assume that partial containers are not dispensed.

11. Ordered: Vantin® 200 mg po bid for 14 days

    On hand: Vantin® 100 mg/5 mL; each bottle contains 100 mL when reconstituted

12. Ordered: Symbicort®; take 2 inhalations q12h for 90 days

    On hand: Symbicort® inhalers; each inhaler contains 120 inhalations

13. Ordered: Advair® Diskus 100/50, 1 puff q12h for 30 days

    On hand: Advair® Diskus 100/50, Advair® Diskus 250/50, and Advair® Diskus 500/50; each Diskus provides 60 puffs

14. Ordered: Novolin® 70/30 (insulin) 25 units subcut 4 times a day, with meals and at bedtime, for 30 days

    On hand: See Label H

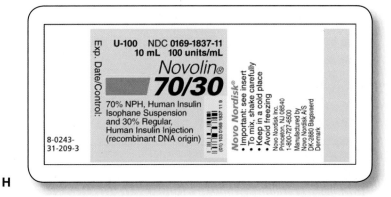

H

15. Ordered: Amoxicillin 200 mg po tid for 14 days

    On hand: See Label I

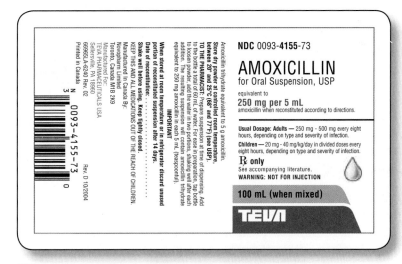

I

This label is for US only, and cannot be altered or translated.

Calculate the days' supply for each of the following medication orders.

16. Ordered: 120 mL Benadryl® 12.5 mg/5 mL; take 3 mL po q6h

17. Ordered: two 1,000 unit vials of Levemir® (insulin); inject 16 units subcut daily

18. Ordered: Lodine 300 mg #20; take 1 cap po bid

19. Ordered: 1 Atrovent® inhaler; take 2 inhalations every 8 hours. Each inhaler contains 120 inhalations.

20. Ordered: Coumadin® 1 mg scored tablets #100; take 1.5 mg po 3 times daily

CHECK UP

For Exercises 1–10, calculate the amount of medication to dispense. When more than one dosage strength is available, choose the most appropriate.

1. Ordered: Zyrtec® 2.5 mg po daily for 60 days
   On hand: Zyrtec® 1 mg/mL syrup

2. Ordered: Ibuprofen 800 mg po tid for 45 days
   On hand: Ibuprofen 400 mg tablets

3. Ordered: Lasix® 60 mg by mouth once a day, in the morning, for 90 days
   On hand: Lasix® 40 mg scored tablets

4. Ordered: Topiramate 25 mg po bid for 21 days
   On hand: See Label A

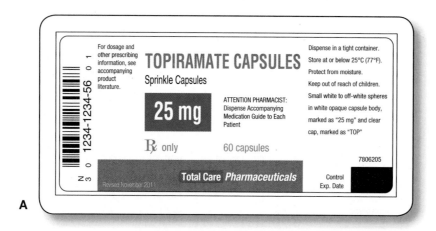

A

5. Ordered: Metformin HCl 1 g po q12h for 30 days
   On hand: See Labels B and C

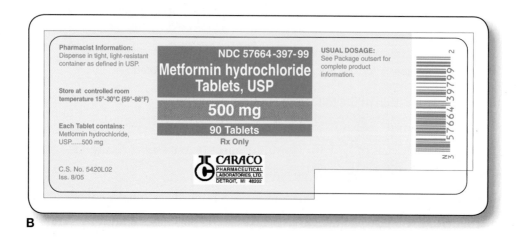

B

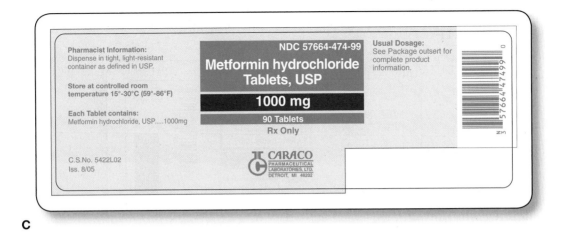

C

6. Ordered: Depakene 250 mg po tid for 60 days
   On hand: See Label D

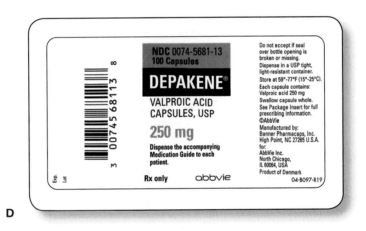

D

7. Ordered: Oxycontin 40 mg orally q12h for 5 days
   On hand: See Label E

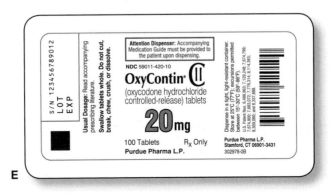

E

8. Ordered: Dilantin 60 mg po tid for 21 days
   On hand: See Label F

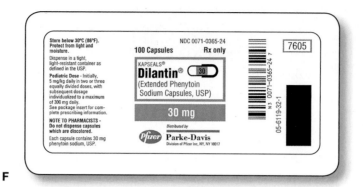

F

9. Ordered: Vistaril 75 mg po qid for 18 days
   On hand: See Label G

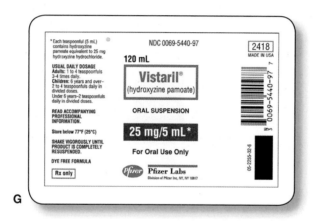

G

10. Ordered: Procardia 20 mg po tid for 30 days
   On hand: See Label H

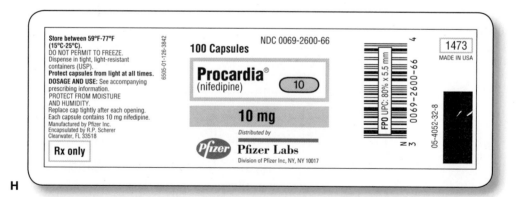

H

For Exercises 11–18, calculate the number of containers of medication to dispense. Assume that partial containers are not dispensed.

11. Ordered: Augmentin® 125 mg/5 mL 125 mg po q8h for 7 days
    On hand: Augmentin® oral suspension 125 mg/5 mL; each bottle contains 75 mL

12. Ordered: Lantus® 14 units subcut once daily for 30 days
    On hand: Lantus U-100, 10 mL vials

13. Ordered: Combivent® 2 inhalations 4 times a day for 90 days
    On hand: Combivent® inhalers; each inhaler contains 120 inhalations

14. Ordered: Penicillin VK 250 mg/5 mL oral suspension; take 2 tsp every 6 hours for 10 days
    On hand: 200 mL bottles of penicillin VK 250 mg/5 mL oral suspension

15. Ordered: Humalog® Mix 75/25; inject 35 units subcut 3 times a day, 15 minutes before meals, for 60 days
    On hand: Humalog® Mix 75/25, 10 mL vials

16. Ordered: Zantac® 37.5 mg IM q8h for 5 days
    On hand: Zantac® Injection 25 mg/mL in 6 mL multidose vials

17. Ordered: Miacalcin 200 international units intranasally daily for 90 days; alternate nostrils daily
    On hand: See Label I

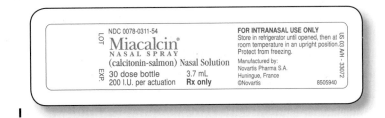

I

18. Ordered: Cephalexin 250 mg po q6h for 10 days
    On hand: Label J

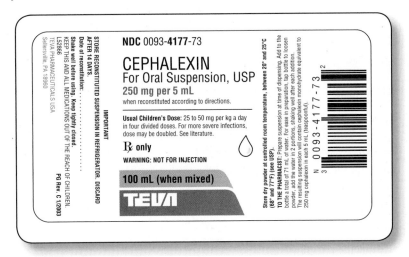

J

This label is for US only, and cannot be altered or translated.

For Exercises 19-27, calculate the days' supply for each of the following medication orders.

19. Ordered: 4 oz doxycycline 50 mg/5 mL; take 1 tsp by mouth every 12 hours

20. Ordered: 180 mL albuterol 2 mg/5 mL syrup; take 2.5 mL by mouth 3 times a day

21. Ordered: Dilaudid® 8 mg #200; take 1 tab q6h

22. Ordered: 1 Symbicort® inhaler; take 2 puffs every 12 hours. Each inhaler contains 100 inhalations.

23. Ordered: two 150 mL bottles of Tussionex®; take 1 tsp q12h

24. Ordered: three 10 mL vials of Humalog® U-100; inject 15 units subcut 4 times a day, before meals and at bedtime

25. Ordered: Ativan® 1 mg tabs #60; 1.5 mg po daily

26. Ordered: two 10 mL vials of human chorionic gonadotropin (HCG); inject 1.5 mL once a day, at bedtime

27. Ordered: Neurontin® 400 mg #100; take 1 capsule by mouth tid

For Exercises 28–30, refer to the information below:

Ordered: See Prescription A

Alan Capsella, MD
Westtown Medical Clinic
989-555-1234

Prescribed Date _April 10, 2014_

Name _Mark Ward_   DOB _8/12/10_

Address _____

Rx: _Amoxil 250 mg/5 mL – oral susp_
    (Generic substitution OK)
QUANTITY: _100 mL_

SIG: _i tsp po q8h_

Refills: _0_

_____MD398475_____   _Alan Capsella MD_
Prescriber ID #   Signature

On hand: See Labels K and L

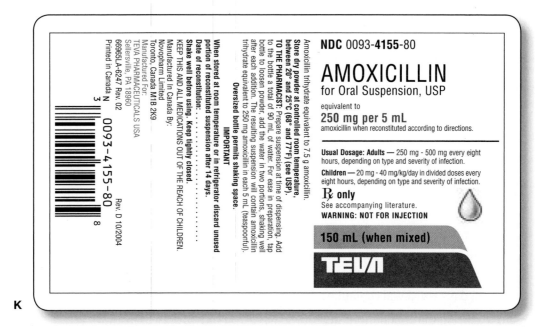

NDC 0093-4155-80

AMOXICILLIN
for Oral Suspension, USP

equivalent to
250 mg per 5 mL
amoxicillin when reconstituted according to directions.

Usual Dosage: Adults — 250 mg - 500 mg every eight hours, depending on type and severity of infection.

Children — 20 mg - 40 mg/kg/day in divided doses every eight hours, depending on type and severity of infection.

℞ **only**
See accompanying literature.
WARNING: NOT FOR INJECTION

150 mL (when mixed)

TEVA

Amoxicillin trihydrate equivalent to 7.5 g amoxicillin.
Store dry powder at controlled room temperature,
between 20° and 25°C (68° and 77°F) (see USP).
TO THE PHARMACIST: Prepare suspension at time of dispensing. Add to the bottle a total of 90 mL of water. For ease in preparation, tap bottle to loosen powder, add the water in two portions, shaking well after each addition. The resulting suspension will contain amoxicillin trihydrate equivalent to 250 mg amoxicillin in each 5 mL (teaspoonful).

Oversized bottle permits shaking space.

IMPORTANT
When stored at room temperature or in refrigerator discard unused portion of reconstituted suspension after 14 days.
Date of reconstitution: . . . .
Shake well before using. Keep tightly closed.
KEEP THIS AND ALL MEDICATIONS OUT OF THE REACH OF CHILDREN.

Manufactured in Canada By:
Novopharm Limited
Toronto, Canada M1B 2K9
Manufactured For:
TEVA PHARMACEUTICALS USA
Sellersville, PA 18960
66965LA-6247 Rev. 02
Printed in Canada N

3
0093-4155-80
Rev. D 10/2004
8

K

This label is for US only, and cannot be altered or translated.

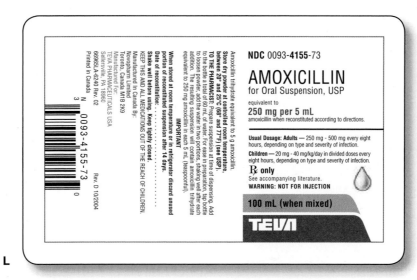

NDC 0093-4155-73

AMOXICILLIN
for Oral Suspension, USP

equivalent to
250 mg per 5 mL
amoxicillin when reconstituted according to directions.

Usual Dosage: Adults — 250 mg - 500 mg every eight hours, depending on type and severity of infection.

Children — 20 mg - 40 mg/kg/day in divided doses every eight hours, depending on type and severity of infection.

℞ **only**
See accompanying literature.
WARNING: NOT FOR INJECTION

100 mL (when mixed)

TEVA

Amoxicillin trihydrate equivalent to 5 g amoxicillin.
Store dry powder at controlled room temperature,
between 20° and 25°C (68° and 77°F) (see USP).
TO THE PHARMACIST: Prepare suspension at time of dispensing. Add to the bottle a total of 60 mL of water. For ease in preparation, tap bottle to loosen powder, add the water in two portions, shaking well after each addition. The resulting suspension will contain amoxicillin trihydrate equivalent to 250 mg amoxicillin in each 5 mL (teaspoonful).

IMPORTANT
When stored at room temperature or in refrigerator discard unused portion of reconstituted suspension after 14 days.
Date of reconstitution: . . . .
Shake well before using. Keep tightly closed.
KEEP THIS AND ALL MEDICATIONS OUT OF THE REACH OF CHILDREN.

Manufactured in Canada By:
Novopharm Limited
Toronto, Canada M1B 2K9
Manufactured For:
TEVA PHARMACEUTICALS USA
Sellersville, PA 18960
66965LA-6240 Rev. 02
Printed in Canada N

3
0093-4155-73
Rev. D 10/2004
0

L

This label is for US only, and cannot be altered or translated.

28. Which label should you choose to fill this medication order?

29. How many bottles will you dispense?

30. Calculate the days' supply.

CRITICAL THINKING APPLICATIONS

Anti-inflammatory steroids, such as prednisone, are often prescribed with a high initial dose that is reduced gradually over the course of several days. The pharmacy receives an order to dispense 20 tablets of prednisone 10 mg. The instructions are to take 4 tablets daily for 2 days, then 2 tablets a day for 2 days, then 1 tablet a day for 4 days, then ½ tablet a day until gone.

1. How many tablets will the patient have left after completing 3 days of treatment?

2. How many days will the medication order last?

CASE STUDY

A patient comes in with a prescription for Humulin® R (insulin). The instructions call for him to inject 20 units subcut 3 times a day with meals and 10 units at bedtime.

1. How many full days will a vial containing 1,000 units last the patient?

2. How many vials will the patient need in order to have a 60-day supply of insulin?

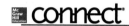

Now that you have completed the materials in the chapter text, go to CONNECT and complete any chapter activities you have not yet done.

Calculations for Compounding

19

CHAPTER

When on the brink of complete discouragement, success is discerning that the line between failure and success is so fine that often a single extra effort is all that is needed to bring victory out of defeat.

Elbert Green Hubbard

LEARNING OUTCOMES

When you have completed Chapter 19, you will be able to:

19.1 Calculate the quantities needed to prepare a liquid compound.

19.2 Calculate the quantities needed to make a solid or semisolid compound.

19.3 Calculate the quantities needed to dilute a stock product.

19.4 Perform calculations using specific gravity.

KEY TERMS

Alligation method
Base
Compound
Compounding
Diluent

QSAD (qsad)
Solute
Solvent
Specific gravity
Stock product

INTRODUCTION

Sometimes it is necessary to mix ingredients together in order to make a solution, cream, ointment, or other product for a patient. This process is known as **compounding**, and the resulting product is a **compound**. In this chapter, you will learn how to calculate the quantities of ingredients needed to prepare compounds.

19.1 Liquid Compounds

Liquid medications include solutions, emulsions, lotions, and tinctures. Liquid mixtures are made up of two main parts: the liquid used to dissolve other ingredients, known as the **solvent** or **diluent**, and the dissolved materials, known as the **solutes**. While manufacturers prepare most of the liquids used in healthcare, it is occasionally necessary to prepare a product for a patient. To do this, you will need to know how concentrations of liquids are expressed.

Prescriptions for liquid compounds are usually written in one of two ways. The prescriber often writes out the quantities of all of the ingredients needed to prepare the product. In this case, calculations are not needed. Sometimes, however, the prescriber indicates the concentration of medication as a percentage. When the order is written as a percentage, it is necessary to perform calculations before you can prepare the product. Remember that *percent* means "per hundred."

RULE 19-1	For liquid mixtures containing a solid medication, the percent strength represents the number of grams of a medication contained in 100 mL of the mixture.
Example	2% hydrocortisone lotion contains 2 g of hydrocortisone in every 100 mL of the lotion.

RULE 19-2	For liquid mixtures containing a liquid medication, the percent strength represents the number of milliliters of a medication contained in 100 mL of the mixture.
Example	50% ethyl alcohol contains 50 mL of ethyl alcohol in every 100 mL of the solution.

Note that both of the previous examples define the amount of an ingredient per 100 mL of the product. You may think that you will need to add the specified amount of medication to 100 mL of the solvent to make these preparations. This, however, would not take into account the volume occupied by the medication. In the example for Rule 19-1, for example, you cannot just add 2 grams of hydrocortisone powder to 100 mL of lotion. To prepare this product, you must first weigh out the hydrocortisone, and then add a sufficient quantity of the lotion to make the final volume of the product 100 mL.

RULE 19-3	When preparing a liquid compound, first measure the medication, then add a sufficient quantity of solvent to bring the final volume to the desired level.
Example	Write a recipe for preparing 100 mL of 2% lidocaine solution from lidocaine powder and water. To prepare this solution, you will need 2 g of lidocaine powder and enough water to bring the final volume to 100 mL. A recipe for preparing this product looks like this:

2% Lidocaine Solution	
Lidocaine	2 g
Water	qsad 100 mL

The abbreviation **QSAD (qsad)** is taken from a Latin phrase meaning "a sufficient quantity to adjust the dimensions to . . . ." In this case, you are adding enough water to make the final volume 100 mL. When you are preparing a liquid solution, the solute and diluent should add up to the desired volume.

These rules can be used when the prescription is for 100 mL of a liquid compound. If the order is for a different volume, however, you will need to calculate the quantity of ingredients to be used. These calculations can be performed using either the proportion method or dimensional analysis.

PROPORTION METHOD

Fractions

Procedure Checklist 19-1

Calculating Quantities for a Percent Strength Liquid Compound by the Proportion Method Using Fractions

1. Refer to Rules 19-1 and 19-2. Write a fraction from the percent strength desired, with the amount of medication (in grams or milliliters) in the numerator and 100 mL in the denominator.

2. Convert the volume ordered to milliliters. Refer to the "Using Systems of Measurement" unit if needed.

3. Write a fraction with the unknown, x, in the numerator and the total volume (in milliliters) of the compound to be prepared in the denominator.

4. Set the two fractions up as a proportion.

5. Cancel units.

6. Cross-multiply and solve for the unknown value.

EXAMPLE 1

Calculate the amount of sodium iodide powder needed to prepare 1 fl oz of a 5% sodium iodide solution, using water as the solvent.

---

1. Applying Rule 19-1, the first fraction for the proportion is:

$$\frac{5 \text{ g sodium iodide powder}}{100 \text{ mL}}$$

2. The volume ordered is 1 fl oz, which is equal to 30 mL.

3. The second fraction for the proportion is:

$$\frac{x}{30 \text{ mL}}$$

4. Setting up the two fractions as a proportion gives you the following equation:

$$\frac{x}{30 \text{ mL}} = \frac{5 \text{ g sodium iodide powder}}{100 \text{ mL}}$$

5. Cancel units.

$$\frac{x}{30 \text{ mL}} = \frac{5 \text{ g sodium iodide powder}}{100 \text{ mL}}$$

6. Solve for the unknown value by cross-multiplying.

$$100 \times x = 5 \text{ g sodium iodide powder} \times 30$$

$$\frac{100 \times x}{100} = \frac{5 \text{ g sodium iodide powder} \times 30}{100}$$

$$x = 1.5 \text{ g sodium iodide powder}$$

Applying Rule 19-3, the recipe for preparing 30 mL of 5% sodium iodide solution looks like this:

5% Sodium Iodide Solution	
Sodium iodide	1.5 g
Water	qsad 30 mL

EXAMPLE 2

Calculate the amount of pure ethanol needed to prepare 500 mL of a 50% ethanol solution, using water as the solvent.

1. Applying Rule 19-2, the first fraction for the proportion is:

$$\frac{50 \text{ mL pure ethanol}}{100 \text{ mL}}$$

2. The volume ordered is already expressed in milliliters.

3. The second fraction for the proportion is:

$$\frac{x}{500 \text{ mL}}$$

4. Setting up the two fractions as a proportion gives you the following equation:

$$\frac{x}{500 \text{ mL}} = \frac{50 \text{ mL pure ethanol}}{100 \text{ mL}}$$

5. Cancel units.

$$\frac{x}{500 \text{ mL}} = \frac{50 \text{ mL pure ethanol}}{100 \text{ mL}}$$

6. Solve for the unknown by cross-multiplying.

$$100 \times x = 50 \text{ mL pure ethanol} \times 500$$

$$\frac{100 \times x}{100} = \frac{50 \text{ mL pure ethanol} \times 500}{100}$$

$$x = 250 \text{ mL pure ethanol}$$

Applying Rule 19-3, the recipe for preparing 500 mL of a 50% ethanol solution looks like this:

50% Ethanol Solution	
Pure ethanol	250 mL
Water	qsad 500 mL

PROPORTION METHOD

Ratios

Procedure Checklist 19-2
Calculating Quantities for a Percent Strength Liquid Compound by the Proportion Method Using Ratios

1. Refer to Rules 19-1 and 19-2. Write a ratio from the percent strength desired, with the amount of medication (in grams or milliliters) before the colon and 100 mL after the colon.

2. Convert the volume ordered to milliliters. Refer to the "Using Systems of Measurement" unit if needed.

3. Write a ratio with the unknown, x, before the colon and the total volume (in milliliters) of the compound to be prepared after the colon.

4. Set the two ratios up as a proportion.

5. Cancel units.

6. Solve for the unknown value by multiplying means and extremes.

EXAMPLE 1

Calculate the amount of sodium iodide powder needed to prepare 50 mL of a 7% sodium iodide solution, using water as the solvent.

1. Applying Rule 19-1, the first ratio for the proportion is:

   7 g sodium iodide powder : 100 mL

2. The volume ordered is already expressed in milliliters.

3. The second ratio for the proportion is:

   x : 50 mL

4. Setting up the two ratios as a proportion gives you the following equation:

   x : 50 mL :: 7 g sodium iodide powder : 100 mL

5. Cancel units.

   x : 50 ~~mL~~ :: 7 g sodium iodide powder : 100 ~~mL~~

6. Solve for the unknown by multiplying means and extremes.

   $100 \times x = 7$ g sodium iodide powder $\times 50$

   $$\frac{100 \times x}{100} = \frac{7 \text{ g sodium iodide powder} \times 50}{100}$$

   $x = 3.5$ g sodium iodide powder

Applying Rule 19-3, the recipe for preparing 50 mL of 7% sodium iodide solution looks like this:

7% Sodium Iodide Solution	
Sodium iodide	3.5 g
Water	qsad 50 mL

EXAMPLE 2

Calculate the amount of pure ethanol needed to prepare 400 mL of a 20% ethanol solution, using water as the solvent.

1. Applying Rule 19-2, the first ratio for the proportion is

   20 mL pure ethanol : 100 mL

2. The volume ordered is already expressed in milliliters.

3. The second ratio for the proportion is:

   x : 400 mL

4. Setting up the two ratios as a proportion gives you the following equation:

   x : 400 mL :: 20 mL pure ethanol : 100 mL

5. Cancel units.

   x : 400 ~~mL~~ :: 20 mL pure ethanol : 100 ~~mL~~

6. Solve for the unknown by multiplying means and extremes.

   $100 \times x = 20$ mL pure ethanol $\times 400$

   $$\frac{100 \times x}{100} = \frac{20 \text{ mL pure ethanol} \times 400}{100}$$

   $x = 80$ mL pure ethanol

Applying Rule 19-3, the recipe for preparing 400 mL of a 20% ethanol solution looks like this:

20% Ethanol Solution	
Pure ethanol	80 mL
Water	qsad 400 mL

Procedure Checklist 19-3

Calculating Quantities for a Percent Strength Liquid Compound by Dimensional Analysis

1. Refer to Rules 19-1 and 19-2. Write a fraction from the percent strength desired, with the amount of medication (in grams or milliliters) in the numerator and 100 mL in the denominator.

2. Convert the volume ordered to milliliters. Refer to the "Using Systems of Measurement" unit if needed.

3. Write an equation with the unknown, x, on one side. Write the volume ordered (in milliliters) multiplied by the fraction from step 1 on the other side.

4. Cancel units.

5. Solve for the unknown.

EXAMPLE 1

Calculate the amount of sodium iodide powder needed to prepare 2 fl oz of a 2.5% sodium iodide solution, using water as the solvent.

1. Applying Rule 19-1, the fraction for the equation is:

$$\frac{2.5 \text{ g sodium iodide powder}}{100 \text{ mL}}$$

2. The volume ordered is 2 fl oz. Recall that 1 fl oz = 30 mL, so $2 \text{ fl oz} \times \frac{30 \text{ mL}}{1 \text{ fl oz}} = 60 \text{ mL}$.

3. Set up the equation, with x on one side and the volume ordered multiplied by the fraction from step 1 on the other side.

$$x = 60 \text{ mL} \times \frac{2.5 \text{ g sodium iodide powder}}{100 \text{ mL}}$$

4. Cancel units.

$$x = 60 \text{ mL} \times \frac{2.5 \text{ g sodium iodide powder}}{100 \text{ mL}}$$

5. Solve for the unknown.

$$x = 1.5 \text{ g sodium iodide powder}$$

Applying Rule 19-3, the recipe for preparing 60 mL of 2.5% sodium iodide solution looks like this:

2.5% Sodium Iodide Solution	
Sodium iodide	1.5 g
Water	qsad 60 mL

EXAMPLE 2

Calculate the amount of pure ethanol needed to prepare 250 mL of a 70% ethanol solution, using water as the solvent.

1. Applying Rule 19-2, the fraction for the equation is:

$$\frac{70 \text{ mL pure ethanol}}{100 \text{ mL}}$$

2. The volume ordered is already expressed in milliliters.

3. Set up the equation, with x on one side and the volume ordered multiplied by the fraction from step 1.

$$x = 250 \text{ mL} \times \frac{70 \text{ mL pure ethanol}}{100 \text{ mL}}$$

4. Cancel units.

$$x = 250 \, \cancel{mL} \times \frac{70 \text{ mL pure ethanol}}{100 \, \cancel{mL}}$$

5. Solve for the unknown.

$$x = 175 \text{ mL pure ethanol}$$

Applying Rule 19-3, the recipe for preparing 250 mL of a 70% ethanol solution looks like this:

70% Ethanol Solution	
Pure ethanol	175 mL
Water	qsad 250 mL

REVIEW AND PRACTICE

19.1 Liquid Compounds

For Exercises 1–10, calculate the quantity of the specified ingredients needed to prepare each solution.

1. Calculate the amount of sodium chloride needed to prepare 500 mL of 0.9% sodium chloride solution, using sodium chloride powder and water.

2. Calculate the amount of lidocaine needed to prepare 50 mL of 2% lidocaine solution, using lidocaine powder and water.

3. Calculate the amount of pure ethanol needed to prepare 350 mL of 70% ethanol solution, using pure ethanol liquid and water.

4. Calculate the amount of sodium iodide needed to prepare 2 fl oz of 3% sodium iodide solution, using sodium iodide powder and water.

5. Calculate the amount of pure ethanol needed to prepare 4 fl oz of 40% ethanol solution, using pure ethanol liquid and water.

6. Calculate the amount of sodium chloride needed to prepare 2 L of 0.45% sodium chloride solution, using sodium chloride powder and water.

7. Calculate the amount of pure isopropanol needed to prepare 750 mL of 60% isopropanol solution, using pure isopropanol liquid and water.

8. Calculate the amount of lidocaine needed to prepare 200 mL of 1% lidocaine solution, using lidocaine powder and water.

9. Calculate the amount of sodium chloride needed to prepare 250 mL of 0.225% sodium chloride solution, using sodium chloride powder and water.

10. Calculate the amount of sodium iodide needed to prepare 50 mL of 1.5% sodium iodide solution, using sodium iodide powder and water.

19.2 Solid and Semisolid Compounds

As with liquid medications, most solid and semisolid products used in healthcare are prepared by manufacturers. Solid products include suppositories and lozenges, while creams and ointments are the most common semisolid products. As with liquids, the concentration of an ingredient in these products is often expressed as a percent. These products, however, are not measured by volume (mL). They are prepared and measured in units of weight, such as grams.

Solid and semisolid mixtures are made up of two main parts: the active ingredient (medication) and the **base**, or inactive material, into which the ingredient is mixed. The base used to prepare a cream is usually a nonprescription cream that can be found in many pharmacies or grocery stores. Examples of cream bases include Dermovan, Velvachol®, and Eucerin®. The base used to prepare an ointment is usually white petrolatum, which is more commonly referred to as petroleum jelly. Vaseline® is a commonly known brand of petroleum jelly. Another common ointment base is Aquaphor®. As with cream bases, these products can be found on the shelf of your pharmacy or grocery store. Suppositories are most often prepared using cocoa butter or glycerin, which are solid at room temperature but melt at body temperature.

As with liquid compounds, orders for these products are usually written in one of two ways. The prescriber often writes out the quantities of all ingredients needed to prepare the product. In this case, calculations are not needed. Sometimes, however, the prescriber indicates the concentration of medication as a percentage. When the order is written in this way, it is necessary to calculate the amounts before you can prepare the product.

RULE 19-4	For solid or semisolid mixtures containing a medication, the percent strength represents the number of grams of a medication contained in 100 g of the mixture.
Example	20% zinc oxide ointment contains 20 g of zinc oxide in every 100 g of the ointment.

In solid and semisolid compounds, you do not need to account for the volume of the medication because the percentage is calculated by weight. You can calculate the amount of base needed by subtracting the amount of medication needed from the total amount of the product needed. In the previous example, 20% zinc oxide equals 20 g of zinc oxide per 100 g of product. In this case, 100 g − 20 g = 80 g, so 80 g of ointment base would be needed to prepare the product.

Rule 19-4 can be used when the prescription is for 100 g of a product. If the order is for a different quantity, however, you will need to calculate the amounts of the ingredients to be used. These calculations can be performed using either the proportion method or dimensional analysis.

PROPORTION METHOD

Fractions

Procedure Checklist 19-4

Calculating Quantities for a Percent Strength Solid or Semisolid Compound by the Proportion Method Using Fractions

1. Refer to Rule 19-4. Write a fraction from the percent strength desired, with the amount of medication (in grams) in the numerator and 100 g in the denominator.
2. Convert the quantity ordered to grams. Refer to the "Using Systems of Measurement" unit if needed.
3. Write a fraction with the unknown, x, in the numerator and the total quantity (in grams) of the compound to be prepared in the denominator.
4. Set the two fractions up as a proportion.
5. Cancel units.
6. Calculate the amount of medication needed for the compound by cross-multiplying and solving for the unknown value.
7. Calculate the amount of base needed for the compound by subtracting the amount of medication needed from the amount of product needed.

EXAMPLE 1

Calculate the amount of hydrocortisone powder and cream base needed to prepare 1 oz of a 2% hydrocortisone cream.

1. Applying Rule 19-4, the first fraction for the proportion is:

$$\frac{2 \text{ g hydrocortisone powder}}{100 \text{ g}}$$

2. The volume ordered is 1 oz, which is equal to 30 g.

3. The second fraction for the proportion is:

$$\frac{x}{30 \text{ g}}$$

4. Setting up the two fractions as a proportion gives you the following equation:

$$\frac{x}{30 \text{ g}} = \frac{2 \text{ g hydrocortisone powder}}{100 \text{ g}}$$

5. Cancel units.

$$\frac{x}{30 \,\cancel{\text{g}}} = \frac{2 \text{ g hydrocortisone powder}}{100 \,\cancel{\text{g}}}$$

6. Calculate the amount of hydrocortisone powder needed by cross-multiplying and solving for the unknown value.

$$100 \times x = 2 \text{ g hydrocortisone powder} \times 30$$

$$\frac{100 \times x}{100} = \frac{2 \text{ g hydrocortisone powder} \times 30}{100}$$

$$x = 0.6 \text{ g hydrocortisone powder}$$

7. Calculate the amount of cream base needed by subtracting the amount of hydrocortisone needed from the amount of product needed.

$$30 \text{ g of product} - 0.6 \text{ g of hydrocortisone powder} = 29.4 \text{ g of cream base}$$

The recipe for preparing 30 g of 2% hydrocortisone cream looks like this:

2% Hydrocortisone Cream	
Hydrocortisone powder	0.6 g
Cream base	29.4 g

EXAMPLE 2

Calculate the amount of triamcinolone powder and Vaseline® needed to prepare 50 g of a 2.5% triamcinolone ointment.

1. Applying Rule 19-4, the first fraction for the proportion is:

$$\frac{2.5 \text{ g triamcinolone}}{100 \text{ g}}$$

2. The quantity ordered is already expressed in grams.

3. The second fraction for the proportion is:

$$\frac{x}{50 \text{ g}}$$

4. Setting up the two fractions as a proportion gives you the following equation:

$$\frac{x}{50 \text{ g}} = \frac{2.5 \text{ g triamcinolone}}{100 \text{ g}}$$

5. Cancel units.

$$\frac{x}{50 \,\cancel{\text{g}}} = \frac{2.5 \text{ g triamcinolone}}{100 \,\cancel{\text{g}}}$$

6. Calculate the amount of triamcinolone powder needed by cross-multiplying and solving for the unknown value.

$$100 \times x = 2.5 \text{ g triamcinolone powder} \times 50$$

$$\frac{100 \times x}{100} = \frac{2.5 \text{ g triamcinolone powder} \times 50}{100}$$

$$x = 1.25 \text{ g triamcinolone powder}$$

7. Calculate the amount of Vaseline® needed by subtracting the amount of triamcinolone needed from the amount of product needed.

50 g of product − 1.25 g of triamcinolone powder = 48.75 g of Vaseline®

The recipe for preparing 50 g of 2.5% triamcinolone ointment looks like this:

2.5% Triamcinolone Ointment	
Triamcinolone powder	1.25 g
Vaseline	48.75 g

PROPORTION METHOD

Ratios

Procedure Checklist 19-5

Calculating Quantities for a Percent Strength Solid or Semisolid Compound by the Proportion Method Using Ratios

1. Refer to Rule 19-4. Write a ratio from the percent strength desired, with the amount of medication (in grams) before the colon and 100 g after the colon.
2. Convert the quantity ordered to grams. Refer to the "Using Systems of Measurement" unit if needed.
3. Write a ratio with the unknown, x, before the colon and the total quantity (in grams) of the compound to be prepared after the colon.
4. Set the two ratios up as a proportion.
5. Cancel units.
6. Calculate the amount of medication needed for the compound by multiplying means and extremes.
7. Calculate the amount of base needed for the compound by subtracting the amount of medication needed for the amount of product needed.

EXAMPLE 1

Calculate the amount of hydrocortisone powder and cream base needed to prepare 1.5 oz of a 0.5% hydrocortisone cream.

1. Applying Rule 19-4, the first ratio for the proportion is:

   0.5 g hydrocortisone powder : 100 g

2. The quantity ordered is 1.5 oz. Recall that 1 oz = 30 g, so $1.5 \text{ oz} \times \frac{30 \text{ g}}{1 \text{ oz}} = 45 \text{ g}$.

3. The second ratio for the proportion is

   $x : 45$ g

4. Setting up the two ratios as a proportion gives you the following equation:

$x : 45 \text{ g} :: 0.5 \text{ g hydrocortisone powder} : 100 \text{ g}$

5. Cancel units.

$x : 45 \text{ g̶} :: 0.5 \text{ g hydrocortisone powder} : 100 \text{ g̶}$

6. Solve for the unknown by multiplying means and extremes.

$100 \times x = 0.5 \text{ g hydrocortisone powder} \times 45$

$$\frac{100 \times x}{100} = \frac{0.5 \text{ g hydrocortisone powder} \times 45}{100}$$

$x = 0.225 \text{ g hydrocortisone powder}$

7. Calculate the amount of cream base needed by subtracting the amount of hydrocortisone needed from the amount of product needed.

$45 \text{ g of product} - 0.225 \text{ g of hydrocortisone powder} = 44.775 \text{ g of cream base}$

The recipe for preparing 45 g of 0.5% hydrocortisone cream looks like this:

0.5% Hydrocortisone Cream	
Hydrocortisone powder	0.225 g
Cream base	44.775 g

EXAMPLE 2

Calculate the amount of triamcinolone powder and Vaseline® needed to prepare 80 g of a 3.5% triamcinolone ointment.

1. Applying Rule 19-4, the first ratio for the proportion is:

3.5 g triamcinolone powder : 100 g

2. The quantity ordered is already expressed in grams.

3. The second ratio for the proportion is:

$x : 80 \text{ g}$

4. Setting up the two ratios as a proportion gives you the following equation:

$x : 80 \text{ g} :: 3.5 \text{ g triamcinolone powder} : 100 \text{ g}$

5. Cancel units.

$x : 80 \text{ g̶} :: 3.5 \text{ g triamcinolone powder} : 100 \text{ g̶}$

6. Solve for the unknown by multiplying means and extremes.

$100 \times x = 3.5 \text{ g triamcinolone powder} \times 80$

$$\frac{100 \times x}{100} = \frac{3.5 \text{ g triamcinolone powder} \times 80}{100}$$

$x = 2.8 \text{ g triamcinolone powder}$

7. Calculate the amount of Vaseline® needed by subtracting the amount of triamcinolone needed from the amount of product needed.

$80 \text{ g of product} - 2.8 \text{ g of triamcinolone powder} = 77.2 \text{ g of Vaseline}^®$

The recipe for preparing 80 g of 3.5% triamcinolone ointment looks like this:

3.5% Triamcinolone Ointment	
Triamcinolone powder	2.8 g
Vaseline	77.2 g

Procedure Checklist 19-6

Calculating Quantities for a Percent Strength Liquid Compound by Dimensional Analysis

1. Refer to Rule 19-4. Write a fraction from the percent strength desired, with the amount of medication (in grams) in the numerator and 100 g in the denominator.

2. Convert the quantity ordered to grams. Refer to the "Using Systems of Measurement" unit if needed.

3. Write an equation with the unknown, x, on one side. Write the quantity ordered (in grams) multiplied by the fraction from step 1 on the other side.

4. Cancel units.

5. Calculate the amount of medication needed for the compound by solving the equation for the unknown.

6. Calculate the amount of base needed for the compound by subtracting the amount of medication needed from the amount of product needed.

EXAMPLE 1

Calculate the amount of hydrocortisone powder and cream base needed to prepare 200 g of a 1% hydrocortisone cream.

1. Applying Rule 19-4, the fraction for the equation is:

$$\frac{1 \text{ g hydrocortisone powder}}{100 \text{ g}}$$

2. The quantity ordered is already expressed in grams.

3. Set up the equation, with x on one side and the quantity ordered multiplied by the fraction from step 1 on the other side.

$$x = 200 \text{ g} \times \frac{1 \text{ g hydrocortisone powder}}{100 \text{ g}}$$

4. Cancel units.

$$x = 200 \, \cancel{\text{g}} \times \frac{1 \text{ g hydrocortisone powder}}{100 \, \cancel{\text{g}}}$$

5. Calculate the amount of hydrocortisone powder needed by solving for the unknown value.

$x = 2$ g hydrocortisone powder

6. Calculate the amount of cream base needed by subtracting the amount of hydrocortisone needed from the amount of product needed.

200 g of product − 2 g of hydrocortisone powder = 198 g of cream base

The recipe for preparing 200 g of 1% hydrocortisone cream looks like this:

1% Hydrocortisone Cream	
Hydrocortisone powder	2 g
Cream base	198 g

EXAMPLE 2

Calculate the amount of triamcinolone powder and Vaseline® needed to prepare 2.5 oz of a 2% triamcinolone ointment.

1. Applying Rule 19-4, the fraction for the equation is:

$$\frac{2 \text{ g triamcinolone powder}}{100 \text{ g}}$$

2. The volume ordered is 2.5 oz. Recall that 1 oz = 30 g, so $2.5 \text{ oz} \times \dfrac{30 \text{ g}}{\text{oz}} = 75 \text{ g}$

3. Set up the equation, with x on one side and the quantity ordered multiplied by the fraction from step 1.

$$x = 75 \text{ g} \times \frac{2 \text{ g triamcinolone powder}}{100 \text{ g}}$$

4. Cancel units.

$$x = 75 \cancel{\text{ g}} \times \frac{2 \text{ g triamcinolone powder}}{100 \cancel{\text{ g}}}$$

5. Solve for the unknown.

$$x = 1.5 \text{ g triamcinolone powder}$$

6. Calculate the amount of Vaseline® needed by subtracting the amount of triamcinolone needed from the amount of product needed.

75 g of product − 1.5 g of triamcinolone powder = 73.5 g of Vaseline®

The recipe for preparing 75 g of 2% triamcinolone ointment looks like this:

2% Triamcinolone Ointment	
Triamcinolone powder	1.5 g
Vaseline®	73.5 g

REVIEW AND PRACTICE

19.2 Solid and Semisolid Compounds

For Exercises 1–10, calculate the quantity of the specified ingredients needed to prepare each product.

1. Calculate the amount of zinc oxide powder needed to prepare 4 oz of 20% zinc oxide ointment.

2. Calculate the amount of cream base needed to prepare 60 g of 1% hydrocortisone cream.

3. Calculate the amount of Aquaphor® needed to prepare 2.5 oz of 20% acyclovir ointment.

4. Calculate the amount of metronidazole powder needed to prepare 30 g of 1% metronidazole cream.

5. Calculate the amount of betamethasone powder needed to prepare 120 g of 0.15% betamethasone ointment.

6. Calculate the amount of cocoa butter needed to prepare 150 g of 2% hydrocortisone suppositories.

7. Calculate the amount of Vaseline® needed to prepare 75 g of 10% zinc oxide ointment.

8. Calculate the amount of lidocaine needed to prepare 30 g of 2% lidocaine cream.

9. Calculate the amount of cholestyramine powder and the amount of Aquaphor® needed to prepare 2 oz of 10% cholestyramine paste.

10. Calculate the amount of betamethasone powder and the amount of cream base needed to prepare 150 g of 0.05% betamethasone cream.

19.3 Diluting a Stock Product

Stock products are commercial products that you have on hand. Medication orders are sometimes written for a concentration that is not commercially available. When this occurs, you will calculate the quantities needed to prepare a compound of the desired concentration. The procedure used to determine these quantities is known as the **alligation method**.

There are two situations in which it is necessary to use the alligation method. If you have a stock product with a concentration that is greater than the desired concentration, you need to calculate the amount of stock product and the amount of diluent to mix. If you have two stock products, and the desired concentration is between the two, you need to calculate the quantities of the two stock products to be mixed. The alligation procedure is the same in either situation.

THE ALLIGATION METHOD

Procedure Checklist 19-7
Calculating Quantities Needed by the Alligation Method

1. Write out a tic-tac-toe grid, and fill in the following values:

higher concentration		
	desired concentration	
lower concentration		

The units of concentration must be the same for all three values, but do not include the units when writing the concentrations on the grid. If you are diluting a single stock product, the lower concentration will be zero.

2. Take the diagonal differences.

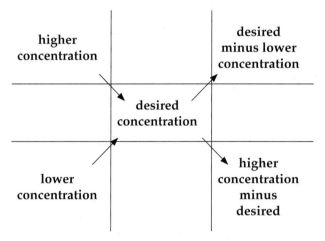

    a. Fill in the upper-right corner with the difference between the desired concentration and the less concentrated stock product. This value tells you how many parts of the more concentrated stock product are needed.

    b. Fill in the lower-right corner with the difference between the more concentrated stock product and the desired concentration. This value tells you how many parts of the less concentrated stock product are needed.

3. Find the total number of parts needed by adding the two values in the right column.

4. Find the size of one part by dividing the total number of parts into the quantity of the product that is needed.

5. Multiply the size of one part (answer from Step 4) by the number in the top right of the grid. The result is the amount of the more concentrated stock product needed.

6. When the product is a liquid, there is no need to calculate the quantity of the less concentrated stock product to use. You add a sufficient quantity (qsad) to achieve the desired volume. When the product is a semisolid, such as a cream or an ointment, subtract the amount of the more concentrated stock product needed (answer from Step 5) from the total amount of product needed. The result is the amount of the less concentrated stock product needed.

EXAMPLE 1 Calculate the amount of 90% ethanol and water needed to prepare 500 mL of 50% ethanol.

1. Fill in the concentrations on the grid. Remember that since you are diluting a single stock product with water, the lower concentration is zero.

2. Take the diagonal differences.

    a. A total of 50 parts of 90% ethanol is needed.

    b. A total of 40 parts of water is needed.

3. Find the total number of parts needed by adding the two values in the right column.

    50 parts 90% ethanol + 40 parts water = 90 parts total

4. Find the size of one part by dividing the total number of parts into the quantity of the product that is needed.

    500 mL needed ÷ 90 parts = 5.56 mL per part

5. Multiply the size of one part (answer from step 4) by the number in the top right of the grid. The result is the amount of the more concentrated stock product needed, in milliliters.

    5.56 mL × 50 = 278 mL of 90% ethanol are needed

6. Since the product in this example is a liquid, there is no need to calculate the amount of water to add. You would dilute 278 mL of 90% ethanol with enough water to bring the total volume of the mixture to 500 mL.

EXAMPLE 2

Calculate the amount of 0.1% and 0.5% triamcinolone creams needed to prepare 60 g of 0.2% triamcinolone cream.

1. Fill in the concentrations on the grid.

0.5		
	0.2	
0.1		

2. Take the diagonal differences.

0.5		0.2 – 0.1 = 0.1 part needed
	0.2	
0.1		0.5 – 0.2 = 0.3 part needed

    a. A total of 0.1 part of 0.5% triamcinolone cream is needed.

    b. A total of 0.3 part of 0.1% triamcinolone cream is needed.

3. Find the total number of parts needed by adding the two values in the right column.

    0.1 part 0.5% + 0.3 part 0.1% = 0.4 part total

4. Find the size of one part by dividing the total number of parts into the quantity of the product that is needed.

    60 g needed ÷ 0.4 part = 150 g per part

5. Multiply the size of one part (answer from step 4) by the number in the top right of the grid. The result is the amount of the more concentrated stock product needed.

    150 g × 0.1 part = 15 g of 0.5% triamcinolone cream needed

6. Subtract the amount of the more concentrated stock product needed (answer from step 5) from the total amount of product needed.

    60 g total − 15 g of 0.5% triamcinolone cream = 45 g of 0.1% triamcinolone cream needed

Paying Attention to Detail

A pharmacy technician is preparing a compound from two stock solutions. One of the stock solutions is labeled 0.5 g per mL, and the other is labeled 100 mg per mL. The product is to contain 300 mg per mL. The technician sets up the following alligation grid:

100		299.5
	300	
0.5		200

 Think! . . . Is It Reasonable? What error did the pharmacy technician make? How could this error have been avoided?

REVIEW AND PRACTICE

19.3 Diluting a Stock Product

For Exercises 1–5, calculate the quantity of the specified ingredients needed to prepare each product. Round your answers to one decimal place, when necessary.

1. Calculate the amount of 50% dextrose solution needed to prepare 500 mL of 40% dextrose solution, using 50% and 10% solutions of dextrose.

2. Calculate the amount of 2% hydrocortisone cream and a cream base needed to prepare 60 g of 1.5% hydrocortisone cream.

3. Calculate the amount of 70% isopropyl alcohol needed to prepare 250 mL of 50% isopropyl alcohol, using water as a diluent.

4. Calculate the amount of 30% and 5% zinc oxide ointments needed to prepare 30 g of 10% zinc oxide ointment.

5. Calculate the amount of 5% sodium chloride solution needed to prepare 1,000 mL of 0.9% sodium chloride solution.

For Exercises 6–15, use the alligation method to calculate the amount of each ingredient needed to compound the following medication orders.

6. Prepare 100 mL of 10% potassium chloride solution using a 5% potassium chloride solution and a 20% potassium chloride solution.

7. Prepare 100 g of 1.5% diphenhydramine hydrochloride cream using 2% diphenhydramine cream and Eucerin® cream.

8. Prepare 1000 mL of a 3% sodium chloride solution using 0.9% sodium chloride solution and 4.5% sodium chloride solution.

9. Prepare 750 mL of D5W using D20W and water.

10. Prepare 500 mL of a 3% lidocaine solution using 5% lidocaine solution and 1% lidocaine solution.

11. Prepare 550 mL of a 2.5% hydrogen peroxide solution using 3% hydrogen peroxide and water.

12. Prepare 250 mL of a 20% ethyl alcohol solution using 50% ethyl alcohol and 10% ethyl alcohol.

13. Prepare 125 g of a 2% hydrocortisone cream using 3% hydrocortisone cream and Eucerin® cream.

14. Prepare 300 g of a 2.5% lidocaine cream using a 1% lidocaine cream and a 5% lidocaine cream.

15. Prepare 1.25 L of a 10% potassium chloride solution using 20% potassium chloride and water.

19.4 Specific Gravity

Specific gravity is a measure of the density of a substance. It is equal to the mass (weight) of the substance divided by the mass of an equal volume of water. Since it is determined by dividing one mass by another, specific gravity has no units. For example, the specific gravity of isopropyl alcohol is 0.78. This means that isopropyl alcohol is less dense than water.

When you have two aqueous solutions containing the same solute, the specific gravities of the solutions are directly related to the concentration of the solute. In a pharmacy, specific gravity is sometimes used to measure the concentration of solutions used for total parenteral nutrition (TPN). TPN is a procedure for administering nutrition intravenously. The specific gravity of patients' urine is also measured to help determine how well the kidneys are functioning.

RULE 19-5	The volume of water, in milliliters, is equal to its mass in grams.
Example	Determine the mass of 150 mL of water. 150 mL of water has a mass of 150 g.

Note: The relationship given in this rule is technically correct only at 4 degrees Celsius. At room temperature, it would be slightly different. The difference is so slight that it is insignificant when performing specific gravity calculations.

SPECIFIC GRAVITY

Procedure Checklist 19-8
Calculating the Specific Gravity of a Solution

1. Convert the mass of the solution to grams.
2. Referring to Rule 19-5, write the mass of an equal volume of water in grams.
3. Enter the values from steps 1 and 2 into the following equation:

$$\text{Specific gravity} = \frac{\text{mass of the solution}}{\text{mass of an equal volume of water}}$$

4. Cancel units.
5. Solve the equation.

EXAMPLE 1	Calculate the specific gravity of a solution if 30 mL of the solution has a mass of 42 g.

1. The mass of the solution is already in grams.

    mass of solution = 42 g

2. Referring to Rule 19-5, we know that 30 mL of water has a mass of 30 g.

3. Enter the values into the equation.

    $$\text{specific gravity} = \frac{42 \text{ g}}{30 \text{ g}}$$

4. Cancel units.

    $$\text{specific gravity} = \frac{42 \cancel{\text{g}}}{30 \cancel{\text{g}}}$$

5. Solve the equation.

    specific gravity = 1.4

The solution has a specific gravity of 1.4.

EXAMPLE 2	Calculate the specific gravity of a solution if 2 mL of the solution has a mass of 1,750 mg.

1. Convert the mass of the solution to grams.

    mass of solution = 1,750 mg = 1.75 g

2. Referring to Rule 19-5, we know that 2 mL of water has a mass of 2 g.

3. Enter the values into the equation.

    $$\text{specific gravity} = \frac{1.75 \text{ g}}{2 \text{ g}}$$

4. Cancel units.

    $$\text{specific gravity} = \frac{1.75 \cancel{\text{g}}}{2 \cancel{\text{g}}}$$

5. Solve the equation.

    specific gravity = 0.875

Procedure Checklist 19-9

Calculating the Volume of a Solution, in Milliliters, from Specific Gravity and Mass

1. Convert the mass of the solution to grams.

2. Divide the mass of the solution by the specific gravity to find the volume of the solution in milliliters.

EXAMPLE 1	Glycerin has a specific gravity of 1.25. Calculate the volume of 50 g of glycerin.

1. The mass of the solution is already in grams.

    mass = 50 g

2. Divide the mass by the specific gravity.

    $50 \div 1.25 = 40$

50 g of glycerin has a volume of 40 mL.

EXAMPLE 2	A 10% solution of acetic acid has a specific gravity of 1.014. Calculate the volume of 1 kg of 10% acetic acid.

1. Convert the mass of the acetic acid to grams.

    mass = 1 kg = 1,000 g

2. Divide the mass by the specific gravity.

$$1{,}000 \div 1.014 = 986.2 \text{ rounded to the nearest tenth}$$

1 kg of 10% acetic acid has a volume of 986.2 mL.

Procedure Checklist 19-10

Calculating the Mass of a Solution, in Grams, from Specific Gravity and Volume

1. Convert the volume of the solution to milliliters.
2. Multiply the volume of the solution by its specific gravity to find its mass in grams.

EXAMPLE 1	Cod liver oil has a specific gravity of 0.925. Calculate the mass of 200 mL of cod liver oil.

1. The volume of the cod liver oil is already in milliliters.

   volume = 200 mL

2. Multiply the volume by the specific gravity.

   $200 \times 0.925 = 185$

200 mL of cod liver oil has a mass of 185 g.

EXAMPLE 2	Ethylene glycol has a specific gravity of 1.125. Calculate the mass of 2 oz of ethylene glycol.

1. Convert the volume to milliliters.

   volume = 2 oz = 60 mL

2. Multiply the volume by the specific gravity.

   $60 \times 1.125 = 67.5$

2 oz of ethylene glycol has a mass of 67.5 g.

REVIEW AND PRACTICE

19.4 Specific Gravity

For Exercises 1–5, find the specific gravity of the solution. Round to four decimal places if necessary.

1. A 200 mL sample of alcohol has a mass of 175 g. Find the specific gravity of the alcohol.

2. 1 oz of Betadine® solution has a mass of 31.2 g. Find the specific gravity of the Betadine® solution.

3. 157 mL of lactic acid has a mass of 160.4 g. Find the specific gravity of the lactic acid solution.

4. 120 mL of glycerol has a mass of 122.8 g. Find the specific gravity of the glycerol.

5. 110 mL of a 0.5% silver nitrate solution has a mass of 110.5 g. Find the specific gravity of the silver nitrate solution.

For Exercises 6–10, find the volume of the solution. Round to the nearest tenth when necessary.

6. Phenol USP has a specific gravity of 1.07. Calculate the volume of 200 g of phenol USP.

7. Normal saline has a specific gravity of 1.0046. Calculate the volume of 4 kg of normal saline.

8. A 3% solution of sodium hydroxide has a specific gravity of 1.0336. Calculate the volume of 150 g of 3% sodium hydroxide.

9. A 10% solution of magnesium sulfate has a specific gravity of 1.1053. Calculate the volume of 75 g of 10% magnesium sulfate.

10. A 5% solution of potassium chloride has a specific gravity of 1.0322. Calculate the volume of 30 g of 5% potassium chloride.

For Exercises 11–15, find the mass of the solution. Round to the nearest tenth when necessary.

11. A 30% solution of hydrochloric acid has a specific gravity of 1.149. Calculate the mass of 0.5 L of 30% hydrochloric acid.

12. Rubbing alcohol has a specific gravity of 0.877. Calculate the mass of 200 mL of rubbing alcohol.

13. A 10% calcium chloride solution has a specific gravity of 1.854. Calculate the mass of 150 mL of the solution.

14. A 4% lactose solution has a specific gravity of 1.016. Calculate the mass of 0.5 L of the solution.

15. A 12% solution of ammonium chloride has a specific gravity of 1.0362. Calculate the mass of 650 mL of the solution.

LEARNING OUTCOME	KEY POINTS
19.1 Calculate the quantities needed to prepare a liquid compound. Pages 563–569	A liquid mixture is a liquid that contains both a solute and a solvent. A solute is a chemical that is dissolved in a solution. A solvent is a liquid used to dissolve or dilute; also known as a *diluent.* Percent concentration for liquid mixtures: ▶ With a solid solute, percent concentration equals the grams of solute dissolved in 100 mL of the mixture. ▶ With a liquid solute, percent concentration equals the milliliters of solute dissolved in 100 mL of the mixture. QSAD (qsad) = quantity sufficient to adjust the solution to a particular volume To prepare a liquid mixture, calculate the amount of solute needed, then add enough solvent to make the desired volume (qsad).
19.2 Calculate the quantities needed to make a solid or semisolid compound. Pages 569–575	The base is the inactive part of a compound with which the active ingredient is mixed. The percent strength for solid and semisolid compounds equals the number of grams of ingredient in 100 g of the compound. To prepare a solid or semisolid compound, first calculate the amount of ingredient needed. Subtract the amount of ingredient needed from the amount of product needed to find the amount of base needed.
19.3 Calculate the quantities needed to dilute a stock product. Pages 575–580	Stock products are commercial products that are available in the pharmacy. The alligation method is a procedure used to calculate the quantities of two materials that need to be mixed in order to prepare a product of a given concentration.
19.4 Perform calculations using specific gravity. Pages 580–583	Specific gravity is a measure of the density of a liquid. When performing calculations using specific gravity, the mass must be converted to grams and the volume to milliliters.

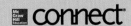
For Exercises 1–5, fill in each blank with the proper term.

1. A(n) _____ is a chemical that is dissolved in a solution.

2. A liquid that is used to dissolve a substance is known as a(n) _____.

3. The _____ method can be used to calculate quantities needed to dilute a stock product.

4. When preparing a cream, an inactive cream _____ is used to dilute a stock product.

5. The abbreviation _____ means to add enough diluent to bring the volume to the desired level.

For Exercises 6–10, calculate the quantities needed to prepare each liquid compound. Round your answers to two decimal places (hundredths) when necessary.

6. Calculate the amount of sodium iodide powder needed to prepare 30 mL of 4% sodium iodide solution, using water as the solvent.

7. Calculate the amount of potassium chloride powder needed to prepare 250 mL of 10% potassium chloride solution, using water as the solvent.

8. Calculate the amount of pure ethanol needed to prepare 200 mL of 60% ethanol solution, using water as the solvent.

9. Calculate the amount of sodium chloride powder needed to prepare 1 liter of 0.45% sodium chloride solution, using water as the solvent.

10. Calculate the amount of dextrose powder needed to prepare 600 mL of 5% dextrose solution, using water as the solvent.

For Exercises 11–15, calculate the quantities needed to prepare the solid and semisolid compounds. Round your answers to two decimal places (hundredths) when necessary.

11. Calculate the amount of salicylic acid powder needed to prepare 150 g of 10% salicylic acid ointment.

12. Calculate the amount of progesterone needed to prepare 240 g of 2% progesterone vaginal suppositories.

13. Calculate the amount of cream base needed to prepare 50 g of 1.5% lidocaine cream.

14. Calculate the amount of zinc oxide powder needed to prepare 20 g of 15% zinc oxide ointment.

15. Calculate the amount of Vaseline® needed to prepare 1.5 oz. of 15% salicylic acid ointment.

For Exercises 16–20, calculate the quantities needed to prepare the indicated compound. Round your answers to two decimal places (hundredths) when necessary.

16. Calculate the amount of 2% lidocaine stock solution needed to prepare 40 mL of 1.5% lidocaine solution, using water as a diluent.

17. Calculate the amount of 40 mg per mL furosemide solution needed to prepare 30 mL of 25 mg per mL furosemide solution, using furosemide solution strengths of 40 mg per mL and 20 mg per mL.

18. Calculate the amount of 50% dextrose solution needed to prepare 300 mL of 7.5% dextrose solution, using water as a diluent.

19. Calculate the amount of ointment base needed to prepare 50 g of 1.5% hydrocortisone ointment from 2% hydrocortisone ointment.

20. Calculate the amount of 5% dextrose solution needed to prepare 200 mL of 10% dextrose solution from 5% and 50% stock solutions.

For Exercises 21–24, calculate the missing value.

	Specific Gravity (round to thousandths)	Mass (round to tenths)	Volume (round to tenths)
21.	1.253	187.5 g	_____ mL
22.	_____	23.7 g	32.5 mL
23.	0.723	_____ g	3.1 L
24.	_____	2.2 oz	65.5 mL

CHECK UP

For Exercises 1–5, match the terms with the definition. (LO 19.1, 19.2, 19.3)

1. A dissolved chemical   a. alligation

2. A liquid used to dissolve other materials   b. base

3. Method used to calculate quantities for dilutions   c. compounding

4. Mixing together ingredients to prepare a product   d. solute

5. The inactive part of a cream, ointment, or suppository   e. solvent

For Exercises 6–16, fill in the blank with the quantity needed. Round your answers to two decimal places (hundredths) when necessary. (LO 19.1, 19.2, 19.3)

6. To prepare 60 g of 0.25% triamcinolone ointment from triamcinolone powder and an ointment base, you need _____ g of triamcinolone powder and _____ g of ointment base.

7. To prepare 500 mL of 5% dextrose in water from dextrose powder and water, you need _____ g of dextrose powder.

8. To prepare 200 g of 20% zinc oxide ointment from zinc oxide powder and Vaseline®, you need _____ g of zinc oxide powder and _____ g of Vaseline®.

9. To prepare 30 g of 1.5% hydrocortisone cream, you need _____ g of 2% hydrocortisone cream and _____ g of 0.5% hydrocortisone cream.

10. To prepare 250 mL of 0.9% sodium chloride solution from sodium chloride powder and water, you need _____ g of sodium chloride powder.

11. To prepare 1,000 mL of 50% isopropanol solution from 70% isopropanol and water, you need _____ mL of 70% isopropanol solution.

12. To prepare 30 g of 2% hydrocortisone cream from hydrocortisone powder and a cream base, you need _____ g of hydrocortisone powder and _____ g of cream base.

13. To prepare 50 mL of 1% lidocaine solution from lidocaine powder and water, you need _____ g of lidocaine powder.

14. To prepare 20 mL of 4% iodide solution from a 10% iodide solution and water, you need _____ mL of 10% iodide solution.

15. To prepare 1 liter of 20% dextrose solution, you need _____ mL of 50% dextrose and _____ mL of 10% dextrose.

16. To prepare 500 mL of 50% ethanol from 90% ethanol and water, you need _____ mL of 90% ethanol.

For Exercises 17–20, calculate the indicated quantity. (LO 19.4)

17. If 1 tsp of cough syrup has a mass of 9.2 g, what is the specific gravity of the cough syrup? Round your answer to three decimal places if necessary.

18. A solution of 50% glycerin in water has a specific gravity of 1.13. Calculate the volume (in milliliters) of 120 g of the solution. Round your answer to one decimal place if necessary.

19. Ethyl alcohol has a specific gravity of 0.789. Calculate the mass (in grams) of 240 mL of ethyl alcohol. Round your answer to one decimal place if necessary.

20. If 50 mL of a boric acid solution has a mass of 52.2 g, what is the specific gravity of the solution? Round your answer to three decimal places if necessary.

CRITICAL THINKING APPLICATIONS

The pharmacy technician is asked to prepare a 10% salicylic acid ointment by using 30 g of a 15% ointment.

1. How much ointment base will be needed to prepare the compound?

2. How much of the 10% ointment will the technician make?

3. The pharmacy technician is doing an inventory and finds a mislabeled bottle of acetic acid that is missing the % concentration. He looks up the specific gravity of acetic acid, and finds the following information:

Concentration of Acetic Acid	Specific Gravity
10%	1.014
50%	1.061
80%	1.075

The technician measures out 15 mL of the acetic acid and weighs it, learning that it has a mass of 15.21 g. What is the concentration of the mislabeled acetic acid?

CASE STUDY

The pharmacy technician is preparing 2% hydrocortisone suppositories. Each suppository will weigh 5 g. Only 1.4 g of hydrocortisone powder are available.

1. How many suppositories can the technician make?

2. How many milligrams of hydrocortisone will each suppository contain?

connect

Now that you have completed the materials in the chapter text, go to CONNECT and complete any chapter activities you have not yet done.

For Exercises 1–4, calculate the amount to dispense for each of the following orders.

1. Ordered: Furosemide 40 mg/4 mL oral solution; take $\frac{1}{2}$ tsp qam for 90 days

   On hand: Furosemide 40 mg per 4 mL oral solution

2. Ordered: Tricor® 48 mg; take 2 tabs qam for 60 days

   On hand: Tricor® 48 mg tablets

3. Ordered: Zemplar 2 mcg three times a week for 8 weeks

   On hand: See Label A

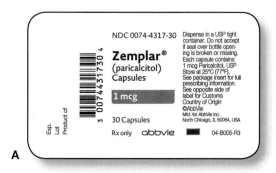

A

4. Ordered: Trileptal® 600 mg bid for 30 days

   On hand: See Label B

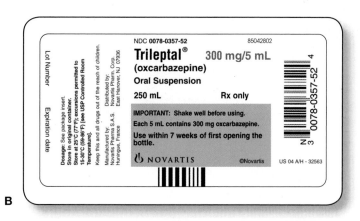

B

For Exercises 5–7, calculate the number of containers to dispense. Assume that partial containers are not dispensed.

5. Ordered: Humulin® 70/30; 36 units subcut qid for 60 days

   On hand: 1,000 unit vials of Humulin® 70/30

6. Atrovent® inhaler; take 2 inhalations q6h for 30 days

   On hand: Atrovent® inhalers; each inhaler contains 120 inhalations

7. Ordered: Omnicef® 125 mg/5 mL oral suspension; take 7 mL every 12 h for 10 days

   On hand: 60 mL bottles of Omnicef® 125 mg/5 mL suspension

For Exercises 8–10, calculate the days' supply for each medication order.

8. Ordered: 3 Flovent® HFA 44 mcg inhalers; take 2 inhalations bid. Each inhaler contains 120 inhalations.

9. Ordered: Lopressor® 50 mg #100; take $1\frac{1}{2}$ tablets every morning

10. Ordered: three 1,000 unit vials of Humulin® 50/50; inject 28 units subcut TID

For Exercises 11–15, calculate the quantities needed to prepare each compound.

11. Using saline as the solvent, calculate the total amount of solute and solvent needed to prepare enough $\frac{1}{4}$ strength hydrogen peroxide to irrigate a wound with 4 oz of $\frac{1}{4}$ strength hydrogen peroxide tid × 3 days.

12. Calculate the amount of Kenalog® 0.5% cream and cream base needed to prepare 150 g of Kenalog 0.3% cream.

13. Calculate the quantities needed to prepare 50 g of a 10% salicylic acid ointment from salicylic acid and Vaseline®.

14. Calculate the amount of 0.5% hydrocortisone ointment and 2% hydrocortisone ointment needed to prepare 4 oz of 1.5% hydrocortisone ointment.

15. Calculate the quantities needed to prepare 350 mL of D5W from dextrose chloride and water.

For Exercises 16–20, calculate the specific gravity, mass, or volume of each solution as directed.

16. 75 mL of a Betadine® solution has a mass of 78 g. Find the specific gravity of the Betadine® solution.

17. A 10% solution of magnesium sulfate has a specific gravity of 1.1053. Calculate the volume of 35 g of 10% magnesium sulfate. Round your answer to the nearest tenth of a milliliter.

18. A 10% solution of calcium chloride has a specific gravity of 1.854. Calculate the mass of 65 mL of the solution. Round your answer to the nearest tenth of a gram.

19. Phenol UPS has a specific gravity of 1.07. Calculate the volume of 1.05 kg of phenol USP. Round your answer to the nearest tenth of a milliliter.

20. A 4% lactose solution has a specific gravity of 1.016. Calculate the mass of 420 mL of the solution. Round your answer to the nearest tenth of a gram.

The following test will help you check your mastery of the major learning outcomes for this text. Applying this information will help prevent dosage calculation and medication administration errors.

For Exercises 1–6, refer to MAR 1.

1. What dose of Neurontin® should be administered? (LO 9.2)

2. By what route should Desyrel® be administered? (LO 9.1)

3. When should Reglan® be administered? (LO 9.3, 9.4)

4. Indicate the time of day, in traditional time, that each medication should be given. Why are no times listed for Ativan? (LO 7.2, 9.1, 9.3, 9.4)

5. Are any of the orders incomplete? If so, what information is missing? (LO 9.2, 11.1)

6. Which order contains an error-prone abbreviation? Correct this abbreviation. (LO 11.3)

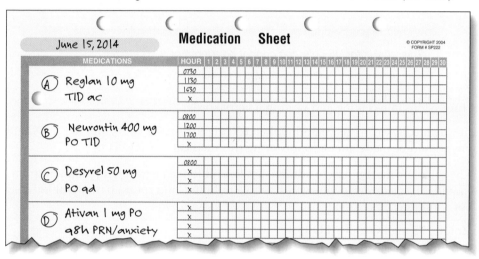

MAR 1

7. Identify the rights of medication administration. (LO 11.5)

8. Describe the three checks of medication administration. (LO 11.4)

For Exercises 9–12, refer to label A. (LO 10.1)

9. What is the generic name of the drug?

10. At what temperature should the drug be stored?

11. What is the dosage strength?

12. If an adult took twice the usual adult dose, how long would the container last?

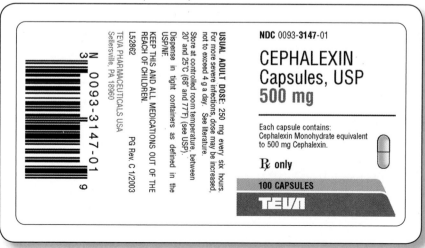

A   *This label is for US only, and cannot be altered or translated.*

For Exercises 13 and 14, refer to label B. (LO 10.1)

13. How much fluid is used to reconstitute the entire container of suspension?

14. If the dosage prescribed for a child is 250 mg, how many doses are in the container?

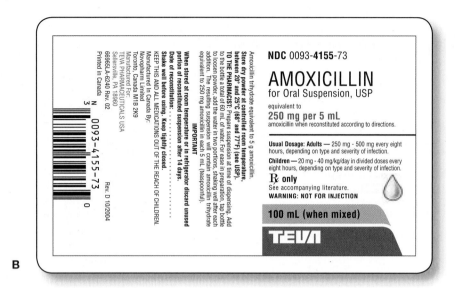

B

This label is for US only, and cannot be altered or translated.

15. Name the three steps in receiving and writing a verbal order. (LO 11.1, 11.2)

16. The patient was medicated with acetaminophen 650 mg for a fever of 102 degrees F. What follow-up observations should be made after administering this medication? (LO 11.6)

For Exercises 17–29, calculate the amount to administer. Round to the nearest tenth of a kilogram. Round answers for oral liquid dosage forms to the nearest whole milliliter, and round parenteral liquid dosage forms to the nearest tenth of a milliliter.

17. Ordered: Zoloft® 75 mg PO daily (LO 13.1)
    On hand: Zoloft® 50 mg scored tablets

18. Ordered: Zovirax® 0.2 g PO q4h for 5 days (LO 13.2)
    On hand: Zovirax® suspension 200 mg/5 mL

19. Ordered: Claforan® 0.6 g IM 30 min pre-op (LO 14.1)
    On hand: Claforan® 300 mg/mL when reconstituted

20. Ordered: Sandostatin® 0.3 mg subcut tid (LO 14.1)
    On hand: Sandostatin® 200 mcg/mL multidose vial

21. The patient is 14 years old and weighs 97 lb. (LO 16.2)
    Ordered: Agenerase® sol 17 mg/kg PO tid
    On hand: Agenerase® Oral Solution, 15 mg/mL

22. The patient is 10 years old and weighs 62 lb. (LO 16.2)
    Ordered: Vancocin® 10 mg/kg IV q6h
    On hand: Vancocin® 500 mg/100 mL

23. Ordered: ampicillin 375 mg IV q6h

On hand: 500 mg vial of ampicillin reconstituted with 1.8 mL sterile water to yield a supply dose of 250 mg/mL. (LO 15.5)

24. The patient is 7 years old and weighs 49 lb. (LO 16.2)

Ordered: Zinacef® 20 mg/kg IM q6h

On hand: Zinacef® 220 mg/mL when reconstituted

25. Ordered: phenytoin extended 300 mg PO daily (LO 13.1)

On hand: Refer to label C.

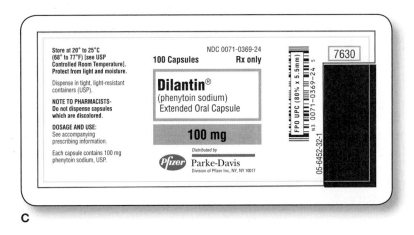

C

26. The patient is 7 years old and weighs 55 lb.

Ordered: Trileptal® 10 mg/kg PO bid. (LO 16.2)

On hand: Refer to label D.

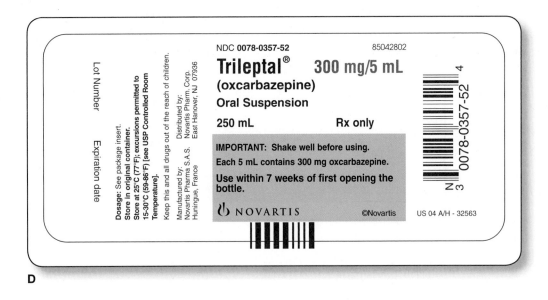

D

27. Ordered: Clarithromycin XL 1 g PO q12h. (LO 13.1)

On hand: Refer to label E.

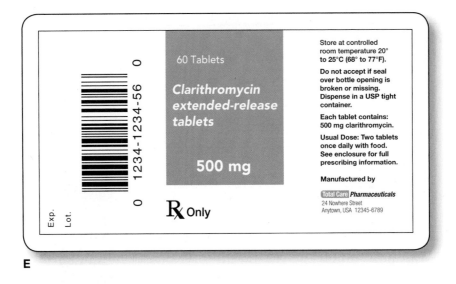

Store at controlled room temperature 20° to 25°C (68° to 77°F).

Do not accept if seal over bottle opening is broken or missing. Dispense in a USP tight container.

Each tablet contains: 500 mg clarithromycin.

Usual Dose: Two tablets once daily with food. See enclosure for full prescribing information.

Manufactured by

Total Care **Pharmaceuticals**
24 Nowhere Street
Anytown, USA 12345-6789

60 Tablets

Clarithromycin extended-release tablets

500 mg

℞ Only

E

28. Ordered: Synthroid® 0.15 mg PO daily. (LO 13.1)

On hand: Refer to label F.

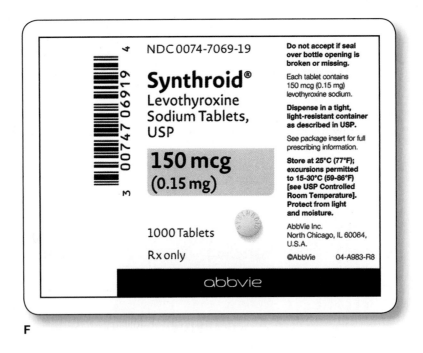

NDC 0074-7069-19

Synthroid®
Levothyroxine
Sodium Tablets,
USP

150 mcg
(0.15 mg)

1000 Tablets

Rx only

Do not accept if seal over bottle opening is broken or missing.

Each tablet contains 150 mcg (0.15 mg) levothyroxine sodium.

Dispense in a tight, light-resistant container as described in USP.

See package insert for full prescribing information.

Store at 25°C (77°F); excursions permitted to 15-30°C (59-86°F) [see USP Controlled Room Temperature]. Protect from light and moisture.

AbbVie Inc.
North Chicago, IL 60064,
U.S.A.

©AbbVie   04-A983-R8

abbvie

F

29. Ordered: morphine sulfate 15 mg subcut q4h prn/pain (LO 14.1)

On hand: morphine sulfate 10 mg/mL vial

What is the amount to administer?

30. You are discharging a patient from the walk-in clinic with a prescription for ear drops, which requires a medicine dropper for administration. What specific patient teaching is required? (LO 8.1, 11.7)

31. Ordered: 1 L D$_5\frac{1}{2}$ NS to infuse at 125 mL/h starting at 0730. At what time will the infusion be complete? (LO 15.4)

32. Which of the following insulins is shorter-acting? (LO 14.5)
  Refer to labels G and H.

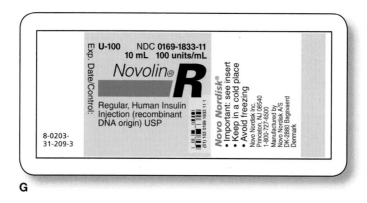

G

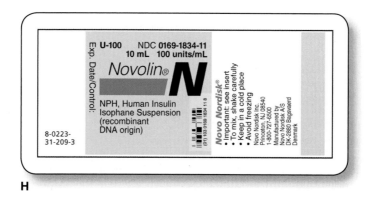

H

33. In what order will you draw the insulin into the syringe for the following order? (LO 14.5)
  Ordered: Humulin® N 46 units and Humulin® R 8 units subcut before breakfast

In Exercises 34–40, find the flow rate.

34. Ordered: 2,000 mL RL over 8 hours, using an infusion pump. (LO 15.3)

35. Ordered: 600 mL 5%D NS over 4 h, 15 gtt/mL tubing. (LO 15.3)

36. Ordered: norepinephrine 4 mg/1,000 mL D5/NS 0.5–30 mcg/min IV. Start infusion at 1 mcg/min and titrate in 1 mcg/min increments to keep systolic BP greater than 90 mm Hg.
  The patient's systolic BP is 86 mm Hg, and the above IV is infusing at 30 mL/h. What should be the new infusion rate? (LO 17.6)

37. Find the flow rate in mL/h for a child who weighs 68 lb. (LO 16.2, 17.5)
  Ordered: Zofran® 0.1 mg/kg IV over 4 min
  On hand: Zofran®, premixed with 32 mg in 5% dextrose, 50 mL, and 10 gtt/mL tubing

38. Ordered: nitroglycerin 18 mcg/min IV
  On hand: nitroglycerin 200 mg/500 mL D5W
  What is the flow rate in mL/h? (LO 17.3)

39. Ordered: ceftriaxone 750 mg in 100 mL NS IVPB over 30 min q8h via infusion pump. (LO 15.5)
On hand: Refer to label I.

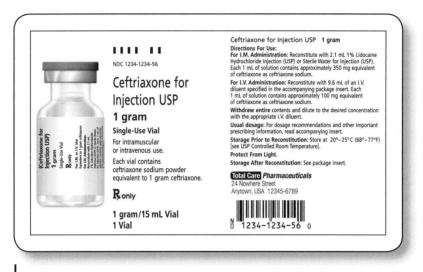

I

40. Ordered: heparin 23 units/kg/h IV
On hand: heparin sodium 25,000 units/500 mL D5W
Patient's weight: 212 lb (LO 17.5)

Determine which concentration of heparin should be used and calculate the amount to be administered.

41. Ordered: heparin 7,500 units subcut q12h (LO 10.2, 14.6)
Refer to labels J, K, and L:

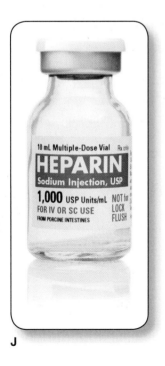

J

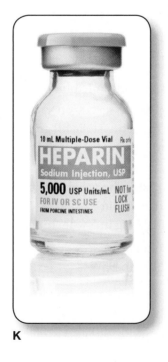

K

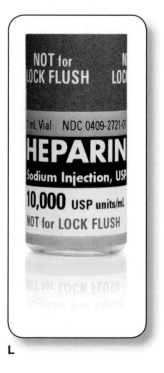

L

42. Find the amount of medication that has already been administered to the patient. (LO 17.5)

Ordered: nitroprusside 40 mg in 500 mL D5W

The patient has received 175 mL.

43. Calculate the ordered flow rate for the following order. Then determine if an adjustment is necessary and calculate the adjusted flow rate. (LO 15.3, 17.3)

Ordered: 650 mL NS over 8 h (15 gtt/mL tubing)

With 5 h remaining, 490 mL of NS remains in the IV bag.

44. Ordered: D_5LR at 80 mL/h started at 1130. At 2245, what volume will be infused? (LO 15.4)

45. Write a recipe for 1,000 mL $\frac{1}{2}$ NS. (LO 15.1, 19.1)

46. The adult patient's height is 150 cm and weight is 61 kg. (LO 16.3)

Ordered: BiCNU 200 mg/m^2 IV over 2 h

How many milligrams of BiCNU should be administered?

47. The adult patient's height is 60 in. and weight is 103 lb. What is the flow rate in mL/h? (LO 14.3, 16.3)

Ordered: leucovorin calcium 200 mg/m^2 IV over 6 min

On hand: Refer to label M.

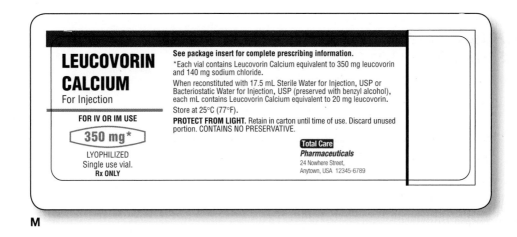

LEUCOVORIN CALCIUM
For Injection

FOR IV OR IM USE

350 mg*

LYOPHILIZED
Single use vial.
Rx ONLY

See package insert for complete prescribing information.
*Each vial contains Leucovorin Calcium equivalent to 350 mg leucovorin and 140 mg sodium chloride.

When reconstituted with 17.5 mL Sterile Water for Injection, USP or Bacteriostatic Water for Injection, USP (preserved with benzyl alcohol), each mL contains Leucovorin Calcium equivalent to 20 mg leucovorin.

Store at 25°C (77°F).

PROTECT FROM LIGHT. Retain in carton until time of use. Discard unused portion. CONTAINS NO PRESERVATIVE.

Total Care
Pharmaceuticals
24 Nowhere Street,
Anytown, USA 12345-6789

M

48. Find the daily maintenance fluid needs for a child who weighs 18 kg. Then find the microdrip tubing flow rate for DMFN. (LO 17.1)

49. The patient: 78-year-old male, 5 ft 7 in. tall, 148 lb, CL_{CR} of 48 mL/min. Determine if the order is safe. If it is, then find the amount to administer. (LO 17.2)

Ordered: Timentin® 1.7 g IV q4h

On hand: Timentin® reconstituted to 20 mg/mL

According to the package insert, for patients with renal impairment, the following maintenance dosages are recommended: for creatinine clearance over 60 mL/min, 3.1 g q4h; for 30 to 60 mL/min, 2 g q4h; for 10 to 30 mL/min, 2 g q8h; for less than 10 mL/min, 2 g q12h. For patients with more advanced impairments, lower dosages are recommended.

50. Ordered: epinephrine 0.1 mg subcut stat (LO 14.2)

On hand: epinephrine 1:1,000 solution

What volume in mL will you administer?

For Exercises 51–54, refer to Prescription 1

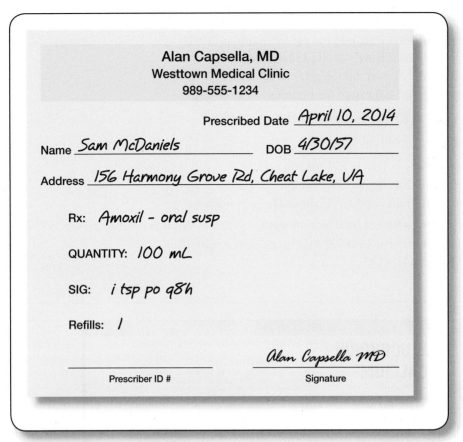

Alan Capsella, MD
Westtown Medical Clinic
989-555-1234

Prescribed Date *April 10, 2014*

Name *Sam McDaniels*   DOB *4/30/57*

Address *156 Harmony Grove Rd, Cheat Lake, VA*

Rx: *Amoxil – oral susp*

QUANTITY: *100 mL*

SIG: *i tsp po q8h*

Refills: *1*

Alan Capsella MD

_____   _____
Prescriber ID #   Signature

Prescription 1

51. How often should the patient take the Amoxil®? (LO 9.3)

52. What is missing from this prescription? (LO 9.3)

53. You have on hand Amoxil® 125 mg/5 mL, 200 mg/5 mL, 250 mg/5 mL, and 400 mg/5 mL. Which one should you dispense? (LO 9.4)

54. What would be the days' supply? (LO 18.2)

55. Name three documents provided by the manufacturer that can be used to look up comprehensive medication information. (LO 10.3)

56. Ordered: acetylcysteine 1.5 g via nebulizer
    On hand: acetylcysteine 20% solution 10 mL vial
    What is the amount to administer? (LO 14.4)

57. What is the hourly dosage for the following heparin order? (LO 17.4)
    40,000 units in 1,000 mL of 5% DW delivered at 25 mL/h

58. Calculate the amount to dispense. (LO 18.1)
    Ordered: Regular insulin 15 units subcut 3 times daily with meals for 90 days
    On hand: 10 mL vials of Regular insulin 100 units/mL

59. Calculate the amount of cream base and hydrocortisone needed to prepare 45 g of 2% hydrocortisone cream. (LO 19.2)

60. Calculate the amount of dextrose solution needed to prepare 1,000 mL of 35% dextrose solution, using a 50% dextrose solution and a 10% dextrose solution. (LO 19.3)

61. Calculate the amount to administer. (LO 13.2)
    Ordered: granisetron 1 mg po 1 hour before chemotherapy
    On hand: granisetron 2 mg/10 mL oral solution

62. Calculate the amount to administer. (LO 13.2)
    Ordered: Amoxicillin 185 mg po q12h
    On hand: Amoxicillin 250 mg/5 mL

63. If 10 mL of a cough syrup has a mass of 18.8 g, what is the specific gravity of the cough syrup? Round your answer to three decimal places if necessary. (LO 19.4)

64. Ethyl alcohol has a specific gravity of 0.789. Calculate the mass of 750 mL of ethyl alcohol. Round your answer to the nearest tenth of a gram if necessary. (LO 19.4)

65. A solution of 50% glycerin has a specific gravity of 1.13. Calculate the volume of 250 g of the solution. Round your answer to the nearest tenth of a milliliter if necessary. (LO 19.4)

24-hour time   A system in which time is indicated with four digits; the first two digits indicate hours since midnight, and the last two digits indicate minutes.

A

Absorption   Movement of a drug from the site where it is given into the bloodstream.

Absorption rate   Movement of a drug from the site where it is given into the bloodstream.

Alligation method   One method for calculating dilutions.

Amount to administer   The volume of liquid or number of solid dosage units that contains the desired dose.

Ampule   Sealed container that usually holds 1 dose of liquid medication.

Antiarrhythmic medications   Medications given to regulate a patient's heart rate and/or rhythm.

Anticoagulant   A class of medication that reduces the blood's ability to clot.

Apothecary system   An older system of measurement based upon a grain of wheat; other common units are the ounce, minim, and dram.

Authorized prescriber (AP)   Licensed healthcare professional who has the authority to write medication orders, or prescriptions.

B

Bar code   Code on a medication label that is used to identify the drug electronically; helps ensure that an individual receives the correct medication.

Base   A substance (such as a liquid, lotion, cream, or ointment) used for compounding that does not contain medication.

Body surface area (BSA)   Surface area of a patient's body, factoring in both height and weight, stated in square meters, or m^2.

Bolus   A volume administered rapidly via IV push to attain a therapeutic blood level of a drug.

C

Calibrated spoons   Specially marked spoons used to administer oral medications with accuracy.

Calibrations   Markings on medication equipment at various intervals.

Caplet   Oval-shaped pill similar to a tablet but having a coating for easy swallowing.

Capsule   Oval-shaped gelatin shell, usually in two pieces, that contains powder or granules.

Cartridge   Prefilled container shaped like a syringe barrel, generally used with a reusable syringe.

Celsius   A temperature scale on which water freezes at 0 degrees and boils at 100 degrees.

Centi (c)   Metric prefix that indicates $\frac{1}{100}$ of the basic unit.

Centigrade   A temperature scale similar to the Celsius scale. Values on this scale are within 0.1 degree of the values on the Celsius scale.

For general purposes, the two scales are used interchangeably; however, Celsius is preferred.

Central line   An IV line that administers large amounts of medications to major veins.

Complex fraction   A fraction in which the numerator and the denominator are themselves fractions.

Compound   A product containing ingredients that were mixed together.

Compounding   To prepare a product by combining ingredients.

Conventional time   A 12-hour system that uses a.m. and p.m. to indicate "before noon" and "after noon," respectively.

Conversion factor   A fraction or ratio made of two quantities that are equal to each other but expressed in different units; for example, 7 days/1 week.

Critical care   Area of a medical facility in which patients are more seriously ill and fast-acting, potent medications are given.

Cross-multiplying   Multiplying the numerator of each fraction by the denominator of the other; for example, cross-multiplying $\frac{A}{B} = \frac{C}{D}$ results in $A \times D = B \times C$.

Cubic centimeter   Measure of volume that is the same as a milliliter (mL).

D

D5W solution   Intravenous solution of 5% dextrose in water.

Daily maintenance fluid needs (DMFN)   Amount of fluids a patient needs over 24 h, including maintenance fluids (both oral and parenteral), medications, diluent for medications, and fluids used to flush the injection port.

Denominator   The bottom number of a fraction; represents the whole.

Desired dose   Amount of drug to be given at one time; the ordered dose.

Diluent   A substance used to dilute; a liquid used to dissolve other chemicals when making a solution; also known as a solvent.

Dilution   A solution created from an already prepared concentrated solution.

Dimensional analysis   A method of dosage calculations that utilizes a series of conversion factors to calculate dosages.

Distribution   Movement of a drug from the bloodstream into other body tissues and fluids.

Dividend   In a division problem, the number you divide into.

Divisor   The number you divide by in a division problem.

Dosage ordered   The amount of drug to be given and how often it is to be given. The desired dose converted to the same unit of measurement as the dose on hand (supply dose).

Dosage strength   Dose on hand per dosage unit; the amount of drug over the form of the drug; for example, 500 mg/tablet or 250 mg/5 mL; ratio strength.

Dosage unit   The quantity of solid or liquid in which the dose is supplied.

Dose on hand   Amount of drug contained in each dosage unit.

Dram   Common unit of volume in the apothecary system; 1 dram = 60 minims

Drip chamber   An area on the IV equipment where the drop of fluid is visualized during an infusion.

Dry weight   Patient's weight when properly hydrated.

Duration   The length of time the effect of a medication, such as insulin, lasts.

E

Eccentric   Off-center.

Electronic medication administration record (eMAR)   Medication administration record that can be viewed and completed on an electronic device.

Elimination   Process in which the drug leaves the body.

Embolism   A traveling blood clot.

Enema   Means of delivering medication or fluids into the rectum.

Enteral   Absorbed through the gastrointestinal tract.

Enteric-coated   Medications that only dissolve in an alkaline environment, such as the small intestine.

Equivalent fractions   Two fractions that have the same value even though they are written differently: $\frac{3}{6} = \frac{5}{10}$

F

Fahrenheit   A temperature scale on which water freezes at 32 degrees and boils at 212 degrees.

Flow rate   A measurement of the amount of fluid entering a patient through an intravenous line per a set amount of time.

Formula   A method of dosage calculation that utilizes a set equation (formula) to calculate the amount to administer; $\frac{D}{H} \times Q = A$

Fraction proportion   Mathematical statement that indicates two fractions are equal.

Frequency   The time(s) of day and how often a medication is to be given.

G

Gelcap   Medication, usually liquid, in a gelatin shell that is not designed to be opened.

Generic name   A drug's official name.

Geriatric   Describes patients who are age 65 and over.

Grain   Basic unit for measurement of weight in the apothecary system.

Gram   Basic unit for measurement of weight in the metric system.

H

Hemodynamics   The study of the circulation of blood in the body.

Heparin   An anticoagulant medication that reduces the blood's ability to clot.

Heparin lock   An infusion port attached to an already inserted catheter for IV access; flushed with heparin.

Heparin protocol   A preprinted order set that guides the administration of IV heparin based on the patient's weight and serum activated partial thromboplastin time (aPTT).

High-alert medication   Medication that has a higher risk of devastating harm or death if the dosage is miscalculated.

Household   Common system of measurement that utilizes the teaspoon, ounce, cup, pint, quart, and gallon.

Hypertonic   Describes fluids that draw fluids from cells and tissues across the cell membrane into the bloodstream, such as 3% saline.

Hypodermic syringe   Syringe used to administer injections.

Hypotonic   Describes fluids that move across the cell membrane into surrounding cells and tissues, such as 0.45% NS and 0.33% NS.

I

Ideal body weight (IBW)   A recommended weight based on criteria such as height, gender, body type, body frame, and age.

Infiltration   Delivery of fluid from an IV infusion outside of a blood vessel into the surrounding tissue.

Infusion pumps   Devices that apply pressure to maintain the rate of an IV infusion, using a sensor to monitor both the rate and when the bag is empty.

Inhalant   Medication that is inhaled; administered directly to the lungs, usually through a metered-dose inhaler or nebulizer.

Instillations   Drops; used to deliver medications to the nose, eyes, and ears.

Institute for Safe Medication Practice (ISMP)   A healthcare organization whose mission includes the promotion of patient safety; devoted to supporting the safe use of medications and preventing medication errors.

Insulin   A pancreatic hormone that stimulates glucose metabolism.

International unit (IU)   Amount of medication needed to produce a certain effect; standardized by an international agreement. Sometimes abbreviated IU, although this abbreviation is on the TJC's Do Not Use list.

Intradermal (ID)   Describes medication administered between layers of the skin.

Intramuscular (IM)   Describes medication administered into a muscle by injection.

Intravenous (IV)   Describes medication delivered directly to the bloodstream through a vein.

Isotonic   Describes fluids that do not affect the fluid balance of the surrounding cells or tissues, such as D5W, NS, and lactated Ringer's.

J

Jejunostomy tube   Tube that delivers medication and nutrients directly into the small intestine.

K

Kilo (k)   Metric prefix that indicates the basic unit times 1,000.

KVO or TKO fluids   "Keep veins open" or "to keep open"; fluids that provide access to the vascular system for emergency situations.

L

Leading ring   The wide ring on the tip of the plunger of a syringe that is closest to the needle; the medication is measured here.

Leading zero   The zero to the left of the decimal point in a decimal number that is less than 1 and therefore has no whole-number part.

Least common denominator   The smallest number that is a common multiple of all the denominators in a group of fractions.

Liter (L)   The basic unit for measurement of volume in the metric system.

Loading dose   An initial bolus dose given to achieve a therapeutic blood level of a drug.

M

Macrodrip tubing   Type of IV tubing that delivers 10, 15, or 20 drops of fluid per milliliter.

Maintenance fluids   Fluids that help patients maintain fluid and electrolyte balance.

Means and extremes   For the equation $A : B = C : D$, A and D are the extremes (ends) and B and C are the means (middle).

Medication administration record (MAR)   A legal document that contains all the information on a medication order, specifies the actual times to administer the medication, and provides a place to document that each medication has been given.

Medication order   Written or computerized form for ordering medications in an inpatient facility; can list multiple medications.

Medicine cup   A calibrated cup used to measure and deliver medications; usually holds 30 mL or 1 oz.

Meniscus   A slight curve in the surface of a liquid.

Metabolism   Chemical changes of a drug in the body; biotransformation.

Meter (m)   Basic unit for measurement of length in the metric system.

Metered-dose inhaler (MDI)   Device to deliver medication into the lungs.

Metric   A widely used system of measurements based upon the meter for length, gram for weight, and liter for volume.

Micro (mc)   Metric prefix that indicates $\frac{1}{1,000,000}$ of the basic unit.

Microdrip tubing   Type of IV tubing that delivers 60 drops of fluid per milliliter.

Milli (m)   Metric prefix that indicates $\frac{1}{1,000}$ of the basic unit.

Milliequivalents (mEq)   A unit of measure based upon the chemical combining power of the substance; defined as $\frac{1}{1,000}$ of an equivalent of a chemical.

Minim   Common unit of volume in the apothecary system.

Mixed number   A fraction with a value greater than 1 that combines a whole number with a fraction.

Monograph   A document of complete and authoritative information about a medication.

N

Nasogastric tube   Type of tube that carries medication through the nose to the stomach.

Nomogram   A special chart used to determine a patient's body surface area (BSA).

Numerator   The top number of a fraction; represents parts of the whole.

O

Official package insert   A package insert for a medication that provides prescribing information to medical professionals.

Onset   Moment when a medication begins its effect, such as when insulin begins to lower the glucose (blood sugar) level.

Ounce   Generally implies a fluid ounce volume when discussing medications; 1 fluid ounce = 8 drams.

P

Package insert   Paper insert that provides complete and authoritative information about a medication.

Package outsert   A document of complete and authoritative information about a medication.

Parenteral   Route of administration other than oral; medications that are delivered outside of the digestive tract; most often refers to injections.

Patient-controlled analgesia (PCA)   Technique that allows the patient to control the amount of pain medication delivered through an IV within limits set by the authorized prescriber.

Patient package insert   An easy-to-understand document provided for patients with each medication.

Peak   The time when a medication has its strongest effect, such as insulin's effect on the glucose level.

Pediatric   Describes patients under the age of 18 years.

PEG tube   Percutaneous endoscopic gastrostomy tube; delivers medication directly into the stomach.

Percent   Per 100 or divided by 100.

Percent strength   Represents the number of grams or milliliters of medication contained in 100 mL of a mixture.

Peripherally inserted central catheter (PICC)   IV line that is inserted in an arm vein and threaded into a central vein, often by a specially trained nurse.

Pharmacokinetics   The study of what happens to a drug after it is administered to a patient.

Phlebitis   Inflammation of a vein, which can be caused by an irritated IV site.

Physician order form   Written or computerized form for medication orders used in an inpatient facility; can list multiple medications.

***Physicians' Desk Reference* (PDR)**   A compilation of information from package inserts of medications; contains information about most currently available prescription drugs.

Polypharmacy   The practice of taking many medications at one time.

Port-A-Cath   A device placed surgically under the skin in the chest in order to deliver drugs into a large, central vein.

Prefilled syringes   Syringes that come from the manufacturer with the medication already inside; usually marked in milliliters (mL) and milligrams (mg).

Prescription   Written or computerized form for medication orders.

Primary line   The main tubing that delivers an IV infusion, usually consisting of a drip chamber, clamp, and injection port(s).

Prime number   Number other than 1 that can be evenly divided by only itself and 1, such as 2, 3, 5, 7, 11, 13, 17, 19, 23, and 29.

Proportion   A mathematical statement that two ratios are equal.

Q

QSAD (qsad)   Abbreviation of a Latin phrase meaning "a sufficient quantity to adjust the dimensions to . . ."; used when preparing solutions.

Quotient   The answer to a division problem.

R

Rate controller   Device that controls the rate of an IV infusion by using a pincher and sensor; the infusion relies on gravity.

Ratio   Expression of the relationship of a part to the whole.

Ratio proportion   Mathematical statement that indicates two ratios are equal.

Ratio strength   The amount of drug in a solution or the amount of drug in a solid dosage such as a tablet or capsule; dosage strength.

Reciprocal   Flipping a fraction so that the numerator becomes the denominator and the denominator becomes the numerator.

Reconstitute   Add liquid to a powder medication; must be done shortly before administering.

Reconstitution   The process of adding liquid to a powder medication.

Rectal   Describes medication administered through the rectum, usually a suppository.

Reduce (simplify)   To divide the numerator and denominator by a common factor. This results in an equivalent fraction with a lower numerator and denominator.

Replacement fluids   Fluids that replace electrolytes or fluids lost from dehydration, hemorrhage, vomiting, or diarrhea.

Roman numerals   A numeral system in which letters indicate numbers; I = 1, V = 5, and X = 10

Route   Path by which a drug is brought into the body.

S

Saline lock   An infusion port attached to an already inserted catheter for IV access; flushed with saline.

Scored   Describes medications having indented lines indicating where they may be broken to divide the medication evenly.

Secondary line   Line used to add medications or other additives to an existing IV or infusion port; also known as piggyback (IVPB).

Sig   Indicates the instructions for the container; found on a prescription.

Simplify   See *Reduce*

Solute   Chemical dissolved in a solvent, making a solution; drug or substance being dissolved in a solution.

Solution   A liquid mixture containing two or more different chemicals.

Solution strength   The amount of dry drug in grams per 100 mL of solution.

Solvent   Liquid used to dissolve other chemicals, making a solution; also called a diluent.

Spansule   Special capsule that contains granules with different coatings that delay the release of some of the medication.

Specific gravity   A measure of the density of a substance relative to the density of water.

Stock product   A product that is already prepared and on hand.

Subcutaneous (subcut)   Describes medication administered under the skin by an injection.

Suspension   A mixture of a solute in a diluent in which the solute does not completely dissolve and is suspended in solvent.

Sustained release   Describes medication that is released slowly into the bloodstream over several hours.

Syringe   Device used to deliver parenteral medications that includes a barrel, plunger, hub, leading ring, and needle.

Syringe pumps   Pumps that provide precise control of IV infusions via a syringe inside of a pump.

T

Tablet   A solid disk or cylinder that contains a drug plus inactive ingredients.

The Joint Commission (TJC)   A healthcare organization whose mission includes the promotion of patient safety. TJC's goal is to continuously improve healthcare by setting standards and by evaluating and accrediting healthcare organizations.

Therapeutic fluids   IV fluids that deliver medication to patients.

Titrate   Adjust the dosage of medication in response to the patient's vital signs.

Titrated medications   Medications that are adjusted or regulated based upon their effect.

Topical medication   Medication applied to the skin.

Trade name   Name of a drug owned by a specific company; also called *brand name.*

Trailing ring   The ring on the plunger of the syringe farthest from the needle. Do *not* measure medication from this ring.

Trailing zero   A zero to the right of the decimal point in a decimal number that follows the last nonzero digit.

Transcription   The process of taking the information from the prescribing practitioner's order (prescription) and transferring it to the prescription label (in outpatient settings) or to the medication administration record (in inpatient settings).

Transdermal   Describes medication administered through the skin.

Tuberculin syringe   A small syringe used for delivering 1 mL of medication or less parenterally.

U

U-100   Common concentration of insulin in which 100 units of insulin are contained in 1 mL of solution.

U-500   Concentration of insulin in which 500 units of insulin are contained in 1 mL of solution.

Unit   Also known as USP unit; amount of a medication required to produce an effect.

United States Pharmacopeia   A medication guide or reference for healthcare professionals.

Universal solvent   Water.

V

Vaporizer   Device that uses boiling water to create a mist from liquid medications; also known as steam inhaler.

Vasoactive medications   Medications that cause the blood vessels to dilate or constrict.

Verbal order   A medication order from an authorized prescriber stated directly, in person or via the telephone, to a nurse or other practitioner whose scope of practice includes the authorization to receive and document such orders.

Vial   Container covered with a rubber stopper, or diaphragm, that holds one or more doses of medication in liquid or powder form.

W

Warnings   Statements found on the medication label that help the healthcare worker to deliver medications safely.

CREDITS

TEXT

Chapter 9

Table 9-1: Adapted from Joint Commission on Accreditation of Healthcare Organizations, 2010; Figure 9-5: Courtesy of Netsmart Technologies (www.ntst.com).

Chapter 10

Figure 10-1 (Provera): Courtesy of Pfizer Inc.; 10-2 (EryPed): Courtesy of Arbor Pharmaceuticals, Inc.; 10-3 (Heparin): Hospira Inc., Lake Forest, IL. USA; 10-4 (Amoxicillin): Courtesy of Teva Pharmaceuticals USA; 10-5 (Ritalin): Copyright © Novartis Pharmaceutical Corp. Used by permission.; 10-6 (Azithromycin): Courtesy of Teva Pharmaceuticals USA; 10-8 (Nitrostat): Courtesy of Pfizer Inc.; 10-13 (Clozaril): Copyright © Novartis Pharmaceutical Corp. Used by permission.; 10-14 (Kaletra): Courtesy of AbbVie Inc.; 10-15 (Valium): Reprinted with the permission of Roche Laboratories, Inc. All rights reserved.; 10-16 (Amoxicillin): Courtesy of Teva Pharmaceuticals USA; 10-17 (Vantin): Courtesy of Pfizer Inc.; 10-18 (Synthroid): Courtesy of AbbVie Inc.; 10-19 (Synthroid): Courtesy of AbbVie Inc.; p. 198 (Erythromycin): Courtesy of Arbor Pharmaceuticals, Inc.; p. 199 (Zithromax): Courtesy of Pfizer Inc.; p. 199 (Cefprozil): Courtesy of Teva Pharmaceuticals USA; p. 199 (Metformin): Courtesy of Caraco Pharmaceutical Laboratories; 10-20 (Depakote): Courtesy of AbbVie Inc.; 10-22 (Vistaril): Courtesy of Pfizer Inc.; 10-24 (Camptosar): Courtesy of Pfizer Inc.; 10-25 (Novolin N): Courtesy of Novo Nordisk Pharmaceuticals, Inc.; 10-26 (Novolin R): Courtesy of Novo Nordisk Pharmaceuticals, Inc.; p. 205 (Metformin): Courtesy of Caraco Pharmaceutical Laboratories; p. 206 (Levoxyl): Courtesy of Pfizer Inc.; p. 206 (Amoxicillin): Courtesy of Teva Pharmaceuticals USA; p. 207 (Flumadine): Courtesy of Caraco Pharmaceutical Laboratories; p. 207 (Premarin): Courtesy of Pfizer Inc.; p. 208 (Novolin): Courtesy of Novo Nordisk Pharmaceuticals, Inc.; p. 209 (Miacalcin): Copyright © Novartis Pharmaceutical Corp. Used by permission.; 10-30 (Alprazolam): Courtesy of Caraco Pharmaceutical Laboratories; Table 10-1: Courtesy of Caraco Pharmaceutical Laboratories; p. 216 (Depakote): Courtesy of AbbVie Inc.; p. 216 (Norvir): Courtesy of AbbVie Inc.; p. 219 (Zemplar): Courtesy of AbbVie Inc.; p. 219 (Novolin R): Courtesy of Novo Nordisk Pharmaceuticals, Inc.; p. 219 (Erythromycin): Courtesy of Arbor Pharmaceuticals, Inc.

Chapter 11

Table 11-1: Copyright, Institute for Safe Medication Practices, Horsham, PA. Reprinted with permission.; p. 249 (Depakene): Courtesy of AbbVie Inc.

Chapter 12

Figure 12-1 (Procardia): Courtesy of Pfizer Inc.; 12-2: Courtesy of Pfizer Inc.; p. 259 (Biaxin): Courtesy of AbbVie Inc.; p. 259 (TriCor): Courtesy of AbbVie Inc.; p. 259 (Synthroid): Courtesy of AbbVie Inc.; p. 259 (Depakote): Courtesy of AbbVie Inc.; p. 260 (Synthroid): Courtesy of AbbVie Inc.; p. 260 (Zithromax): Courtesy of Pfizer Inc.; p. 260 (Amoxicillin): Courtesy of Teva Pharmaceuticals USA; p. 260 (Levothroid): Courtesy of Forest Laboratories, Inc.; p. 260 (Prandin): Courtesy of Novo Nordisk Pharmaceuticals, Inc.; p. 261 (Metformin): Courtesy of Caraco Pharmaceutical Laboratories; 12-3 (Erythromycin): Courtesy of Arbor Pharmaceuticals, Inc.; 12-4 (Famvir): Copyright © Novartis Pharmaceutical Corp. Used by permission.; 12-5 (Norvir): Courtesy of AbbVie Inc.; 12-6 (Metformin): Courtesy of Caraco Pharmaceutical Laboratories; 12-7 (Amicar): Courtesy of Clover Pharmaceuticals Corp; p. 275 (Amoxicillin): Courtesy of Teva Pharmaceuticals USA; p. 275 (Tricor): Courtesy of AbbVie Inc.; p. 275 (Procardia): Courtesy of Pfizer Inc.; p. 276 (Kaletra): Courtesy of AbbVie Inc.; p. 276 (Synthroid): Courtesy of AbbVie Inc.; p. 277 (Erythromycin): Courtesy of Arbor Pharmaceuticals, Inc.; p. 277 (Provera): Courtesy of Pfizer Inc.; p. 277 (Vistaril): Courtesy of Pfizer Inc.; p. 278 (Ritalin): Copyright © Novartis Pharmaceutical Corp. Used by permission.; p. 278 (Camptosar): Courtesy of Pfizer Inc.; p. 282 (Amoxicillin): Courtesy of Teva Pharmaceuticals USA; p. 282 (Depakene): Courtesy of AbbVie Inc.; p. 282 (Gleevec): Copyright © Novartis Pharmaceutical Corp. Used by permission.; p. 283 (Procardia): Courtesy of Pfizer Inc.; p. 283 (Zemplar): Courtesy of AbbVie Inc.; p. 283 (Zoloft): Courtesy of Pfizer Inc.; p. 283 (Cefprozil): Courtesy of Teva Pharmaceuticals USA; p. 283 (Trileptal): Copyright © Novartis Pharmaceutical Corp. Used by permission.; p. 285 (Depakote): Courtesy of AbbVie Inc.; p. 285 (Lexapro): Courtesy of Forest Laboratories, Inc.; p. 285 (Erythromycin): Courtesy of Arbor Pharmaceuticals, Inc.; p. 286 (Depakene): Courtesy of AbbVie Inc.; p. 286 (Dilantin): Courtesy of Pfizer Inc.; p. 286 (Lisinopril): Courtesy of Teva Pharmaceuticals USA; p. 287 (Erythromycin): Courtesy of Arbor Pharmaceuticals, Inc.; p. 287 (Amoxicillin): Courtesy of Teva Pharmaceuticals USA; p. 287 (Metformin): Courtesy of Caraco Pharmaceutical Laboratories; p. 288 (Cefprozil): Courtesy of Teva Pharmaceuticals USA; p. 288 (Sandostatin): Copyright © Novartis Pharmaceutical Corp. Used by permission.; p. 289 (Lipitor): Courtesy of Pfizer Inc.; p. 289 (Cephalexin): Courtesy of Teva Pharmaceuticals USA.

Chapter 13

Page 296 (Depakote): Courtesy of AbbVie Inc.; p. 305 (Clozaril): Copyright © Novartis Pharmaceutical Corp. Used by permission.; p. 305 (Xanax): Courtesy of Pfizer Inc.; p. 305 (Famvir): Copyright © Novartis Pharmaceutical

Corp. Used by permission.; p. 306 (Aricept): Used with permission from Eisai Inc.; p. 306 (Prandin): Courtesy of Novo Nordisk Pharmaceuticals, Inc.; p. 307 (Synthroid): Courtesy of AbbVie Inc.; p. 307 (Lipitor): Courtesy of Pfizer Inc.; p. 307 (Zoloft): Courtesy of Pfizer Inc.; p. 307 (Gleevec): Copyright © Novartis Pharmaceutical Corp. Used by permission.; Figure 13-9 (Erythromycin): Courtesy of Arbor Pharmaceuticals, Inc.; 13-10 (Amoxicillin): Courtesy of Teva Pharmaceuticals USA; 13-11 (Amoxicillin): Courtesy of Teva Pharmaceuticals USA; 13-12 (Amoxicillin): Courtesy of Teva Pharmaceuticals USA; p. 319 (Erythromycin): Courtesy of Arbor Pharmaceuticals, Inc.; p. 319 (Amoxicillin): Courtesy of Teva Pharmaceuticals USA; p. 319 (Zithromax): Courtesy of Pfizer Inc.; p. 320 (Vistaril): Courtesy of Pfizer Inc.; p. 321 (Erythromycin): Courtesy of Arbor Pharmaceuticals, Inc.; p. 321 (Amoxicillin): Courtesy of Teva Pharmaceuticals USA; p. 321 (Zithromax): Courtesy of Pfizer Inc.; p. 322 (Cefprozil): Courtesy of Teva Pharmaceuticals USA; p. 322 (Trileptal): Copyright © Novartis Pharmaceutical Corp. Used by permission.; p. 324 (OxyContin): © 2014 Purdue Pharma L.P., used with permission.; p. 325 (Zemplar): Courtesy of AbbVie Inc.; p. 325 (Cefprozil): Courtesy of Teva Pharmaceuticals USA; p. 327 (Synthroid): Courtesy of AbbVie Inc.; p. 327 (Metformin): Courtesy of Caraco Pharmaceutical Laboratories; p. 327 (Cefprozil): Courtesy of Teva Pharmaceuticals USA; p. 328 (Cephalexin): Courtesy of Teva Pharmaceuticals USA; p. 328 (Vistaril): Courtesy of Pfizer Inc.; p. 328 (Norvir): Courtesy of AbbVie Inc.; p. 331 (Prandin): Courtesy of Novo Nordisk Pharmaceuticals, Inc.; p. 331 (Erythromycin): Courtesy of Arbor Pharmaceuticals, Inc.; p. 331 (Tricor): Courtesy of AbbVie Inc.; p. 332 (Depakote ER): Courtesy of AbbVie Inc.; p. 332 (Vistaril): Courtesy of Pfizer Inc.; p. 332 (Cephalexin): Courtesy of Teva Pharmaceuticals USA; p. 333 (Cefprozil): Courtesy of Teva Pharmaceuticals USA.

Chapter 14

Page 345 (Heparin): Hospira Inc., Lake Forest, IL. USA; p. 345 (Sandostatin): Copyright © Novartis Pharmaceutical Corp. Used by permission.; p. 346 (Heparin): Hospira Inc., Lake Forest, IL. USA; p. 347 (Zemplar): Courtesy of AbbVie Inc.; 14-9 (Zyprexa): © Copyright Eli Lily and Company. All rights reserved. Used with permission.; 14-10 (Package insert for Zyprexa): © Copyright Eli Lily and Company. All rights reserved. Used with permission.; p. 369 (Synagis): Courtesy of Medimmune, Inc.; 14-24 (Novolin): Courtesy of Novo Nordisk Pharmaceuticals, Inc.; 14-25 (Humalog): © Copyright Eli Lily and Company. All rights reserved. Used with permission.; 14-26 (Humalog): © Copyright Eli Lily and Company. All rights reserved. Used with permission.; p. 384 (Novolin N): Courtesy of Novo Nordisk Pharmaceuticals, Inc.; p. 384 (Novolin R): Courtesy of Novo Nordisk Pharmaceuticals, Inc.; p. 385 (Novolin): Courtesy of Novo Nordisk Pharmaceuticals, Inc.; p. 389 (Heparin): Hospira Inc., Lake Forest, IL. USA; p. 396 (Heparin): Hospira Inc., Lake Forest, IL. USA; p. 399 (Heparin): Hospira Inc., Lake Forest, IL. USA; p. 403 (Heparin): Hospira Inc., Lake Forest, IL. USA; p. 405 (Sandostatin): Copyright © Novartis Pharmaceutical Corp. Used by permission.; p. 406 (Zyprexa label and package insert): © Copyright Eli Lily and Company. All rights reserved. Used with permission. p. 407 (Novolin N): Courtesy of Novo Nordisk Pharmaceuticals, Inc.; p. 407 (Novolin R): Courtesy of Novo Nordisk

Pharmaceuticals, Inc.; p. 408 (Novolin): Courtesy of Novo Nordisk Pharmaceuticals, Inc.; p. 410 (Heparin): Hospira Inc., Lake Forest, IL. USA; p. 411 (Sandostatin): Copyright © Novartis Pharmaceutical Corp. Used by permission.; p. 412 (Sandostatin): Copyright © Novartis Pharmaceutical Corp. Used by permission.

Chapter 15

Figure 15-1 (Lactated Ringer's): Courtesy of Baxter International Inc.; 15-2 (5% dextrose injection): Courtesy of Baxter International Inc.; 15-3 (0.9% sodium chloride injection): Courtesy of Baxter International Inc.; 15-4 (5% dextrose and 0.45% sodium chloride): Courtesy of Baxter International Inc.; 15-20 (5% dextrose injection): Courtesy of Baxter International Inc.; 15-22 (Eloxatin): The oxaliplatin PI is available with permission from Sanofi US, as licensor. It is subject to change and HCPs should independently verify that the PI remains current and up to date prior to the treatment of patients. Current PI is publically available from DailyMed. http://dailymed.nlm.nih.gov/dailymed/lookup.cfm?setid=3c740b43-f396-4998-bc66-6964a21f7161; 15-23a (Heparin): Hospira Inc., Lake Forest, IL. USA; 15-23b (0.9% sodium chloride injection): Hospira Inc., Lake Forest, IL. USA; p. 454 (Heparin): Hospira Inc., Lake Forest, IL. USA.

Chapter 16

Figure 16-4 (Erythromycin): Courtesy of Arbor Pharmaceuticals, Inc.; 16-5 (Amoxicillin): Courtesy of Teva Pharmaceuticals USA; p. 480 (Amoxicillin): Courtesy of Teva Pharmaceuticals USA; p. 480 (Kaletra): Courtesy of AbbVie Inc.; p. 481 (Kaletra): Courtesy of AbbVie Inc.; p. 481 (Cephalexin): Courtesy of Teva Pharmaceuticals USA; p. 482 (Erythromycin): Courtesy of Arbor Pharmaceuticals, Inc.; p. 492 (Gammagard): Images courtesy of Baxter Healthcare Corporation. All rights reserved.; p. 492 (Camptosar): Courtesy of Pfizer Inc.; p. 494 (Trileptal): Copyright © Novartis Pharmaceutical Corp. Used by permission.; p. 494 (Erythromycin): Courtesy of Arbor Pharmaceuticals, Inc.

Chapter 17

Page 504 (Zosyn): Courtesy of Pfizer Inc.; p. 505 (Zosyn): Courtesy of Pfizer Inc.; p. 519 (Heparin): Hospira Inc., Lake Forest, IL. USA; p. 533 (Heparin): Hospira Inc., Lake Forest, IL. USA.

Chapter 18

Figure 18-1 (Erythromycin): Courtesy of Arbor Pharmaceuticals, Inc.; p. 542 (Amoxicillin): Courtesy of Teva Pharmaceuticals USA; p. 543 (Cephalexin): Courtesy of Teva Pharmaceuticals USA; p. 544 (Cephalexin): Courtesy of Teva Pharmaceuticals USA; p. 545 (Clozaril): Copyright © Novartis Pharmaceutical Corp. Used by permission.; p. 545 (Lexapro): Courtesy of Forest Laboratories, Inc.; p. 546 (Vistaril): Courtesy of Pfizer Inc.; p. 546 (Prandin): Courtesy of Novo Nordisk Pharmaceuticals, Inc.; p. 546 (Zemplar): Courtesy of AbbVie Inc.; p. 547 (Norvir): Courtesy of AbbVie Inc.; p. 547 (Vantin): Courtesy of Pfizer Inc.; p. 548 (Cefprozil): Courtesy of Teva

Pharmaceuticals USA; p. 548 (Amoxicillin): Courtesy of Teva Pharmaceuticals USA;. p. 549 (Cephalexin): Courtesy of Teva Pharmaceuticals USA; p. 553 (Xanax): Courtesy of Pfizer Inc.; p. 554 (Trileptal): Copyright © Novartis Pharmaceutical Corp. Used by permission.; p. 554 (Zoloft): Courtesy of Pfizer Inc.; p. 555: (Novolin): Courtesy of Novo Nordisk Pharmaceuticals, Inc.; p. 555 (Amoxicillin): Courtesy of Teva Pharmaceuticals USA; p. 556 (Metformin): Courtesy of Caraco Pharmaceutical Laboratories; p. 557 (Metformin): Courtesy of Caraco Pharmaceutical Laboratories; p. 557 (Depakene): Courtesy of AbbVie Inc.; p. 557 (OxyContin): © 2014 Purdue Pharma L.P., used with permission.; p. 558 (Dilantin): Courtesy of Pfizer Inc.; p. 558 (Vistaril): Courtesy of Pfizer Inc.; p. 558 (Procardia): Courtesy of Pfizer Inc.; p. 559 (Miacalcin): Copyright © Novartis Pharmaceutical Corp. Used by permission.; p. 559 (Cephalexin): Courtesy of Teva Pharmaceuticals USA; p. 561 (Amoxicillin): Courtesy of Teva Pharmaceuticals USA.

Chapter 19

Page 589 (Zemplar): Courtesy of AbbVie Inc.; p. 589 (Trileptal): Copyright © Novartis Pharmaceutical Corp. Used by permission.

Comprehensive Evaluation

Page CE-1 (Cephalexin): Courtesy of Teva Pharmaceuticals USA; p. CE-2 (Amoxicillin): Courtesy of Teva Pharmaceuticals USA; p. CE-3 (Dilantin): Courtesy of Pfizer Inc.; p. CE-3 (Trileptal): Copyright © Novartis Pharmaceutical Corp. Used by permission.; p. CE-4 (Synthroid): Courtesy of AbbVie Inc.; p. CE-5 (Novolin): Courtesy of Novo Nordisk Pharmaceuticals, Inc.; p. CE-6 (Heparin): Hospira Inc., Lake Forest, IL. USA.

PHOTO

Design Elements

Light Bulb: © Photodisc/Getty Images RF; Learning Link: © Gyro Photography/Getty Images RF.

Front Matter

Page v: © Burazin/Photographer's Choice/Getty Images RF; p. vi: © Radius Images/Getty Images RF; p. vii: © Jack Hollingsworth/Getty Images RF; p. viii: © Steve Cole/ Digital Vision/Getty Images RF; p. ix: © Image Source/ Getty Images RF; p. xiv: © Burazin/Photographer's Choice/ Getty Images RF; p. xxii: © Chris Stein/Digital Vision/Getty Images RF; p. xxiii: © Fred Tanneau/AFP/Getty Images; pp. xxiv–xxvii (blank page background): © Stockbyte/Getty Images RF; p. xxviii: © Stockbyte/PunchStock RF.

Units 1-6

Opener (Colorful pills on spoon): © ma-k/Getty Images RF.

Chapter 8

Figure 8.4: © Total Care Programming, Inc.; 8.5 (both): Courtesy of Apothecary Products LLC; 8.8: © Total Care Programming, Inc.; 8.9a: © 2014, Retractable Technologies, Inc. All rights reserved; 8.9b: © Medline Industries, Inc. All rights reserved, 2014; 8.10: Courtesy and © Becton, Dickinson and Company; 8.11 8.12, 8.14, 8.15, 8.17: © Total Care Programming, Inc.; 8.18: Courtesy and © Becton, Dickinson and Company; 8.19: © Total Care Programming, Inc.; 8.20: Courtesy of Schreiner MediPharm; 8.22: © Royalty-Free/Corbis; 8.23: Photo by Susan Sienkiewicz and Jennifer F. Palmenen; 8.25: © Total Care Programming, Inc.

Chapter 13

Figures 13.1, 13.2, 13.5–13.7: © Total Care Programming, Inc.

Chapter 14

Figure 14.28: © Excelsior Medical.

Chapter 15

Figure 15.5: © Chris Gallagher/Science Source; 15.6, 15.7: © Total Care Programming, Inc.; 15.8: © Imageroller/Alamy RF; 15.9-15.12, 15.15, 15.21: © Total Care Programming, Inc.; 15.23c & p. 454 (Label E): © Excelsior Medical.

Chapter 16

Figure 16.1: © McGraw-Hill Education/Jill Braaten, photographer; 16.2: © Creatas/PunchStock RF; 16.3: © Total Care Programming, Inc.

Chapter 17

Figure 17.1: Photo by Susan Sienkiewicz and Jennifer F. Palmenen.

INDEX

Goethe, Johann Wolfgang, 104
gr, 95, 96, 100, 100t
Grain (gr), 95, 96, 100, 100t, 105t
Gram (g), 86t, 90, 100t
Granulex—Regranex, 222
Grapefruit juice, 301
GT, 160t
gt, 99t
gtt, 99t
gtt/min, 426

H

h, 161t
H₂O, 415t
Haloperidol, 302t
Handwritten physician orders, 223f
Hartmann's solution, 415t
HCl, 229t
HCT, 229t
HCTZ, 229t
Hemodynamics, 525
Heparin, 350, 388–392
Heparin—Hespan, 222
Heparin dosages, 513–518
Heparin flush, 444, 444f
Heparin lock, 438, 439f, 443
Heparin lock flush solution, 388
Heparin protocol, 513
High-alert medication, 374, 497
Highlights (package insert), 211t
Hourly dose, 517–518
Hourly flow rates (dosage per time infusions), 506–512
Household system of measurement, 98–99
  abbreviations, 99t
  equivalent household measures, 98t
  equivalent measures, 100t
  units of measure, 98, 99t
HS, 227t
hs, 227t
Hubbard, Elbert Green, 563
Humalog, 375t
Humalog 50/50, 375t, 380, 381f
Humalog Mix 75/25, 375t, 380
Humulin 50/50, 375t
Humulin 70/30, 375t
Humulin—Novolin, 222
Humulin N, 375t, 376f
Humulin R, 375t, 376f
Hypertonic, 417
Hypodermic syringe, 133
Hypotonic, 417

I

i/d, 228t
Ibuprofen, 187
IBW. *See* Ideal body weight (IBW)
ID, 160t

ID administration. *See* Intradermal (ID) administration
Ideal body weight (IBW), 502
IJ, 227t
IM, 160t
IM administration. *See* Intramuscular (IM) administration
Improper fraction, 32
IN, 227t
Incompatible IV solutions, 418t
Inderal—Adderall, 222
Indications and usage (package insert), 211t
Infiltration, 423–424, 423f, 424t
Infusion Nurses Society IV infiltration scale, 423f, 424t
Infusion pump, 421, 421f
Inhalants, 146m 363
Injection routes, 133, 334, 335f
Insomnia, 466t
Instillations, 146
Institute for Safe Medication Practices (ISMP), 161, 227
Insulin, 203, 374–383
  brand/generic names, 375t
  coffee, and, 302t
  combinations, 380–382
  label, 203f, 376f, 379f
  measuring a single insulin dose, 380
  pen device, 381f
  syringes, 135–136, 136f, 377–379
  timing of action, 375, 375t
  vial, 541
Insulin combinations, 380–382
Insulin label, 203f, 376f, 379f
Insulin pens, 381f
Insulin syringe, 135–136, 136f, 377–379
Intermittent IV flush, 444, 444f
Intermittent IV infusion, 438–444
Intermittent peripheral infusion devices, 438
International time (24-hour clock), 118, 119f, 120
International units, 101
Intestinal conditions, 462t
Intradermal (ID) administration, 191, 335f
Intramuscular (IM) administration, 191, 192f, 335f
Intravenous (IV) administration, 191, 192f, 335f
Intravenous (IV) calculations, 413–453, 497–536
  abbreviations, 414, 415t
  additives, 417, 418t
  adjusting the flow rate, 428–431, 524
  calculate amount to administer/flow rate, 439–443
  categories of IV solutions, 414
  central IV therapy, 422

compatibility, 417, 418t
daily maintenance fluid needs (DMFN), 498–501
dry weight, 525
embolism, 423
flow rate, 425–431, 506–512, 519–522
flow rate adjustments, 428–431, 524
flow rate based on body weight per time, 519–522
heparin dosages, 513–518
heparin flush, 444, 444f
hourly flow rates (dosage per time infusions), 506–512
infiltration, 423–424, 423f, 424t
infusion time, 433–435
infusion volume, 435–437
intermittent IV infusion, 438–444
isotonic, hypotonic, hypertonic, 417
IV concentrations, 415–417
IV labels, 414, 415t
macrodrip/microdrip tubing, 419, 426, 426f, 427f
patient education, 443
peripheral IV therapy, 422
phlebitis, 424
primary line, 419, 419f
regulating IV infusions, 420–422
saline/heparin lock, 438, 439f, 443
secondary line, 420, 420f, 438
titrated medications, 525–528
volume of solution received, 522
Intravenous (IV) fluids, 413
Iodine—Lodine, 222
ISMP. *See* Institute for Safe Medication Practices (ISMP)
ISMP's List of Error-Prone Abbreviations, Symbols, and Dose Designations, 227–230t
Isotonic, 417
IU, 227t
IV, 160t. *See also* Intravenous (IV) calculations
IV push, 514
IV solution bag, 419f
"IV Vanc," 230t
IVP, 161t
IVPB, 160t, 420
IVSS, 160t

J

Jejunostomy tube, 130
Johnson, Samuel, 497

K

kg, 86t, 90t, 100t
Kidney disease/dysfunction, 462t, 464–465
kilo-, 85, 86t, 89t
Kilogram (kg), 86t, 90, 100t, 105t